Clinical Arrhythmology

Clinical Arrhythmology

Second Edition

Antoni Bayés de Luna
Emeritus Professor of Cardiology, Universitat Autònoma de Barcelona Honorary Director, Cardiology Service,
Hospital de la Santa Creu i Sant Pau, Barcelona Senior Consultant, Hospital Universitari Quirón,
Barcelona, Spain

Adrian Baranchuk MD FACC FRCPC FCCS
Professor of Medicine, Queen's University, Kingston, Ontario, Canada,
Editor-in-Chief, Journal of Electrocardiology
President, International Society of Electrocardiology

With the collaboration of:
Diego Goldwasser, Xavier Viñolas, Miquel Fiol, Iwona Cygankiewicz, Javier García Niebla, Andrés Pérez Riera,
Pedro Iturralde, Ramon Oter, Antoni Bayés Genís, Ramon Brugada, Wojciech Zareba, Usama Boles,
Aldo G. Carrizo, Andrés Enriquez, Benedict Glover, and Dario de Toro.

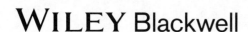

Registered Office(s)
John Wiley & Sons, Inc., 111 River Street, Hoboken, NJ 07030, USA
John Wiley & Sons Ltd, The Atrium, Southern Gate, Chichester, West Sussex, PO19 8SQ, UK

Editorial Office
The Atrium, Southern Gate, Chichester, West Sussex, PO19 8SQ, UK

For details of our global editorial offices, customer services, and more information about Wiley products visit us at www.wiley.com.

Wiley also publishes its books in a variety of electronic formats and by print-on-demand. Some content that appears in standard print versions of this book may not be available in other formats.

Library of Congress Cataloging-in-Publication Data

Names: Bayés de Luna, Antoni, 1936- author. | Baranchuk, Adrian, author.
Title: Clinical arrhythmology / Antoni Bayés de Luna, Adrian Baranchuk.
Description: Second edition. | Hoboken, NJ : John Wiley & Sons, Inc., 2017. |
  Includes bibliographical references and index. |
Identifiers: LCCN 2017014000 (print) | LCCN 2017014650 (ebook) | ISBN
  9781119212836 (pdf) | ISBN 9781119212768 (epub) | ISBN 9781119212751
  (cloth)
Subjects: | MESH: Arrhythmias, Cardiac--diagnosis | Arrhythmias,
  Cardiac--physiopathology | Arrhythmias, Cardiac--therapy | Cardiac
  Electrophysiology | Electrocardiography--methods
Classification: LCC RC685.A65 (ebook) | LCC RC685.A65 (print) | NLM WG 330 |
  DDC 616.1/28--dc23

LC record available at https://lccn.loc.gov/2017014000

Cover Design: Wiley
Cover Image: Courtesy of Antoni Bayés de Luna

Set in 10/12pt WarnockPro by SPi Global, Chennai, India

Printed in Singapore by C.O.S. Printers Pte Ltd

10 9 8 7 6 5 4 3 2 1

Contents

Foreword by Dr. Valentin Fuster

When I received the manuscript from Antoni Bayés de Luna and his collaborators to write a foreword for this book, I realized at a glance what a great opportunity this work provides. This has been the rule with books published by Antoni Bayés de Luna – they appear when they are needed most. I still remember his book on electrocardiology, which explained the technique of "Electrocardiography" for beginners in a way that was not only concise but very thorough. This book has been translated into eight languages and remains very successful throughout the world. This also occurred with his book on "Sudden death", as well as his correlations between electrocardiography and cardiovascular magnetic resonance imaging. But for now I would like to talk about *Clinical Arrhythmology*, which is what interests us most. The current books on arrhythmias mainly explain the great technological advances being achieved in diagnosis and, in particular, the interventionist treatment of cardiac arrhythmias. However, most of these books fail to examine the clinical aspects closely enough and do not emphasize the crucial role in diagnosis of the surface electrocardiogram, nor do they discuss how the clinical cardiologist or family doctor, or even the emergency medicine doctor, might proceed once this diagnosis is performed, in order to rapidly and efficiently treat the specific arrhythmias in the clinical context in which they appear. The book is full of the experience of Antoni Bayés de Luna teaching electrocardiology and arrhythmias in the style of Paul Puech, Leo Schamroth, and Charles Fisch, with an updated state-of-the-art view of the management of arrhythmias.

This book is filled with advice on how to diagnose and effectively treat arrhythmias with classic knowledge that, at the same time, is up-to-date, using many references from 2010. Antoni Bayés de Luna emphasizes the necessity to consult and use the medical guidelines of the scientific societies, while at the same time giving a personal touch derived from his considerable experience. This is especially present in Chapter 1, where he emphasizes the importance that history taking and physical examination still have when diagnosing and treating arrhythmias. He gives a series of recommendations that state the necessity to know heart anatomy and physiology well, in addition to outlining how to approach a case with arrhythmias. I also consider the updated physiopathologic mechanisms of arrhythmias to be of great interest. Later on, in the second part of the book, all the different clinical, electrocardiographic, prognostic, and management aspects of different arrhythmias are clearly commented on. The third part deserves close study because it is where sudden death, being the most important complication of arrhythmia, is examined and discussed in different heart diseases and situations.

I feel that this book demonstrates the great authority of the author, as well as his deep knowledge of clinical arrhythmia and electrocardiography, great didactic capabilities, and many years of experience in this field. I am sure it will be extremely useful for doctors who are first faced with cardiac arrhythmias, not only in the diagnosis but also in obtaining a clear idea on how to focus management of the condition, including the last advances in the treatment through ablation techniques and pacemaker and defibrillator implantation in different types of arrhythmias.

I would like to offer my wholehearted congratulations to Antoni Bayés de Luna for providing all his personal experience in a subject of great clinical importance and based on the crucial value placed on the history taking and, especially, the surface electrocardiogram in the diagnosis and management of cardiac arrhythmias.

I predict that this book will be a huge success because of its usefulness and timeliness. It will make diagnosis and treatment of different cardiac arrhythmias much easier for students, doctors, and even specialists, without the apprehension often generated in the medical community.

Dr. Valentin Fuster
Director, Mount Sinai Heart Center, New York
Professor of Medicine, Mount Sinai School of Medicine
Past President, American Heart Association
Past President, World Heart Federation

Foreword by Dr. Pere Brugada i Terradellas

When Professor Antoni Bayés de Luna placed 3 kg of printed material in my hands, I immediately knew what was happening: the "master of masters" had struck again. Undoubtedly, it was a new book. And, undoubtedly, it was a book related to electrocardiology, the great love of his life. Knowing him as I have for so many decades, I did not doubt that the manuscript I was now holding had been written to fill a gap in medical knowledge. But what could Antoni have written now that he had not already written? His various books on electrocardiography, published in the most common languages, are known by every admirer of the electrical activity of the heart. No cardiologist has described the electrocardiogram in as much detail as he. His daily work has consisted of the nearly impossible job of dissecting the electrical activity of the heart. And this all without electrocuting himself!

I looked carefully at the title on the first page and those 3 kg soon became lighter: *Clinical Arrhythmology*. Here was the big secret. Finally, the book that describes the mechanisms, diagnostic clues, and management of cardiac arrhythmias, written by the clinical cardiologist for the clinical cardiologist. Thanks to great advances in the study of cardiac electrophysiology, arrhythmia mechanisms are well understood today. However, the general cardiologist, the internist, and the general practitioner must depend continuously on the electrocardiogram to define the swelling mechanism in any cardiac rhythm disorder. Combining clinical and electrophysiologic knowledge with an updated approach of medical management, to produce an integrated textbook of clinical arrhythmology is a challenge few would take on. For this, a clinical and scientific tenacity is required that only a chosen few possess, one of whom is Professor Antoni Bayés de Luna.

These thoughts crossed my mind during the minutes I took to look through the manuscript. Antoni, aware of my love for his work, asked if I would like to write a foreword for this book. Absolutely! I said, I would do it with great pleasure, in order to thank him on behalf of myself and many others for his great efforts in teaching, and for the numerous hours of pleasant reading he has given us. To thank him for the great care he has always taken with his books, including this one, naturally, to offer us clear outlines accompanied by greatly didactic diagrams, which are a pleasure to read and study.

Clinical Arrhythmology is obligatory reading for any physician directly or indirectly related to disorders of cardiac rhythm, including cardiologists, internists, sports medicine doctors, and general practitioners. They will find in this book that a combination of clinical experience and great electrocardiographic skills is the best way to approach successfully the diagnosis and treatment of cardiac arrhythmias. It is also a superb resource for paramedics who may be faced with cardiac arrhythmias.

Professor Bayés de Luna must be congratulated on his magnificent effort and the excellent end result of this book.

Dr. Pere Brugada i Terradellas
Scientific Director, Centro UZ Brussel
Cardiovascular Centre, Brussels, Belgium

Preface

A few years ago, I, Antoni Bayés de Luna, wrote a book on *Clinical Arrhythmology*. The title was chosen to express that my aim was to share with the reader my point of view, as a clinical cardiologist, of what are the most important concepts related to arrhythmias, including genetic, epidemiological, and diagnostic aspects that may be useful to treat these patients. My objective was to ensure that the clinician who is facing a patient with a possible or already established arrhythmia has gained, after reading the book, all the information necessary to diagnose arrhythmias, understand ECG tracings, and obtain a good clinical history. I also aimed to teach about the prognosis of certain conditions, including the risk of possible complications such as stroke, cognitive impairment, and sudden death, so that the clinician could decide what the most appropriate treatment is.

In order to reach this goal, the book is divided into three sections.

In the first section, the concept, classification, and clinical aspects of arrhythmias are presented, with emphasis on its relation to sudden death, as well as the most interesting information still relevant today on the great utility of anamnesis and physical examination. The characteristics of each type of cardiac cell are described and, finally, the most important electrophysiological mechanisms associated with cardiac arrhythmias are also discussed.

The second section describes the key elements used to carry out an electrocardiographic diagnosis of the various active and passive arrhythmias, their clinical and prognostic implications, and the best available treatments, using a practical approach. The current use of antiarrhythmic agents and the various techniques (cardioversion and ablation) and implantable devices (pacemakers, defibrillators, etc.) available are also briefly discussed (these topics are discussed more extensively in the Appendix).

In Chapter 7, the reader will find out how to perform an analytical study and differential diagnosis of different arrhythmias.

The third section deals with the most frequent arrhythmological syndromes, including pre-excitation and channelopathies, as well as other electrocardiographic patterns suggestive of increased risk of sudden death.

Finally, in the Appendix, a few concepts that are necessary to understand the literature are expanded on: sensitivity, specificity, and predictive values. In this section, new antiarrhythmic agents and novel techniques for diagnosis and treatment are covered. Guidelines issued by the most important scientific societies are also mentioned.

Throughout the book, emphasis is placed on the importance of surface electrocardiography as the basic technique to diagnose arrhythmias at a clinical physician's level.

All the information is presented in a cohesive way, although at times it may result in repetition of some aspects and concepts. I am aware of this, but believe it to be useful, particularly to the nonexpert, in order to reinforce basic knowledge and ideas. At the same time, the reader is very often referred to further information, either by cross-references related to other sections of the book or by reference to sections just before ("see before") or after ("see after") in the same chapter. I believe that this makes the book more harmonious and allows to the reader to interact better with other parts of the book. Additionally, at the end of each chapter, there are self-evaluation questions, the answers to which may be found on the pages of the book where the corresponding "letter tag" appears in the margin.

In terms of bibliography, a list of updated recommended texts for general reference is provided after this preface. In addition, at the end of each chapter, there is a list of specific references pertaining to each particular subject. The name of the first author of each of these articles has been cited in the text in an appropriate position.

I am sure, therefore, that after reading this book the reader will have learned all the basic concepts needed to face the often difficult problems of immediate diagnosis based on electrocardiographic tracings. I hope the reader will not only understand the most important clinical, prognostic, and therapeutic implications of the diagnosis in every case but also will acquire more confidence in this task.

This book is the result of many years of teaching cardiology, especially electrocardiography and arrhythmias. It is a source of pride for me to have Valentin Fuster and Pedro Brugada, two of the greatest representatives of cardiology in the world on both sides of the Atlantic, Catalans like me and good friends of mine since the beginning of time, honor me by writing glowing forewords for the book. I feel that their words not only complement the work but also express its meaning for the general cardiologists, cardiology residents, and internists.

I am very pleased that the book was very well received by general practitioners and clinical cardiologists, and when the Publisher decided to produce a second edition I suggested that an update of all the information given in the text, especially in relation to diagnostic criteria, new types of drugs and devices, and new prognostic implications, was needed. It was also very important to provide an update on new electrophysiological techniques, such as all types of pacemaker, new Holter devices, ICDs, CRT, and, especially, ablation techniques, including the new devices for LAA closure, and so on. This update had to be not only related to the technical aspects of the procedures but especially devoted to a discussion of when each technique should be indicated and the most characteristic aspects of each one of them.

In order to help this book evolve into a classic "*Textbook of Clinical Arrhythmology*", we decided that it was necessary for the new edition, and especially for future editions, to incorporate a co-author who would bring a new flavor but maintain the philosophy of a *book of one author* (not a book written by many authors each with different points of view and one editor-in-chief). This was for me a crucial point.

In order to do this, we decided to invite Professor Adrian Baranchuk, Head of the Heart Rhythm Service from Queen's University, Kingston, Ontario, Canada, to become a co-editor of the book. Adrian has demonstrated to me all the requirements that I have explained before: he is a very good clinician and an excellent and up-to-date invasive electrophysiologist, with a great teaching vocation and an extraordinary capacity to transmit knowledge. Therefore, he was for me the best person to transform a second edition of the book into an updated one that includes all the new aspects of our profession developed during the last five years whilst simultaneously maintaining all the characteristics of an authoritative author book. I have worked with him in different projects for the last few years and I was very confident that he has, without any doubt, the adequate scientific profile to perform this task.

I hope that the scientific community will receive the book enthusiastically as a "textbook" for cardiology fellows, internal medicine and emergency residents, medical students, general practitioners and allied professionals.

Lastly, I thank very much all the collaborators that have contributed to the first edition and that continue to contribute in this second edition. I also welcome the new contributors to this second edition. Additionally, thanks very much to our mentors and many other collaborators that have supported us in many aspects. Great appreciation must be shown to the amazing secretarial support from our beloved Montse Saurí and Esther Gregoris, and especially to my family, my wife María Clara for her constant support and all my five children and their families.

Preface to the Second Edition by Dr Adrian Branchuk

Now, I will introduce Adrian Baranchuk to write the second part of this foreword.

It is certainly not "common place" when an opportunity arises like the one Professor Bayés de Luna has given me to join him as co-author of the second edition of *Clinical Arrhythmology*. I am thrilled, honored, and challenged by this offer. I have carried out all my medical education in Argentina, reading from Professor Bayés de Luna's books and listening to him delivering talks and teaching large audiences all around the world. To me, he represents all that I wanted to achieve in my academic career. I still cannot believe that I have the opportunity to discuss electrocardiography, arrhythmias, and cardiovascular diseases with him. Dr Bayés de Luna is a super active physician, an avid researcher, and a spectacular mentor.

When he invited me to co-author this amazing book (the first edition of which I had on my shelf), I accepted immediately without knowing what I was getting into.

I have read and revised each line of this incredible treasure. There is so much to learn from this book!

He asked me to look at it with my "young eyes" (he called it "young blood") to be sure that we were not missing any new relevant information. I did my best to accommodate summaries of all new techniques, both for diagnosis and treatment. I am sure that I have missed a few important issues, and I hope we will correct these omissions in the next edition.

The last five years of my career have been enlightened by the constant presence of Professor Bayés de Luna. His advice both in the areas of academic medicine and also in more personal aspects of my life, have produced a change in how I face medicine, and how I balance my academic career and my personal life. For that, I will always be grateful and I hope to be able to transmit the same "spirit" to my students.

Clinical Arrhythmology is a book for anyone interested in clinical arrhythmias and electrocardiology. It is written in the very special way that Professor Bayés de Luna does it: mixing evidence-based medicine with his profuse clinical experience. One can find "tips" and "pearls of wisdom" in almost every page.

I invite you to enjoy this "book of the author", where you will be able to navigate through the lessons of one of the *ECG Masters of the World*. I am sure that you will enjoy it as much as I did in collaborating to produce this amazing second edition.

I would like to dedicate this book to all those in the world who, despite personal difficulties and limitations, wake up every day with the certainty that a better world is possible. My recognition to my mentors and students, the force behind every project I face. My love and gratitude to my wife and daughter, Barbara and Gala, for the joy of life.

Antoni Bayés de Luna
ICCC-St. Pau Hospital, Barcelona, Spain

Adrian Baranchuk
Queen's University, Kingston, Ontario, Canada
June 2017

Recommended General Bibliography

American Guidelines: www.americanheart.org.

Bayés de Luna A. *Tratado de electrocardiografía clínica.* Científico-Médica, Barcelona, 1978.

Bayés de Luna A, Cosín J, eds. *Cardiac Arrhythmias.* Pergamon Press, Oxford, 1978.

Bayés de Luna A. *Textbook of Clinical Electrocardiography,* 5th updated edn. Wiley-Blackwell, Oxford, 2011.

Braunwald E, Zipes D, Libby P. *Heart Diseases,* 6th edn. WB Saunders, Philadelphia, 2001.

Cosín J, Bayés de Luna A, García Civera R, Cabadés A, eds. *Cardiac Arrhythmias. Diagnosis and Treatment.* Pergamon Press, Oxford, 1988.

Elizari M, Chiale P. *Arritmias Cardíacas.* Panamericana, Buenos Aires, 2003.

Fisch C, Knoebel S. *Electrocardiography of Clinical Arrhythmias.* Futura NJ, New York, 2000.

European Guidelines: www.escardio.org.

Fuster V. Ed. *The Heart.* McGraw-Hill, New York, 2010.

Goldstein S, Bayés de Luna A, Guindo J. *Sudden Cardiac Death.* Futura NJ, New York, 1994.

Gussak I, Antzelevitz C. *Electrical Diseases of the Heart.* Springer Verlag, London, 2008.

Issa Z, Miller J, Zipes D. *Clinical Arrhythmology and Electrophysiology.* WB Saunders, Philadelphia, 2009.

Iturralde P. *Arritmias Cardíacas.* McGraw-Hill Interamericana, México, 2002.

Josephson ME. *Clinical Cardiac Electrophysiology.* Wolters- Kluwer, Philadelphia, 2008.

Zipes D, Jalife J. Cardiac *Electrophysiology: from Cell to Bedside,* 4th edn. WB Saunders, Philadelphia, 2004. xii

Part I

Anatomical and Electrophysiological Considerations, Clinical Aspects, and Mechanisms of Cardiac Arrhythmias

1

Clinical Aspects of Arrhythmias

Definition of Arrhythmia

Arrhythmias are defined as **any cardiac rhythm other than the normal sinus rhythm.** Sinus rhythm originates in the sinus node. The electrocardiographic characteristics of normal sinus rhythm are:

- An impulse originated in sinus node initiates a positive P wave in I, II, VF, V_2-V_6, and positive or ± in leads III and V_1 that is transmitted through the atria, the atrio-ventricular (AV) junction, and the intraventricular specific conduction system (ISCS).
- In the absence of pre-excitation, the PR interval ranges from 0.12 to 0.20 s.
- At rest, the sinus node discharge cadence tends to be regular, although it presents generally slight variations, which are usually not evident by palpation or auscultation. However, under normal conditions, and particularly in children, it may present slight to moderate changes dependent on the phases of respiration, with the heart rate increasing with inspiration.
- In adults at rest, the rate of the normal sinus rhythm ranges from 60 to 80 beats per minute (bpm). Thus, sinus rhythms over 80 bpm (sinus tachycardia) and those under 60 bpm (sinus bradycardia) may be considered arrhythmias. However, it should be taken into account that sinus rhythm varies throughout a 24-h period, and sinus tachycardia and sinus bradycardia usually are a physiologic response to certain sympathetic (exercise, stress) or vagal (rest, sleep) stimuli. Under such circumstances, the presence of these heart rates is normal.
- As already stated, it is normal to observe a certain variation of the heart rate during 24 hours. Thus, the evidence of a completely fixed heart rate both during the day and at night is suggestive of arrhythmia. In addition, it is important to remember that:

  (i) **The term arrhythmia does not mean rhythm irregularity**, as regular arrhythmias can occur, often with absolute stability (flutter, paroxysmal tachycardia, etc.), sometimes presenting heart rates in the normal range, as is the case with the flutter 4×1. On the other hand, some irregular rhythms should not be considered arrhythmias (mild to moderate irregularity in the sinus discharge, particularly when linked to respiration, as already stated).

  (ii) **A diagnosis of arrhythmia in itself does not mean evident pathology**. In fact, in healthy subjects, the sporadic presence of certain arrhythmias, both active (premature complexes) and passive (escape complexes, certain degree of AV block, evident sinus arrhythmia, etc.) is frequently observed.

Classification

There are different ways to classify cardiac arrhythmias:

- **According to the site of origin**: arrhythmias are divided into supraventricular (including those having their origin in the sinus node, the atria, and the AV junction), and ventricular arrhythmias.
- **According to the underlying mechanism**: arrhythmias may be explained by (i) abnormal formation of impulses, which includes increased heart automaticity (extrasystolic or parasystolic mechanism) and triggered electrical activity, (ii) reentry of different types, and (iii) decreased automaticity and/or disturbances of conduction (see Chapter 3).
- **From the clinical point of view** arrhythmias may be **paroxysmal, incessant, or permanent**. In reference to tachyarrhythmias (an example of an active arrhythmia, see later), paroxysmal tachyarrhythmias occur suddenly and usually disappear spontaneously (i.e., AV junctional reentrant paroxysmal tachycardia); permanent tachyarrhythmias are always present (i.e., permanent atrial fibrillation); and incessant tachyarrhythmias are characterized by short and repetitive runs of supraventricular (Figure 4.21) or ventricular (Figure 5.4) tachycardia. Extrasystoles may also occur in a paroxysmal or incessant way (see Chapter 3, Mechanisms Responsible for Active Cardiac Arrhythmias). Some bradyarrhythmias,

such as advanced AV block (an example of passive arrhythmia, see later), may also occur in a paroxysmal or permanent form.

- **From an electrocardiographic point of view**, arrhythmias may be divided into two different types: active and passive (Table 1.1):
  - **Active arrhythmias** due to increased automaticity, reentry, or triggered electrical activity (see Chapter 3 and Table 3.1) generate isolated or repetitive premature complexes on the electrocardiogram (ECG), which occur before the cadence of the regular sinus rhythm. The isolated premature complexes may be originated in a parasystolic or extrasystolic ectopic focus. The extrasystolic mechanism presents a fixed coupling interval, whereas the parasystolic presents a varied coupling interval. Premature complexes of supraventricular origin (p') are generally followed by a narrow QRS complex, although they may be wide if are conducted with aberrancy. The ectopic P wave (P') is often not easily seen as it may be hidden in the preceding T wave. In other cases the premature atrial impulse remains blocked in the AV junction, initiating a pause instead of a premature QRS complex (Figures 4.1C and 7.3). The premature complexes of ventricular origin are not preceded by an ectopic P wave, and the QRS complex is always wide (≥ 0.12 s), unless they originate in the upper part of the intraventricular specific conduction system (see Chapter 5, Electrocardiographic Diagnosis).

    Premature and repetitive complexes include all types of supraventricular or ventricular tachyarrhythmias (tachycardias, fibrillation, flutter). In active cardiac arrhythmias due to reentrant mechanisms, a unidirectional block exists in some part of the circuit (Figure 3.6).
  - **Passive arrhythmias** occur when cardiac stimuli formation and/or conduction are below the range of normality due to a depression of the automatism and/or a stimulus conduction block in the atria, the AV junction, or the specific intraventricular conduction systems (ICS).

    From an electrocardiographic point of view, many passive cardiac arrhythmias present isolated late complexes (**escape complexes**) and, if repetitive, slower than expected heart rate (bradyarrhythmia). Even in the absence of bradyarrhythmia, some type of conduction delay or block in some portion of the specific conduction system (SCS) may exist, for example, first-degree or some second-degree sinoatrial or AV blocks, or atrial or ventricular (bundle branch) blocks. The latter encompasses the aberrant conduction phenomenon (see Chapter 3, Aberrant Conduction). Thus, the electrocardiographic diagnosis of passive cardiac arrhythmia can be made because it may be demonstrated that the ECG changes are due to a depression of automatism and/or conduction in some part of the SCS, without this manifesting in the ECG as a premature complex, as it does in reentry (Figure 3.6).
- Atrial or ventricular blocks are not usually considered arrhythmias. But in our opinion, they should be included as passive cardiac arrhythmias like other types of blocks (sinoatrial or AV). This is why they have been included in this book (see Chapter 3, Heart Block, and Chapter 6, Atrial Blocks, and Ventricular Blocks).

Table 1.1 Classification of arrhythmias according to their electrocardiographic presentation.

Active arrhythmias	Passive arrhythmias
Supraventricular	Escape complex
• Premature complexes	Escape rhythm
• Tachyarrhytmias	Sinus bradycardia
– Different types of tachycardia	Sinoatrial block
– Atrial fibrillation	Atrial block
– Atrial flutter	Atrioventricular block
• Ventricular	Ventricular block
• Premature complexes	Aberrant conduction
• Different types of tachycardia	Cardiac arrest
• Ventricular flutter	
• Ventricular fibrillation	

Clinical Significance and Symptoms

The incidence of the majority of arrhythmias increases progressively with age and arrhythmias are not frequent in children. Data from the Holter ECG recordings (see Appendix A-3, Holter electrocardiographic monitoring and related techniques) have demonstrated that isolated premature ventricular complexes (PVC) are present in about 10–20% of young people in 24-h recordings, and their presence is nearly a rule in the 80+ age group. Similarly, sustained chronic arrhythmias, such as atrial fibrillation, are exceptional in children and are present in about 10% of subjects over 80 years of age. However, **there are arrhythmias that arise particularly in children**, such as some paroxysmal and incessant AV junctional reentrant tachycardias (AVJRT), as well as some monomorphic ventricular tachycardias (idiopathic) and polymorphic ventricular tachycardias (catecholaminergic).

In this book devoted to providing the basis for the diagnosis, prognosis, and treatment of arrhythmias, **active and passive classification of arrhythmias** is used (Table 1.1):

- Active cardiac arrhythmias include isolated or repetitive impulses that command heart rhythm, instead of the basic normal sinus rhythm. They are recorded on the ECG tracing as isolated (premature supraventricular or ventricular complexes), repetitive (named runs), or sustained complexes (different types of tachyarrhythmias).
- Many passive cardiac arrhythmias show isolated or repetitive sinus or escape complexes in the ECG tracings with an abnormally slowed heart rate (bradyarrhythmias). This may be due to depression of automaticity or sinoatrial or AV block. However, in some cases the mechanism responsible for the passive cardiac arrhythmia is delayed conduction, which may modify the ECG pattern (first-degree AV block, or atrial or ventricular bundle branch block), but this does not mean that the heart rate has to be slow.

The most important clinical significance of arrhythmias is related to an association with sudden cardiac death (Goldstein *et al.*, 1994; Recommended General Bibliography p. xvii). It is also important to remember that frequently arrhythmias (especially atrial fibrillation) may lead to embolism, including cerebral emboli, often with severe consequences. Also, it must be remembered that sometimes fast arrhythmias may trigger or worsen heart failure (HF). These aspects will be commented on.

Arrhythmias and Sudden Death (SD)

Some of the most important aspects of SD, a true epidemic of the twenty-first century, will now be examined here. In other parts of the book (Chapters 8–11) specific

aspects of SD in relation to different heart diseases or situations are discussed in more detail.

Epidemiology

Sudden death is probably the most challenging issue in modern cardiology, taking into account the remarkably high number of SD cases (the estimated number of SD in the United States is approximately 400 000 cases per year, although in Mediterranean countries, such as Spain, the incidence is lower) (Keys and Keys, 1975; Masiá *et al.*, 1998; Marrugat *et al.*, 1999; Sans *et al.*, 2005) and the important social impact of SD events.

Even though SD has been reported in newborns, in whom it has been related to repolarization disorders, alterations of the autonomic nervous system (ANS), and an increase of vagal tone (see Chapter 11, Sudden Infant Death Syndrome), it is indeed very rare in the first decades of life. At this age it often occurs during sports activities (Bayés de Luna *et al.*, 2000) and is often associated with inherited heart disease (hypertrophic cardiomyopathy, arrhythmogenic right ventricular dysplasia/cardiomyopathy, and channelopathies). The incidence of SD gradually but significantly increases after 35–40 years of age and is particularly high during the acute phase of myocardial infarction (MI). It is also frequent during the chronic phase of ischemic heart disease (IHD), as well as in subjects with any heart disease, especially when heart failure (HF) is present (Myerburg *et al.*, 1997) (Figure 1.1).

Associated Diseases

As previously discussed, acute IHD is frequently associated with SD in adults. In the majority of cases of SD outside acute IHD or channelopathies, HF, or at least left ventricular dysfunction, is present. HF may be idiopathic or present in patients with chronic IHD, hypertension, cardiomyopathies, and so on. More details on this association are shown in Chapter 11 (see Chapter 11, Ischemic

Figure 1.1 Relationship between the incidence of sudden death (SD) and age. Note that the sudden death may also be associated with different diseases along the life period (Myerburg *et al.*, 1992).

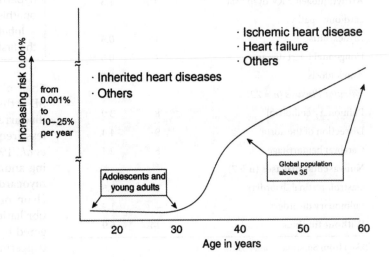

Heart Disease, and Heart Failure). Inherited heart disease (InHD) can cause SD at any age but the overall impact is small (Figure 1.1). It should be emphasized, however, that it is responsible for the majority of cases of SD that occur before the age of 35 years. InHD appears more in men and may occur during exercise (cardiomyopathies) or sleep or rest (channelopathies) (see Chapter 9).

We performed a study (the EULALIA trial) that included 204 cases of SD occurring in the Mediterranean area (Subirana *et al.*, 2011). In this study, the epidemiological and pathological aspects of diseases associated with SD were analyzed. Table 1.2 shows the diagnosis obtained by the pathologists. When compared with other similar Anglo-Saxon studies (Burke *et al.*, 1997), what caught our attention was that the number of cases presenting with IHD found at autopsy, as well as the incidence of acute thrombosis, as an anatomopathologic expression of MI, was lower than in previously published Anglo-Saxon studies (80–90% vs 58% and 52% vs 40% for IHD and acute thrombosis, respectively) (Figure 1.2). Our findings are concordant with previously known evidence (Keys and Keys 1975; de Lorgeril *et al.*, 1999;

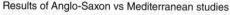

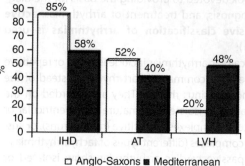

Figure 1.2 Comparative study on the incidence of ischemic heart disease (IHD), acute thrombosis (AT), and left ventricular hypertrophy (LVH) in the EULALIA trial.

Marrugat *et al.*, 1999; Sans *et al.*, 2005) that the incidence of IHD in Mediterranean regions is lower, probably related to diet, lifestyle, and environment (Mediterranean culture). In contrast, SD victims from the Mediterranean region presented left ventricular hypertrophy more frequently than other studies (48% vs 20%) (Virmani *et al.*, 2001; Subirana *et al.*, 2011). From a clinical point of view, the victims of SD in the EULALIA trial presented anginal episodes less frequently (20% vs 37%), which was in agreement with the reduced number of cases with IHD found at autopsy, when compared with the Maastricht study (de Vreede-Swagemakers *et al.*, 1997). In our series, the incidence of associated InHD was 3% (hypertrophic cardiomyopathy and arrhythmogenic right ventricular cardiomyopathy). In approximately 7% of cases autopsy did not reveal any changes. Some of these cases might be explained by channelopathies (Table 1.2).

Table 1.2 Sudden death victims: pathological abnormalities found in necropsy.

Sudden death victims (n = 204)	N	%
Cardiovascular diseases (n = 183)		
Heart diseases (n = 161)		
Ischemic heart disease	119	58.4
Hypertensive heart disease	20	9.9
Valvular diseases	5	2.4
Idiopathic left ventricular hypertrophy	4	1.9
Dilated cardiomyopathy	4	1.9
Hypertrophic cardiomyopathy	3	1.5
Arrhythmogenic RV dysplasia/ cardiomyopathy	3	1.5
Myocarditis	1	0.5
Congenital heart disease	1	0.5
Amyloidosis	1	0.5
Vascular diseases (n = 22)		
Pulmonary embolism	8	3.9
Dissection of the aorta	9	4.4
Cerebral hemorrhage	5	2.4
Nonvascular diseases (n = 7)		
Gastrointestinal disorders	3	1.5
Pulmonary disorders	4	1.9
Without findings	14	6.9

Taken from Subirana *et al.*, 2011.

> The majority of SD cases occur in subjects with ischemic heart disease and/or heart failure. It must be emphasized that heart failure is most frequently related to hypertension, chronic ischemic heart disease, cardiomyopathies, and valvular heart disease.
>
> Inherited heart diseases are the main cause of SD in the first decades of life.

Chain of Events Leading to Final Arrhythmias and SD

SD is the final stage of a chain of events that ends in cardiac arrest, usually due to ventricular fibrillation (VF) or, less frequently, extreme bradyarrhythmia (Bayés-Genis *et al.*, 1995). In all cases there are a number of modulating and/or triggering factors that act on the vulnerable myocardium precipitating SD. Figure 1.3 shows this chain of events in different heart diseases. Ventricular fibrillation (VF) can appear without previous VT, triggered by a PVC in the presence of other modulating or triggering factors (including genetic and environmental),

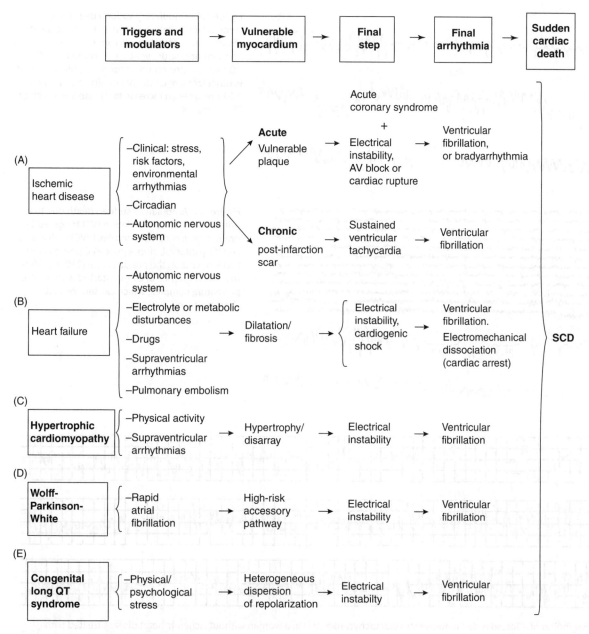

Figure 1.3 Chain of events that trigger cardiac sudden death (CSD) and parameters that different diseases present at the different stages leading to CSD (adapted from Bayés-Genis *et al.*, 1995).

and/or the sympathetic overdrive secondary to physical or mental stress. Usually under normal circumstances, probably all of these factors would not be of any consequence, but in the presence of acute ischemia they may trigger SD (Figure 1.5). The VF may be secondary to classic monomorphic sustained VT (Figure 1.4) or Torsades de Pointes VT (Figure 1.6). Sudden death is seldom a consequence of bradyarrhythmia (Figure 1.7).

Therefore, the final arrhythmias that precipitate SD are not always the same (Figures 1.4–1.8). In a study that we performed revising the final causes of SD in 157 ambulatory patients who died suddenly while wearing a Holter recorder (Bayés de Luna *et al.*, 1989), it was found that in two-thirds of patients SD was caused by **sustained VT that precipitated** VF (Figure 1.8, Table 1.3). This was generally accompanied by fast baseline heart rate (sinus tachycardia or rapid atrial fibrillation), which may be considered a sign of sympathetic overdrive (Figure 1.4). VF without previous VT, usually associated with acute IHD, is more frequently seen as a consequence of PVCs with an R/T phenomenon. In our experience with ambulatory patients this pattern was observed in less than 10% of cases (Figure 1.5). Curiously, in 13% of cases, SD was due to Torsades de Pointes VT precipitating VF, generally

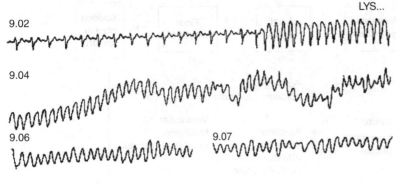

Figure 1.4 Ambulatory sudden death due to a ventricular fibrillation (VF) in an ischemic heart disease patient treated with amiodarone for frequent premature ventricular complexes. At 9:02 a.m. he presented a monomorphic sustained ventricular tachycardia (VT), followed by a VF at 9:04 a.m. after an increase in VT rate and width of QRS complex.

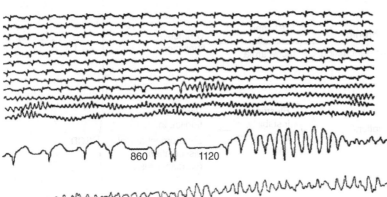

Figure 1.5 Ambulatory sudden death due to a primary ventricular fibrillation (VF) triggered by a premature ventricular complex (PVC) with a short coupling interval, after a post-PVC pause (1120 ms) longer than the previous one (860 ms). Note that the sequence of events started with an atrial premature complex, which caused the first shorter pause.

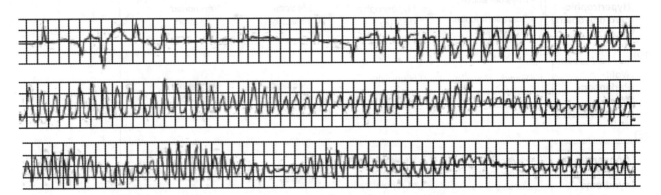

Figure 1.6 Beginning of a Torsades de Pointes ventricular tachycardia (VT) in a woman without ischemic heart disease treated with quinidine for runs of nonsustained VT. The Torsades de Pointes VT triggered a ventricular fibrillation (VF).

in patients without severe heart disease but taking antiarrhythmic Class I type drugs because of nonfrequent ventricular arrhythmias, sometimes isolated PVCs (proarrhythmic effect). We believe that if this study were performed now, the number of cases would be much smaller due to the evidence shown by the CAST study (Echt *et al.*, 1991) demonstrating that class I antiarrhythmic agents are dangerous, especially in patients with heart disease. Thus, currently the prescription of class I antiarrhythmic drugs in post-MI patients is much lower. Finally, cases of SD due to extreme bradyarrhythmia (≈15% in our study) (Figure 1.8B) were related more to

progressive depression of the sinus node and AV node automatism (Figure 1.7) than to AV block.

Figure 1.8 shows the final arrhythmias that cause SD in patients with different clinical settings: (A) in a mobile coronary care unit on route to hospital due to an acute coronary syndrome (Adgey *et al.*, 1982), (B) in ambulatory patients (Holter recording) (Bayés de Luna *et al.*, 1989), and (C) in patients hospitalized because of severe HF (Luu *et al.*, 1989). In the first situation (A), there are more cases of without previous VT than in our ambulatory cohort (B), most probably because patients in group A were in the acute phase of a MI. On the other hand,

Figure 1.7 Sudden death due to a progressive bradycardia in a patient with acute infarction and electromechanical dissociation.

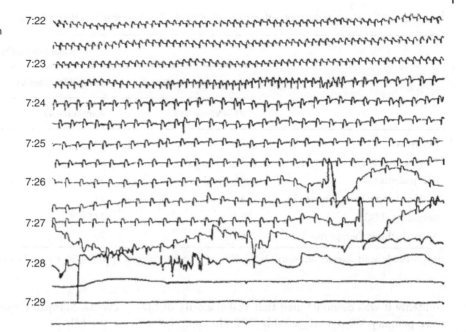

Figure 1.8 Sudden death: final arrhythmias. (A): in patients with acute ischemic heart disease (Adgey *et al.*, 1982). (B): in ambulatory patients wearing a Holter monitor, in whom a depressed ejection fraction was present in 80% of cases (Bayés de Luna *et al.*, 1989). (C): in patients with advanced heart failure (Luu *et al.*, 1989).

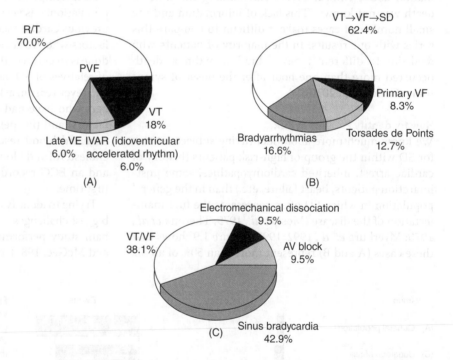

patients with severe HF (group C) presented extreme bradyarrhythmias more frequently as a cause of SD. This could be the reason why antiarrhythmic drugs are not efficient in preventing SD in patients with severe HF. In our series (Figure 1.8B), 80% of patients had a depressed ejection fraction (EF), although their functional class was acceptable. These patients were "too healthy to die", and many of these cases of SD could have been prevented with adequate therapy that sometimes consists of not prescribing an antiarrhythmic agent. The

Hippocratic Oath must be remembered: "c", "First, do no harm".

Our results were similar to those demonstrated in patients treated with implantable cardioverter defibrillators (ICD) with or without cardiac resynchronization therapy (CRT) (ICD-CR). In these cases, fast VTs also frequently appeared and were treated by antitachycardia pacing (Leitch *et al.*, 1991; Grimm *et al.*, 2006). In contrast, in a small series of post-MI patients with an EF <40%, using an insertable loop recorder, who died

Table 1.3 Clinical characteristics of patients who died suddenly while wearing a Holter device.

	Ventricular tachyarrhythmias		
	Group I Primary VF and	Group II Torsades de	Group III
	VT → VF n = 143	Pointes n = 43	Bradyarrhythmias n = 48
Age (years)	70	60	70
Gender (males) (%)	76	40	39
IHD patients (%)	84	50	70
With no known heart disease (%)	4	22	10
Resuscitated (%)	20	28.5	4
Antiarrhythmic therapy (%)	64	76	–

IHD, ischemic heart disease; VF, ventricular fibrillation; VT, ventricular tachycardia. Taken from Bayés de Luna *et al.*, 1989.

suddenly it was demonstrated that vast majority of SD were primary VF not triggered by VT. However, information about clinical events surrounding the time of death was not known. This lack of information and the small number of cases make it difficult to compare this series with our results. In the majority of patients who died due to different types of bradyarrhythmia, death occurred more than one hour after the onset of symptoms (Gang *et al.*, 2010).

How to Identify Patients at Risk

We know much more about identifying subjects at risk for SD within the group of high-risk patients (history of cardiac arrest, inherited cardiomyopathies, some post-infarction patients, heart failure, etc.) than in the general population in which SD often represents the first manifestation of the disease (Moss *et al.*, 1979; Théroux *et al.*, 1979; Myerburg *et al.*, 1992, 1997). Figure 1.9 shows that these cases (A and B) represent more than 50% of all SD

events. Many of these cases represent patients with first acute MI.

As it is impossible to carefully screen the entire general population, it is very difficult to identify subjects with no previous cardiovascular symptoms and no apparent risk factors who are at risk for SD. Currently, what should be done is to perform the following tasks: (i) a detailed study of relatives of SD patients; (ii) when seeing a patient for whatever reason, ask whether there are any family members who have had IHD, InHD, or present evident risk factors; and (iii) perform a complete physical examination and blood test (testing for risk factors, especially cholesterol and blood glucose) and take a blood pressure and an ECG recording when an adult is visited for the first time.

Trying to identify the subjects at risk for SD is one of the biggest challenges of modern cardiology. In the Framingham study performed on a general population (Kannel and McGee, 1985), two things were demonstrated: (i) the

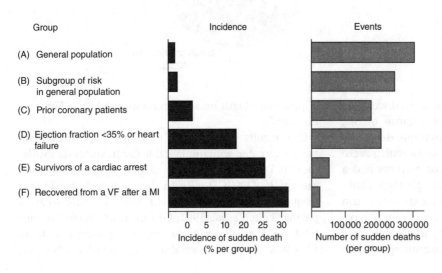

Figure 1.9 Left: the percentage of patients with SD is much higher in the high-risk groups (D–F) than in the general population (A, B). The total amount of cases occurring in the general population is greater than the number of all other subgroups of patients at risk (Myerburg *et al.*, 1997).

Figure 1.10 Risk of sudden death (SD) in the Framingham study according to multivariate risk (see inner note) in males and females (Kannel and McGee, 1985).

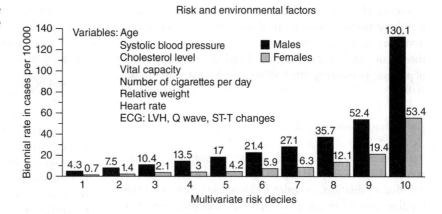

presence of alterations in the ECG, especially the bundle branch block, and left ventricular hypertrophy significantly increases the risk of SD, mainly in men; and (ii) in a multivariate analysis, the risk of SD increased especially in men, in relation to the amount of risk factors they had (Figure 1.10). Recently, it has been demonstrated that an increase of N-terminal prohormone brain natriuretic peptide (NT-proBNP) levels suggest, more than other previously described biochemical risk factors (dyslipidemia), an increased risk of sudden death in women (Korngold *et al.*, 2009) and in patients with heart failure (Vazquez *et al.*, 2009).

Risk stratification by an estimated calcium "score" by multislice computed tomography (CT) scan may help to identify patients with asymptomatic IHD. Nevertheless, this method is not currently recommended as a routine test (Greenland *et al.*, 2000), although it might be useful in patients with multiple risk factors (ATP III Guidelines 2001). The latest ACC and Associated Societies statement does not support the application of this technique in the general population and raises doubts as to whether this test should even be performed in medium- and high-risk patients (Hendel *et al.*, 2006). Also, its indiscriminate use is not recommended by other authors (Bonow 2009). In our opinion, in middle-aged patients with significant family history and/or multiple risk factors, it may be useful to perform the calcium "score" and, if positive, use a noninvasive coronarography by means of the latest generation multislice CT scan, which currently emits less radiation. Magnetic resonance imaging (MRI) offers more information on heart anatomy and function in a single test, and in a safer manner.

The difficulties in identifying subjects at risk for cardiac arrest are increased by the fact that the general population is more willing to perform medical examination to detect certain malignancies (colon, breast in women, and prostate in men). Adequate examinations, such as a multislice CT (in patients with a positive family history, and/or positive exercise test without symptoms

or other risk factors) or genetic tests in special situations (young patients with a family history of SD, suspicion of channelopathies, etc.), to determine apparently silent patients at risk for SD have to be performed more frequently.

The third part of this book deals with different aspects related to SD in different heart diseases and situations. The mechanisms that trigger fatal arrhythmias and the characteristics of an anatomic or electrophysiologic substrate, if known, that make the myocardium vulnerable to VF/SD will be explained.

How to Prevent SD

Obviously, the best way to prevent SD is to identify subjects at risk (see above). In the group with the highest risk (Figure 1.9D–F) it may be necessary, even compulsory, to implant an ICD, (see Chapters 5, 8, and 9, and Appendix A-4). This alone does not prevent SD but may help to avoid it when the final arrhythmia appears.

Thus, it is known how to prevent sudden death in patients at high risk (Myerburg *et al.*, 1992). It is much more difficult, however, to prevent SD events in the general population. The true prevention of SD is fighting the associated diseases, such as IHD, HF, and InHD Prevention of IHD should start in childhood, with an adequate health education promoting a healthy lifestyle, including controlled exercise, and an adequate diet to avoid overweight and obesity, preventing the development of risk factors. Of course, it is crucial to fight and treat high cholesterol, hypertension, diabetes, and other risk factors when they are present because they are, at least in part, responsible for the presence of atherosclerotic plaques. Also it is important, if possible, to avoid and treat HF adequately from the moment it starts, and it is necessary to diagnose and manage InHD This includes detailed personal and family history (history of syncope/SD), as well as the knowledge that a simple ECG pattern can identify a patient at risk for SD (see Chapter 9). When looking to the future, what is needed to reduce the burden of SD is an arteriosclerotic plaque stabilizer, preferably a chemical additive to food or water, that may be given to the global population, to stabilize the fibrous cap of the plaque and reduce the probability of plaque erosion/rupture and SD (Moss and Goldenberg, 2010).

The Management of a Patient Resuscitated (Survivors) from a Cardiac Arrest

Patients resuscitated from an out-of-hospital cardiac arrest should be referred to a reference center for a detailed evaluation, in order to identify the cause of the cardiac arrest, using an exhaustive examination that includes noninvasive and, if necessary, invasive tests. This is the routine approach for patients who suffered a cardiac arrest with and without evident heart disease. A report (Krahn *et al.*, 2009) recommends genetic testing only when a genetic disease appears to be responsible for cardiac arrest in the clinical test results. In our opinion, genetic studies need to be more accessible and cheaper. This would encourage their use and would be of great benefit regardless of their current limitations, in addition to studying the relatives of patients with InHD (see Chapter 9).

Ventricular fibrillation is the cause of cardiac arrest in most of the cases (Figure 1.8). Therefore, it is necessary to prevent the first episode and, in any case, to organize a proper plan to prevent future episodes. If VF appears to be associated with ischemia, the possibility of revascularization has to be considered (see Chapter 11, Chronic Ischemic Heart Disease). Other possible mechanisms involved in the triggering of VF have to be ruled out, that is, in rapid AF in patients with Wolff–Parkinson–White syndrome (WPW) in whom ablation of the accessory pathway is mandatory.

In many other cases of cardiac arrest due to VT/VF, if no trigger is found, it is usually necessary to implant an ICD with a resynchronization pacemaker (CRT), only if needed (see Chapters 9–11).

Obviously, in cardiac arrest due to passive arrhythmias, an urgent pacemaker implantation is required (see Chapter 6).

For more details about ICD indications/implantation see Chapters 5 (Ventricular Tachycardias, and Ventricular Fibrillation), 9, and 11 (Ischemic Heart Disease and Heart Failure), as well as Appendix A-4 (Automatic Implantable Cardioverter Defibrillator (ICD)), and guidelines of scientific societies (Recommended General Bibliography p. xvii).

Arrhythmias and Severe Clinical Complications

The relationship of active/passive arrhythmias with SD has been mentioned. Now, the other important clinical complications of tachy/bradyarrhythmias not associated to SD will be exposed. Tachyarrhythmias may induce severe consequences on the patient's clinical and hemodynamic status, which may appear as:

o A crisis of left ventricular failure, and also a congestive HF (tachycardiomyopathy).
o A crisis of angina (hemodynamic angina).
o A low cardiac output with dyspnea and weakness.
o Hypotension that may be significant, even resulting in cardiogenic shock.
o Embolism, more often systemic, frequently cerebral, sometimes with severe consequences. It has been recently demonstrated that not only a complete stroke but also cognitive impairment may be caused by cerebral microembolism in patients with sluggish left atrium related to AF or may be even in its absence but with stagment LA due to advanced IAB (Bayés de Luna *et al.*, 2017).
o Dizziness, pre-syncope, syncope. Syncope may be benign or may be a marker of life-threatening arrhythmia (see later).

The most frequent symptoms related to bradyarrhythmia are a low cardiac output, dizziness, syncope, and even SD.

All the symptoms related to brady or tachyarrhythmias are especially important in relation to:

o The presence or absence of heart disease. An association with either acute ischemia or HF is of utmost importance.
o Duration of the arrhythmia; the longer it is, the greater the risk of not being well tolerated.
o Heart rate (fast tachycardia or severe bradycardia) during the arrhythmia. Consequently, an episode of short duration, with a not very fast heart rate in subjects without heart disease, does not affect the cardiac output, and it will not result in significant hemodynamic impairment. On the other hand, very rapid episodes, especially in patients with heart disease and poor ventricular function, may cause evident hemodynamic impairment resulting in dyspnea, hypotension (Figure 1.11), angina, syncope, and even shock and congestive HF if the arrhythmia is sustained.
o The presence or absence of AF dissotiation.

Some aspects of syncope, the most alarming symptom associated with arrhythmias, which may be of practical interest to the reader, will now be examined.

Syncope: Serious or Innocent Symptom?
Concept

Syncope is the sudden and transient loss of consciousness caused by an important reduction in cerebral

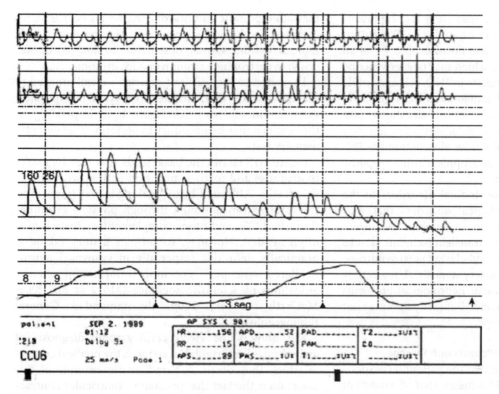

Figure 1.11 Note the drop of blood pressure coinciding with an abrupt rise of heart rate during a paroxysmal tachycardia.

perfusion. It is accompanied by loss of muscular tone and a total spontaneous recovery in a short period of time. At times there is only a feeling of dizziness or unsteadiness (pre-syncope) (Garcia Civera *et al.*, 1989).

This is the most worrying symptom of patients with arrhythmias. It can be either the expression of an innocent process or a marker of evident risk of SD. From clinical and prognostic points of view, there are three types of syncope: (i) neuromediated via vagal reflex and those due to orthostatic hypotension that are usually benign; (ii) related to heart diseases, such as severe tachy- or bradyarrhythmia, or those due to obstruction of flow (aortic stenosis, or mixoma for example) (see later), which are usually malignant; and (iii) very short crisis of cerebral ischemia or epilepsies. In fact, clear transient ischemic attack (TIA) has to be excluded as one type of syncope (see later). These different types of syncope are examined, as are the ways to cope with them. It must be remembered that syncope represents 1% of all cases attended to in an emergency department.

Mechanisms

- **Neuromediated reflex syncope.** A high percentage of syncopal episodes (>50%) are neuromediated via a vasovagal reflex, often with triggering factors related to increased vagal tone, such as cough, micturition,

venous puncture, orthostatism, and so on. Recent studies have shown that some polymorphism of protein G is associated with family history and may explain the susceptibility to vasovagal syncope (Márquez *et al.*, 2007; Lelonek *et al.*, 2009). **Hypotensive orthostatic syncope** is frequent (10–20%). It is caused by a dysautonomy reflex during orthostatism, which produces a loss of vaso-constrictive reflexes in the vessels of the lower extremities, reducing baroreceptor sensitivity and producing reactive hypotension to such a degree that it decreases cerebral flow and induces syncope. **Hypersensitivity of the carotid sinus** (a pause >3 s, or a decrease in blood pressure >30 mm, that occurs after carotid sinus massage for 10 s with or without syncope) may also induce a neuromediated syncope via a vagal stimulus from a sick carotid sinus, and may be the cause of an unexplained fall, especially in the elderly. This syncope is often related to some accidental pressure on the carotid sinus (while shaving, for instance). Patients referred to a tilt test should have a carotid sinus massage performed. The association between neuromediated syncope and carotid sinus hypersensitivity is approximately 30%.

- **Syncopes of cardiac origin** include all syncopes related to arrhythmias (5–10%); they encompass bradyarrhythmias (sick sinus syndrome and advanced

AV block) and tachyarrhythmias (very fast supraventricular arrhythmias, i.e., pre-excited atrial fibrillation with WPW, sustained VT, and polymorphic VT of all types). These arrhythmias, which may trigger syncope and VF/SD, are seen especially in IHD, HF, and InHD (cardiomyopathies and channelopathies), as well as in other heart diseases and clinical situations (see Chapters 8–11). Also, syncopes of cardiac origin may be related to obstruction of flow obstruction (2–3%), as in aortic stenosis, hypertrophic cardiomyopathy (CM), mixoma, and so on.

- **Syncopes related to neurological disorders** in the past included the neurological disorders that may induce a brusque reduction in cerebral perfusion, which may happen in some transient ischemic attacks with loss of consciousness (subclavian steal syndrome or bilateral severe carotid artery stenosis). Usually they are accompanied by transient neurological problems (transient ischemic attack, etc.) but really they may not be considered a true syncope.

Diagnosis and Management of Patients with Syncope

Firstly, we have to be certain that the patient has experienced a syncopal episode. This means that all aspects of the definition of syncope must be present: abrupt and transient loss of consciousness, caused by a brusque reduction in cerebral flow, accompanied by a loss of muscular tone, followed by a total spontaneous recovery. The group of Bob Sheldon, in Canada, has published a series of articles in how to differentiate neuromediated syncope from seizures, and from other arrhythmic forms of syncope. The Calgary score helps physicians to discriminate benign from malignant forms of syncope using only interrogation tools (Sheldon *et al.*, 2002, 2006, 2010).

Next, we must always rule out factors that may provoke prolonged unconsciousness, such as hysterical attacks, hypoglycemia, intoxication including alcohol (heavy drinkers), or dizziness and vertigo among others. We must also exclude epileptic episodes that sometimes produce problems of differential diagnosis, although history taking is very useful in general (see above). During epileptic attacks there is no reduction in cerebral perfusion; however, some infrequent epileptic forms may present arrhythmias with syncopal episodes and even SD following an epileptic convulsion (Rugg-Gunn *et al.*, 2004; Tomson *et al.*, 2008).

Syncopes may be accompanied by seizures (pallor, no pulse, rapid recovery with facial flush – Stokes–Adams crisis) and may occur at rest or, typically, during exercise (see Chapter 9). It must be emphasized that it is extremely important to differentiate neuromediated vasovagal syncopes, including orthostatic syncope, which are generally benign, from syncope due to cardiac origin

that often present an unfavorable prognosis. The latter includes (see before) syncope due to very slow or very rapid arrhythmias, or an obstruction to flow (aortic stenosis, hypertrophic cardiomyopathy, myxoma, etc.).

To recognize the origin of syncope we will proceed to the basal study that includes history taking, physical examination, and an ECG (Figure 1.12). Depending on the results it may be necessary to perform other complementary tests.

Figure 1.12 shows the basal study that may be useful to diagnose and further manage a patient with syncopal attacks. Although history taking is very important, the information obtained through physical examination, the ECG, and other complementary tests is also often needed. However, sometimes history taking is practically definitive (especially in vasovagal neuromediated syncopes). For more information see the guidelines of scientific societies (Moya *et al.*, 2009; McCarthy *et al.*, 2009; Recommended General Bibliography p. xvii).

Not only is the electrocardiographic diagnosis of arrhythmias important, but so too is the medical context in which they occur. A paradigmatic example of this assertion is the fact that premature ventricular contractions having similar clinical and electrocardiographic characteristics are usually benign in healthy patients, whereas in patients with ischemic heart disease and poor ventricular function they represent an evident risk of sudden death, especially in the presence of acute ischemia.

Units of cardiac syncope have to be prepared to perform a tilt test. Indications for a tilt test have been limited to cases of syncope where the cause is not clear through extensive interrogation of triggers, clinical scenarios, and physical examination. It is still useful as an integral part of the study of the autonomic nervous system. A tilt test should not replace clinical judgement:

○ It is important **to obtain a comprehensive history** (Colman *et al.*, 2009), including: (i) family antecedents of syncope or SD, which is very important in attempting to rule out InHD; (ii) antecedents of previous heart disease (MI, history of valve heart disease, etc.); (iii) the number of prior syncopes, and in adults whether they also occurred during childhood; and (iv) the evaluation of: (a) the prodromal symptoms or circumstance of appearance (exercise, movements, digestion, emotions, etc.); (b) the onset (abrupt or slightly gradual); (c) the position in which they occur, such as standing (orthostatic hypotension) or sitting; (d) what the patient was doing before (cough, defecation, micturition, carotid sinus massage, neck movements, venous puncture, etc.); (e) the recovery

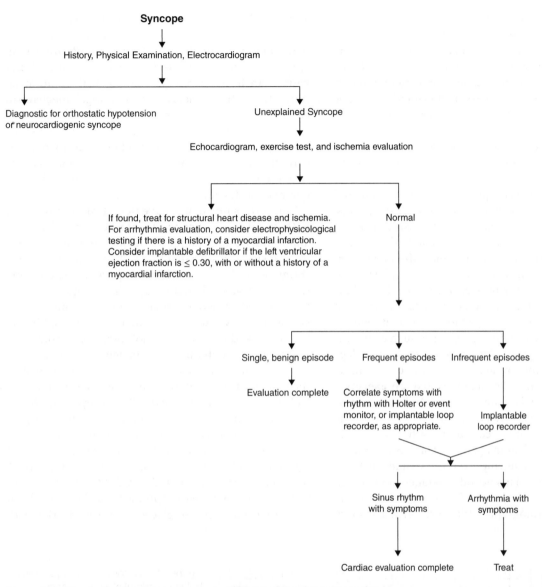

Figure 1.12 Algorhythm for the management of patients with syncope (see text).

of consciousness (rapid or gradual); (f) associated events (tongue biting); and (g) appearance (pallor), and so on.

- With all the data it will be possible, in many cases, to have already an impression of the etiology of syncope. Obviously, it is very important to proceed to **physical examination** (auscultation of the heart and arteries of the neck, and palpation of the heart and vessels).
- In addition, **correct interpretation of the ECG** is of the utmost importance, particularly AV or bundle blocks, LVH, Q waves, and so on, the correct measurement of the QT interval, and the recognition of possible ECG Brugada patterns, as well as the slight alteration of repolarization seen in V1–V3 that may be

considered normal variant but correspond to different inherited heart diseases (see Chapter 9).

Neuromediated syncope usually occurs at rest, although some exceptions exist (see later), with a tendency to occur in standing position or after digestion. Three types of response can be observed during a tilt test (see Appendix A-3, Tilt Table Test): vasodepressor, cardioinhibitory, and mixed. In general, the vasodepressor component is predominant over the cardioinhibitory type (especially in the young and in the very elderly). However, on some occasions, long pauses corresponding to malignant vagal syncopes can be observed. Profound cardioinhibitory responses, including progressive heart rate lowering due to depressed automatism and/or depressed AV conduction (Figure 1.13), may be life-threatening or contribute to life-threatening situations like motor vehicle accidents. Changes in blood pressure and heart rate are continuously recorded during a tilt test. In the case of significant cardioinhibitory component response, pacemaker implantation may be considered occasionally (see later). Nevertheless, studies using implantable loop recorders demonstrate that even syncope due to serious cardioinhibitory pauses (>15–20 s) do not usually induce permanent cardiac arrest and SD.

Exercise syncope is frequently of cardiac origin and tends to occur abruptly with no prodromal symptoms. Patients may present a Stokes–Adams crisis (see previously). Nevertheless, some syncopes of cardiac origin, including some channelopathies, may often appear at rest. In addition, some exercise syncope may be neuromediated (oftenly in the post-exercise period) (Calkins *et al.*, 1995) (see later). It is very important to rule out neuromediated vasovagal syncope in patients with a syncope that occurred during exercise, such as in athletes. However, syncope during exercise is a "red flag" and should prompt immediate actions to determine the cause of syncope. As already stated, **an exercise-provoked syncope is usually associated with a serious structural heart disease**, such as severe aortic stenosis, hypertrophic cardiomyopathy, or acute ischemia or some channelopathies. For this reason, all syncopes presented during exercise should be thoroughly investigated. This includes detailed clinical and family history to search for SD history, ECG during exercise, echocardiography, tilt test, MRI, coronary angiography, and even electrophysiology studies (EPS) and genetic tests, in order to rule out associated pathology. **Usually the continuation of practicing sports is contraindicated, unless the underlying cause can be resolved** (i.e., WPW with rapid atrial fibrillation). If the neuromediated vagal mechanism can be proven, in the absence of structural heart disease and channelopathies, it is not necessary to discontinue sports activity, but it should be performed under careful control (Calkins *et al.*, 1995). Some patients may require "extra" studies in order to allow them to compete professionally.

Currently, **some drugs have been tested in patients with vasovagal syncopes** (β blockers, dihydroergotamine, midodrine, fluhidrocortisone, etc.) but no definitive answer to all patients has been established yet (Brignole *et al.*, 1992; Sheldon *et al.*, 2010). At the same time, pacemakers do not always offer adequate protection (see later). Nonpharmacological treatment, consisting of lifestyle advice (adequate fluid and salt intake is advised and excessive alcohol intake is discouraged) and physical counter pressure maneuvers (leg-crossing, handgrip and arm tensing, etc.) are recommended as the first-line treatment to avoid vasovagal syncope (Van Dijk *et al.*, 2006; Brignole *et al.*, 2004; Moya *et al.*, 2009). Also, autonomic nervous system training, such as a progressively prolonged time in standing position leaning back on the wall, may be useful avoiding neuromediated syncope, and some promising results have been reported (Reybrouck and Ector, 2006). This difficult to undertake therapeutic approach has been validated in a first randomized placebo-controlled trial with

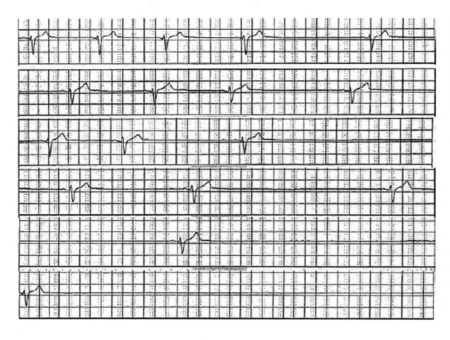

Figure 1.13 Six continuous strips (from a Holter recording) of a patient aged 35 years who presented a syncope after venous puncture. Sinus automaticity is progressively depressed in the absence of an escape rhythm, and a pause lasting 15 s arose leading to syncope.

promising results that hopefully will be confirmed in the future in a larger randomized trial (Tan *et al.*, 2010). The authors of this book are not using this approach (tilt training) very much, as most of the patients fail to do it in a systematic manner. It may be used in some doubtful cases and, if positive, help to assume that the syncope is neuromediated.

In orthostatic hypotensive syncope, fluorocortisone may be effective and some drugs (α- and β-blockers, diuretics, angiotensin converting enzyme inhibitors (ACE-I), sublingual nitrates, etc.) should be avoided. It may be beneficial to use long elastic stockings. When spending a long period of time in standing position cannot be avoided, it is advisable to perform the physical counterpressure maneuvers (see before) as a preventive measure to favor venous blood return. It is also helpful to drink plenty of water before prolonged standing position (lectures, etc.). Ideally, one has to avoid and/or control triggering factors, like prolonged standing or venous puncture (Figure 1.13).

Clinical findings suggesting a diagnosis of "syncope" account for around 1% of urgent care clinic visits (see before). Therefore, there is a need for consensus on risk stratification (Benditt and Can, 2010). One of the last proposed is the ROSE rule (Reed *et al.*, 2010), which has an excellent sensitivity and negative predictive value (NPV) in the identification of high-risk patients with syncope.

For the management of syncope, we refer to *The Integrated Strategy for Syncope Management* by the European Society of Cardiology (Brignole *et al.*, 2004; McCarthy *et al.*, 2009; Moya *et al.*, 2009). From these guidelines, we will comment on some relevant aspects (Morady 2009):

- Neuromediated and hypotensive syncopes are the most common.
- The examination of a ≥40-year-old patient with syncope must include the compression of the carotid sinus on either side for 10 s. The provocation of pauses of >3 s and/or a decrease in blood pressure of >30 mm is indicative of syncope due to carotid sinus hypersensitivity (see before).
- The tilt test is used to confirm a diagnosis of neuromediated syncope but is not to be used for evaluating the efficacy of treatments. It is acknowledge that proper interrogation may result in fewer tilt tables, reducing costs and diagnostic tests (Sheldon *et al*, 2006, 2010).
- Implantable loop recorders may be more cost effective than external recorders or the conventional Holter recorder in the diagnosis of infrequent syncope (see Appendix A-3, Tilt table test, Figure 1.12). Patients with recurrent unexplained syncope and major structural

heart diseases that have received a therapy guided by means of an implantable loop recorder, had a significantly lower number of recurrences (RAST trial) (Krahn *et al.*, 2001).

- In patients with syncope and an EF <30%, the implantation of an ICD without prior invasive EPS may be considered. However, in our opinion, neuromediated vasovagal syncope needs to be ruled out in this group of patients. A more complete clinical study is advisable.
- Electrophysiology study may be of help in patients with syncope due to suspected severe bradyarrhythmia (bundle branch block especially with long PR) or history of palpitations (possible associated tachyarrhythmia). Some groups may implant a pacemaker in patients with syncope and bifascicular block. Currently, the group of Shendon in Calgary is running the SPRITELY study, which is randomizing patients with syncope and bifascicular block to receive either an implantable loop recorder or a pacemaker.
- As first-line therapy, to prevent neuromediated syncope, the following measures are advisable: (i) a regular intake of water (minimum of 2.5 liters/day) and salt (2 g/day) unless contraindicated, (ii) the avoidance of triggers (i.e., venous puncture to be standing for long periods of time), (iii) performing muscular contractions in arms and legs, especially standing, (iv) avoiding alcohol, and (v) if prodromal symptoms appear, laying down in dorsal decubitus with the legs raised.
- There is no evidence from any study supporting the efficacy of drugs (β-blockers, disopyramide, midodrine, chloridin, etc.) in preventing neuromediated syncope (see before).
- The usefulness of pacemakers depends on the type of syncope. It is mandatory in the majority of cases of advanced AV block (see Chapter 6, Clinical, Prognostic, and Therapeutic Implications of the Passive Arrhythmia), and also in most cases of sick sinus syndrome and bradycardia–tachycardia syndrome. Obviously, in the majority of cases of VT/VF an ICD has to be implanted. However, **in neuromediated syncope the usefulness of a pacemaker is not universally recommended.** It has even been suggested that the positive results found in some studies may be biased by the placebo effect (Raviele *et al.*, 2004). The VPS II Study (Connolly *et al.*, 2003), which removed the placebo effect by implanting pacemakers to patients with neuromediated syncope and comparing ON and OFF groups, demonstrated that pacemakers are not useful for the treatment of neuromediated syncope. However, since the INVASY trial (Occhetta *et al.*, 2004), it is thought that physiologic pacing starting early, when the decrease in heart rate is detected (e.g., using a Medtronic VERSA), may help to

avoid syncope from recurring. Some patients with profound cardioinhibitory syncope may benefit from pacemaker implantation. In those cases, "rate-drop" pacemakers (Medtronic) are recommended because they can be activated early at the beginning of the pause, avoiding the patient to become symptomatic. Finally, in patients with hypersensitive carotid sinus syncope, implantation of bicameral pacemaker has been shown to be effective (Kenny *et al.*, 2001).

o The occurrence of a recent (i.e., within the last 6 months) unexplained syncope in patients with hypertrophic cardiomyopathy is a risk factor for SD (see Chapter 9, Hypertrophic Cardiomyopathy).

Arrhythmias and Unpleasant but not Serious Symptoms

Many active arrhythmias, whether isolated (premature atrial or ventricular complexes) or sustained (atrial fibrillation, tachycardias), do not result in evident hemodynamic disturbances but are subjectively uncomfortable, appearing in the form of precordial discomfort, regular or irregular palpitations (to feel the heart beat), and dyspnea. The sensation of anticipated beats is typical for premature complexes, whereas fast regular or irregular palpitations suggest paroxysmal tachycardias or atrial fibrillation, especially if the onset is sudden. A sensation of very rapid neck pulsations is typical for paroxysmal AV junctional reentrant tachycardia (see Chapter 4, Junctional Reentrant (Reciprocating) Tachycardia: Clinical Presentation). In contrast, sinus tachycardia is characterized by regular, gradually increasing palpitations. Also, nonsevere bradyarrhythmias may induce dizziness and fatigue, especially if the heart rate does not increase properly with exercise.

The patient may be concerned about these symptoms, but they usually do not represent a severe concern. However, this does not mean that they are not potentially dangerous symptoms and that no treatment has to be prescribed. It will depend essentially on the patient's clinical context.

Asymptomatic Arrhythmias

Finally, there are other cases in which the patient may be unaware of the presence of an arrhythmia, including frequent PVCs or relatively rapid atrial fibrillation. It should be borne in mind that, in general, PVCs are detected more easily in healthy subjects than in subjects with severe heart disease. However, it could be necessary to treat these arrhythmias if prognosis could be improved. The presence of asymptomatic PVCs with special characteristics are markers of risk in many cases, such as post-MI (Bigger *et al.*, 1984; Moss *et al.*, 1979), HF (Van Lee *et al.*, 2010) hypertrophic CM (McKenna *et al.*,

2002), and other inherited heart diseases, and so on., and sometimes need to be treated (see Chapters 5, 9 and 11). Some passive arrhythmias, such as severe bradycardia, second-degree Wenckeback type AV block in athletes, or vagal overdrive, may be completely asymptomatic, and usually do not require specific treatment (see Chapter 6, Clinical, Prognostic, and Therapeutic Implications of the Passive Arrhythmia).

The Importance of Clinical History and Physical Examination in Diagnosis and Assessment of Arrhythmias
(Bellet, 1969; Knoebel et al., 1993; Recommended General Bibliography p. xvii)

It must be remembered that it is not an electrocardiographic tracing with a heart rhythm disorder that is being dealing with but a patient with a special clinical context who presents an arrhythmia. History taking and physical examination will help us to determine the type of arrhythmia with which we are dealing and to make an overall assessment based on the following facts:

o An arrhythmia may or may not be suspected before an ECG is performed. Sometimes a patient describes a change in heart rhythm suggestive of an arrhythmia, but nothing appears on the ECG tracing, even if an arrhythmia is detected during the physical examination. These cases need complementary testing (an exercise test, and especially a Holter ECG recording) for a clear diagnosis and evaluation. Alternatively, it may be possible to detect an arrhythmia during a physical examination when the patient does not present any suggestive symptoms.

o Bear in mind that the prognostic importance and the therapeutic implications of arrhythmias depend to a large extent on the clinical setting in which they occur.

o Moreover, there are special situations (athletes with syncope, patient's relatives with a history of SD) in which it becomes important to integrate the family history, physical examination results, and surface ECG with other special electrocardiographic techniques (exercise testing, Holter ECG recording, EPS) and imaging techniques (echocardiography, cardiac MRI, and coronarography), as well as genetic tests, to reach a correct diagnosis, to determine the patient's prognosis, and to be able to take the most appropriate therapeutic decision. It is important to emphasize the value of extensive electrocardiographic knowledge, as minor changes (i.e., repolarization abnormalities), such as the presence of negative T waves in leads V1 to V3–V4 in the case of arrhythmogenic right ventricular dysplasia, or a slight ST-segment elevation with r′, usually seen in lead V1 in the case of Brugada syndrome, may be essential to suggest a diagnosis.

Management of a Patient with Suspected Arrhythmias

In order to make a diagnosis of arrhythmia, two factors in particular should be taken into consideration by a physician when examining a patient: (i) the rate of the heart rhythm and (ii) heart rhythm regularity or irregularity.

The study of these two characteristics of the heart rhythm through history taking and physical examination (especially arterial pulse palpation and auscultation) is very important for the presumptive diagnosis of arrhythmias, even though electrocardiography remains the definitive and key technique for such diagnoses. It should be emphasized that the arrhythmia should not be viewed as an isolated ECG recording, but as a tracing taken within a given clinical setting.

History Taking

The patient may present symptoms: palpitations, dyspnea, angina, dizziness, or syncope (Stokes–Adams attack). However, it is advisable to remember that the patient is often not aware that they present any type of arrhythmia. Sometimes, not only does the patient not take notice of the onset of arrhythmia, but they are also not aware of the presence of a rapid/slow, regular/irregular rhythm. This happens particularly in atrial fibrillation with relatively slow rates and in many cases of premature complexes. If the patient feels the arrhythmia, history taking and the physical examination will inform if isolated irregularities of the pulse, typical of premature complexes, are present, or if regular or irregular episodes of rapid or slow rhythm are present.

The onset of an episode in a patient with a rapid heart rate may be progressive (sinus tachycardia) or sudden, from one second to the next (paroxysmal tachyarrhythmia). When tachycardias appear and disappear in a sudden but repetitive way, they are called incessant tachycardias. It should be noted that a characteristic of supraventricular paroxysmal tachycardias is that not only are the onset and cessation abrupt (paroxysmal), but also polyuria may occur at the end if the episode is long. In the presence of a paroxysmal AV junctional reentrant tachycardia (AVJRT), with the circuit exclusively in the AV junction (AVNRT), the patient may feel a rapid regular pounding in the neck due to the transmission of atrial activity contracting against the closed AV valves. This does not happen when an accessory pathway participates in the reentry circuit (junctional reentrant tachycardia with accessory pathway (AVRT)) (see Chapter 4, Junctional Reentrant (Reciprocating) Tachycardia).

In fact, the feeling that the heart beat exist is the demonstration that the heart contraction is strong and presumably in a failing heart usually the presence of strong contraction is not frequently felt. Patients with acute AM present frequently PVC but often are not aware of that.

The Physical Examination

The physical examination (especially palpation and auscultation) obviously allows the heart rate to be checked and determines whether the rhythm is regular or irregular (see above).

It may also be useful to verify the presence of AV dissociation (atria and ventricles contract separately and independently). The presence of AV dissociation practically ensures that a wide QRS complex tachycardia is of ventricular origin (AV dissociation by interference). If the rhythm is slow, it corresponds to an advanced AV block (AV dissociation by block). In these cases, the first heart sound varies in intensity in accordance with the relationship between the P wave (atrial contraction) and the QRS complex (ventricular contraction) (Figure 1.14).

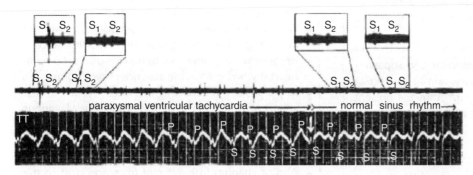

Figure 1.14 Differences in the intensity of the first heart sound during a ventricular tachycardia (VT). Note how, when it reverts, after quinidine administration, the intensity of the first sound is unchanged (Bellet, 1969).

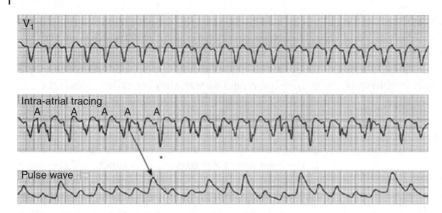

Figure 1.15 Ventricular tachycardia with atrioventricular (AV) dissociation. The dissociation between atrial (A) and QRS complexes is very evident in the intra-atrial tracing. Furthermore, when the A wave precedes the QRS, the AV synchrony provokes a vigorous pulse wave (arrow). Meanwhile, when the A wave overlaps with the QRS, the pulse wave is weaker, yet the contraction against closed AV valves causes a cannon wave in the intra-atrial recording (asterisk).

Be reminded that the AV valves open with the atrial contraction (P wave), and the first heart sound is recorded when the AV valves close. A long P-QRS interval means that the first heart sound has been generated at the time that the leaflets of the AV valve are nearly closed, as a long time has passed since the atrial contraction, and they tend to get back to this previous position spontaneously. Therefore, when closing, no intense heart sound may be detected. Meanwhile, if the closure happens immediately following the atrial contraction, the leaflets of the AV valves are separate and the first heart sound is louder. Thus, in AV dissociation, when the P-QRS interval is short, the first heart sound is more intense, like cannon shot (Bellet, 1969). In practice, AV dissociation produces a first heart sound of varying intensity in the clinical auscultation (Figure 1.14).

The presence of cannon A waves (A wave of high amplitude) in the venous pulse, which occurs when the atrial and the ventricular contractions eventually coincide, and the verification of variable systolic pressure may also help to diagnose AV dissociation (Figure 1.15).

tool, because they are difficult to obtain and to record, and an ECG, which is the key tool for diagnosis, may be performed immediately at any medical center. However, it will be of interest to readers to know that, as just stated, the auscultation of the first heart sound (Figure 1.14) may be useful for a differential diagnosis of wide QRS complex tachycardia and slow rhythms (sinus bradycardia vs advanced AV block). In patients with regular tachycardia and a wide QRS of uncertain origin, the usefulness of the physical examination, so well studied in the nineteenth century by McKencie and Wenckebach, in particular the auscultation of the first heart sound and the examination of the venous pulse, has been confirmed (Garrat *et al.*, 1994).

> Arrhythmias may be suspected after history taking or physical examination in any of the following circumstances:
>
> - Subjective feeling of heart rhythm anomalies (regular or irregular palpitations, anticipated beat, etc.).
> - History of episodes of tachycardia characterized by abrupt onset, sometimes with pounding in the neck, and concomitant polyuria.
> - Dizziness with slow or very rapid rhythm.
> - Past history of pre-syncope or syncope, even without knowledge of coinciding heart rhythm disturbances.
> - Irregular or very slow (<40 bpm) or rapid (>100 bpm) heart rhythm, even in the absence of symptoms.
> - Any transient variation in the intensity of the first sound at auscultation, in the amplitude of venous pulse A wave, and in the blood pressure levels.
> - Absence of changes in heart rate during exercise, or during the day and night.
> - Abrupt changes in heart rate from one beat to the next.

> Monitoring and recording of the venous pulse, blood pressure monitoring, and especially auscultation of the first sound may help to make a diagnosis of atrioventricular (AV) dissociation.
>
> These classical signs may still be useful to make a differential diagnosis between ventricular and supraventricular tachycardia with aberrancy, and to suspect an advanced AV block when bradyarrhythmia is present. Undoubtedly, when the patient is in critical condition, the most important thing is to give therapeutic assistance as soon as possible.

Today, data obtained from the physical examination in a patient with arrhythmia are scarcely used as a diagnostic

The Importance of Surface ECG and Other Techniques

Surface ECG recording is the key technique used for diagnosis of a cardiac arrhythmia. Carotid sinus massage with electrocardiographic recording may help in the differential diagnosis of the different types of tachyarrhythmias, according to the results of this maneuver (Figures 1.16 and 4.70) (Table 1.4).

On some occasions, however, conventional surface electrocardiography cannot confirm an arrhythmia suggested by history taking or physical examination, or it cannot confirm the correct diagnosis. In searching

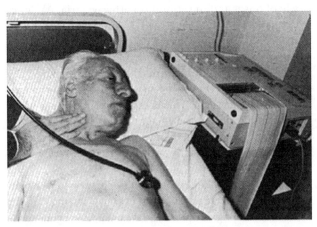

(A). Sinus tachycardia: usually present a transient delay

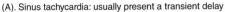

(B). Paroxysmal reentrant supraventricular tachycardia: frequently ceases

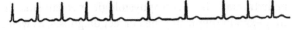

(C). Atrial fibrillation increase of AV block

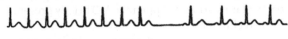

(D). Flutter 2:1: the degree of AV block usually increases

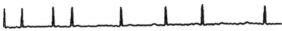

(E). Ventricular tachycardia: usually there is no modification

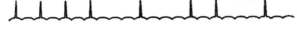

Figure 1.16 Note the correct procedure for carotid sinus massage (CSM). The force applied with the fingers should be similar to that required to squeeze a tennis ball, during a short time period (10–15 s), and the procedure should be repeated four to five times on either side, starting on the right side. Never perform this procedure on both sides at the same time. Caution should be taken in older people and in patients with a history of carotid sinus syndrome. The procedure must include continuous ECG and auscultation. (A–E): examples of how different arrhythmias react to CSM. See Table 1.4 for more information.

Table 1.4 Response of the different arrhythmias elicited by carotid sinus massage (CSM).

Arrhythmia	Response
1. Sinus tachycardia	Without evident effect on the tachycardia, but appears to cause a transient slowing down. If the mechanism is reentry, no changes are observed
2. Monomorphic focal atrial tachycardia	Depends on mechanism: without effect if the mechanism is micro-reentry; sometimes transitory suppression if occurs by increased automatism; frequently suppression if by triggered activity
3. AV junctional tachycardia due to an ectopic focus	Without effect on the tachycardia
4. AV junctional reentrant tachycardia (AVJRT)	The tachycardia can finish. If not tachycardia continues without changes in the heart rate
5. Atrial fibrillation	Without effect on the fibrillation rate, but there is a slowing down of the ventricular rate due to AV block
6. Atrial flutter (including the atrial macro-reentrant tachycardia)	Without effect on the arrhythmia, but frequently more atrial waves are blocked by vagal action on the AV node. This is useful when the atrial waves are not visible.
7. Ventricular tachycardia	In general, without effect on the arrhythmia. However, exceptionally, some cases of ventricular tachycardia have stopped with vagal maneuver

for the arrhythmia, some other tests have to be used (Holter ECG recording, event loop recorder, exercise ECG testing, tilt test, etc.). To reach the correct diagnosis, it may be necessary to perform intracavitary EPS or use amplified waves (Bayés de Luna, *et al.*, 1978) and filtering systems (Goldwasser *et al.*, 2011), which are not available in commercial devices. Through these latter techniques, it is possible to see the P wave or ectopic atrial activity when it is not visible or is hidden in the precedent T wave (see Appendix A-3, Other Surface Techniques to Register Electrical Cardiac Activity, Figures A.13 and 4.62). It will also sometimes be necessary to have radiologic and echocardiographic data, as well as other imaging techniques (isotopes, MRI), coronarographic studies (conventional and/or noninvasive), and even genetic tests to determine the presence of associated diseases and to be able to better assess the prognosis of the arrhythmias (see Appendix A-3, Other Nonelectrocardiographic Techniques).

Electrocardiographic Diagnosis of Arrhythmias: Preliminary Considerations

To make a valid electrocardiographic interpretation of an arrhythmia and understand the electrophysiologic mechanism that may explain its presence, it is necessary to take into account the following:

o It is advisable to have a magnifying glass and calipers (alternatively, the use of available commercial semi-automatic calipers, i.e., ICONICO, USA). They may be used to accurately measure the wave duration, the distance between P waves or QRS complexes, the differences in the coupling interval (distance between a premature P wave or QRS complex and the P wave or QRS complex of the preceding basal rhythm), and so on. With current digitalized ECGs saved as PDF files: magnification ×8 or ×10 is also beneficial.

o It is helpful to take a long strip of the ECG tracing, especially important in the case of possible parasystole, and record 12-lead ECGs. This will help to perform the differential diagnosis of ventricular versus supraventricular tachycardias with aberrancy, and also will help to determine the site of origin and mechanisms of supraventricular and ventricular arrhythmias.

o In the case of paroxysmal tachycardias, a long strip should be recorded during carotid sinus massage, and some maneuvers (deep respiration and Valsalva, as well as other vagal maneuvers) performed for diagnostic and therapeutic purposes (Figures 1.16 and 4.70, Table 1.4).

o It is advisable to obtain ECG recordings during exercise testing, both in patients with premature complexes, in order to verify if they increase or decrease, and in patients with bradyarrhythmias, to identify an abrupt or gradual acceleration. If acceleration is abrupt, and

the heart rate is doubled or even more, this indicates a 2:1 sinoatrial block. If acceleration is gradual, this indicates a bradycardia due to depression of automatism.

o It is useful to have the overall patient history and previous ECGs. This is especially necessary in patients with potential pre-excitation syndrome or in patients with wide QRS complex tachycardias.

o **The "secret" to making a correct diagnosis of arrhythmia is to properly detect and analyze the atrial and ventricular activity and to determine the AV relationship.** For this purpose, over 90 years ago (Johnson and Denes, 2008), Lewis created some diagrams that are still considered very useful today. In most cases, only three areas are required to explain the site of onset and the stimulus pathway: atria, AV junction, and ventricles (Figures 1.17 and 1.18). Figure 1.19 shows how to outline Lewis diagrams in order to define the AV relationship.

o It is advisable to **determine the sensitivity, specificity, and predictive value of the different signs and diagnostic criteria.** This is especially important when performing differential diagnosis in the case of wide QRS tachycardia, between ventricular tachycardia and supraventricular tachycardia with aberrancy (see Appendix A-2).

o As previously stated, **it is often necessary to perform special techniques,** such as exercise testing, Holter ECG recording, amplified waves, EPS, imaging techniques, etc., to better understand the prevalence of arrhythmias, the electrophysiologic mechanisms that may explain them, and the correct diagnosis, as well as for prognostic evaluation and the prescription of a particular treatment. Appendix A-3 briefly presents all these techniques.

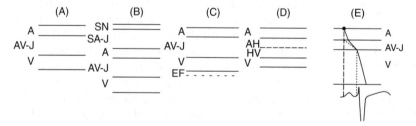

Figure 1.17 A, B, C and D: several examples of Lewis diagrams including: (A) only the atrioventricular (AV) junction, (B) the AV and sinoatrial (SA) junctions, (C) a ventricular arrhythmogenic focus, and (D) a division of the AV junction in two parts, (AH–HV). (E) it depicts the way of the sinus impulse (•) through the atria and AV junction as per the diagram shown in (A). The solid line shows the real way of the impulse across the heart. In general the dashed line is used instead, because it is the place at which the atrial and ventricular activity starts. Thus, the time that the sinus impulse spends to arrive and to cross the AV junction, the most important information, is more visible. EF: ectopic focus.

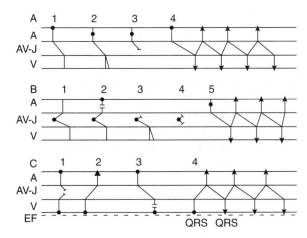

Figure 1.18 (A): 1: normal atrioventricular (AV) conduction of sinus impulse; 2: premature atrial impulse (complex) with aberrant ventricular conduction; 3: premature atrial impulse blocked at the AV junction; 4: sinus impulse with slow AV conduction that initiates an AV junctional reentrant tachycardia.
(B): 1: premature junctional impulse with an anterograde conduction slower than the retrograde; 2: premature junctional impulse sharing atrial depolarization with a sinus impulse (atrial fusion complex); 3: premature junctional impulse with exclusive anterograde conduction and, in this case, with aberrancy (see the two lines in ventricular space); 4: premature junctional impulse concealed anterogradely and retrogradely; 5: premature atrial impulse leading to AV junctional reentrant tachycardia.
(C): 1: sinus impulse and premature ventricular impulse that cancel mutually at the AV junction; 2: premature ventricular impulse with retrograde conduction to the atria; 3: sinus impulse sharing ventricular depolarization with a premature ventricular impulse (ventricular fusion beat); 4: premature ventricular impulse triggering an AV junctional reentrant tachycardia. EF: ectopic focus.

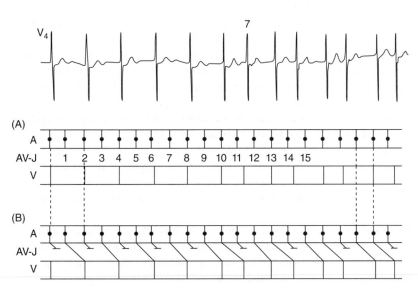

Figure 1.19 Placement of atrial waves and ventricular waves within the atrial and ventricular spaces, as seen at first glance (A). Although at first glance we do not see two atrial P waves for each QRS, we presume that atrial waves are ectopic (negative in V4 and probably very fast), and have to be double the QRS complexes, one visible and the other hidden in the QRS. This is confirmed when we check carefully the bigeminal rhythm. Later on we joined the atrial and ventricular waves through the AV junction (B). These data come from a patient with cardiomyopathy and digitalis intoxication, showing an atrial rate of 150 bpm and a first ventricular rate of 75 bpm. Later on, there are coupled bigeminal complexes. This is an example of ectopic atrial tachycardia with 2×1 AV block and later Wenckeback 3×2 AV block. The atrial waves are ectopic because their morphology differs from sinus P waves seen in previous ECG, and because it is very narrow (0.05 s) and negative in V4. The digitalis intoxication explains the presence of AV block. The first, third, fifth, seventh, and ninth P' waves conduct with long PR interval (0.40 s). The seventh QRS complex (7) is premature and precedes a series of coupled complexes (bigeminal rhythm). This complex is probably not caused by the eleventh atrial wave, as the corresponding P'R lasts only 0.18 s, whereas the other previous conducted atrial waves (P'), with the same coupling interval, show a P'R of 0.40 s. Instead, the tenth atrial wave (P') may be conducted with a P'R of 0.56 s; and therefore the eleventh P' is not conducted. The sequence: P'R = 0.40 s, P'R = 0.56 s, P' not conducted is afterwards repeated, perpetuating the Wenckebach sequence where the twelfth and thirteenth P' waves are conducted, whereas the fourteenth is not, etc.

Self Assessment

A. What is an arrhythmia?
B. How are arrhythmias classified in this book?
C. What is the essential significance of arrhythmias?
D. What are the diseases most frequently associated with sudden death (SD)?
E. What are the final arrhythmias preceding SD?
F. How can we identify subjects at high risk for SD?
G. How can SD be prevented?
H. Describe the most important mechanism of syncope.

I. Describe the first-line measures to prevent neuromediated syncope.
J. Why does the first sound vary in intensity?
K. When may an arrhythmia be suspected after history taking and physical examination?
L. What are the previous considerations to be taken into account when making a diagnosis of arrhythmia?
M. What are the Lewis diagrams?

References

Adgey AA, Devlin JE, Webb SW, Mulholland HC. Initiation of ventricular fibrillation outside the hospital in patients with acute ischemic heart disease. Br Heart J 1982;47:55.

ATP III Guidelines. Executive Summary of the Third Report of The National Cholesterol Education Program (NCEP) Expert Panel on Detection, Evaluation, and Treatment of High Blood Cholesterol in Adults (Adult Treatment Panel III). JAMA 2001;285:2486.

Bayés de Luna A, Boada Fx, Casellas A, *et al*. Concealed atrial electrical activity. J Electrocardiol 1978; 11: 301.

Bayés de Luna A, Coumel P, Leclercq JF. Ambulatory sudden cardiac death: mechanisms of production of fatal arrhythmia on the base of data from 157 cases. Am Heart J 1989;117:151.

Bayés de Luna A, Baranchuk A, Martínez-Sellés M, Platonov PG. Anticoagulation in patients at high risk of stroke without documented atrial fibrillation. Time for a paradigm shift? Ann Noninv Electrocardiol 2017; 22(1): doi: 10.1111/anec.12417.

Bayés-Genis A, Viñolas X, Bayés de Luna A, *et al*. Electrocardiographic and clinical precursors of ventricular fibrillation: chain of events. J Cardiovasc Electrophysiol 1995;6:410.

Bayés de Luna A, Furlanello F, Maron BJ, Zipes DP. Arrhythmias and sudden death in athletes. Kluwer Academic Publishers. Dordrecht, The Netherlands, 2000.

Bellet S. Clinical disorders of the heartbeat. Lea & Febiger. Philadelphia, PA, 1969.

Benditt DG, Can I. Initial evaluation of "syncope and collapse" the need for a risk stratification consensus. J Am Coll Cardiol 2010;55:722.

Bigger JT, Fleiss JL, Kleiger R, *et al*. The relationships among ventricular arrhythmias, left ventricular dysfunction, and mortality in the 2 years after myocardial infarction. Circulation 1984;69:250.

Bonow RD. Should coronary calcium screening be used in CV prevention strategies? N Engl J Med 2009;361:990.

Brignole M, Menozzi C, Gianfranchi L, *et al*. A controlled trial of acute and long-term medical therapy in tilt-induced neurally mediated syncope. Am J Cardiol 1992;70:339.

Brignole M, Alboni P, Benditt DG, *et al*. Guidelines on management (diagnosis and treatment) of syncope – update 2004. Europace 2004;6:467 and Eur Heart J 2004:25:2054.

Burke AP, Farb A, Malcom GT, *et al*. Coronary risk factors and plaque morphology in men with coronary disease who died suddenly. N Engl J Med 1997;336:1276.

Calkins H, Seifert M, Morady F. Clinical presentation and long-term follow-up of athletes with exercise induced vasodepressor syncope. Am Heart J 1995;129:1159.

Colman N, Bakker A, Linzer M, *et al*. Value of history-taking in syncope patients: in whom to suspect long QT syndrome? Europace 2009;11:937.

Connolly SJ, Sheldon R, Thorpe KE, *et al*. Pacemaker therapy for prevention of syncope in patients with recurrent severe vasovagal syncope: Second Vasovagal Pacemaker Study (VPS II): a randomized trial. JAMA, 2003;289(17):2224.

Echt DS, Liebson PR, Mitchell LB, *et al*. Mortality and morbidity in patients receiving encainide, flecainide, or placebo. The Cardiac Arrhythmia Suppression Trial. N Engl J Med 1991;324:781.

Gang UJ, Jøns C, Jørgensen RM, *et al*. CARISMA investigators. Heart rhythm at the time of death documented by an implantable loop recorder. Europace 2010;12:254.

Garcia Civera R, Sanjuan R, Cosin J, Lopez Merino V. Síncope. Editorial MCR. Barcelona, 1989.

Garrat CJ, Griffith MJ, Camm J, *et al*. Value of physical signs in the diagnosis of ventricular tachycardia. Circulation 1994;90:3103.

Goldstein S. Identification of patients at risk for sudden death in congestive heart failure. J Clin Pharmacol 1991;31(11):1085.

Goldwasser D, Serra G, Bayés de Luna A, *et al.* New computer algorithm to improve P wave detection during supraventricular tachycardia. Europace 2011;13:1028.

Greenland P, Abrams J, Aurigemma GP, *et al.* Prevention Conference V: Beyond secondary prevention: identifying the high-risk patient for primary prevention: noninvasive tests of atherosclerotic burden: Writing Group III. Circulation 2000;101:E16.

Grimm W, Plachta E, Maisch B. Antitachycardia pacing for spontaneous rapid ventricular tachycardia in patients with prophylactic cardioverter-defibrillator therapy. Pacing Clin Electrophysiol 2006;29:759.

Hendel RC, Patel MR, Kramer CM, *et al.* ACCF/ACR/SCCT/SCMR/ASNC/NASCI/SCAI/SIR 2006 appropriateness criteria for cardiac computed tomography and cardiac magnetic resonance imaging: a report of the American College of Cardiology Foundation Quality Strategic Directions Committee Appropriateness Criteria Working Group, American College of Radiology, Society of Cardiovascular Computed Tomography, Society for Cardiovascular Magnetic Resonance, American Society of Nuclear Cardiology, North American Society for Cardiac Imaging, Society for Cardiovascular Angiography and Interventions, and Society of Interventional Radiology. J Am Coll Cardiol 2006;48:1475.

Johnson NP, Denes P. The ladder diagram (A 100+ year history). Am J Cardiol 2008;101:1801.

Kannel WB, McGee DL. Epidemiology of sudden death: insights from the Framingham Study. Cardiovasc Clin 1985;15(3):93.

Kenny RA, Richardson DA, Steen N, *et al.* Carotid sinus syndrome: a modifiable risk factor for nonaccidental falls in older adults (SAFE PACE). J Am Coll Cardiol 2001;38:1491.

Keys AB, Keys M. How to eat well and stay well the Mediterranean Way. Doubleday. New York, 1975.

Knoebel SB, Williams SV, Achord JL, *et al.* Clinical competence in ambulatory electrocardiography. A statement for physicians from the AHA/ACC/ACP Task Force on Clinical Privileges in Cardiology. Circulation. 1993l;88(1):337.

Korngold EC, Januzzi JL Jr, Gantzer ML, *et al.* Amino-terminal pro-B-type natriuretic peptide and high-sensitivity C-reactive protein as predictors of sudden cardiac death among women. Circulation 2009;119:2868.

Krahn AD, Klein GJ, Yee R, *et al.* Randomized assessment of syncope trial: conventional diagnostic testing versus a prolonged monitoring strategy. Circulation 2001;104:46.

Krahn AD, Healey JS, Chauhan V, *et al.* Systematic assessment of patients with unexplained cardiac arrest: Cardiac Arrest Survivors With Preserved Ejection Fraction Registry (CASPER). Circulation 2009;120:278.

Leitch JW, Gillis AM, Wyse DG, *et al.* Reduction in defibrillator shocks with an implantable device combining antitachycardia pacing and shock therapy. J Am Coll Cardiol 1991;18:145.

Lelonek M, Pietrucha T, Matyjaszczyk M, *et al.* A novel approach to syncopal patients: association analysis of polymorphisms in G-protein genes and tilt outcome. Europace 2009;11:89.

de Lorgeril M, Salen P, Martin JL, *et al.* Mediterranean diet, traditional risk factors, and the rate of cardiovascular complications after myocardial infarction: final report of the Lyon Diet Heart Study. Circulation 1999;99:779.

Luu M, Stevenson WG, Stevenson LW, *et al.* Diverse mechanisms of unexpected cardiac arrest in advanced heart failure. Circulation 1989;80:1675.

Márquez MF, Hernández-Pacheco G, Hermosillo AG, *et al.* The Arg389Gly beta1-adrenergic receptor gene polymorphism and susceptibility to faint during head-up tilt test. Europace 2007;9:585.

Marrugat J, Elosua R, Gil M. Epidemiology of sudden cardiac death in Spain. Rev Esp Cardiol 1999;52:717.

Masiá R, Pena A, Marrugat J, *et al.* High prevalence of cardiovascular risk factors in Gerona, Spain, a province with low myocardial infarction incidence. REGICOR Investigators. J Epidemiol Community Health 1998;52:707.

McCarthy F, McMahon CG, Geary U, *et al.* Management of syncope in the Emergency Department: a single hospital observational case series based on the application of European Society of Cardiology Guidelines. Europace 2009;11:216.

McKenna WJ, Behr ER. Hypertrophic cardiomyopathy: management, risk stratification, and prevention of sudden death. Heart 2002;87:169.

Morady F. Review of guidelines. J Am Coll Cardiol 2009;54:1819.

Moss AJ, Davies HT, De Camilla J, *et al.* Ventricular ectopic beats and their relation to sudden and non sudden cardiac death after myocardial infarction. Circulation 1979;60:998.

Moss AJ, Goldenberg I. Prevention of sudden cardiac death: need for a plaque stabilizer. Am Heart J 2010;159:1.

Moya A, Sutton R, Ammirati F, *et al.* Guidelines for the diagnosis and management of syncope (version 2009): the Task Force for the Diagnosis and Management of Syncope of the European Society of Cardiology (ESC). Eur Heart J 2009;30:2631.

Myerburg RJ, Kessler KM, Castellanos A. Sudden cardiac death. Structure, function, and time-dependence of risk. Circulation 1992;85(1 Suppl):I2.

Myerburg RJ, Interian A Jr, Mitrani RM, *et al.* Frequency of sudden cardiac death and profiles of risk. Am J Cardiol 1997;80(5B):1F.

Occhetta E, Bortnik M, Audoglio R, *et al*. INVASY Study Investigators. Closed loop stimulation in prevention of vasovagal syncope. Inotropy Controlled Pacing in Vasovagal Syncope (INVASY): a multicentre randomized, single blind, controlled study. Europace 2004;6:538.

Raviele A, Giada F, Menozzi C, *et al*. Vasovagal Syncope and Pacing Trial Investigators. A randomized, double-blind, placebo-controlled study of permanent cardiac pacing for the treatment of recurrent tilt-induced vasovagal syncope. The vasovagal syncope and pacing trial (SYNPACE). Eur Heart J 2004;25:1741.

Reed MJ, Newby DE, Coull AJ, *et al*. The ROSE (risk stratification of syncope in the emergency department) study. J Am Coll Cardiol 2010;55:713.

Reybrouck T, Ector H. Tilt training: a new challenge in the treatment of neurally mediated syncope. Acta Cardiol 2006;61:183.

Rugg-Gunn FJ, Simister RJ, Squirrell M, *et al*. Cardiac arrhythmias in focal epilepsy: a prospective long-term study. Lancet 2004;364:2212.

Sans S, Puigdefábregas A, Balaguer-Vintró I, *et al*. Increasing trends of acute myocardial infarction in Spain: the MONICA-Catalonia Study. Eur Heart J 2005;26:505.

Sheldon R, Rose Ritchie D, *et al*. Historical criteria that distinguish syncope from seizures. J Am Coll Cardiol 2002; 40(1):142.

Sheldon R, Rose S, Connolly S, *et al*. Diagnostic criteria for vasovagal syncope based on a quantitative history. Eur Heart J 2006;27(3):344.

Sheldon R, Hersi A, Ritchie D, *et al*. Syncope and structural heart disease: historical criteria for vasovagal syncope and ventricular tachycardia. J Cardiovasc Electrophysiol 2010;21(12):1358.

Subirana MT, Babot J, Bayés de Luna A, *et al*. Specific characteristics of sudden death in Mediterranean area. Am J Cardiol 2011;107(4):622.

Tan MP, Newton JL, Chadwick TJ, *et al*. Home orthostatic training in vasovagal syncope modifies autonomic tone: results of a randomized, placebo-controlled pilot study. Europace 2010;12:240.

Théroux P, Waters DD, Halphen C, *et al*. Prognostic value of exercise test soon after myocardial infarction. N Engl J Med 1979;301:341.

Tomson T, Nashef L, Ryvlin P. Sudden unexpected death in epilepsy: Current knowledge and future directions. Lancet Neurol 2008;8:1021.

Van Dijk N, Quartieri F, Blanck JJ, *et al*. Effectiveness of physical counterpressure maneuvers in preventing vasovagal syncope: the physical counterpressure maneuvers trial. J Am Coll Cardiol 2006;8:1652.

Van Lee V, Mitiku T, Hadley D, *et al*. Rest premature ventricular contractions on routine ECG and prognosis in heart failure patients. Ann Noninvasive Electrocardiol 2010;15:56.

Vazquez R, Bayes-Genis A, Cygankiewicz I, *et al*. The MUSIC risd score: a simple method for predicting mortality in ambulatory patients with chronic heart failure. Eur Heart J 2009;30(9):1088.

Virmani R, Burke AP, Farb A. Sudden cardiac death. Cardiovasc Pathol 2001;10:211.

de Vreede-Swagemakers JJ, Gorgels AP, Wellens HJ, *et al*. Out-of-hospital cardiac arrest in the 1990s: a population-based study in the Maastricht area on incidence, characteristics and survival. J Am Coll Cardiol 1997;30:1500.

2

Anatomic and Electrophysiologic Basis

In this chapter, the anatomic and electrophysiologic basis needed to better comprehend the mechanisms of cardiac arrhythmias is presented. This is a crucial part in learning how to make a well-reasoned diagnosis of arrhythmia and in understanding its most important clinical, prognostic, and therapeutic implications.

Anatomic Basis

Ultrastructural Characteristics of Cardiac Muscle Cells

There are two types of cells in the heart: (i) cardiac contractile cells, responsible for the cardiac pump function, that is, the atrial and ventricular contraction, and (ii) specific conduction system (SCS) cells, which are responsible for the impulse formation (automatism) and impulse transmission to the contractile myocardium, initiating the excitation–contraction coupling. The ultrastructural aspects of these cells will be commented on first before the electrophysiologic characteristics are described.

Contractile Cells

From an ultrastructural point of view, contractile myocardial cells, having no automatic capacity, are long and narrow and include three different components with specific functions (Figure 2.1).

o **Activation/Relaxation system**. This is made up of: (a) the cellular membrane, or sarcolemma, a structure formed by two lipid layers along which there are pores with a radius of about 3.5 Å through which individual ions permeate the so-called ion channels (Figure 2.1C(1), see also Slow and Fast Response Cells); (b) the T system, where the cell membrane invaginates into the sarcomeres at the Z-band level to promote electrical excitation inside the cell; and (c) the sarcoplasmic reticulum, where the calcium necessary for cell contraction is to be found. The sarcoplasmic reticulum is a specialized structure through which the T system comes into contact with the sarcomere.

o **The contractile system is organized into sarcomeres** (Figure 2.1A, 2.1C(2) and 2.1C(3)). A sarcomere is a structure capable of generating a force for muscle contraction. It is the contractile unit of myocardial cells, as well as the basic component of myofibrils. Myofibrils are composed of sarcomeres and are interconnected through intercalated disks (Figure 2.1C(2)). Each individual sarcomere has dark and light bands that overlap (actin and myosin bands), and is composed of proteins. Actin filaments are anchored to lateral stripes, which delimit the sarcomeres and are called Z bands (Figure 2.1A and 2.1C(3)).

o **The mitochondrial system** (Figure 2.1C(2)) provides energy to the cells. The mitochondria, which together with the sarcoplasmic reticulum take up a great part of the intermyofibrillar space, are cell organoids of complex structure in which the high energy compounds (ATP) necessary to initiate the contraction are formed.

Specific cells

(Eriksson and Thornell, 1979; Martínez-Palomo et al., 1970)

From an ultrastructural point of view, there are three types of noncontractile specific cells: P cells, transitional cells, and Purkinje cells (Figure 2.2).

o **P cells** are so-called because of the simplicity of their structure (primitive), their appearance (pale), and their automaticity-pacemaker function (pacing) (Figure 2.2A). P cells present a polyhedric morphology and are principally clustered at the center of the sinus node. Their number decreases from the center to the peripheral area. They are also present in the atrioventricular (AV) node, particularly at the lower part, in the junction area with the bundle of His (NH nodal–Hisian zone). P cells have contact only with other P cells and with transitional cells. This contact is direct, with no intercalated disks connecting them, as in sarcomeres. This fact may have an influence on the slow conduction speed of electrical stimuli within the sinus node.

Clinical Arrhythmology, Second Edition. Antoni Bayés de Luna and Adrian Baranchuk.
© 2017 John Wiley & Sons Ltd. Published 2017 by John Wiley & Sons Ltd.

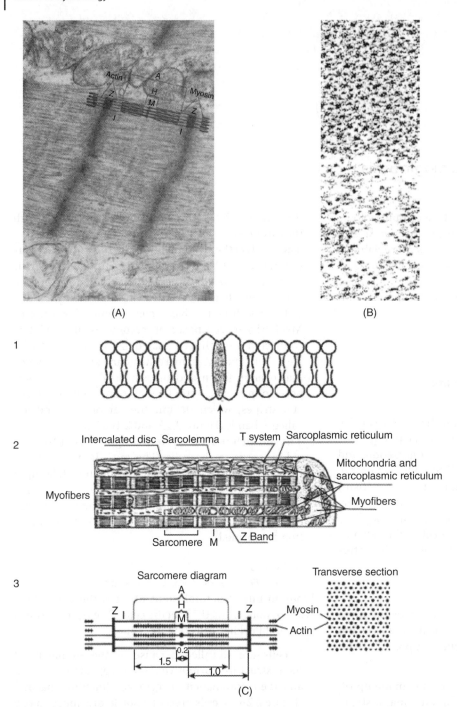

Figure 2.1 (A) Microphotography of a sarcomere where actin and myosin filaments are observed (see C). (B) Transverse section of the sarcomere. (C) 1: Structure of the cellular membrane (or sarcolemma) showing an ionic channel; 2: section of a myocardial contractile cell including all different elements; 3: enlarged sarcomere scheme.

○ **Transitional cells** constitute a group of heterogeneous cells interposed between the P cells, the Purkinje cells, and the contractile cells. They are usually present in the sinus node as well as the AV node, the bundle of His and the Purkinje–muscle junction (Figure 2.10). Transitional cells present a long and narrow morphology and, compared to contractile cells, have a T system and intercalated disks, but no sarcoplasmic reticulum. This hinders intercellular junctions, which are scarce (Figure 2.2D). This, along with the long and narrow cell morphology (the longer and narrower, the slower the conduction), accounts for the slow conduction speed of stimuli through the sinus node, AV node, atrionodal (AN) and N zone, as well as the Purkinje–muscle junction.

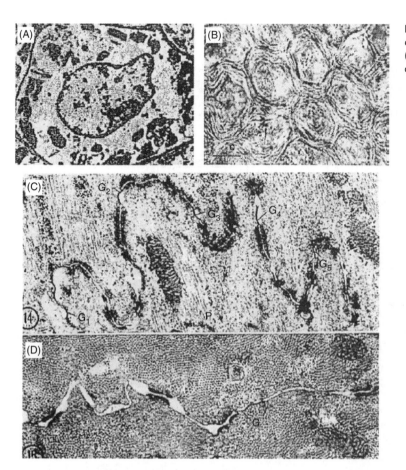

Figure 2.2 (A) P cells. (B) Purkinje cells. (C) Purkinje cells show many intercalated discs (G1–G5). (D) Transitional cells show few intercellular connections (G).

o **The Purkinje cells** are more frequently found in the bundle of His and branches, as well as in the internodal bundles, although less numerously. They are also found around the two nodes. They are mainly present at the NH zone of the AV node, leading to a faster conduction in this area compared to the superior and central areas of the AV node (see Atrioventricular Junction; Figures 2.3 and 2.23). From a functional point of view, these cells constitute the link with the contractile cells through the transitional cells of the two nodes and the bundle of His and branches (Figure 2.10). They are short, wide cells (Figure 2.2B), linearly aligned with many intercalated disks (Figure 2.2C). This explains why, although they have a certain automatic activity, their principal function is to rapidly conduct stimuli. A Y-shaped association of three Purkinje cells is frequently observed, which could be the anatomic basis explaining micro-reentry.

Anatomy of the Specific Conduction System

The specific conduction system consists of the sinus node, the internodal conduction pathways, the AV junction, and the intraventricular conduction system (Figure 2.3).

Sinus Node

The sinus node is a bean-sized structure 1–2 cm long located at the junction of the inferior vena cava with the right atrium (Figure 2.4). The sinus node is the structure within the SCS that contains the greatest amount of P cells. P cells have the greatest automatism capacity, thus the automaticity of the sinus node is greater than that of the AV junction, where a lower number of P cells is observed, and much greater than that of the ventricular Purkinje fibers, where P cells are rarely present. Later, the electrophysiologic characteristics of heart cells will be dealt with (see Electrophysiologic Characteristics); these explain how the major automaticity of P cells is due to the fact that their transmembrane diastolic potential (TDP), or Phase 4, has the steepest slope, therefore ensuring that they reach the threshold potential earlier (Figures 2.3 and 2.9). As more P cells are clustered at the sinus node, it becomes the source of normal heart automaticity.

The sinus node is traversed by the sinus node artery originating from the right coronary artery or the circumflex artery (approximately 50%). The relatively large dimensions of the sinus node artery are really striking, especially considering that its function is to perfuse the small-sized sinus node and that the inlet and outlet calibers are similar (Figure 2.4). This may be due to the

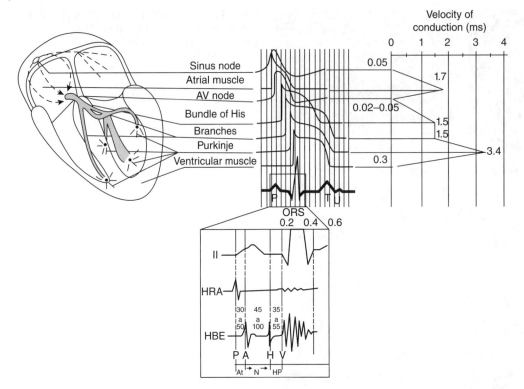

Figure 2.3 Scheme of the morphology of the transmembrane action potential (TAP) of the different structures of the specific conduction system, as well as the different conduction speeds (ms) through these structures. Below, there is an enlarged depiction of the PR interval with the His bundle electrogram recording. HRA: High right atria; HBE: ECG of the Bundle of His; PA: from start of the P wave to the low right atrium; AH: from low right atrium to the bundle of His; HV: from bundle of His to the ventricular Purkinje.

fact that when the sinus node artery passes along the inner part of the sinus node, it is probably helping to modulate the heart rate, as P cells can sense its pulsations and act as a regulating mechanism for the next sinus impulse.

The sinus node is innervated by vagal and sympathetic fibers, which are responsible for the physiologic changes of the heart rate 24 h a day (emotions, efforts, rest). An excessive increase of vagal activity accounts for many bradyarrhythmias, and an excessive increase of the sympathetic activity, sometimes associated with a decreased

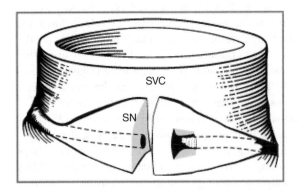

Figure 2.4 Shape and location of the sinus node (SN) with the artery that crosses it. SVC: superior vena cava.

vagal activity, explains the presence of sinus tachycardia, including the so-called inappropriate sinus tachycardia (see Chapter 4, Sinus Tachycardia: Concept).

Internodal and Interatrial Activation

For many years it has been considered that the sinus impulse was transmitted toward the AV node mainly through three intermodal tracts: the anterior branch of superoanterior tract (Bachmann's bundle), the middle (Wenckebach's tract), and the inferoposterior tract (Thorel's tract). Today is known that the activation is transmitted like a wave from sinus node to AV node (Figure 2.5), but that the conduction from sinus node to the left atrium is performed preferentially through the superior tract of Bachmann, although it also takes place in the area of the fossa ovalis and, in a few cases, in the lower atrial zone at the Koch triangle (Holmqvist *et al.*, 2008; Recommended General Bibliography p. xvii). This explain the P wave morphology (± in this case) in II, III, and VF in the presence of a pathologic block of the stimulus in the upper part of the atrium (Bachmann's bundle area) (Bayés de Luna *et al.*, 1985) (see Figures 3.19 and 10.4).

The atrial activation arrives to the AV node in the so-called transitional zone through four different cellular groups (see below; Figure 2.6). The whole atrial tissue

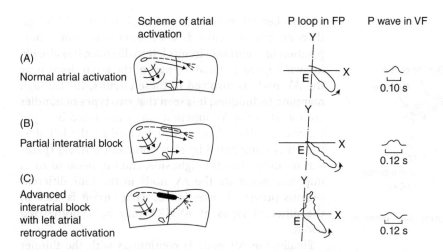

Figure 2.5 Left: Scheme of atrial activation in a normal P wave (A), in presence of partial IAB (C). Right: Characteristics of the P loop and P wave in each case. Note that in normal conditions the breakthrough in left atrium also occurs at the level of coronary sinus. The dotted line shows that the Bachmann bundle is the preferential way of interatrial conduction. The remaining atrial activation is performed without preferential pathways. The primary left atrium breakthrough is in the Bachmann bundle and also often in the fossa ovalis area (see arrow).

presents a significant vagal innervation, which is greater than in the ventricles. This explains the importance of the vagus triggering certain episodes of atrial fibrillation (see Chapter 4, Atrial Fibrillation: Mechanisms).

Atrioventricular Junction (Figure 2.6)

The term atrioventricular (AV) junction should be applied to the entire area encompassing the compact AV node, the specialized tissue of the low atrium close to the AV node up to the coronary sinus (AN junction), and the tissue from which His potentials are recorded on the atrial side of the fibrous skeleton (NH area). The AV junction is followed by the bundle of His, leading to the intraventricular conduction system (Figures 2.6–2.8). The lower atrial part of the AV junction comes into contact with the AV node in four particular areas (Figure 2.6): two superior-left areas (1, 2) and two inferior-right areas (3, 4). The AV node is

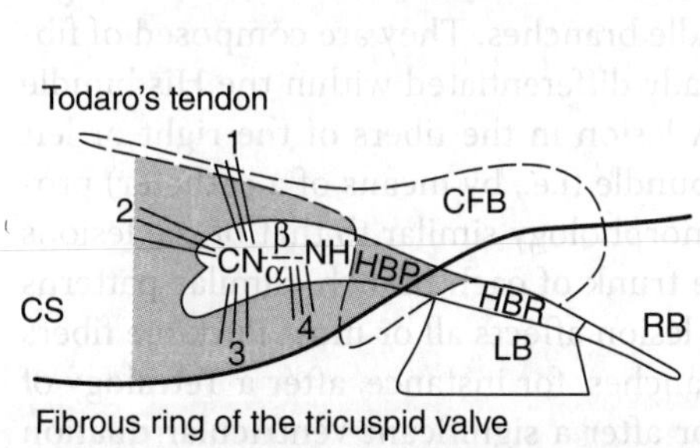

Todaro's tendon

Figure 2.6 Structure of the atrioventricular (AV) junction extending further than the AV node (the compact node). The zone shaded in grey is included in the AV junction, and may be involved in the reentry circuits exclusive of the AV junction: CFB: central fibrous body; CN: compact AV node; HBP: bundle of His – penetrating portion; HBR: bundle of His – ramifying portion; LB: left branch; RB: right branch. Slow conduction (α) and rapid conduction (β) pathways; 1–4: entry of fibers of atrial pathways entering the AV node: NH: node–His transition zone; CS: coronary sinus.

directly above the septal leaflet insertion of the tricuspid valve and is lateral to and in front of the coronary sinus ostium (Figure 2.6). P cells are found in the AV junction (lower atria and perinodal AV node area) and bundle of His; they account for the subsidiary automatism in this region, which is of great clinical value when a sinus function depression occurs. However, in the compact AV node (CN), there are more transitional cells, which together with the P cells and the Purkinje cells compose a network of fibers (Figure 2.7A). A greater number of Purkinje cells can be found in the node–His junction (NH), and the bundle of His and branches.

The function of the AV junction is to transmit the cardiac impulses from the atria toward the ventricles, with some delay in the impulse conduction. This is particularly due to the predominant presence of transitional cells in the AN junction, and in the compact AV node itself. Through transmembrane action potential (TAP) recordings, a decrementing conduction (slow-response TAP formation) in this zone has been shown (Figure 2.23). Cardiac impulses, however, do not extinguish, because, when they arrive at the bundle of His, the rate of conduction increases due to a greater number of Purkinje fibers. The TAP then shows a rapid response. The decreased rate of conduction explains the presence of an isoelectric line recorded after the P wave (a bundle of His deflection may be recorded with intracavitary ECG) (Figure 2.3). This is teleologically very important if atrial fibrillation occurs, in order to prevent a massive and disastrous conduction of f waves toward the ventricles.

Atrioventricular junctional reentrant tachycardias (AVJRT or JRT) were once thought to originate from a functional circuit located within the AV node itself. It was believed that there was a longitudinal dissociation

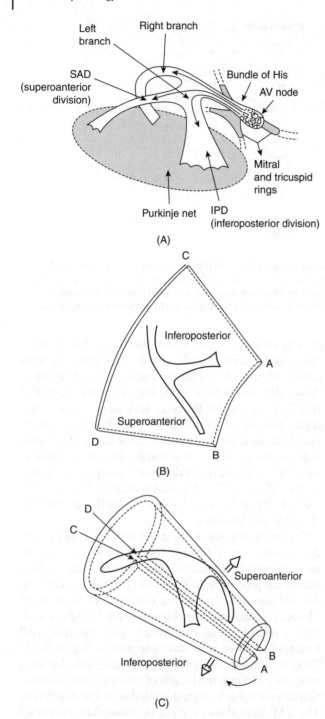

Figure 2.7 (A) Scheme of the intraventricular conduction system, starting at the AV node with its network cells, and the bundle of His, with its parallel fibers heading for the right or the left branches. The latter is divided into two fascicles: superoanterior and inferoposterior fascicles. (B) Left ventricle open and (C) left ventricle closed (trifascicular concept).

of the AV node with fast conduction on the left side (β pathway) and slow conduction on the right side (α pathway) (Figures 3.9 and 3.10).

At present, it is known that these conduction pathways have an anatomic basis (Wu and Yeh, 1994; Inoue

and Becker, 1998; Katritsis and Becker, 2007). Although there are still particular details about the anatomic composition of reentrant circuits left to discover, it is already known (Figure 2.6) that: (i) part of the atrial tissue near the AV node is involved in these circuits; (ii) through mapping techniques, it is seen that two types of bundles are found in the AV junction, one constituted by rapid conduction fibers (pathway β), located on the left side, the other constituted by slow conduction fibers (pathway α), located on the right side; and (iii) because atrial impulses penetrate the AV node in the four different regions previously mentioned, what circuit is used in the different types of AVNRT may be hypothesized about.

Finally, the AV node is continuous with the thinner bundle of His, which penetrates the central fibrous body (penetrating part). After the "branching" part of the bundle of His reaches the superior border of the muscular septum, the His bundle bifurcates (Figure 2.6). Fibers in the bundle of His are arranged in a parallel and linear fashion. The left branch detaches from the branching bundle, and the straight fibers of this branching region give rise to the right branch (Figures 2.6 and 2.7A).

The blood supply to the AV node usually originates (>90%) from a branch of the right coronary artery, the AV nodal branch. The rest originate from a branch of the left circumflex. This explains why inferior myocardial infarctions may present with advanced AV block (see Chapter 11, Passive Arrhythmias).

Regarding innervation, there is a varied network of vagal (cholinergic) fibers and sympathetic (adrenergic) fibers. This AV node network, in particular vagal innervation, is present to a greater extent than in the ventricles.

Intraventricular Conduction System
The bundle of His is divided into two branches, the right and the left bundle branches. They are composed of fibers that are already differentiated within the His bundle (Figure 2.7A). A lesion in the fibers of the right or left side of the His bundle (i.e., by means of a catheter) produces an ECG morphology similar to that of the lesions produced in the trunk of each branch. Similar patterns occur when the lesion affects all or most Purkinje fibers of one of the branches, for instance, after a Tetralogy of Fallot surgery, or after a significant ventricular dilation due to pulmonary embolism in the case of the right branch; in the case of the left ventricle (LV), the pattern is the result of a significant ventricular dilation (dilated cardiomyopathy), or a severe electrolytic disorder (i.e., hyperkalemia). In summary, an ECG tracing showing a right (RBBB) or left (LBBB) bundle branch block pattern usually reflects a compromise in the trunk of the left and right bundle branches. However, it is possible to observe a similar morphology when the injury is more proximal

(bundle of His) or more distal (ventricular Purkinje fibers).

The right bundle branch may be divided into three different parts (Sodi-Pallarés and Calder, 1956): the subendocardial, which becomes intramyocardial, then once again subendocardial. Then, at the level of the right anterior papillary muscle, it divides into several branches, which usually constitute two selectively delimited Purkinje areas: the superoanterior, and the inferoposterior regions. The ECG recording resulting from the right bundle branch block (RBBB) are described later (Figures 3.26 and 6.24).

The trunk of the left bundle branch (5–7 mm in length) is divided into two anatomically well-defined fascicles: the superoanterior and the inferoposterior (Rosenbaum *et al.*, 1968). This explains why the intraventricular conduction system is generally considered a **trifascicular system** (Figure 2.7). The ECG recording that originates when a LBBB is present is shown in Figures 3.27 and 6.25.

○ The superoanterior division (SA), longer and narrower, goes through the LV outflow tract until the left anterior papillary muscle base is reached. It may be easily affected by the pathologies that occur frequently in this area (Figures 2.7 and 2.8). The inferoposterior (IP) division, shorter and wider, leads to the base of the posterior papillar muscle, an area where less hemodynamic stress exists. Therefore, an isolated injury in the inferoposterior division is much less frequent. A block in these two divisions originates typical morphologies in the ECG tracing, as defined by Rosenbaum *et al.* (1968) as hemiblocks, now more frequently known or named as superoanterior or inferoposterior blocks (see Figures 3.28 and 3.29).

○ From an anatomic point of view, there are usually some middle fibers (Figure 2.8A) located between the two fascicles. In some cases, they form a true third fascicle. In other cases, they are found in the form of a fiber fan or protrude from one of the two divisions. The ventricular quadrifascicular theory is based on the existence of these fibers (right bundle branch, SA and IP divisions, and medial fibers) (Uhley 1973, 1979; Bayés de Luna *et al.*, 2012) (Chapter 6).

The initiation and spread of ventricular activation has been known since the pioneering work of Durrer *et al.* (1970). He demonstrated that left ventricular activation starts at three distinct points of the left ventricular endocardium (Figure 2.8B): two are part of the papillary muscles receiving the electrical impulse through the aforementioned divisions, and the third is located in the middle anterior septal region, approximately where the medial fibers are located (Figure 2.8A). These works support the previously mentioned **quadrifascicular theory**. Following these observations, the Josephson group (Cassidy *et al.*, 1984; Josephson, 2008; Recommended General Bibliography p. xvii) analyzed ventricular activation by means of the CARTO system. They confirmed that LV activation is initiated at the endocardium of the mid-septum and at the superior region of the LV free wall, as described by Durrer *et al.* (1970). They also consider it possible that the activation may be initiated at the third point as suggested by Durrer.

A complete AV block may occur when a lesion occurs at the AV level or at both branches of the bundle of His. It may also occur when the right bundle branch and the two left divisions are blocked. In this situation, it has been suggested that the left ventricle, exceptionally, may be activated through the middle fibers. In the case of a LBBB occurring due to a compromise of both fascicles, there is a transseptal global activation of the LV, although perhaps some activation originating in the middle fibers may exist. This would account for a wide QRS in the

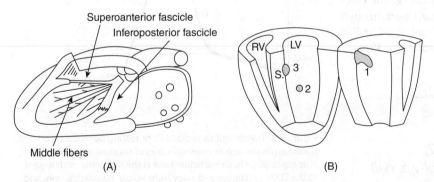

Figure 2.8 (A) Left lateral view of the specific conduction system. The superoanterior (SA) division, longer and narrower, reaches the superior papillary muscle base, and the inferoposterior (IP) division, shorter and wider, stretches to the posterior papillary muscle base. In the middle there is usually a fiber network, generally fan-shaped (medial or middle fibers). (B) According to Durrer, left ventricular activation starts in three different points: points 1 and 2 are located at the insertion of the SA and IP divisions, whereas point 3 could be placed at some part of the zone of the medial or middle fibers. This may support the quadrifascicular theory of the intraventricular conduction system.

presence of a fine q wave in I, VL, and V6. In some cases, before a complete block of the right bundle branch and the two divisions occurs (trifascicular block), the ECG may show a RBBB with an intermittent block in both fascicles (Rosenbaum-Elizari's syndrome) (Rosenbaum *et al.*, 1968) (see Chapter 10, Right bundle branch block plus alternating block in the two divisions of the left bundle branch, and also Figure 10.13).

Blood supply to the intraventricular conduction system is as follows: (i) the right bundle branch and the SA division of the left bundle branch are supplied by the left anterior descending (LAD) artery; (ii) the IP division of the left bundle branch receives a dual blood supply (septal branches of the LAD artery, and branches of the right coronary (RC) artery, or sometimes the circumflex (Cx) artery; and (iii) the trunk of the left bundle branch also receives a dual blood supply (LAD and RC arteries).

As far as innervation is concerned, the sympathetic fibers generally run along the coronary arteries and penetrate periodically into the epicardium until they reach the subendocardium. Meanwhile, vagal fibers are mainly present in the subendocardial region and reach the subepicardium in the basal ventricular region at the level of the AV groove. Sympathetic disturbances produce more arrhythmogenic effects on the ventricular myocardium than those produced by vagal disturbances, which usually act by modulating the sympathetic drive.

Purkinje Network
(Figures 2.7 and 2.8)

Purkinje fibers are present throughout the SCS, especially in the bundle of His and branches (Purkinje network), and, to a lesser extent, in the atrial muscle. Purkinje fibers connect the SCS to the contractile myocardial fibers through the transitional cells, forming a real network (Figure 2.7A). The number of these cells decreases in the ventricle from the endocardium to the epicardium. In humans they are not present in the epicardium, in contrast to other mammals. Purkinje fibers deliver the electrical impulse to the contractile myocardial fibers through excitation–contraction coupling (see Chapter 2, Cardiac Activation: Excitation–Contraction Coupling, p. 45).

Electrophysiologic Characteristics
(Hofman and Cranefield, 1960; Paes de Carvalho and Hofman, 1966; Markus et al., 1998; Issa et al., 2012; Recommended General Bibliography p. xvii)

Slow and Fast Response Cells

From an electrophysiologic point of view, the cardiac cells already discussed may be grouped into two different categories (Figure 2.9):

(i) The automatic slow response cell are the sinus node P cells and, to a lesser extent, some of the AV junction cells, and the fast response cells are the contractile cells. Purkinje cells are fast response cells, too, but they also have a certain automatic potential (Figures 2.3 and 2.16). Transitional cells display, as the name suggests, an intermediate TAP, among the Purkinje cells, the contractile cells, and the P cells (Figures 2.2 and 2.10).

(ii) The electrophysiologic characteristics during diastole, or resting phase TDP, and systole, or activation, phase (depolarization plus repolarization-TAP) of each cell type are different. This explains why one type of cell has an automatic behavior whereas the other type does not (Figures 2.13, 2.16, and 2.19). Table 2.1 shows the different characteristics of both

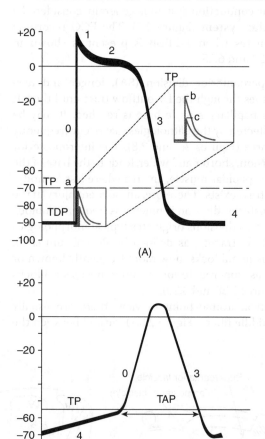

Figure 2.9 Transmembrane diastolic or resting potential (TDP) and transmembrane action potential (TAP) of contractile (A) and automatic (B) cells. Of particular note is the difference with regard to the TDPs, rectilinear and away from zero in contractile cells, and with ascending slope and closer to zero in automatic cells. A TAP is generated only if the stimulus reaches the threshold potential (TP), after it is excited by a neighboring cell (a in A) or because it features an automatic capacity (B). It should be observed that in the rapid response cells (with no automatic capacity) a stimulus not reaching the TP (b and c in A) does not generate a TAP (see box).

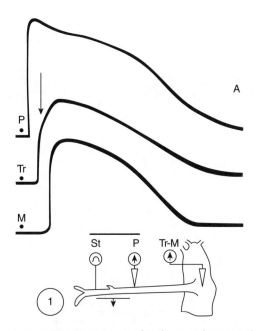

Figure 2.10 Preparation of Purkinje and contractile myocardium tissues. The morphology of the transmembrane action potential (TAP) of Purkinje (P), transitional (Tr), and contractile myocardial cells (M) is shown. The location of the stimulation electrode (St) and the recording micropipette in the three cell groups (P, Tr, and M) are also shown. Depending on the depth of the micropipette penetration, the TAP of a transitional cell (Tr) or a typical TAP of the contractile myocardial cell is recorded (M).

fast and slow response cells. A distinctive characteristic of these cells is how they recover excitability. In rapid response cells, recovery is voltage dependent, whereas in slow response cells recovery is time dependent.

First, the morphologic constitution of cells and how ion channels work are described. These channels are structures facilitating the ion interchange and are responsible for the TDP and the TAP, and, consequently, cellular activation (depolarization plus repolarization) of both types of cells. Thus, it is possible to infer how cardiac activation occurs (see Conduction of Stimuli, p. 43, and Figure 2.3).

Ion Channels

Ion flow across the cell membrane is through channels, which are macromolecular structures located in the bilipid layer of the cell membrane (Figures 2.1 and 2.11). Na^+, Ca^{++} and K^+ play a major role in cell activation; these are discussed here at length. The channels through which these ions flow have a similar, but not identical, basic macromolecular structure. The basic structure, which may be considered the functional unit (repeating units along the cell membrane) of the Na^+ channels found in the voltage-dependent contractile cells (Table 2.1), will be described. This functional unit

Table 2.1 Comparative characteristics of slow and fast response cells.

		Rapid response cells	Slow response cells
1.	Location	Mainly in atrial and ventricular muscles and in cells of the intraventricular conduction system	Cells from the sinus node, AV node, and mitral and tricuspid rings
2.	TDP level and types of TDP (stable or unstable)	Ranges from –80 to –95 mV. TDP is stable in contractile cells. However, in His–Purkinje cells there is a slight diastolic depolarization, resulting in a TDP with mild ascending slope	Approximately –70 mV (initial value). Unstable TDP showing an ascending slope, which initiates the TAP in automatic structures (sinus node, etc.)
3.	TP level	Approximately –70 mV	<–55 mV
4.	Rise of phase 0	Rapid	Slow
5.	Height of phase 0	High: from +20 to +40 mV	Low: from 0 to +15 mV
6.	Conduction velocity	Rapid (0.5–5 m/s)	Slow (0.01–0.1 m/s)
7.	Na^+ rapid channels	Present	Present
8.	Slow channels (mainly Ca^{++} channels, some Na^+ channels)	Present	Present
9.	Depolarization inhibition	By means of tetrodoxine, which inhibits the rapid Na^+ rapid channels	Manganese, cobalt, nickel, verapamil, etc., which inhibit the slow channels
10.	Effective refractory period duration (and, therefore, restoration of excitability); AB: distance during which the cell is unexcitable	AB: a little shorter than the TAP duration (excitability recovery is voltage dependent)	AB: longer than the TAP duration (excitability recovery is time dependent)

AV, atrioventricular; TAP, transmembrane action potential; TDP, transmembrane diastolic potential; TP, threshold potential.

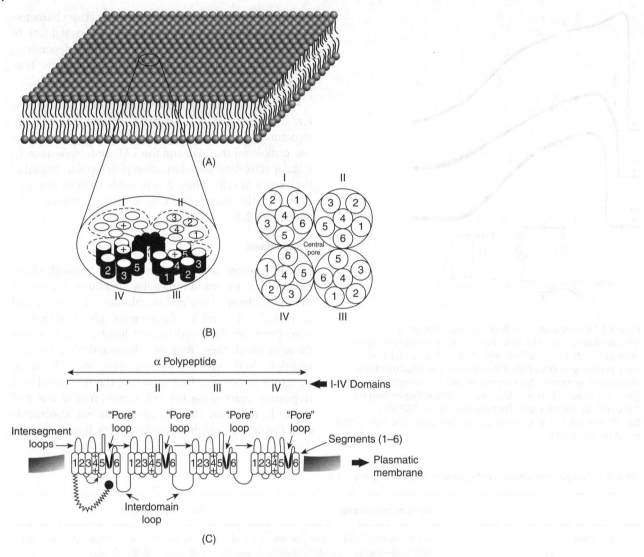

Figure 2.11 (A) Molecular composition of the cellular membrane, comprising a lipid bilayer where the different ionic channels are embedded, with pores (Figure 2.1C). (B) Schematic composition of an ionic channel with its domains, each of which comprises six segments. (C): The domains are displayed. A voltage sensor is found in segment 4 of each domain. See also the ball-and-chain mechanism for channel inactivation (*).

(Figure 2.11) is made up of four domains, each domain comprising six segments of hydrophobic amino acids (Figure 2.11C). The voltage sensor is located in the S4 segment, and the pore zone of each domain is found in the peptide chain, which joins segments S5 and S6. The four domains wrap around themselves so that the pore zones of each individual domain stay in the center, creating the central channel pore (Figure 2.11B). The Ca^{++} channels comprise a similar group, although they have some special characteristics, particularly in the central pore. The K^+ channels have a similar domain composition formed by six segments, although the formation of these domains into functional units is different.

The rapid inactivation of voltage-dependent cell channels (contractile and Purkinje cells) takes place by means of a gating mechanism in each domain, comprising an N-terminal peptide in the form of a chain-like structure, ending with a ball (ball-and-chain model) (asterisk in Figure 2.11) that occludes the pore zone.

Several hypothetic models have been described (Coraboeuf, 1971) to explain the ion inward current and its inactivation throughout the cell membrane. It has been suggested (Figure 2.12) that two gates exist: the activation gate (m), which rapidly opens to permit Na^+ flow, and the inactivation gate (h), which closes slowly, in particular for Ca^{++}, when the membrane has already been depolarized, first by Na^+ and later by Na^+ Ca^{++}. Therefore, there is a greater Na^+ ion flow overall. The abovementioned ball-and-chain model corresponds to gate h.

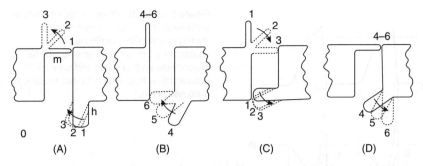

Figure 2.12 Highly schematic representation of sodium (or calcium) channels. The channel is controlled by an activation gate (m) and an inactivation gate (h). (A) Activation (opening of gate m; gate h starts to close); (B) inactivation (gate m is still open; gate h is closed); (C) and (D) recovery from an inactivated state is determined by the slow reopening of gate h and close of gate m. According to this, inactivation and recovery kinetics (closing and opening of the same gate) should be the same for a given potential (Bayés de Luna and Cosin, 1978).

Before describing how ion interchange through these channels allows the formation of the TDP and the TAP in both automatic cells (slow response cells) and contractile cells (fast response cells), it must be remembered that some genetically mediated changes in activity (mutations and polymorphisms of the channels) constitute a new group of diseases: the "channelopathies" (long QT and short QT syndromes, Brugada's syndrome, etc.) (see Chapter 9, Ionic Channel Disorders in the Absence of Apparent Structural Heart Disease: Channelopathies). From an electrocardiographic point of view, they all have a characteristic phenotypic expression, and clinically they represent an increased risk for fatal arrhythmia.

> Na^+, K^+, and Ca^{++} ion channels have a similar macromolecular structure, constituted by functional units comprising four domains of six segments each. These four domains assemble by wrapping around themselves so that the pore zones of each individual domain stay in the center, forming the central channel pore (Figure 2.11).

Transmembrane Diastolic Potential and Transmembrane Action Potential of Fast and Slow Response Cells
(Table 2.1)

TDP and TAP in both cell types are discussed here, as is their origin and the ionic mechanisms accounting for them.

Transmembrane Diastolic Potential

Contractile cells are polarized during the diastolic phase. This means that there is a balance between the positive charges outside the cell (Na^+, Ca^{++}, and, to a lesser extent, K^+) and the negative charges inside the cell (mainly, the nondiffusible anion negative charges A^-, which outnumber the K^+ ion, the most important positive intracellular ion (Figure 2.14). When two separate microelectrodes are placed on the external surface of a contractile cell in the resting phase, a horizontal line is recorded (baseline line, at zero level), suggesting that there is no potential difference on the cell surface. However, if an electrode is placed inside the cell, the recording will shift downwards (Figure 2.15), showing the potential difference between the outside (+) and the inside (–) of the cell. This potential difference should not have a positive or negative sign, although an upward shift is indicated by a positive sign, whereas a downward shift is shown by a negative sign. **In contractile cells this line, called the TDP, is stable** (rectilinear Phase 4 at –90 mV) (Figure 2.9). Even though not all ionic currents in the diastole are well known, it is known that contractile cells show an equilibrium between inward diastolic currents of Na^+, Ca^{++} (Ibi) and outward K^+ current (IK2). This explains why TDP is not modified and remains stable (Figure 2.16A). Here, TDP does not reach the threshold potential (TP) ($\approx$ –70 mV) by itself but requires the impulse delivered by a neighboring cell (Figures 2.9 and 2.13B).

The automatic cells of the SCS have a TDP (Phase 4) with an initial value of –70 mV and an ascending slope line, which rises to reach the TP by itself ($\approx$ –55 mV). At this time, the downward K^+ conductance (gK) and the upward Na^+ and Ca^{++} conductance (gNACa) cross over, initiating the automatic formation of the TAP (Figures 2.9 and 2.13A). Figure 2.16C shows how the inward diastolic Na^+, Ca^{++}, and K^+ currents, including the If current, remain stable in the automatic cell during diastole, rapidly inactivating the outward currents of K ions (Ipk). This is depicted by a reduced size of the arrows representing the outward Ip(k) current. As a consequence of the mild diastolic depolarization due to outward current Ip(K) inactivation, especially by the inward If current, the sinus node TDP slope increases progressively and reaches the TP sooner, showing the greatest automatism. If the If current is inactivated, for example, with ivabradine, the TDP slope will decrease and the sinus automatism will be reduced (see Chapter 4, Sinus Tachycardia: Prognostic and Therapeutic Implications).

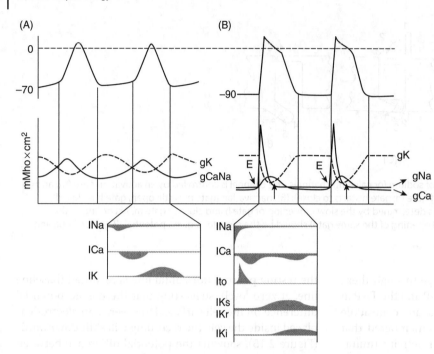

Figure 2.13 Most relevant ionic currents in automatic (A) and contractile (B) cells during systole. Contractile cells are characterized by an early and abrupt Na$^+$ inward flow and an initial and transient K$^+$ outward flow (Ito), which are not present in automatic cells.

In Purkinje cells (Figure 2.16B), the rate of the TDP ascending shift is lower, as the dominant inward ionic current of Na$^+$ Ca^{++} (Ibi) is much less capable of inactivating the dominant outflow ionic current (IK$_2$), and therefore shows a much lesser automatism than that of slow response cells. In Figure 2.16B, the IK$_2$ current arrows are thicker than the Ip(K) current arrows (Figure 2.16C). Finally, the contractile cells (Figure 2.16A) present a diastolic equilibrium between the inward (Ibi) current and the outward (IK2) current of NaCa (similar arrows). This explains why TDP remains stable and no automatic capacity is observed.

Transmembrane Action Potential
Depolarization (Phase 0) In diastole in automatic cells, there is an imbalance between the ionic inward currents (Na$^+$, Ca^{++}, and K$^+$, especially the If current of K) and

the ionic outward current (Ip). Thus, the level of TDP decreases progressively, as K$^+$ (gK) conductance decreases and Na$^+$ and Ca^{++} (gNa-Ca) conductance increases until they cross over (see before) (Figure 2.13). The intersection of conductance occurs at the TP level and is lower (about −55 mV) than that of the contractile cells (about −70 mV) (Figures 2.9 and 2.13). The TAP, which was first recorded by Draper and Weidman (1951), originates in the automatic cells at the moment that the TDP reaches the TP, and has a slow rising rate and less abrupt Phase 0 rise, because depolarization occurs essentially through the Na and Ca slow channels (Isi) (Figure 2.16C). Moreover, because the initial TDP is closer to 0 (Figure 2.9), the lower the TDP, the slower the dv/dt of response, according to the membrane response curve (Figures 2.17 and 2.18).

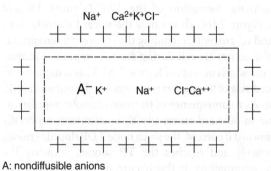

A: nondiffusible anions

Figure 2.14 The predominant negative charges inside the cell are due to the presence of significant nondiffusible anions, which outweigh the ions with a positive charge, especially K$^+$.

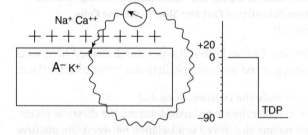

Figure 2.15 Two microelectrodes placed at the surface of a myocardial fiber record a horizontal reference line during the resting phase (zero line), meaning that there are no potential differences on the cellular surface. When one of the two electrodes is introduced inside the cell, the reference line shifts downwards (−90 mV). This line (the TDP) is stable in contractile cells, but with a more or less ascending slope in the specific conduction system cells.

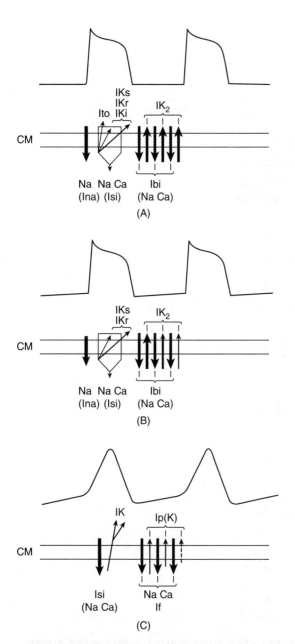

Figure 2.16 Ionic current during systole and diastole through the cellular membrane (CM) in a contractile cell (fast response cell) (A), Purkinje cell (B), and automatic cell (slow response cell) (C). During diastole, the IK₂ current is constant in contractile cells (A) but this is not so in Purkinje cells (B) (represented by a reduction of the IK₂ current arrow thickness). The K current (Ip) in automatic cells is even more rapidly inactivated (greater reduction or even disappearance, broken arrows representing the Ip current (C)). In a fast response cell (contractile cell) (A), the TDP is stable during diastole, and the NaCa current (Ibi) does not predominate over the K current (this explains why in this case Ibi and IK₂ arrows are generally the same size). The ionic currents of automatic and contractile cells during systole may also be seen (Figure 2.13).

Meanwhile, in the fast response cells, the prototype of which are the contractile cells, the TDP is –90 mV and stable, as in diastole there is an equilibrium between the inward NaCa currents (Ibi) and the outward K currents (IK2) (the voltage-clamp technique is used to analyze ionic changes at different voltage levels (Coraboeuf, 1971)) (Figure 2.16A). When the TDP receives a propagated impulse of a sufficient strength to reach the TP, a TAP is initiated (Figure 3.2). The TAP in these cells is abrupt on the initial Phase (start of Phase 0), as the TDP is lower (–90 mV). According to what we already know about the membrane response curve, when the TDP is lower, the TAP ascending velocity is greater (Figure 2.18).

This first phase of the TAP – abrupt rise of Phase 0 in the fast response cells – corresponds to the QRS recording in the clinical ECG (Figure 2.19). It does not occur spontaneously because the fast response cells have a stable (contractile cells) or a slightly ascending (Purkinje cells) TDP. It only initiates when the impulse delivered by the automatic cells triggers the abrupt Na⁺ entrance of an inward Na⁺ current, and the first part of TAP is formed (Figure 2.13).

At the end of Phase 0 in contractile cells (fast response cells), depolarization has already occurred as a result of the initial abrupt inward Na⁺ current into the cell (rapid Na⁺ channels), followed by a slow inward Ca⁺⁺ Na⁺ current (slow channels). The dominant inward Na⁺ and Ca⁺⁺ currents induce the presence of negative charges at one side outside the cell, originating a pair of charges (–+), known as the depolarization dipole (Figure 2.19).

Repolarization (Phases 1, 2, and 3) Once depolarization has occurred (Phase 0), both contractile and Purkinje cells (fast response) and automatic cells (slow response) have to repolarize. Every depolarized cell has the intrinsic capacity to recover or repolarize, the same way a rubber band is capable of returning to its original shape when the stretching factor has ceased. Similarly, cells have to recover the electric charges they maintain in the resting phase.

In contractile cells (Figure 2.19), the onset of repolarization corresponds to Phase 1 and the initial part of Phase 2 of the TAP. During this period, after transient and early abrupt outward K⁺ current (Ito), a slow outward ionic K⁺ current begins to flow outside the cell to compensate the abrupt inward Na⁺ current, although Na⁺ and Ca⁺⁺ ions are still entering the cell through the slow channels. In this phase, however, the TAP curve goes from Phase 0 to the maximum reverse polarity (+20 mV). This phase corresponds to the J point and the onset of ST segment in the clinical ECG.

o At some point during the TAP Phase 2, the ionic permeability of the membrane for K⁺ and Na⁺ Ca⁺⁺ coincides with the intersection of the Na⁺ Ca⁺⁺ and K⁺ conductance (g) (the conductance represents an inverse value of the membrane resistance against an ion flow) (Figure 2.13; see arrows). This corresponds

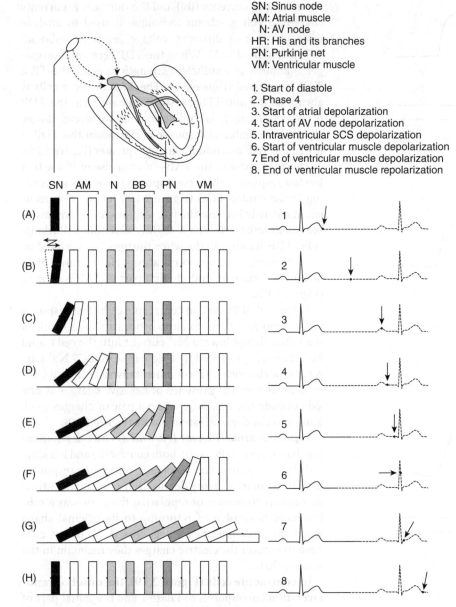

SN: Sinus node
AM: Atrial muscle
 N: AV node
HR: His and its branches
PN: Purkinje net
VM: Ventricular muscle

1. Start of diastole
2. Phase 4
3. Start of atrial depolarization
4. Start of AV node depolarization
5. Intraventricular SCS depolarization
6. Start of ventricular muscle depolarization
7. End of ventricular muscle depolarization
8. End of ventricular muscle repolarization

Figure 2.17 Sequence of cardiac activation: a comparison with dominoes, where the first domino topples the one next to it and so on. This occurs in the heart, when the heart structure with the most automatic capacity (the first black domino) has moved enough (C) to transmit its impulses to the neighboring cells. The black domino represents the heart pacemaker (sinus node: SN) and the striped dominoes represent the cells with less automaticity, which, in fact, does not usually manifest, as these cells are depolarized by the propagated impulse transmitted by the black domino (SN). White dominoes usually do not feature automaticity. The point dividing the continuous from the broken line in the ECG curve indicates the time point of the cardiac cycle corresponding to these different electrophysiologic situations.

to the isoelectric ST segment in the ECG (Figure 2.19). When the K^+ outflow is greater than the Na^+ inflow (Figure 2.19), a repolarization dipole (or pair of charges $(+-)$) is formed outside the cell.

o At a certain point in Phase 2, and especially in Phase 3, when the ECG T wave is recorded, the K^+ outflow is quite significant and Na^+ Ca^{++} can no longer enter. Thus, at the end of Phase 3 the electric polarity of the cell membrane is identical to that at the end of Phase 4 (start of Phase 0), with the TDP being −90 mV. However, the ionic conditions are not the same as those observed at the beginning of the TAP: inside the cell there is an increased level of Na^+ and Ca^{++}, whereas the K^+ level has decreased. This ionic imbalance is corrected at the beginning of Phase 4 through an active mechanism (ionic pump) (Figure 2.19). This ionic

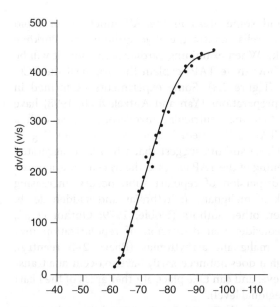

Figure 2.18 Membrane response curve. The response dv/dt depends on the transmembrane diastolic potential (TDP) at each time point.

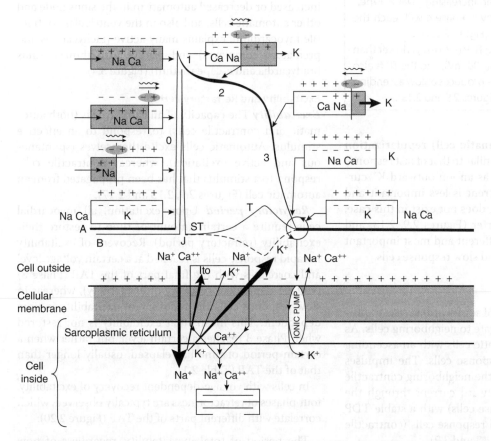

Figure 2.19 Diagram of the electroionic changes occurring during cellular depolarization and repolarization of contractile myocardium cells. In Phase 0 the depolarization dipole (−+) is formed, when the Na inward flow occurs. In Phase 2, when an important and constant K outward flow is observed, the repolarization dipole is formed (−+). Depending on whether a unique cell or the whole left ventricle is examined, a negative repolarization wave (broken line) or a positive repolarization wave (continuous line) is recorded (see text).

pump transports Na$^+$ and Ca^{++} from the inside of the cell to the outside, whereas K$^+$ is transported in the reverse. To carry out this process, energy is obtained from ATP hydrolysis by ATPase activity.

- The TDP of contractile cells is stable, with no diastolic depolarization observed, as there is a diastolic equilibrium between the ionic inward and outward currents. When an impulse delivered by a neighboring cell is received, an abrupt inward Na$^+$ current [Ina] is initiated, the gNa exceeds the gK, the TP is reached, and the TAP is originated (Figure 2.13B).
- Contractile cells have a resting stable TDP of −90 mV. When the TP is reached as a result of the impulse propagated by neighboring cells, they initiate a fast ascending TAP (Figure 2.13B).
- Meanwhile, in automatic cells the TDP shows a slight diastolic depolarization caused by an imbalance between the ionic inward current, especially the If current (rather stable), and the K+ ion outward current (Ip), which is rapidly deactivated. This results in a TDP (Phase 4) with a slight ascending slope associated with a decreasing gK and an increasing gNaCa. When both conductances cross over, Phase 4 will reach the TP and the TAP will initiate (Figure 2.13A).
- In automatic cells the resting TDP (−70 mV) is lower than that of the contractile cells (−90 mV), and the TP is also reached at a lower level. This produces a slow ascending TAP (slow response cells) (Figures 2.9 and 2.13).

Slow response cell (automatic cell) repolarization shows an ionic mechanism similar to that of fast response cells (contractile cells), such as an ion outward K$^+$ current, although this ionic current is less important and less persistent. Thus, Phase 1 does not exist in this case, and Phases 2 and 3 are shorter (Figures 2.9, 2.13, and 2.16). Table 2.1 shows the different and most important characteristics of the rapid and slow response cells.

Automaticity

Automaticity is the capacity of some cardiac cells to produce stimuli that may propagate to neighboring cells. As previously discussed, automatic cells with an ascending TDP (Phase 4) are slow response cells. The impulses received from these cells by the neighboring contractile cells cause an abrupt Na$^+$ inward current through the rapid channels (rapid response cells) with a stable TDP and trigger the TAP of rapid response cells (contractile and Purkinje cells) (Figures 2.13 and 3.2).

The different structures of the heart have different TDP and TAP curves according to the cells that predominate in them: slow response cells (automatic cells) (sinus node and some areas in the AV junction) or rapid response cells (contractile myocardium and Purkinje network). When examining cardiac activation, it will be shown how these TAPs explain the origin of the ECG tracing (Figure 2.3). Some experiments performed in wedge preparations (Yan and Antzelevitch, 1998) have shown that the ventricular myocardium area with a longer TAP is the medial zone (M cell zone) (Figure 2.24). These authors suggest that when an exaggerated lengthening of the TAP exists in the M cell zone, a transmural dispersion of repolarization occurs, increasing the risk of malignant arrhythmias and sudden death. However, other authors (Noble, 1979; Opthof *et al.*, 2007) consider that dispersion of repolarization may explain malignant arrhythmias (Phase 2–3 reentry), although it does not necessarily have to occur at a transmural level and can take place at other areas of the heart (transregional level).

The sinus node is, under normal conditions, the structure showing the greatest automatism, followed by the AV node and, to a lesser degree, the ventricular Purkinje network (Figure 2.3). As discussed later on (see the section regarding the mechanism of arrhythmias, Chapter 3), the increased or decreased automatism in the sinus node and other automatic cells, and also in the ventricular contractile myocardium, explains many active (tachycardias and premature complexes) and passive arrhythmias (sinus bradycardia and escape rhythm) (Figure 3.4).

Excitability and Refractory Period

Excitability The capacity of all cardiac cells (both automatic and contractile cells) to respond to an effective stimulus. Automatic cells excite themselves (spontaneous and active excitation), whereas contractile cells respond to a stimulus that has been propagated from an automatic cell (Figures 2.9, 2.13 and 2.17).

Refractory period Upon excitation, all myocardial cells require a certain amount of time to restore their excitability (refractory period). Recovery of excitability in rapid response cells is reached at a certain voltage level and correlates with the final part of the TAP (Phase 3) (voltage-dependent recovery of excitability), whereas in slow response cells the recovery of excitability is time dependent. This means that excitability is not restored when Phase 3 reaches a certain level, but rather when a certain period of time has elapsed, usually longer than that of the TAP (Table 2.1).

In cells with voltage-dependent recovery of excitability, four phases of refractoriness are typically observed, which correlate with different parts of the TAP (Figure 2.20):

o The period of total inexcitability, regardless of how great the stimulus applied is, corresponds to the absolute refractory period (ARP), and covers most parts of systole.

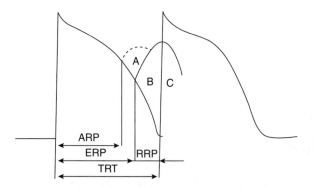

Figure 2.20 Cellular excitability phases and refractory periods in cells where excitability recovery is voltage-dependent (rapid response). ARP: absolute refractory period. There is no response. At the end of this period there is a response zone with local potentials (A). ERP: effective refractory period. At the end of this period a propagated response zone is initiated, but only when suprathreshold stimuli are applied (B). RRP: relative refractory period. It corresponds to the zone of response to suprathreshold stimuli. TTR: time of total recovery. It is equivalent to the ERP + RRP. At the end of the RRP a normal response is initiated (C), corresponding to a TAP with a morphology equal to basal morphology.

○ The period of local responses (Figure 2.20A) is a very short period, during which potentials are initiated in the cell but are not able to propagate. The effective refractory period (ERP) of the cell corresponds to the sum of the ARP and the phase (A) of local potentials.
○ The period of partial excitability, which corresponds to the end of TAP Phase 3, occurs when suprathreshold stimuli are required to produce the propagated response. This phase corresponds to the relative refractory period (RRP) of the cell. The sum of the ERP and the RRP corresponds to the total recovery time (TRT).
○ The period of supernormal excitability (PSE) takes place at the end of the TAP and at the start of diastole (Phase 4). During this period the cells respond to infra-threshold stimuli (Figures 2.21 and 3.15).

In a zone or tissue of the SCS, the functional and effective refractory period is measured through the application of increasingly premature atrial extra stimuli (see Appendix, Figure A.6).

Clinically, in a conventional ECG, the RRP (Figure 2.21) begins at the time when the stimulus is conducted more slowly than normal. For example, in the AV junction a baseline PR interval of 0.20 s is prolonged to 0.26 s, with shortening of the RR interval (tachycardia or premature complexes) (Figure 2.22B). The ARP (Figure 2.21) begins at the time when a stimulus is not conducted. In the AV junction, it originates a pause (Figure 22C). In patients with tachycardization or atrial premature complexes, a stimulus falling during the onset of RRP will be conducted at a slower rate, and if it falls during ARP it will not be conducted at all (Figure 2.22, left, B and C). Moreover, a

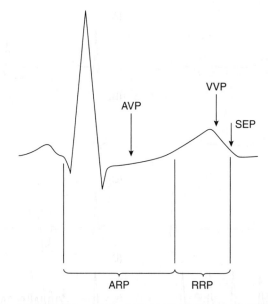

Figure 2.21 Location of refractory periods at atrioventricular (AV) level, the supernormal excitability period and vulnerable periods at atrial and ventricular level in the human ECG. ARP: absolute refractory period; RRP: relative refractory period; AVP: atrial vulnerable period. VVP: ventricular vulnerable period; SEP: supernormal excitability period.

ventricular premature complex may impair the conduction of the next P wave, or even prevent conduction (Figure 2.22, right, B and C).

The existence of different refractory periods at different structures of the SCS may cause a stimulus to be blocked in only one of its zones. Later, aberrant conduction, which is related to this concept and is of significant clinical interest (see Chapter 3, Concealed Conduction), is discussed.

Vulnerable Period

The ventricular vulnerable period (VVP) is a small zone located around the peak of the T wave. A stimulus falling in this zone may trigger a ventricular fibrillation (R/T phenomenon) (Figure 2.22, right, D). The atrial vulnerable period (AVP), a zone where the atrial stimuli may trigger an atrial fibrillation, is located at the beginning of the ST segment (Figure 2.22, left, D).

Conduction of Stimuli

Conductivity is the capacity of cardiac fibers to transmit stimuli from automatic cells to neighboring cells. The stimulus originates in the sinus node and propagates through the SCS (see Cardiac Activation: Excitation–Contraction Coupling).

The normal conduction of stimuli is made along the cell membrane through an electroionic phenomenon. Although there is no chemical mediator directly involved, some chemical compounds (cate-cholamines, acetylcholine, antiarrhythmic agents, etc.) may have an effect on the rate at

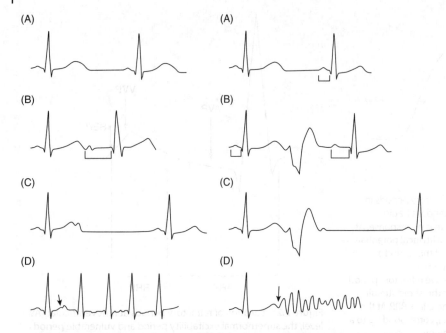

Figure 2.22 Left: (A) Normal sinus rhythm; (B) premature atrial complex (PAC) conducted with long PR as it falls in the atrioventricular (AV) junction relative refractory period (RRP); (C) PAC not conducted as it falls in the AV junction absolute refractory period (ARP); (D) when a PAC falls into the atrial VP, it may trigger an AF (Figure 4.34). Right: (A) Normal sinus rhythm; (B) interpolated premature ventricular complex (PVC) followed by a long PR interval because of concealed conduction of PVC in AV junction (Figure 5.7C); (C) PVC preventing conduction of next P wave, as the AV junction is in the ARP due to concealed conduction of PVC in AV junction (Figure 5.7A); (D) when a PVC falls in the ventricular VP, especially in the case of acute ischemia, a VF may be triggered (Figures 5.42–5.44).

which stimuli propagate. It should be noted that most of the components of the cardiac fibers have a low resistance and are good conductors of electric currents. The cell membrane shows variable resistance to the transmission of the electrical impulse, depending on the ultrastructural characteristics of the different cardiac cells (see Anatomy of Specific Conduction System, and Figures 2.1 and 2.2).

Conduction differs in the fast response cells (contractile and His–Purkinje system cells) (regenerative conduction) and in the slow response cells (particularly in the AN and N zones of the AV junction, and in the sinoatrial junction) (decrementing conduction) (Figure 2.23).

The rate of conduction in the heart is essentially determined by two factors:

(i) The rate of TAP ascending (dv/dt of Phase 0), which is rapid in the rapid response fibers and slow in the slow response fibers.
(ii) Ultrastructural characteristics. Narrow fibers (contractile and transitional cells) and those without intercalated disks (P cells) conduct stimuli slower than wide fibers with many intercalated disks (Purkinje cells) (Figure 2.2). When passing from a narrow fiber zone to a wide fiber zone, the conduction increases (from the AV node to the His–Purkinje system), and vice versa (Figure 2.23).

In the sinoatrial junction and the AV node, particularly in the upper part, the slow conductance is caused by the great number of P and transitional cells within these structures (see Anatomy of Specific Conduction System).

The disturbances of the normal conduction of stimuli may include the following:

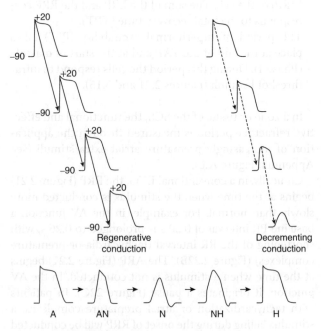

Figure 2.23 Stimulus conduction of regenerative-type (contractile cells – myocardium) and decrementing-type (areas with slow response cells – AV junction below and sinoatrial junction).

o **Conduction** through **accessory pathways**, as in pre-excitation syndromes, and this explains many supraventricular arrhythmias, which may occasionally trigger ventricular malignant arrhythmias (see Chapter 8).

o A premature stimulus is conducted while later stimuli are blocked. This phenomenon is known as **supernormal conduction** (Figure 3.15). In this case, a differential diagnosis should be made with the **gap phenomenon** (Gallagher *et al.*, 1973), which also involves the conduction of a premature stimulus when a later stimulus is not propagated (see Chapter 3, Active Cardiac Arrhythmias with Fixed Coupling Interval: Other Mechanisms) (Figure 3.16).

o **Unidirectional block occurs in a reentrant circuit**, which causes many active arrhythmias (see Chapter 3, Active Cardiac Arrhythmias with Fixed Coupling Interval: Reentry). A unidirectional entrance or exit block from an ectopic focus may also explain the parasystole (see Chapter 3, Active Cardiac Arrhythmias with Variable Coupling Interval: The Parasystole).

o **Conduction is slow in some areas of the SCS**, accounting for many passive arrhythmias. This includes the different types of **heart block**, as well as **aberrant conduction** phenomena (see Chapter 3, Aberrant Conduction) and **concealed conduction** (see Chapter 3, Concealed Conduction).

Cardiac Activation: Excitation-Contraction Coupling
(Figure 2.3)

It is already known that slow response cells show automaticity. This means that they are able to excite themselves and transmit this excitation to neighboring cells. Figure 2.3 shows the activation of the heart starting in sinus node and going through the atria, the AV junction, and the intraventricular conduction system it reaches the contractile myocardium. It demonstrates how the successive superimposition of TAPs of the different structures gives rise to the human ECG (P-QRS-T). Figure 2.3 also shows the correlation between the human surface ECG and the intracavitary ECG. The passage of the stimulus through the bundle of His (H) not detected in the surface ECG may be observed in an intracavitary recording, which helps in better recognizing the exact location of the AV block.

> Normal conduction velocities in the different heart structures are: atria 1–2 m/s (ratio 20); AV node 0.05 m/s (ratio 1); His–Purkinje system 1.5–4 m/s (ratio 40); ventricle 0.3 m/s (ratio 6) (Figure 2.3).

Electrical activation is followed by a mechanical contraction at the Purkinje–muscle junction (**excitation–contraction coupling**). When a cell is excited by an electrical stimulus, calcium is released from the sarcoplasmic reticulum, thus inducing the actin–myosin interaction. In the presence of calcium, the inhibition by troponin over this interaction is removed. As a result, ATPase is released, converting ATP into ADP, generating strength and bringing the actin and myosin filaments closer. This is the basis for sarcomere shortening and, therefore, is essential to myocardial contraction. When calcium is reabsorbed into the sarcoplasmic reticulum, the contractile capacity becomes inactive.

From Cellular Electrogram to Human ECG
(Figures 2.24–2.29) (Sodi–Pallarés and Calder, 1956; McFarlane and Lawrie, 1989; Bayés de Luna, 2011)

Why Cellular Electrogram and Human ECG have Different Polarities of the Repolarization Wave?

When a microelectrode is placed on the outside of a cell with another microelectrode placed inside, a stable TDP is recorded in the contractile cells. If the cell is conveniently stimulated, a monophasic curve called a TAP is recorded, which corresponds to cell depolarization and repolarization [(Figures 2.3 and 2.19). Both the cellular electrogram and human ECG represent the sum of cell or ventricular depolarization plus repolarization (not taking the atria into account (these generate the P wave, as discussed later on) and considering the ventricles as a large cell – left ventricle (LV) – which generates the QRS complex). Although in both cases the depolarization (QRS) is similar ($\bigwedge$), repolarization is different: negative ($\smile$) in the cellular electrogram, and positive ($\frown$) in the human ECG. The reason for this is that in humans

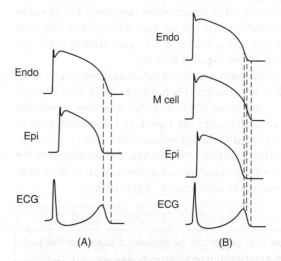

Figure 2.24 (A) The TAPs of subendocardium and subepicardium are shown. The latter, according to the theory used to explain the normal ECG, is the last to depolarize and the first to repolarize. (B) According to Yan and Antzelevich (1998), the epicardium repolarizes first (coincides with the peak of T wave) and the endocardium later, but the area that repolarizes the latest is the M cell area (coincides with the end of T wave) (see text).

the epicardial TAP completes repolarization earlier than that of the subendocardial TAP (area far from the electrode), which is not the case at a cellular level.

Since Wilson *et al.* (1943), it is accepted that the discordance between cellular electrogram and human ECG can be explained by the fact that in humans the dipole of the repolarization wave (T wave) is originated in the left ventricle, in a zone opposite to where the dipole of the depolarization wave (QRS) starts, whereas in the cellular electrogram it originates in the same place (Figures 2.25–2.27).

This means that some zones of the heart activated earlier show a longer TAP than those activated later. Different experimental works on animals (Burgess and Abildskov, 1972; Burnes *et al.*, 2001) and humans, based on epicardial and endocardial TAP recording during angiogram and cardiac surgery (Franz *et al.*, 1987), have demonstrated that **the zone of shorter TAP and subsequently earlier repolarization is located in the epicardium**, even though it is well known that the epicardial zone depolarizes after the endocardial zone (Durrer *et al.*, 1970; Cassidy *et al.*, 1984). Therefore, it seems evident that a transmural gradient exists. There are different opinions on the zones of the heart in which this repolarization gradient is present. Some authors (Noble, 1979; Opthof *et al.*, 2007) believe that this does not take place at a transmural level, but rather at a transregional one (at an apical-basal level, according to Noble). Some authors, primarily the Antzelevitch group (Yan and Antzelevitch, 1998), have carried out studies in wedge preparations, which have proven that the epicardium is repolarized earlier and that the end of the epicardial TAP corresponds to the T wave peak. However, they found that in the middle portion of the ventricular wall (M cell area) repolarization takes longer when compared to the endocardium, and showed that the end of the TAP in this zone corresponds to the end of the T wave (Figure 2.24) (see Chapter 3, Other Types of Reentry).

There is no consensus about the area experiencing a longest TAP of left ventricle (Opthof *et al.*, 2007). Nevertheless, it is clear that there is a myocardial zone that repolarizes earlier, coinciding with the T peak and, according to most authors, located in the epicardium. Also, there is undoubtedly another zone that repolarizes later, coinciding with the end of the T wave, and located in the endocardium or middle portion of the ventricular wall (M cells).

Human ECG origin can be explained based on the fact that the epicardium repolarizes before the endocardium (Figure 2.26).

At a cellular level, it occurs in the opposite way, as the area far from the electrode (equivalent to the endocardium) repolarizes before the area proximal to the electrode (the epicardium) (Figure 2.25).

Two Theories to Explain the Origin of Cellular Electrogram and Human ECG

Cellular electrogram and human ECG are explained by two different theories. The first theory suggests that the curves of the cellular and human electrograms are the result of successive recordings of cellular and human (left ventricle) depolarization and repolarization, taken from an electrode located opposite the initial stimulation site (depolarization). The second theory suggests that the cellular and human electrograms are the sum of the subendocardial (or cellular area most distal to the recording electrode) and subepicardial (or cellular area most proximal to the recording electrode) TAPs. It should be noted that the TAP Phase 0 corresponds to QRS, Phases 1 and 2 to ST segment, and the end of Phase 2 and Phase 3 to the T wave (Figure 2.19).

The Cellular Electrogram and the Human ECG are the Result of Successive Recordings of Cellular or Ventricular Depolarization and Repolarization

The curve of the cellular electrogram (Figure 2.25) is the result of the sum of the cellular depolarization and repolarization recordings taken at the site opposite from where the stimulus reaches the cell.

As seen in Figure 2.25A, cell depolarization initiates a depolarization dipole (−+) when positive Na charges begin to enter the inside of the cell, the expression of which is a vector (→) with the arrowhead representing the dipole positive charge. The recording electrode (A), located at the side opposite to where the depolarization started, records a positive deflection, as it faces the positive part of the dipole, or head of the vector. When the cell is completely depolarized (negative charges on the outside of the cell), a positive complex is recorded. In the contractile cell, depolarization and repolarization start in the same place (same sense phenomena); therefore, because the repolarization dipole (+−) and its vectorial expression (←) move to the area opposite to where the recording electrode is located with the negative charge facing the recording electrode, it is recorded as a negative deflection at the end of the repolarization (Figure 2.25B). Thus, the cellular electrogram has a positive depolarization and a negative repolarization (Figure 2.25A + B).

The human ECG is characterized by a positive repolarization (T wave) similar to that of the QRS complex. This is because the human ECG recording may be considered equivalent to that of the left ventricular electrogram, as if it were a "large cell" responsible for the human ECG (Figure 2.26). Here, depolarization is similar to that of an isolated cell, and therefore a positive QRS complex is recorded from the corporal surface equivalent to the epicardium (Figure 2.26C). However, the repolarization dipole begins at the opposite side compared to

(A)   Cellular depolarization

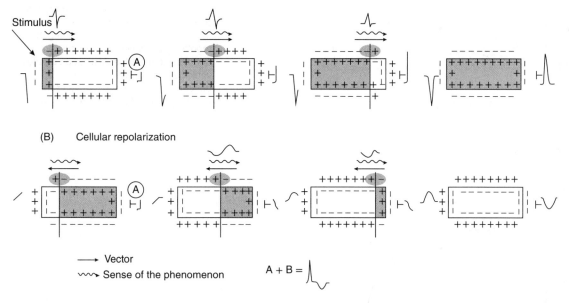

(B)   Cellular repolarization

→ Vector
〰〰 Sense of the phenomenon

$A + B =$

Figure 2.25 Diagram showing how the cellular electrogram curve (A + B) is originated, according to the dipole theory. (A) Cellular depolarization; (B) cellular repolarization (see text).

Figure 2.26 Explanatory diagram of depolarization (QRS) and repolarization (T) morphology in the normal human heart. Figures on the left show a view of the left ventricular free wall (from the outside); therefore, only the charge distribution on the external surface of the "large left ventricular cell" may be seen. Figures on the right show profile diagrams in which intracellular and extracellular changes of electric charge are depicted. When electrode A is located close to the epicardium, a normal electrocardiographic curve is recorded (see text).

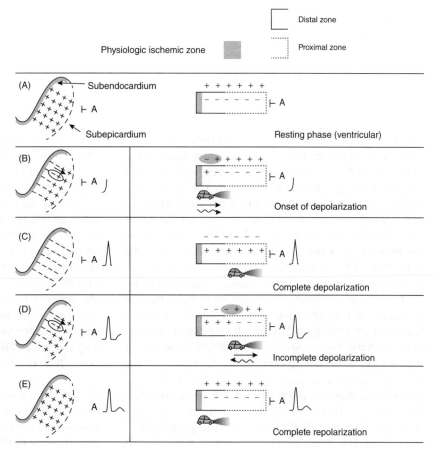

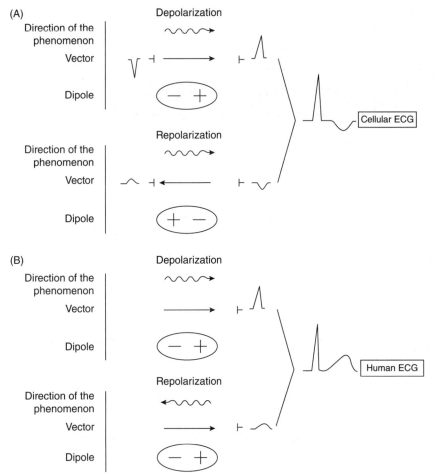

(A)

Depolarization

Direction of the
phenomenon

Vector

Dipole

Repolarization

Direction of the
phenomenon

Vector

Dipole

Cellular ECG

(B)

Depolarization

Direction of the
phenomenon

Vector

Dipole

Repolarization

Direction of the
phenomenon

Vector

Dipole

Human ECG

Figure 2.27 (A) Cellular depolarization and repolarization dipoles with the corresponding vectors (→) and direction (~ ~>) of the phenomenon, which give rise to the cellular electrogram with negative repolarization wave. (B) Ventricular depolarization and repolarization dipoles, with the corresponding vectors and direction of the phenomenon and the resulting human ECG curve (QRS-T curve).

that of an isolated cell, the epicardium (next to the electrode) instead of the endocardium (distal area), as repolarization in the human heart (LV) begins in the area with relatively greater blood perfusion, the epicardium, and moves from this area to a lower perfusion area, the endocardium. It is known that the endocardium has lesser blood perfusion compared to the epicardium, as the endocardium has a terminal circulation (Bell and Fox, 1974). This facilitates a perfusion gradient from a low-perfusion area to a high-perfusion area (from endocardium to epicardium). Additional support for the low perfusion of the subendocardium is the fact that the endocardium is subjected to the left ventricular telediastolic pressure. Consequently, the repolarization vector moves away from the epicardium to the endocardium, although the positive charge of the dipole (head of the vector) continues to point toward the recording electrode (similar to car headlights shining while driving in reverse (Figure 2.26D)). As the recording electrode is located in the epicardium, a positive deflection is

recorded (positive T wave) (Figure 2.26E). Figure 2.27 shows how the correlation between dipole, vector, and the direction of phenomenon of activation may explain the ECG curve, both at cellular and human levels.

This is actually a simplification of how the ECG recording is generated. The LV has been considered to be the only factor responsible and depolarization to be represented by one vector. In practice, this is not so. The human ECG requires at least one vector to express the sum of all atrial vectors responsible for the way the stimulus depolarize the atria, known as the atrial depolarization loop, or P loop (Figure 2.28A), and three vectors responsible for ventricular depolarization, or the QRS loop (Figure 2.28B). Additionally, ventricular depolarization (QRS) is followed by the ventricular repolarization wave (T wave), through which the ventricles give rise to the repolarization loop, or T loop (Figure 2.28C). **The projection of the P, QRS, and T loops over the positive and negative hemifields of each lead explains the morphology of the ECG** (Bayés de Luna, 2011).

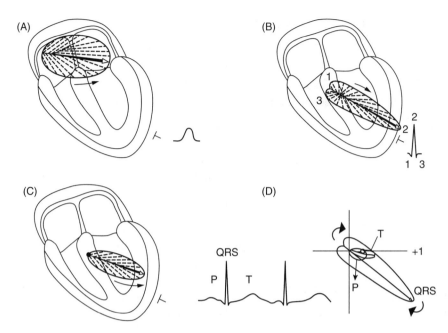

Figure 2.28 (A) Atrial depolarization loop; (B) ventricular depolarization loop with three vectors; (C) ventricular repolarization loop; (D) note the loop–ECG correlation.

The Cellular Electrogram and the Human ECG are the Result of the Sum of the TAPs of the Subendocardium (or Distal Cellular Area) and the Subepicardium (or Proximal Cellular Area)

According to this theory, there is no need to consider the dynamic activation of the heart or to question how the depolarization and repolarization dipole is formed. This theory discusses the activation of the left ventricle of the heart and also the activation of an isolated cell (A and B in Figure 2.29) under three situations: (i) at resting phase, (ii) when depolarization is completed, and (iii) when repolarization is completed. In accordance with Ashman and Hull (1947) and other authors (Cabrera, 1958; Cooksey *et al.*, 1977) the activation of a cell or the LV, as the expression of the human ECG, equals the sum of the TAPs of the most distal cellular part (subendocardium in

the LV), plus the TAPs of the most proximal cellular or ventricular part (subepicardium in the LV). By doing this sum (Figure 2.29), we may understand how the cellular electrogram shows a negative T wave and the human ECG a positive T wave.

> Dipole → Vector → Loop → Hemifield → ECG

This theory, which explains the basis of the human ECG based on the sum of TAPs in two different areas of the heart (generally, the endocardium and the epicardium) is very useful in understanding the repolarization alterations observed during myocardial ischemia (changes in T wave, ST segment depression and elevation).

---

1. There is considerable evidence that the epicardium (most proximal area to the electrode) is the first area of the human heart to repolarize.
2. Cellular electrogram and human ECG result from the sum of TAP from the distal (endocardium in the heart) and proximal (epicardium in the heart) areas to the recording electrode.
3. According to another theory, both the cellular electrogram and the human ECG are the result of the succes-

sive recordings of cellular or ventricular depolarization and repolarization.
4. The correlation between the contractile cell TAP and the human ECG is as following (Figure 2.19):
   o Phase 0: QRS
   o Phase 1 and start of Phase 2: J point and onset of ST segment
   o Phase 2 (mid-part): ST segment isoelectric line
   o End of Phase 2 and Phase 3: T wave.

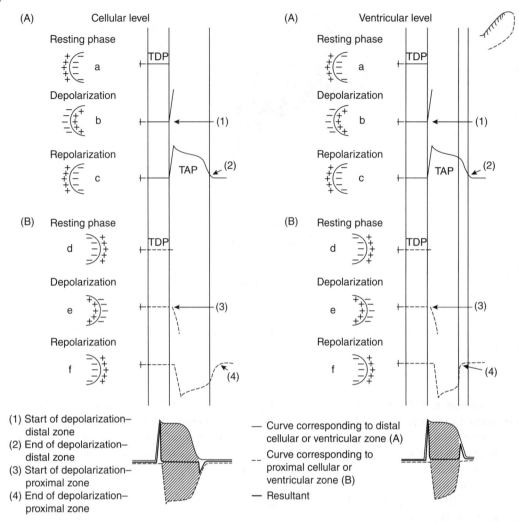

(A)   Cellular level

Resting phase

a   TDP

Depolarization

b   (1)

Repolarization

c   TAP   (2)

(B)   Resting phase

d   TDP

Depolarization

e   (3)

Repolarization

f   (4)

(A)   Ventricular level

Resting phase

a   TDP

Depolarization

b   (1)

Repolarization

c   TAP   (2)

(B)   Resting phase

d   TDP

Depolarization

e   (3)

Repolarization

f   (4)

(1) Start of depolarization–
     distal zone
(2) End of depolarization–
     distal zone
(3) Start of depolarization–
     proximal zone
(4) End of depolarization–
     proximal zone

— Curve corresponding to distal
    cellular or ventricular zone (A)

-- Curve corresponding to
    proximal cellular or
    ventricular zone (B)

— Resultant

Figure 2.29 Both at cellular and ventricular level, the sum of the transmembrane action potentials (TAPs) from the area distal (A) and proximal (B) to the electrode initiates the cellular and human (ventricular) ECG. We see the human ECG (right) for which we consider ventricular activation (actually left ventricle activation) responsible for the ECG. The subendocardium TAP corresponds to the TAP of the left ventricular area distal to the electrode. At the end of depolarization (b) the electrode is facing the inner positivity of the distal area, as that area is depolarized and has negative charges on the outside and positive charges on the inside, giving rise to an ascending Phase 0 of the TAP. At the end of repolarization (c), which occurs at a later time than in the subepicardium, the electrode is facing the inner negativity, as the outer repolarized area is already positive. Therefore, the curve returns to the isoelectric line, although, as the subendocardium repolarization ends later, its TAP also ends at a time later than that of the subepicardium. The opposite is true in the case of the subepicardium TAP. Its TAP corresponds to the TAP of the left ventricular area proximal to the electrode. When it depolarizes, which occurs later than in the subendocardial area, this zone is negatively charged on the outer side, so the electrode faces a negative charge, thus recording the Phase 0 as negative (e). When this zone is repolarized (f), which occurs sooner than in the subendocardial area, the electrode faces outer positive charges, as the repolarization is already complete, and the subepicardium TAP curve returns to the isoelectric line. By adding together both TAPs (below) it may be inferred how the human ECG is originated with a positive depolarization (QRS) and repolarization (T) waves. On the left, a cellular electrogram is shown, which has a negative repolarization wave because the proximal zone of the isolated cell has a longer TAP compared with that of the distal zone (contrary to what is observed at the ventricular level). This is due to the fact that there is no perfusion gradient favoring the proximal zone (in the LV the subepicardium, see text); thus repolarization starts at the distal zone (equivalent to the subendocardium) and ends later in the proximal zone (equivalent to the epicardium).

Self Assessment

A. What are the three components of contractile cells?

B. From an ultrastructural point of view, how many types of specific cells do you know?

C. What are the most outstanding anatomic characteristics of the sinus node?

D. How many internodal tracts are there? How do they reach the atrioventricular (AV) node?

E. What anatomic structures comprise the AV junction?

F. What are the characteristics of the circuit that constitute the base of the AV junctional reentrant tachycardias with circuit exclusively within the AV junction?

G. What is the trifascicular theory of the intraventricular specific conduction system (SCS)?

H. What is the quadrifascicular theory?

I. From an electrophysiologic point of view, how many types of cells are there in the heart?

J. What is the basic structure of the ion channels, i.e. the Na channels?

K. Describe how the transmembrane diastolic potential (TDP) originates.

L. Describe how the transmembrane action potential (TAP) originates.

M. Describe the automaticity.

N. Describe the refractory period.

O. Describe the vulnerable period.

P. Describe the conductivity. Is it the same in every cell?

Q. Explain the sequence of cardiac activation from the sinus impulse until complete heart activation is achieved.

R. How does the sequence dipole–vector—loop–hemifield explain the electrocardiogram (ECG)?

S. Explain how the ECG is a result of the sum of the TAPs of the subepicardium and subendocardium.

T. Explain the correlation between the phases of the ventricular myocardial TAP and human ECG morphology.

References

Ashman R, Hull E. Essentials of electrocardiography. The McMillan Co., New York, 1947.

Bayés de Luna A. Electrocardiography. John Wiley & Sons Ltd, 2011.

Bayés de Luna A, Cosin J (eds). Cardiac Arrhythmias. Pergamon Press, Oxford 1978

Bayés de Luna A, Fort de Ribot R, Trilla E, *et al*. Electrocardiographic and vectorcardiographic study of interatrial conduction disturbances with left atrial retrograde activation. J Electrocardiol 1985;18:1.

Bayés de Luna A, Pérez Riera A, Baranchuk A, *et al*. Electrocardiographic manifestation of the middle fibers/septal fascicle block: a consensus report. J Electrocardiol 2012;45:454.

Bell JR, Fox AC. Pathogenesis of subendocardial ischemia. Am J Med Sci 1974;268:2.

Burgess JM, Abildskov J. The sequence of normal ventricular recovery. Am Heart J 1972;84:660.

Burnes J, Waldo A, Rudy Y. Imaging dispersion of ventricular repolarization. Circulation 2001;104:1299.

Cabrera E. Teoria y práctica de la electrocardiografía. Instituto Nacional de Cardiología. La Prensa Médica Mexicana, México, 1958.

Cassidy D, Vasallo J, Marchlinski F, *et al*. Endocardial mapping in humans: activation patterns. Circulation 1984;70:37.

Cooksey I, Dunn M, Massie E. Clinical ECG and VCG. The Year Book Medical Pub, Chicago, IL, 1977.

Coraboeuf E. Membrane ionic permeabilities and contractile phenomena in the heart. Cardiovascular Res 1971;1:55.

Draper M, Weidman S. Cardiac resting and action potentials recorded with an intracellular electrode. J Physiol 1951;115:74.

Durrer D, Van Dam R, Freud G, *et al*. Total excitation of the isolated human heart. Circulation 1970;41:899.

Eriksson A, Thornell LE. Intermediate myofilaments in heart Purkinje fibers. J Cell Biol 1979;80:231.

Franz MR, Bargheer K, Rafflenbeul W, *et al*. Monophasic action potential mapping in human subjects with normal electrocardiograms: direct evidence for the genesis of the T wave. Circulation 1987;75:379.

Gallagher JJ, Damato AN, Caracta AR, *et al*. Gap in the AV conduction in man; types I and II. Am Heart J 1973;85:78.

Hofman B, Cranefield P. Electrophysiology of the heart. McGraw-Hill Book Co., New York, 1960.

Holmqvist F, Husser D, Tapanainus J, *et al*. Interatrial conduction can be accurately determined using standard 12 lead ECG. Heart Rhythm 2008;5:413.

Inoue S, Becker A. Posterior extension of human AV node. Circulation 1998;97:188.

Issa ZP, Miller JM. Zipes DP. Clinical, arrhythmology and electrophysiology, 2nd edn. Elsevier-Saunders, 2012.

Josephson ME. Clinical cardiac electrophysiology. Wolters-Kluwer, Philadelphia, PA, 2008.

Katritsis D, Becker A. The AV nodal re-entrant circuit. A proposal. Heart Rhythm 2007;4:1354.

Markus E, Yamagishi T, Tomaselli G. Structure and function of voltage gated channels. J Physiol 1998;508:647.

Martínez-Palomo A, Aleanis J, Benítez D. Transitional cardiac cells of the conductive system of the dog heart. J Cell Biol 1970;47:1.

McFarlane P, Lawrie T (eds). Comprehensive electrocardiography. Pergamon Press, Oxford, 1989.

Noble D. The initiation of the heart beat. University Press, Oxford, 1979.

Opthof T, Coronel R, Plotnikov AN, *et al.* Dispersion of repolarization in canine ventricle and the ECG T wave: T interval does not reflect transmural dispersion. Heart Rhythm 2007;4:341.

Paes de Carvalho A, Hofman BF, Langan WB. Two components of cardiac action potential. Nature 1966;211:938.

Rosenbaum M, Elizari M, Lazzari J. Los hemibloqueos. Edit. Paidos, Buenos Aires, Argentina, 1968.

Sodi-Pallarés D, Calder R. New basis of electrocardiography. Mosby, St. Louis, IL, 1956.

Uhley H. The quadrifascicular nature of the peripheral conduction system. In: Dreyfus L, Likoff W (eds). Cardiac arrhythmias. Grune-Stratton, New York, 1973.

Uhley H. The concept of trifascicular intraventricular conduction: historical aspects and influence on contemporary cardiology [review]. Am J Cardiol 1979;43:643.

Wilson F, Hill I, Johnston F. The interpretation of the galvanometric waves when one electrode is distant from the heart and the other in contact with its surface. Am Heart J 1943;4:807.

Wu D, Yeh S. Double loop figure of eight reentry as a mechanism of multiple AV reentry. Am Heart J 1994;127:83.

Yan GX, Antzelevitch C. Cellular basis for the normal T wave and the electrocardiographic manifestations of the long-QT syndrome. Circulation 1998;98:1928.

3

Electrophysiologic Mechanisms

Mechanisms Responsible for Active Cardiac Arrhythmias

When talking about the mechanisms responsible for active cardiac arrhythmias it should be taken into account that quite frequently the arrhythmia is triggered by one mechanism and perpetuated by another. Additionally, it must be borne in mind that there are modulating factors (unbalanced autonomic nervous system (ANS), ischemia, ionic and metabolic alterations, stress, alcohol and coffee consumption, etc.) that favor the appearance and maintenance of arrhythmias. It is useful to compare tachyarrhythmias (Table 3.1) to a burning forest. The fire may be triggered with a match (premature impulse) but for the fire to perpetuate the bushes and trees should be dry enough (substrate). There are many modulating factors having an impact on the fire [arrhythmia] starting sooner and perpetuating, such as wind or heat [equivalent to tachycardia, instability of the ANS, ischemia, etc.], or extinguishing sooner, such as rain or cold (equivalent to the stability of the ANS, sympathetic nervous system integrity, etc.).

In this chapter the specific mechanisms that initiate and perpetuate different arrhythmias are examined. Further discussed are the triggering and/or modulating factors when each particular arrhythmia is examined in the following chapters.

Active arrhythmias may be related to the basal rhythm or occur independently. In the first case, the premature isolated P′ or QRS complex, or the first P′ wave or QRS complex in rapid rhythms, presents a fixed or nearly fixed coupling interval in the electrocardiogram (ECG). This is because the arrhythmia is initiated by a mechanism depending on the previous basal rhythm. The coupling interval is defined as the time from the onset of the preceding QRS complex (if the active arrhythmia is a ventricular arrhythmia), or the P′ wave (if it is an atrial arrhythmia), to the beginning of the ectopic P′ or QRS complex (Figures 3.1A and B).

Active arrhythmias not associated to the baseline rhythm are much less frequent. Usually they are isolated complexes of parasystolic origin and nearly always have a frankly variable coupling interval (Figures 3.1 C and D). These arrhythmias may also occur as sustained tachycardias (see Chapter 5, Other Monomorphic Ventricular Tachycardias). The electrocardiographic features of these two types of active arrhythmias will now be discussed.

The different mechanisms of both active and passive cardiac arrhythmias are shown in Table 3.1. The majority of isolated active arrhythmias (supraventricular or ventricular complexes) or repetitive arrhythmias (tachycardias, fibrillation, and flutter) show a fixed coupling interval and are usually caused by a reentrant mechanism or an abnormal generation of the stimulus (increased automaticity or triggered activity) (see the next section Active Cardiac Arrhythmias with Fixed Coupling Interval). Rare active parasystolic arrhythmias are due to increased automaticity of a protected ectopic focus (see Active Cardiac Arrhythmias with Variable Coupling Interval: the Parasystole). Other less frequent mechanisms of active arrhythmias are shown in the same table. Passive arrhythmias are explained by depressed automatism or conduction disturbances.

Active Cardiac Arrhythmias with Fixed Coupling Interval

Active arrhythmias appearing as isolated complexes or repetitive runs of various complexes (non-sustained tachycardia) usually show a fixed coupling interval of the first complex (Figure 3.1A and B). Actually, only parasystolic active arrhythmias (see Active cardiac arrhythmias with variable coupling interval: the parasystole) present a variable coupling interval of the first complex (Figure 3.1.C and D, and page 77).

The coupling interval can be measured in the presence of isolated or repetitive runs of premature ectopic complexes, so that the coupling intervals of the first complex of each run can be compared. In sustained tachycardias the initial complexes are not usually seen and, if they were, they could not be compared with another episode in most cases. Nevertheless, the majority of the supraventricular and ventricular tachycardias are related

Clinical Arrhythmology, Second Edition. Antoni Bayés de Luna and Adrian Baranchuk.
© 2017 John Wiley & Sons Ltd. Published 2017 by John Wiley & Sons Ltd.

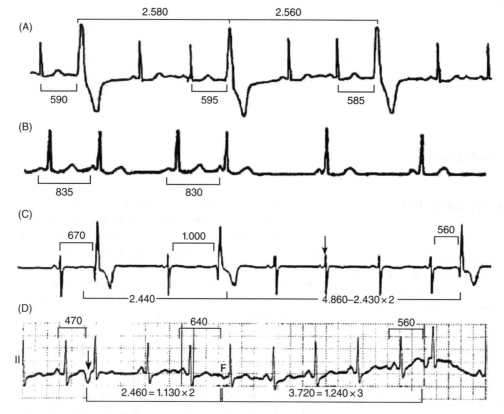

Figure 3.1 (A) Ventricular extrasystole; (B) atrial extrasystole; (C) ventricular parasystole; (D) atrial parasystole (see text). All numbers are expressed in ms.

Table 3.1 Arrhythmia mechanisms.

Active arrhythmias	B. Variable coupling interval
A. Fixed coupling interval	Parasystole
Abnormal generation of stimulus	*Passive arrhythmias*
• Increase of automaticity	Due to the depression of automaticity
• Triggered electrical activity	Due to a conduction disturbance
○ Premature post-potentials	• Block
○ Late post-potentials	• Aberrant conduction
Reentry	• Concealed conduction
• Classical: anatomic circuit	
• Functional:	TAP: transmembrane action potential.

Other less frequent mechanisms under column A:

Reentry
- Classical: anatomic circuit
- Functional:
  - ○ Circular movement:
    - ○ Leading circle
    - ○ Spiral wave (rotors)
  - ○ Different TAP duration and/or morphology in different myocardial areas, including the Phase 2 reentry: long and short QT syndromes and Brugada's syndrome

Other less frequent mechanisms
- Supernormal excitability and conduction
- Gap phenomenon
- Concealed conduction
- Wedensky effect

to the baseline rhythm, as the incidence of tachycardias of parasystolic origin, independent of the baseline rhythm, is very low. The mechanisms of supraventricular and ventricular tachyarrhythmias and heart rate are shown in Table 3.2. Each of these different mechanisms will now be looked at in more detail.

Abnormal Generation of Stimulus
Increase of Automaticity

Automaticity is the capacity of some cardiac cells (the automatic slow response cells present in the sinus node and to a lesser degree in the atrioventricular (AV) node)

Table 3.2 Mechanisms involved in the main supraventricular and ventricular tachyarrhythmias.

Arrhythmia	Main mechanism	Heart rate (bpm)
Sinus tachycardia	↑ Automaticity	>90
	Sinoatrial reentry	100–180
Monomorphic atrial tachycardia (Tables 4.4–4.6)	Focus origin (micro-reentry, ↑ Automaticity or triggered activity)	90–140 (incessant tachycardia) Till 200–220 (macroreentrant paroxysmal tachycardia)
	Macroreentry	If >220, it is considered an atypical flutter
Junctional ectopic tachycardia	Abnormal generation of stimuli	100–180
Junctional paroxysmal reentrant		
● Reentry only through AV junctional circuit	Reentry in circuit exclusively limited to the AV junction	140–200
● Reentry circuit with anomalous pathway involvement	Reentry in circuit involving also an anomalous pathway	(paroxysmal tachycardia, AVRT, associated to W–P–W)
Incessant tachycardia		Atrial ectopic focus junctional reentrant Generally <140 (incessant tachycardia)
Chaotic atrial tachycardia	Multiple atrial foci	100–200
Atrial fibrillation	Micro-reentry	400–700 (atrial waves)
	Automatic focus with fibrillatory conduction	
	Rotors with fibrillatory conduction	
Atrial flutter	Macroreentry	Generally, 240–300 with AV conduction mainly 2 × 1
Classic VT with structural heart disease	Reentry with anatomic or functional circuit (rotors)	From 110 to >200
VT/VF in channelopathies	In most of the cases (long and short QT, and Brugada's syndrome) due to differences in the duration and/or the morphology of TAP at different myocardial areas	From 140 to >200
Idioventricular rhythm	Increase of automaticity	60–100
VT with narrow QRS	Usually reentry (verapamil-sensitive)	120–160
Parasystolic VT	Protected automatic focus	Generally <140
Torsades de Pointes VT	Post-potentials and/or rotors	160–250
VT with no evident heart disease	Triggered activity, reentry or automaticity increase (Table 5.3)	110–200
Ventricular flutter	Macroreentry	250–350
Ventricular fibrillation	Micro-reentry with fibrillatory conduction	>400
	Automatic focus with fibrillatory conduction	
	Rotors with fibrillatory conduction	

AV, atrioventricular; TAP, transmembrane action potential; VF, ventricular fibrillation; VT, ventricular tachycardia, AVRT: atrio-ventricular reentrant tachycardia, W–P–W: Wolf–Parkinson–White syndrome.

to not only excite themselves but also to produce stimuli that can propagate (Figure 3.2). Therefore, automatic cells excite themselves and produce stimuli that may propagate, whereas contractile cells are only excited by a stimulus from a neighboring cell, transmitting it to the nearest cell (domino effect theory) (see Figure 2.17). Under normal conditions, contractile cells are not automatic cells because they do not excite themselves.

Certain electrophysiologic characteristics of the automatic cells derived from the ionic currents responsible for

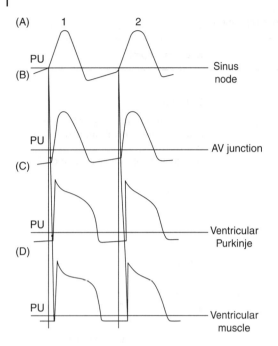

Figure 3.2 Sinus node transmembrane action potential (TAP) (A) transmitted to the atrioventricular (AV) junction (B), the ventricular Purkinje (C) and ventricular muscle (D).

the ascending slope of transmembrane diastolic potential (TDP) (Phase 4). In particular, the rapid inactivation during diastole of the outward K(Ip) current by the if has an impact on discharge rate (see Chapter 2, Transmembrane Diastolic Potential; Figures 2.13 and 2.16). The most important characteristics are (Figure 3.3):

○ The rate of rise of TDP (Phase 4): the faster the rise, the faster the discharge rate and vice versa (Figure 3.3A).
○ The level of threshold potential (TP): the lower (further from O), the faster the discharge rate and vice versa (Figure 3.3B)
○ The baseline level of the previous TDP: The more negative (further from 0), the lower the discharge rate and vice versa (Figure 3.3C).

The modifications of these three factors account, in general, for the increase or decrease of the heart automaticity (Figure 3.4). Under normal conditions, the sinus automaticity is transmitted to the AV node (see arrow in Figure 3.4B(1)) and then to the ventricle (see arrow in

Figure 3.4C(1)), immediately after which these two structures depolarize.

The top part of Figure 3.4 shows how the normal sinus automaticity (1 and 2) originates a transmembrane action potential (TAP) capable of propagating itself (B1 and C1). If for any of the reasons previously mentioned (Figure 3.3) (reduced rate of the TDP rise (b and b′), a lower baseline TDP level (c) or a TP level nearer 0 (d)), the normal sinus automaticity (a) decreases, the TAP curve will not form in due time (Figure 3.4A: continuous line (2) but later decreasing the sinus automaticity (A: broken line 2b). On the other hand, through an opposite mechanism the sinus automaticity will increase and the TAP generation will take less time. The increase of a Phase 4 slope of AV node or ventricle cells (B(h) and C(i)), or any of the other two mechanisms that increase the discharge rate of a cell (Figure 3.3B and C), explains the occurrence of active arrhythmias due to an increased automaticity. The effect of all these phenomena on the ECG becomes evident with the presence of heart rate variations under sinus rhythm and the presence of premature or late supraventricular and ventricular QRS complexes (see right side of Figure 3.4 and legend).

About 10% of paroxysmal supraventricular tachycardias, as well as some ventricular tachycardia and supraventricular and ventricular premature complexes (extrasystoles) with fixed or nearly fixed coupling intervals, are due to an increased automaticity. Recently (Haïssaguerre *et al.*, 2005), it has been proven that premature atrial impulses arising around the pulmonary veins trigger most of the paroxysmal atrial fibrillations, in the absence of significant heart disease. It has been shown (Morel and Meyronet, 2008) that the increased automaticity in pulmonary veins is due to the presence of the interstitial cells of Cajal, the main function of which, it was believed until now, was to control the motility of the digestive tract cells.

Triggered Electrical Activity

Another mechanism that can originate active arrhythmias with fixed or nearly fixed coupling intervals due to an abnormal generation of stimulus is the triggered electrical activity (Antoons *et al.*, 2007; Wit and Boyden, 2007). This is due to the presence of early or late postpotentials significant enough that their oscillatory

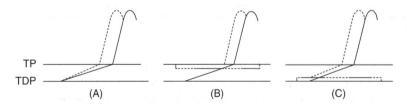

Figure 3.3 Factors influencing the increase of automaticity (broken lines). (A) Faster diastolic depolarization; (B) threshold potential (TP) decrease; (C) transmembrane diastolic potential (TDP) less negative than normal.

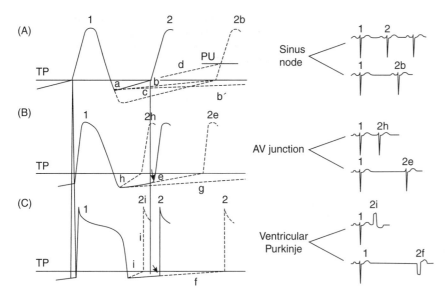

Figure 3.4 (A) Sinus node transmembrane action potential (TAP) curve; (B) atrioventricular (AV) junction TAP curve; (C) ventricular Purkinje TAP curve. It is observed how under normal conditions the stimulus is propagated from the sinus node to the AV junction and to the ventricular Purkinje system, before these structures reach the threshold potential (TP) by means of their own automaticity. Left: See the lines joining the TAPs of the sinus node, the AV junction and the ventricular Purkinje system. This figure shows the generation of active and passive arrhythmias due to disturbances of automaticity: (a) normal diastolic depolarization curve of the sinus node; (b) diminished diastolic depolarization curve; (b′) very diminished diastolic depolarization curve; (c) normal diastolic depolarization curve with a lower initial TDP; (d) normal diastolic depolarization curve with a less negative TP; (e) normal diastolic depolarization curve of the AV junction; note that before this curve is complete (i.e., before it reaches the TP), the sinus stimulus (arrow) initiates a new TAP (end of the continuous line in "e"); (f) normal diastolic depolarization curve of a ventricular Purkinje fiber (the same as in "e" applies); (g) marked decrease of the automaticity of the AV junction; (h) increase of automaticity of the AV junction; (i) increased automaticity in ventricular Purkinje fibers. Therefore, under pathologic conditions, the increased automaticity of the AV junction (h) and the ventricular Purkinje system (i) may be greater than that of the sinus node (active rhythms). Alternatively, the normal automaticity of the AV junction (broken lines in "e" and "g") or the ventricle (broken line in "f") may substitute the sinus depressed automaticity (b and b′) (passive rhythms). Right: Electrocardiographic examples of the different electrophysiologic situations commented (normal sinus rhythm: 1–2; sinus bradycardia: 1–2b; junctional extrasystole: 1–2h; junctional escape complex: 1–2e; ventricular extrasystole: 1–2i and ventricular escape complex: 1–2f).

vibrations initiate a response that may be propagated (Figure 3.5). Early post-potentials originate in the beginning of Phase 3 before repolarization has been completed (Figure 3.5A–C) and late post-potentials are explained by the presence of oscillatory diastolic depolarizations (Figure 3.5D and E). Some post-potentials originating at the end of Phase 3 have also been described (Zipes, 2003).

- **Early post-potentials** are related to polymorphic ventricular Torsades de Pointes type tachycardias (T de P–VT). However, rotors may also be involved in the generation of T de P-VT. Different agents and situations favor the triggering of early post-potentials (hypoxia, acidosis, drugs, ionic alterations, etc.), inhibiting the outward K^+ ionic currents or increasing the inward Na^+ Ca^{++} ionic current. The net Ca^{++} currents also play a certain role. All these mechanisms may result in a prolongation of the TAP and, consequently, the QT interval.
- **Late post-potentials** are generated in certain pathologic situations, for example, when due to dysfunction of the ryanodin receptor there is a Ca^{++} ion overload expelled from the sarcoplasmic reticulum during diastole. This Ca^{++} current can depolarize the cell and initiate a TAP when the TP is reached during the diastole (late post-potentials). Tachyarrhythmias of this origin are induced by catecholamines and exercise, and may be interrupted by adenosine and vagal maneuvers.

Reentry

Reentry is the mechanism that explains many active arrhythmias (the majority of premature complexes and tachyarrhythmias, including atrial and ventricular fibrillation). The classical concept of reentry (Moe and Méndez, 1966) involves an active wave front propagating around an anatomic circuit in such a way that the wave front loops back on itself (reentry). There are other types of reentry, which will be described later.

Classical Reentry
(Figures 3.6–3.10)

According to the concept described by Moe and Méndez (1966), for this phenomenon to occur three conditions

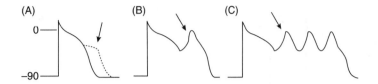

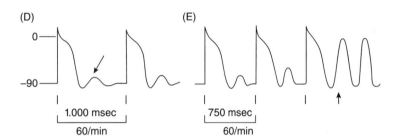

Figure 3.5 The presence of early (A–C) and late (D and E) post-potentials is the mechanism addressing the occurrence of early stimuli (complexes) due to triggered activity.

are necessary: **(i) the presence of a circuit, (ii) a unidirectional block** in part of the circuit, and **(iii) an appropriate conduction velocity** (Bayés de Luna 2011; Josephson 2008; Zipes-Jalife 2004; Recommended General Bibliography p. xvii).

i) **The presence of an anatomic circuit** through which the stimulus may circulate (reentry). Regardless of the reentrant circuit, for this phenomenon to occur and perpetuate there must be a unidirectional block together with an adequate conduction velocity somewhere in the circuit. The reentrant circuit may:

- **Be initiated in a small area** (micro-reentry) of the Purkinje network or the Purkinje–muscular junction, both in the atrial or ventricular muscle (Figure 3.6A(a,b)). As discussed (see Chapter 2, Purkinje Cells), it has been postulated that just three Purkinje cells (Y-shaped) may constitute a microcircuit. This mechanism explains the majority of the premature atrial and ventricular complexes. Traditionally, it was also believed that most cases of atrial fibrillations (AF) were caused by multiple micro-reentries. Recently, it has been proven that the "rotor theory" (Jalife *et al.*, 2000) and the increase of automaticity, especially at the pulmonary vein level (Haïssaguerre *et al.*, 1998) (see previously), may account for many cases of AF, in particular paroxysmal AF in healthy individuals (Figure 3.14).

- **Be located in more extensive areas** of the ventricle (i.e., an area surrounding a post-infarction scar) or through the specific intraventricular conduction system (branch–branch reentry) (Figure 3.6B(1 and 2)) (see Chapter 5, Ventricular Tachycardias).

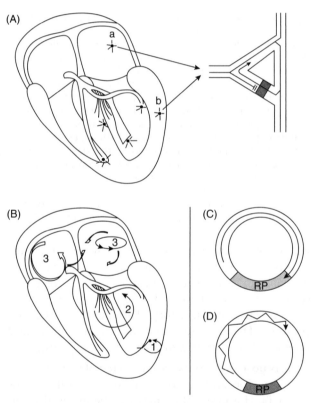

Figure 3.6 Examples of circuits involved in classical reentrant atrial and ventricular arrhythmias. (A) The circuit is usually located in the Purkinje–atrial muscle junction (a) or Purkinje–ventricular muscle junction (b) (micro-reentry). (B) It may also be located in a necrotic area of the ventricle (1) or in a circuit involving the left specific intraventricular system (2), or in the atria (3) (flutter or macro-reentrant tachycardia) (see Figure 3.7). (C) and (D) Perpetuation of a reentry depends on the refractory period (RP) duration and the conduction velocity (CV). If the RP is long and the CV is fast, reentry is not perpetuated (C), whereas it is perpetuated if the RP is short and the CV slow.

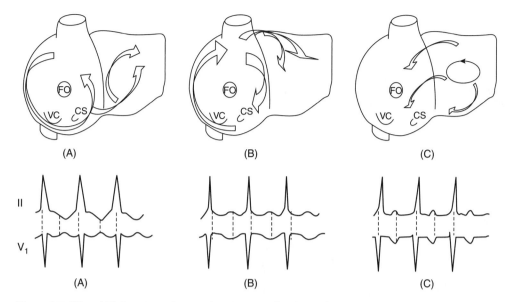

Figure 3.7 (A) and (B) Circuits explaining the presence of common flutter with counter clockwise rotation and noncommon (reverse) flutter with clockwise rotation. (C) Possible macro-reentrant circuit in the case of an atypical flutter, as well as macro-reentrant atrial tachycardia.

- **Be macrocircuits** localized preferably in the right atrium causing typical or common flutter (counterclockwise rotation) and reverse flutter (clockwise rotation) (Figure 3.7A and B). The atypical flutter and the macro-reentrant atrial tachycardia usually originate in the left atrium and, less frequently, in the right atrium (Figure 3.7C). We use the term atrial tachycardia if the heart rate is <200–220 bpm and atypical flutter if the heart rate is >220 bpm. In fact, both arrhythmias are the same and are only differentiated by the atrial rate (see Chapter 4, Flutter F Waves).
- **Involve the AV junction.** Here there are two types of circuits:
  (a) **A circuit comprising the AV junction exclusively** (Figure 3.8A). It was previously believed that this circuit was functional and located within the AV node (intranodal). It was presumed that the AV node had a longitudinal dissociation, with a slow conduction tract (α) and fast conduction tract (β) (Figure 3.8A). Now it is known (Wu and Yeh, 1994; Katritsis and Becker, 2007) that these circuits have an anatomic basis in which tissue of the lower atrium is also involved (AV junction) (Figure 2.6). This results in several possible circuits accounting for the different types of reentrant tachycardias with exclusive involvement of the AV junction structures.

  o **Slow-fast type**. Tachycardias originating in this type of circuit are reentrant (reciprocating) paroxysmal tachycardias and constitute approximately 50% of paroxysmal tachycardias involving the AV junction (paroxysmal junctional reentrant tachycardia exclusively, P-AVNRT, or paroxysmal tachycardias originated in a circuit involving an accessory pathway, P-AVRT). In a few cases the tachycardia is due to the abnormal generation of stimuli.

  In the case of a P-AVNRT, a premature stimulus (atrial premature impulse) is blocked in the fast pathway (β) still in the absolute refractory period (ARP). It may go through the α pathway with a shorter refractory period, albeit with a lower conduction velocity. As a result, this stimulus is conducted to the ventricles (1 in Figure 3.9A) with a longer P'R than the baseline PR interval. At some point as the fast pathway (β) is out of the refractory period, the premature stimulus retrogradely invades this pathway and rapidly reaches the atrium (P'), while at the same time entering again into the slow pathway (α), and is conducted to the ventricles to generate the QRS-2 complex (2 in Figure 3.9A). Conduction to the atrium is very fast, and the ectopic P' is concealed in

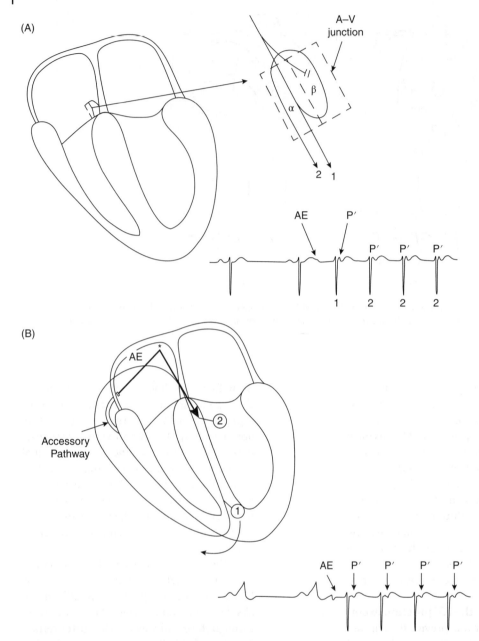

(A)

A–V junction

β

α

2 1

AE   P′

P′ P′ P′

1 2 2 2

(B)

AE

Accessory
Pathway

②

①

AE P′ P′ P′ P′

Figure 3.8 (A) Example of reentrant arrhythmias with circuit involving the AV junction (A) exclusively, or also involving an accessory pathway (B). In the first case (A), the premature atrial extrasystole (AE), which does not undergo anterograde conduction on the β pathway is conducted through the α pathway. Then, it facilitates a reentry through the β pathway, with fast atrial retrograde activation (P′), which may be concealed within or at the end of the QRS complex (it may mimic an r′ or S wave). In the second case (B), the circuit has the following composition: His–Purkinje system – ventricular muscle – accessory pathway – atrial muscle – His–Purkinje system. An atrial extrasystole (AE) is blocked in the accessory pathway that presents a unidirectional block, thus being conducted through the normal pathway. Consequently, the resulting complex (1) does not present a δ wave. This impulse reenters retrogradely over the accessory pathway activates the atria, and initiates a reentrant tachycardia with narrow QRS complexes (2) (without δ wave). In this case, due to longer conduction over the accessory pathway, the P′ is recorded close but at a short distance from the QRS (RP′ < P′R).

the QRS complex or stuck at the end of it, simulating an "S" or "r" wave.

In summary, in slow-fast tachycardia (Typical AVNRT) in which the circuit is exclusively in the AV junction (Figures 3.8A and 3.9A), a slow and anterograde conduction follows the α pathway, whereas a fast and retrograde conduction takes place on the β pathway.

o **Fast-slow type**. This tachycardia is much less frequent in adults. The episodes are incessant and nonparoxysmal (Coumel *et al.*,

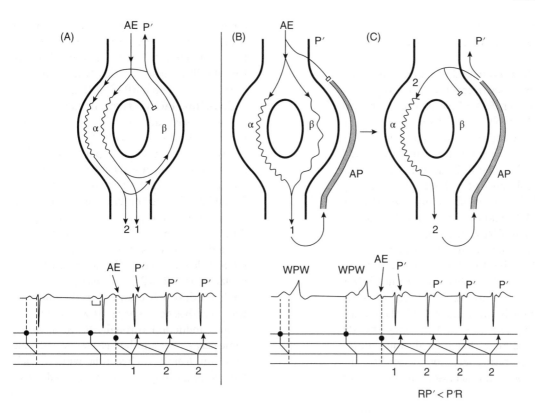

Figure 3.9 Example of slow-fast tachycardia with exclusive involvement of the AV junction (A) (AVNRT), or with the involvement of an accessory pathway (AP) (AVRT) in the circuit (B). (C) shows now the reentry is completed (2). In both cases, the tachycardia circuit, the Lewis diagram, and an example of the onset of tachycardia with an atrial extrasystole (AE) are shown.

1974). It was thought to imply an inverted AV junctional circuit, with a stimulus going down through the fast pathway (β) and slowly up through the slow pathway (α). Currently, it is known that this type of tachycardia use a circuit in which an anomalous bundle takes part (see later and Chapter 4, Junctional Reentrant Tachycardia: Mechanism). The stimulus is anterogradely conducted through the (β) pathway and is retrogradely conducted through an anomalous pathway (AP) with long conduction times (Figure 3.10).

o Special cases of paroxysmal junctional reentrant tachycardia with a circuit involving the AV junction only (AVNRT) (see p. 105) that have pathways with similar anterograde and retrograde conduction velocities behaving as intermediate pathways (fast-fast tachycardias or slow-slow tachycardias). Occasionally, more than one type of tachycardia is seen in the same patient (Wu and Yeh, 1994). Slow-slow tachycardias are usually found after ablation, as a consequence of characteristic modifications of some "fast fibers" that have turned into "slow fibers". The determination of these slow-slow circuits must be done with

electrophysiologic studies (Yamabe *et al.*, 2007).

(b) **A reentrant circuit with the involvement of the AV junction and an accessory pathway** (macro-reentry) (Figure 3.8B). Conduction through an accessory pathway in sinus rhythm accounts for early ventricular activation (short PR + δ wave) of Wolff–Parkinson–White type pre-excitation (see Chapter 8). The presence of an accessory pathway allows a macrocircuit to be configured (specific conduction system (SCS) + accessory pathway) (Figures 3.8B, 3.9B and 3.10); this is the reason why reentrant arrhythmias can originate when a unidirectional block is present somewhere along the circuit and an adequate conduction velocity exists. In this situation two types of tachycardias may be observed:

o **Tachycardias with retrograde conduction over the accessory pathway** (AVRT-AP). In this case the QRS is narrow. There can also be a slow-fast tachycardia and a fast-slow tachycardia, as in the case of reentrant tachycardia with a circuit that exclusively involves the AV junction. However as we have already commented (p. 59) the current mechanism that explains all cases of fast-slow tachycardia is probably one that involves an accessory pathway.

Slow-fast type tachycardia. These are paroxysmal tachycardias and represent approximately 50% of paroxysmal tachycardias with involvement of the AV junction. The onset of this tachycardia usually occurs with an atrial premature impulse (atrial extrasystole). The P′R interval of this atrial extrasystole present in both cases is a long interval, but is usually longer in AVNRT (Figure 3.9A and B). This occurs because in paroxysmal AVNRT the atrial extrasystole is conducted only by the α pathway as it is blocked in the β pathway used as a retrograde arm of the tachycardia (Figure 3.9A). In the case of paroxysmal AVRT, the atrial extrasystole is not completely blocked in the β pathway and this explains why the PR interval is not lengthened too much. Elsewhere, retrograde conduction to the atrial through the accessory pathway lasts

longer than in the reciprocating (reentrant) tachycardia with exclusive involvement of the AV junction (AVNRT) and, for this reason, the P′ is close but clearly located after the QRS, but with a RP′<P′R (Figure 3.9B).

Fast-slow tachycardia. In these infrequent cases in adults (<5%), the tachycardia is incessant (incessant AVRT) (Coumel *et al.*, 1974). The circuit is made up usually of a fast arm through the normal SCS (β pathway) and a slow arm that was first thought to be formed by slow retrograde conduction over the α pathway but now it is known (Figure 3.10) (see Chapter 4, and before) to be formed by an accessory pathway with slow retrograde conduction (Figure 3.10 B). This explains the P′R<RP′ relationship.

○ **Tachycardias with anterograde conduction over one accessory pathway** and retrograde conduction through the SCS, or, in some cases, over another accessory pathway. This antidromic tachycardia with a *wide QRS* complex may use, as an antegrade arm,

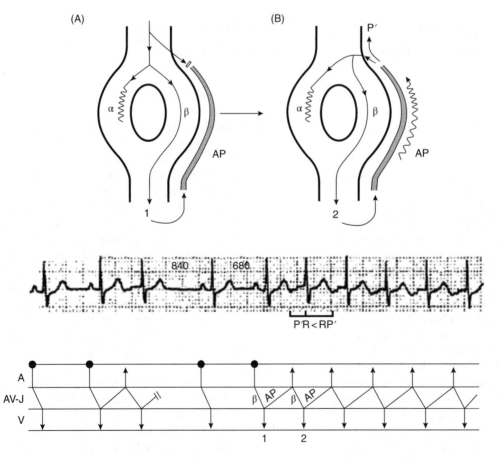

Figure 3.10 Top: the mechanism of fast-slow tachycardia – (A) onset reentrant tachycardia (ß), (B) retrograde conduction through accessory pathway (AP). Middle and bottom: onset and end of an episode. β: β pathway, AP: accessory pathway.

an accessory pathway-type Kent bundle (see Figure 5.26). In the case of atypical pre-excitation, the antegrade arm is usually a right atriofascicular bundle (see Figure 4.22, and Chapter 4, Paroxysmal Junctional Re-entrant Tachycardia: The ECG During the Tachycardia). These tachycardias should be distinguished from ventricular tachycardia (VT) and supraventricular tachycardia (SVT) with bundle branch block aberrancy (see Chapter 5, Differential Diagnosis of Wide QRS Complex Tachycardias).

ii) **A zone of the circuit has a unidirectional block**. In this situation, the stimulus may be conducted in one direction only (see || in Figures 3.6, 3.9, and 3.10).

iii) **The conduction velocity through the circuit is adequate**. Conduction of a stimulus through a circuit depends on the circuit length, conduction velocity, and the refractory period originated by the stimulus. It should be noted that wave length is equal to the refractory period by the conduction velocity (Figure 3.6C and D). The conduction velocity must be slow to improve the probability that all segments of the circuit are out of the refractory period when the reentrant stimulus reaches them (Figure 3.6D). If the conduction velocity is very high, and especially if the refractory period is relatively long, the stimulus cannot pass through the zone (Figure 3.6C). On the other hand, if the conduction velocity is too slow, the next sinus stimulus would enter the circuit and prevent reentry from occurring.

Regarding surface ECG, there are two principal forms of AV junctional reentrant tachycardias (JRT) with narrow QRS:

- Slow-fast type. These are paroxysmal AV junctional reentrant tachycardias, either without (AVNRT) (Figure 3.8A) or with accessory pathway involvement (AVRT) (Figure 3.8B). If the circuit exclusively involves the AV junction (Figure 3.9A), the P′ is masked at the end of QRS or hidden within the QRS complex. If an accessory pathway is involved in the circuit (AVRT), the P′ is separated from the QRS but with RP′<P′R (Figure 3.9B).
- Fast-slow type. These rare tachycardias are incessant and it has been demonstrated that the retrograde arm of the circuit is an anomalous pathway (Figure 3.10).

Other Types of Reentry

There are other types of reentry with a functional, rather than anatomic, basis. Some are related to a circular movement like: (i) Allesie's leading circle reentry (Allesie

et al., 1977) (Figure 3.11B); (ii) reentry by double spiral wave (El-Sherif *et al.*, 1997) or from a single spiral wave (rotors) (Jalife *et al.*, 2000; Vaquero *et al.*, 2008) (Figure 3.13C and D); (iii) reentries related to the dispersion of repolarization between two areas of the myocardium (Phase 2 reentry) – these two areas may lie between different layers of the left ventricle (intramural dispersion) (Yan and Anzelevitch, 1998) (Figure 3.11E) (TAP longer in the endocardium/M cells than in the epicardium) or between different areas of myocardium (transregional dispersion) (Noble, 1979; Opthof *et al.*, 2007) (see Chapter 2, From Cellular Electrogram to Human ECG). Other types of reentry include anisotropic reentry, reflection reentry, and so on (see Recommended General Bibliography p. xvii). The following are the most frequently reported types of functional reentry:

- **Leading circle reentry** (Figure 3.11B): this concept, coined by Allesie *et al.*, (1977), is characterized by the fact that the tissue around which the stimulus travels is constantly bombarded by the excitation wave, and therefore is only partially excitable. This model, compared with the classical reentry model, is characterized by: (i) the conduction velocity (CV) and the refractory period (RP) being more important than the anatomic obstacle itself, (ii) the impulse partially penetrating the circuit, and (iii) the head of the excitation wave being very close to the refractory tail, making the excitable zone very narrow and often incomplete.
- **Reentry by spiral wave (rotors)**: a "rotor" is a source of energy that manifests itself as a rotatory excitatory wave (spiral wave), which, when encountering and interacting with an unexcitable obstacle (scar, hole) or with the surrounding tissue with heterogeneous electrophysiologic properties, may be split into two spiral waves (Figure 3.11C). Each spiral wave is fixed to a point called a "singular point", around which they start rotating (reenter) in a way that resembles whirlpools (figure-of-eight reentry) (Figure 3.11C) (El-Sherif *et al.*, 1997).
  - **A reentry may also originate from the rotation of only one spiral wave** with an activation front bending towards the center (core) of rotation (singular point) (Jalife *et al.*, 2000; Vaquero *et al.*, 2008). This generates a voltage gradient between the activation front and the cells in the center of rotation, which facilitates a stable rotational movement of the rotor, perpetuating the reentry (Figure 3.11D). The tissue near the singular point (center of rotation) may have a very fast wave length (refractory period × conduction velocity), which results in a 1 × 1 conduction. This is explained because in this area the TAP has shortened to a large extent, chiefly because of

an increased functioning of K⁺ currents. The hyperfunction of the IK currents shortens the TAP sufficiently enough to maintain a high-frequency rotor. Nevertheless, away from the singular point, the TAP is not very short (Figure 3.11D) and the myocardial tissue cannot conduct at the velocity of the rotor. This results in a nonuniform conduction, which is different from the 1 × 1 conduction. This

may lead to the spiral wave break-up and fibrillatory conduction starts (Figure 3.12 and 3.13D).

o Qu and Gurfinkel (2004) have suggested a **classification system for ventricular arrhythmias based on the different types of dynamic activity of a spiral wave**. It is generally accepted that the stable and linear rotation movement of a spiral wave could explain the generation of a sustained VT (Figure 3.13A). It

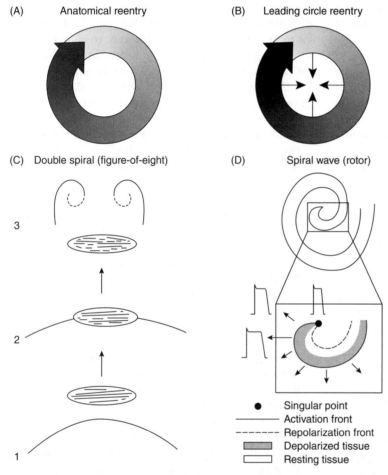

Figure 3.11 (A) Classical reentry (anatomical obstacle) (Figure 3.6). (B) Allesie's model – leading circle – (functional obstacle). In the classical circuit the tip of the activation wave is far away from the refractory tail (A), whereas in Allesie's model it is very close to the refractory tail (B). This justifies how in (B) the excitability zone is narrow (and, in most cases, incomplete). In A, the presence of an anatomic obstacle prevents the activation wave entering the circuit, whereas in B the wave can penetrate the circuit, at least partially. (C) Double spiral (rotors): figure-of-eight model: (1) an activation front approaches an obstacle (either anatomic or functional) in its refractory period, reaches it (2), and under the appropriate conditions it splits into two fixed fronts resembling a figure-of-eight (continuous line: activation front; broken line: circular movement of singular points) (3). (D) Single spiral wave (rotor) theory. The activation front of the rotor (continuous black line) adopts a spiral shape and its curvature bends towards the rotation center. A voltage gradient (VG) exists between the rotation center (singular point), which is in passive status (short TAP), and the neighboring areas (activation front), which are active and show a longer TAP. The depolarized area

(gray) and the resting area (white) are shown. The TAP is shortened as it approaches the singular point due to the hyperfunction of K currents. Although the TAP shortening is necessary to establish a high-frequency rotor, if it becomes too short the areas more distal to the singular point (with a longer TAP) cannot conduct at the speed of the rotor, with a high discharge rate. This may lead to the disruption of the spiral wave and may initiate fibrillatory conduction. (E) Example of Phase 2 reentry due to heterogeneous dispersion of repolarization (HDR). According to Antzelevitch, dispersion takes place at a transmural level and the TAP of M cells is the longest compared with the TAP of the rest of the wall areas. This HDR originates a ventricular gradient (VG) between the areas with longer TAP and the area with shortest TAP (epicardium) and accounts for the possible occurrence of VT/VF in patients with long QT syndrome (2) and short QT syndrome (3). In Brugada's syndrome (4), the HDR takes places between the endocardium and the epicardium of the RV at the beginning of Phase 2 (VG), because of the transient predominance of outward Ito current. Epi: Epicardium; M: M cells (see Chapter 9).

(E)
Reentry due to hetereogenous dispersion of repolarization (phase 2)*
1
2
3
4
M
Epi
GV
M
Epi
GV
M
Epi
GV
Endo
Epi
Normal
Long QT
Short QT
Brugada's syndrome
*According to Antzelevitch at transmural level

Figure 3.11 (*Continued*)

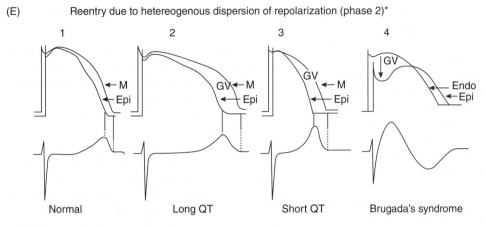

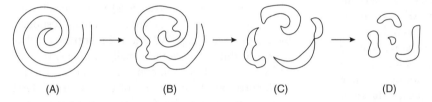

(A)
(B)
(C)
(D)

Figure 3.12 Here we see how a spiral wave (rotor) (A) (Figure 3.11) is disrupted and turned into a meandering (B) and, later, increasingly chaotic conduction until it completely breaks up, resulting in a fibrillatory conduction (C and D).

has also been postulated based on considerable evidence that changes in the rotation characteristics of this spiral wave tip (i.e., a meandering rotation) would account for the T de P-VT (petal meandering rotation) (Figure 3.13B) and polymorphic VT (anarchic meandering rotation) (Figure 3.13C). Experimental studies have demonstrated that a system displaying different kinds of oscillation is unstable. An unstable system tends to be chaotic, and this leads the spiral wave to break up (Figures 3.12 and 3.13D). From an

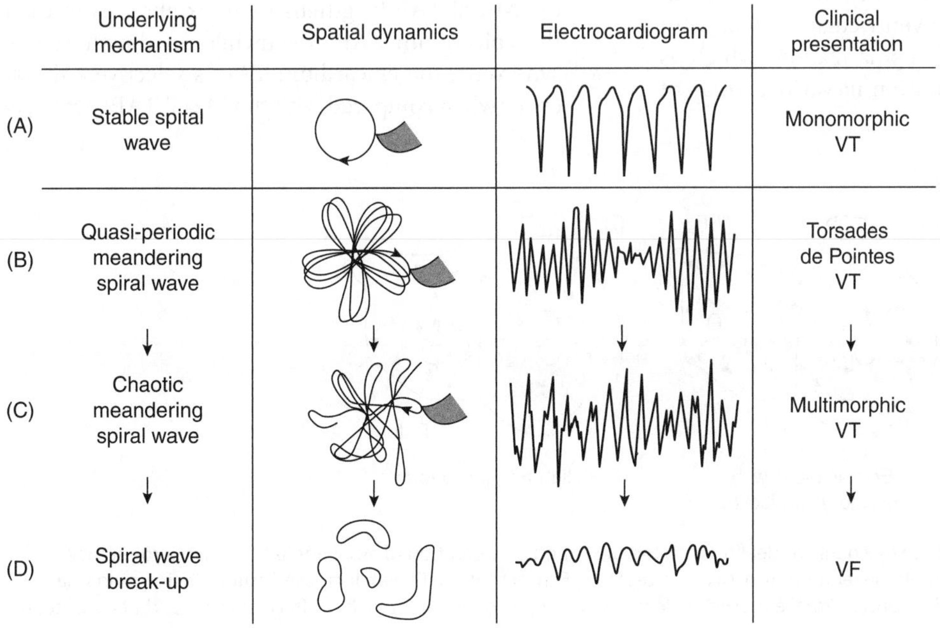

Underlying mechanism
Spatial dynamics
Electrocardiogram
Clinical presentation
(A)
Stable spital wave
Monomorphic VT
(B)
Quasi-periodic meandering spiral wave
Torsades de Pointes VT
(C)
Chaotic meandering spiral wave
Multimorphic VT
(D)
Spiral wave break-up
VF

Figure 3.13 Different spiral wave (rotor) modalities, with their ECG phenotypic expression and clinical presentation (adapted from Qu and Gurfinkel, 2004) (see text).

arrhythmological point of view, the transition to chaotic activation waves constitutes a triggering mechanism for ventricular fibrillation (VF). This is an appealing explanation, because it includes, in a sequential manner, the generation of the different types of ventricular tachycardias and VF. Nevertheless, it should also be borne in mind the classical mechanism that develops and perpetuates the VF, repetitive micro-reentry, which generally originates from a premature ventricular complex falling in the vulnerable ventricular period (see Chapter 5, Ventricular Fibrillation).

o **Atrial fibrillation** (AF) may also be initiated and perpetuated by a **"rotor" mechanism** (Figure 3.14C). The initiating mechanism of this type of AF is a premature atrial impulse initiated by a high frequency rotor that converts itself into fibrillatory conduction (as previously described). A **second mechanism** that could explain the AF is an **automatic focus**, usually located in the surrounding area of the pulmonary veins, which also has fibrillatory conduction (Haïssaguerre *et al.*, 1998) (Figure 3.14B). However, as in VF, there is a lot of evidence supporting the theory that in many cases **classical multiple micro-reentries** may be responsible for initiating and maintaining atrial fibrillation, especially in patients with heart disease (Figure 3.14A).

The most significant similarities and differences between the mechanisms that initiate and maintain AF and VF are discussed later (see Chapter 5, Ventricular Fibrillation: Mechanism and Figure 5.45).

• **Heterogeneous dispersion of repolarization** (Figure 3.11E): this section includes: (i) transmural dispersion of repolarization (TDR), shown by different TAP durations in various areas of the ventricular wall, and (ii) transregional dispersion of repolarization, which is caused by different TAP duration in various areas of the heart (i.e., baseapex). Different aspects related to these facts are discussed here.

o We have already commented (see Chapter 2, From Cellular Electrogram to Human ECG) that in the human heart there is a dispersion of repolarization. Considerable evidence shows that the epicardium is the first area to repolarize, whereas the endocardium is the last area to repolarize (Burgess *et al.*, 1972; Franz *et al.*, 1987). Nevertheless, we have also said (see before and Chapter 2, From Cellular Electrogram to Human ECG) that some authors have demonstrated, in isolated wedge preparations (Yan and Anzelevitch, 1998), that the middle layer of the ventricle – M cells zone (see Figure 2.24) – is repolarized even later than the endocardium. These repolarization differences between the three layers of the left ventricle (endocardium, epicardium, and middle – zone of the so-called M cells) are responsible for the TDR. This explains the voltage gradient responsible for the triggering TAP Phase 2 reentrant mechanism leading to some malignant ventricular arrhythmias. It has been confirmed that the T wave peak corresponds to the end of the epicardial TAP, whereas the end of the T wave corresponds to the end of M' cell TAP. The Antzelevitch group (Yan and Anzelevitch, 1998) considers **the T peak–T end interval to be an index of the transmural dispersion of repolarization (TDR)**. Several studies have documented that an increase in the T peak–T end distance constitutes a marker of possible ventricular arrhythmias in channelopathies (Gussak-Antzelevitch, 2008). According to these authors, in the long QT syndrome the TDR is produced because the M cell TAP lengthens to an extent greater than the epicardium TAP. Meanwhile, in the short QT syndrome, the epicardium TAP is selectively shortened (when compared with the M cell TAP), whereas

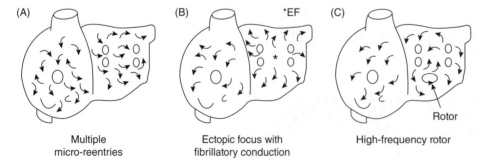

Figure 3.14 This figure shows the three mechanisms dealing with the onset and perpetuation of atrial fibrillation. (A) Micro-reentry located in an ectopic focus induces multiple reentries (classical concept). (B) Ectopic focus (EF) with increased automaticity (pulmonary veins) (asterisk) and fibrillatory conduction. (C) Atrial extrasystole located in ectopic focus initiates a high-frequency rotor that perpetuates the arrhythmia with fibrillatory conduction.

in Brugada's syndrome a selective shortening of the epicardial TAP of the right ventricle is observed (Figure 3.11E-GV). TDR may also contribute to the triggering of the catecholaminergic VT (Chapter 9).

o Although it is accepted that the increase in the T peak–T end interval is a marker of arrhythmogenesis, not all investigators agree on the mechanisms involved. In a study performed in an intact heart, the M cell zone did not present the longest lasting TAP (Voss *et al.*, 2009). Instead, the same authors have demonstrated, in anesthetized dogs (Opthof *et al.*, 2007), that the T wave peak does not coincide with the end of left ventricle epicardial repolarization, but rather with the earliest ventricular repolarization area. Similarly, the T wave end does not correspond to the end of the endocardium/middle layer of the ventricular wall (M cell) repolarization, but to the end of the global ventricular repolarization.

Consequently, many authors believe **that the T peak–T end interval** constitutes an indicator of the total dispersion of the ventricular repolarization, rather than the transmural dispersion of the repolarization. Regardless of this, **it is believed to have a greater prognostic value than the QTc and the QT dispersion with regard to the occurrence of T de P-VT in patients with long QT syndrome**

(Takenaka *et al.*, 2003; Watanabe *et al.*, 2004; Yamaguchi *et al.*, 2003).

o It has been suggested that **in Brugada's syndrome the triggering of VT**, which subsequently degenerates into VF, may be **due to significant transregional and not transmural dispersion**. These differences are supported by a marked conduction delay and by some kinetic repolarization alterations in different zones of the right ventricle (Lambiasse *et al.*, 2009) (see Chapter 9).

o Therefore, it seems evident that a repolarization dispersion between two myocardial zones, either transmural (Franz *et al.*, 1987; Yan and Anzelevitch, 1998) or transregional (Noble, 1979; Opthof *et al.*, 2007; Lambiasse *et al.*, 2009) exists. This dispersion, which according to several authors occurs between the epicardium and endocardium, is very useful to explain the origin of the normal ECG (see Chapter 2, From Cellular Electrogram to Human ECG).

o **In heart diseases other than channelopathies, it is necessary to validate whether the T peak–T end interval is equivalent to the repolarization dispersion** between different myocardial zones, as well as compare its prognostic value with the conventional parameters used in the clinical evaluation of repolarization (e.g., QTc interval and the QT dispersion).

- The most frequent mechanism associated with active arrhythmias with fixed coupling intervals, whether isolated – premature impulses – or repetitive – tachyarrhythmias – is reentry in different variations: classical reentry, due to a movement around an anatomic obstacle, functional reentry, due to a circular movement without an anatomic obstacle (leading circle and spiral wave "rotors"), reentry due to a heterogeneous increase in the TAP dispersion, whether intramural or in other parts of the myocardium, and so forth (Table 3.1).
- The increase of the T peak–T end interval as a result of the heterogeneous dispersion of repolarization, regardless of the zones at which it takes place (Figure 3.11E), may be considered a marker of arrhythmogenesis, at least in some channelopathies.

- Active arrhythmias are also explained by an abnormal generation of impulses, including the triggered electrical activity and pure increase of automaticity.
- Thus, we should remember the old Chinese proverb: "Black cat or white cat? Doesn't matter: what is important is that it can catch mice."
- Frequently, some type of reentry and an abnormal generation of impulses interact. The triggered electrical activity or increase in automaticity being the initiating mechanisms of the arrhythmia, and some type of reentry the mechanism sustaining the arrhythmia.

Other Mechanisms
Unexpected Conduction

- **Supernormal excitability and conduction**. In some circumstances, premature stimuli are blocked even when earlier stimuli are conducted. This interesting phenomenon, classically know as supernormal conduction, is believed to occur when the earliest stimulus is conducted because it falls in the supernormal excitability phase (Childers, 1984). In fact, it does not represent a faster than normal conduction, but rather the unexpected conduction of a stimulus, which can only

reach the TP if it falls in the supernormal excitability phase. The supernormal conduction probably only exists in the His–Purkinje system. Through this mechanism, a subthreshold stimulus falling in the supernormal excitability phase of the ventricular Purkinje can initiate a premature impulse (premature ventricular complex) (Figure 3.15A, arrow).

The clearest evidence of supernormal conduction in clinical electrocardiography is probably the disappearance of the right bundle branch block morphology in earlier QRS complexes, for example, in atrial

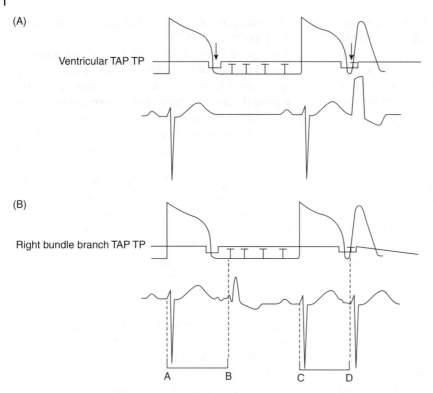

(A)

Ventricular TAP TP

(B)

Right bundle branch TAP TP

A   B   C   D

Figure 3.15 Apart from the reentrant mechanisms, there are other mechanisms accounting for the existence of early stimuli triggered by a preceding stimulus (extrasystole). In this figure it may be observed how the subthreshold stimuli (T) originated in an ectopic focus may generate a transmembrane action potential (TAP) and turn into a premature complex (supernormal conduction) only when they fall into the supernormal phase of ventricular excitability (arrow) (A). On the other hand, an atrial extrasystole (which is usually conducted with a right bundle branch block morphology) may be normally conducted when it occurs earlier, when the right bundle branch is in a supernormal phase of excitability (AB>CD, in part B of the figure).

premature complexes with a shorter RR interval (Figure 3.15B).

Some other explanations justifying this apparently supernormal conduction of a stimulus are now examined.

o **Gap phenomenon** (Figure 3.16). Electrophysiologic studies have shown, in many cases, the conduction of a premature impulse through the AV junction, when other less premature stimulus is blocked, is due to the fact that the earlier stimulus (A2 in C) causes a greater delay in a proximal zone (A2 H2) than the less premature stimulus (A2 in B), which has not been distally conducted. This results in the unexpected conduction of the earliest stimulus (A2 in C) through the more distal zone that is already out of its refractory period when the earlier stimulus (A2 in C) reaches this zone with a delay (Gallagher *et al.*, 1973). In this case, conduction of the earliest stimulus is due to the proximal delay, whereas in supernormal conduction it is independent of the delay while being associated with the supernormal excitability. This is known as a "gap" phenomenon.

o **Concealed conduction**. It has been suggested that the unexpected narrow QRS complex, following a short RR in a patient with AF who presents some wide QRS complexes with longer RR intervals (compare complexes 3 and 6 in Figure 4.51), is due to a supernormal conduction in the blocked branch. However, it is more likely (see Concealed conduction) to be caused by a concealed conduction of "f" waves in both bundle branches, which facilitate the switch from a long-short cycle (originating a wide QRS complex due to aberrant conduction) to a short-short cycle, thus explaining the presence of a narrow QRS (see complex 3 in Figure 4.51 and see Chapter 4, Differential Diagnosis Between Aberrancy and Ectopy in Wide QRS Complexes).

o **The Wedensky phenomena**. It is worth commenting that more than 100 years ago, Wedensky described three phenomena (effect, facilitation, and inhibition) related to changes in cell excitability (nerve cells) secondary to previous stimulation (Bayés de Luna, 1978, see Recommended General Bibliography p. xvii).

The Wedensky effect, described in the heart by Castellanos more than 50 years ago (Castellanos *et al.*, 1966), consists of a subthreshold stimulus with the potential to produce an efficient response if preceded by a strong stimulus. This would explain the presence of some premature ectopic complexes with a long and fixed coupling interval, which cannot be adequately explained by reentry.

Active Arrhythmias with Variable CouplingInterval: the Parasystole

There are premature impulses not related to the basic rhythm, which therefore have a variable coupling interval

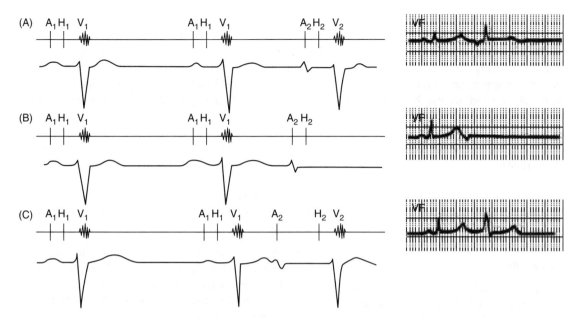

Figure 3.16 Left: (A), (B), and (C): Diagrams showing the gap phenomenon. (A): The extrastimulus A_2 is normally conducted. (B): The extrastimulus A_2 is not conducted to the ventricles, and it is blocked in the area below the His fascicle (normal A_2-H_2 conduction). (C): If the extrastimulus A_2 occurs earlier, it may be conducted with some delay through the atrioventricular (AV) node (long A_2-H_2), getting to the His fascicle later than in the previous case (B), and therefore being possibly conducted through the His–Purkinje system. Right: Three examples of VF lead, in the same patient featuring different atrial impulses with variable coupling intervals (increasingly premature from top to bottom (0.50, 0.40, and 0.32)) and different impulse conduction. (A): The atrial extrasystole is normally conducted. (B): The atrial extrasystole is not conducted. (C): The atrial extrasystole is conducted with aberrancy. If no His bundle electrogram recording is performed, there are no objective data supporting whether a phenomenon like this is a gap phenomenon or explained by supernormal conduction.

(Figure 3.1B). This is caused by an ectopic focus that is prevented from being depolarized by the impulses from the basic rhythm, usually because of a unidirectional entrance block (Figure 3.17). However, when the surrounding tissue is out of the refractory period, the ectopic stimuli originated in this so-called parasystolic focus may come out, resulting in variable premature complexes (independent of the basal rhythm–parasystolic complexes).

From an electrocardiographic point of view, the parasystolic complex not only has a variable coupling interval but also interectopic intervals that are multiples of each other, although there are some exceptions (see Chapter 5, Extrasystole Compared to Parasystole), giving rise to fusion complexes if the sinus and parasystolic complexes occur simultaneously (see Chapter 5, Premature Ventricular Complexes: Concept, Premature Ventricular Complexes: Mechanisms, and Figure 5.2). If there is an exit block of the impulse from the focus, the parasystolic rhythm will be blocked totally or partially, although it may still keep its intrinsic rate (see Figure 5.35) (Koulizakis *et al.*, 1990). This can be confirmed if the exit block disappears and it makes visible the real rate of arrhythmia.

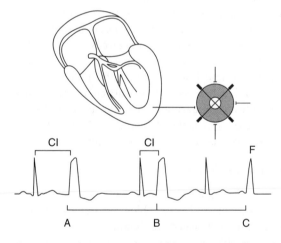

Figure 3.17 The parasystolic mechanism is generally explained by an entry block in the ectopic focus. The central point represents the parasystolic focus, surrounded by an area with an entry block (shaded area). Parasystolic stimuli may be conducted out of this zone but external stimuli cannot get into it. Usually, some degree of exit block also exists (see Figure 5.35). Bottom: Scheme of parasystolic ventricular premature complexes with the characteristic three electrocardiographic features: variable coupling interval (CI), multiple interectopic intervals, and fusion complexes (F) (see Figure 5.2).

Tachycardias initiated by an increase in parasystolic automaticity are infrequent, their discharge rate is not very high and they usually occur in runs (see Chapter 5, Other Monomorphic Ventricular Tachycardias).

In very few cases, for example, when the parasystolic focus is mathematically related to the basal rhythm (basal rhythm 90 bpm and parasystolic focus rhythm 30 bpm), it is possible for the parasystolic rhythm to have a fixed or nearly fixed coupling interval (modulated parasystole) (Oreto *et al.*, 1988).

Mechanisms Leading to Passive Arrhythmias

Depression of Automaticity

If passive arrhythmia is caused by a decrease in sinus automaticity for any of the previously mentioned reasons (Figure 3.4), its discharge rate falls below the normal discharge rate of the AV junction (40–60 beats per min (bpm)), which is the subsidiary structure with the highest discharge rate, a pacemaker of this AV junction will command the heart rhythm when its TAP reaches the TP (defensive mechanism that may explain some passive arrhythmias) (Figure 3.4B). If the AV junction automaticity is also depressed, the ventricular Purkinje fibers will act as a pacemaker at a discharge rate generally incompatible with life (15–30 bpm) (Figure 3.4C).

Therefore, when the sinus automaticity is depressed, an ectopic subsidiary rhythm from the AV junction or ventricles takes over control of the heart rhythm at the natural discharge rate (e and f in Figure 3.4C). This discharge rate is lower when the pacemaker is in the ventricular Purkinje fibers, because the junctional AV pacemaker is also depressed. The ventricular or AV junctional complexes appearing as a result are called QRS escape complexes, if isolated (Figure 3.4(2e) and (2f)), and escape rhythms, if repetitive (see Figure 6.1).

Depression of Conduction

Conduction alterations that may explain many passive arrhythmias include: (i) heart block, (ii) aberrant conduction, and (iii) concealed conduction.

Heart Block

The slowing down of the stimulus conduction can take place at the sinoatrial junction, the atria, the AV junction, and the ventricles. Blocks occurring at the sinoatrial junction and AV node are those usually studied in arrhythmology. Nevertheless, the concepts explained here relative to the different degrees of blocks are also applicable to blocks that occur in the atria and ventricles. Therefore, these types of blocks will also be discussed.

Generally, we refer to the block as an anterograde stimulus block, although it is evident that the blocks may be unidirectional (anterograde or retrograde) and bidirectional.

Three degrees of block may be distinguished (Bayés de Luna, 2011): (i) first-degree block, when there is a delay in the stimulus conduction but the stimuli may cross the zone; (ii) second-degree block, when only some stimuli are blocked; and (iii) third-degree block, when all stimuli are blocked and not exiting the area in question.

First-degree Block

All stimuli are conducted, although with a delay in conduction.

o *First-degree sinoatrial block.* This cannot be diagnosed by conventional surface electrocardiography, as neither the sinus activity nor the conduction from the sinus node to the atria can be recorded with this technique (Figure 3.18A).

o *First-degree interatrial block.* This is shown by a wide and notched P wave (Figure 3.19B). It frequently coincides with left atrial enlargement (LAE), which also causes a wide P wave due to a concomitant interatrial block. In both cases the P wave is ≥0.12 s, but in the isolated interatrial block the negative part of the P wave in V1, unlike in LAE, is usually shorter because the P wave loop shows a smaller backwards location (Figure 3.20B).

o *First-degree AV block.* The electrocardiographic manifestation of this type of block in the AV junction is a long PR interval with 1:1 conduction (Figure 3.21A).

o *First-degree bundle branch block.* The ECG pattern of a first-degree right bundle branch block is rsr' in lead V1, qr in VR and qRs in lead V6, but with a QRS complex <0.12 s. The ECG pattern of a first-degree left bundle branch block is QS in V1 and an isolated R wave in lead V6 with QRS complex <0.12 s (Figure 3.22). The diagnosis of first-degree hemiblocks will not be discussed here (Rosenbaum *et al.*, 1968; Bayes de Luna *et al.*, 2011).

Second-degree Block

This occurs when some stimuli are blocked. It is classified as type I (Mobitz I) or Wenckebach type if a progressive conduction delay occurs before the block of stimuli occurs, and type II or Mobitz II if the block appears suddenly.

o *Second-degree block at sinoatrial and AV level.* In second-degree Wenckebach type block the conduction delay is progressively longer but the total delay are progressively shorter. This explains, both at the AV junction (Figure 3.21B) and at the sinoatrial junction (Figure 3.18B), why the RR intervals are increasingly shorter (AB>BC) after the pause initiated as a result of

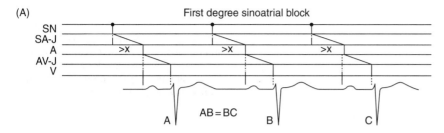

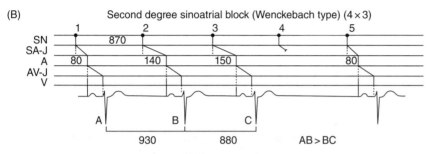

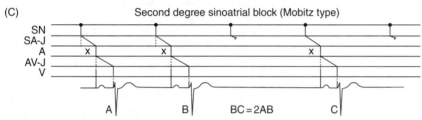

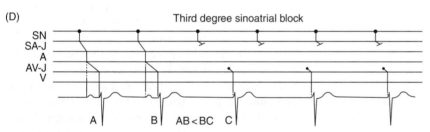

Figure 3.18 (A) First-degree sinoatrial block. The sinoatrial conduction is consistently slowed down (> x), but this does not translate onto the surface ECG (x = normal sinoatrial conduction time). (B) Second-degree sinoatrial block (Wenckebach type, 4 × 3). The sinoatrial conduction time progressively increases from normality (80 ms) to absolute block (80 = x, x + 60, x + 70) and block. The distance between the first two RR (930 ms) is greater than that between the second and the third RR (880 ms). The sinoatrial conduction cannot be determined. However, considering that distances 1–2, 2–3, 3–4, and 4–5 are the same, and assuming that the sinus rhythm cadence is 870 ms, 1, 2, 3, 4 and 5 theoretically represent the origin of the sinus impulses. Therefore, as we have assumed that the first sinoatrial conduction time of the sequence is 80 ms, the successive increases in the sinoatrial conduction, which explain the shortening of RR duration and the subsequent pause, should be 80 + 60 (140) and 140 + 10 (150). Thus, it is explained that in the Wenckebach sinoatrial block the greatest increase occurs in the first cycle of each sequence, after each pause (AB > BC). The PR intervals are constant. The second RR interval is 50 ms shorter, as this is the difference between the increases of sinoatrial conduction between the first and the second cycles. Actually, the first RR of the cycle equals 870 + 60 = 930 ms, whereas in the second cycle it equals 930–50 (50 is the difference between the first increment, 60, and the second one, 10) = 880 ms. (C) Second-degree sinoatrial block (Mobitz type). Sinoatrial conduction (normal or slowed down) is constant (x) before the stimulus is completely blocked (BC = 2AB). (D) Third-degree sinoatrial block. An escape rhythm appears (in this case, in the junction) with no visible P waves in the ECG. The escape rhythm may retrogradely activate the atria (not seen in the scheme) (AB < BC) (see Figures 6.9–6.13).

the total block of stimuli, until a complete conduction block occurs and another pause is observed. This phenomenon, implying progressively shorter RR due to the increasingly smaller increment in the absolute block delay, is known as the Wenckebach phenomenon (Figure 3.18B and 3.21B).

In the AV junction, apart from the previously mentioned phenomenon related to the RR intervals, which is the only diagnostic clue to determine a second-degree sinoatrial Wenckebach-type block, the increasing delay of conduction is observed by measuring the PR interval, which progressively lengthens, although the increases

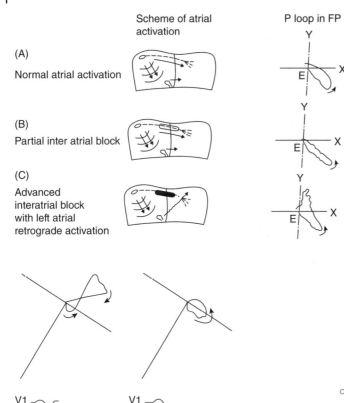

Scheme of atrial activation

(A) Normal atrial activation

(B) Partial inter atrial block

(C) Advanced interatrial block with left atrial retrograde activation

P loop in FP

P wave in VF

0.10 s

0.12 s

0.12 s

Figure 3.19 Scheme of atrial activation under normal conditions (A), in first-degree interatrial block (B) and in third-degree interatrial block (C), with the corresponding P loops and the P morphology in II, III, and VF (see Figure 6.14). Orthogonal leads x and y are equivalent to leads I and VF.

V1

(A)

V1

(B)

Figure 3.20 (A) and (B) Morphology of P wave in V1 and P loop, when a partial isolated interatrial block exists (B), or when it is associated with the enlargement of the left atrium (A).

are smaller each time (x + 60, x + 80 ms) (Figure 3.21B). These rules frequently do not apply in blocks at AV level, where the increases are greater or smaller than expected (atypical Wenckebach phenomena). Figure 3.21E shows two examples, one caused by concealed conduction and the other by a reciprocal complex.

In rare cases, the Wenckebach phenomenon in the AV junction occurs in the presence of a 2×1 fixed AV block. In this case, the blocked P wave of the 2×1 fixed AV block remains unchanged, whereas the conducted P wave presents the characteristics of the Wenckebach phenomenon with the PR interval increasing until the P wave is blocked (alternating Wenckebach phenomenon) (Figure 3.21F). This probably occurs because the two block types appear at two different levels of the AV junction: the 2×1 fixed block at a proximal level and the Wenckebach-type AV block at a more distal level (Figure 3.21F) (Halpern *et al.*, 1973; Amat y Leon *et al.*, 1975). This phenomenon was called "Wenckebach of alternate periods."

In second-degree Mobitz II-type block, the non-conducted stimulus is preceded by a fixed or nearly fixed conduction. At the AV junction this is shown by

a blocked P wave without previous PR lengthening, which leads to a pause equaling approximately twice the baseline RR (Figure 3.21C, BC = 2AB). This unexpected pause, which approximately doubles the baseline RR interval, is the only diagnostic evidence of this block at a sinoatrial junction level (Figure 3.18C, BC = 2AB).

o *Second-degree block at the atrial level.* This corresponds to the transient presence of the first or third degree interatrial block. This concept may include also the transient presence of abnormal P wave morphology different of the morphology of first or third degree interatrial block. The appearance of these changes may be ectopically induced, in which case the change in the P wave morphology occurs after an atrial or ventricular premature systole (Figures 3.22 and 6.15) and nonectopically induced. In the latter case it is manifest by the presence of a P wave of differing morphology and polarity, but sinus in origin, which can be seen in the same recording (see Figure 6.15) or in different recordings (Figure 3.24). This is due to the fact that at some point an area of the atria is temporarily in refractory period. This explains the transitory change in the morphology of the P wave, caused by the change in direction of the atrial activation vector as a result of part of the atria being in refractory period (Figure 3.23) these transient changes of P wave may be included in the term of atrial aberrancy (Chung, 1972; Julia *et al.*, 1978).

o *Second-degree block at a ventricular level.* It is the so-called ventricular aberrancy, and corresponds to transient presence of first or third degree ventricular block (Singer and Ten Eick, 1971; Rosenbaum *et al.*, 1973; El-Sherif *et al.*, 1974) (see Aberrant Conduction and Figures 3.31–3.37).

One rare type of second-degree block at a ventricular level is the bundle branch block of Wenckebach type (type I or Mobitz I). This block may be diagnosed from a repetitive sequence of progressive appearance

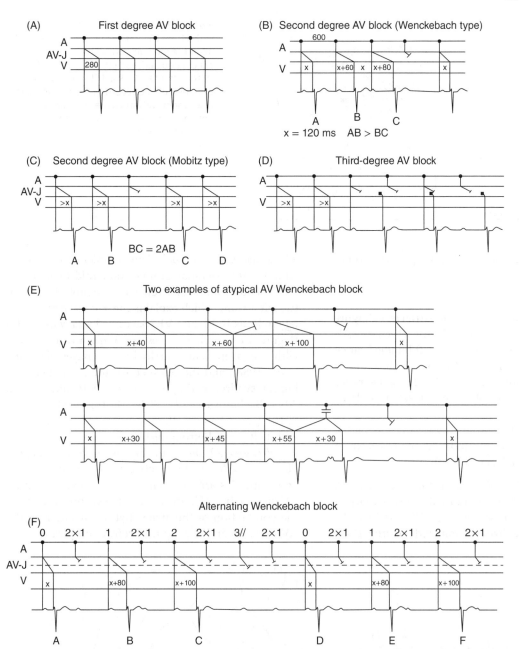

Figure 3.21 (A) First-degree atrioventricular (AV) block. The PR interval is always prolonged (>200 ms). (B) Second-degree AV block 4 × 3 (Wenckebach type). The criterion AB > BC also applies in this case (see text and Figure 3.18B). (C) Second-degree AV block (Mobitz type) (BC = 2AB). (D) Third-degree AV block. A clear AV dissociation may be seen. After two QRS complexes have been conducted there is a pause, followed by wide QRS (at slow frequencies) dissociated from P waves. In this case, the wide QRS complexes are junctional. (E) Atypical Wenckebach blocks. Top: With abnormal lengthening of the increase preceding the pause (PR = x + 100) due to a concealed retrograde conduction of the preceding complex in the AV junction. Bottom: The abnormal PR shortening is due to the existence of a reciprocal complex in the AV junction. (F): Example of an alternating Wenckebach block.

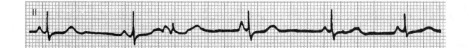

Figure 3.22 Example of aberrant atrial conduction ectopically induced by an atrial extrasystole. Note that the next P wave, after the atrial extrasystole, presents transient different P wave morphology with the same PR interval as the other P waves. This makes it improbable that it may be due to atrial escape beat.

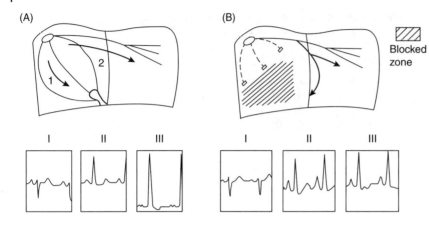

Figure 3.23 Top: (A) normal atrial activation with ÂP ≈ +30° (flat P in III); (B) when a block in part of the right atria exists, the blocked zone is depolarized with some delay, right-shifting the ÂP (flat P in I). Bottom (A) and (B): examples of ECG recorded a few days apart in a patient with subacute cor pulmonale and different P waves (morphology and P axis) in the frontal plane due to second-degree atrial block.

of more advanced bundle branch block pattern (Brenes *et al.*, 2006) (Figure 3.24).

Third-degree Block

Here, all stimuli are blocked at the sinoatrial level (Figure 3.18D), the Bachman bundle area (Figure 3.19C), the AV junction (Figure 3.21D), the right and left bundle branch (Figures 3.25 and 3.26), or in the divisions of the left bundle (hemiblocks) (Figures 3.27 and 3.28). The appearance of a pattern of third degree block may develop suddenly or progressively.

See in Figure 3.29 the progressive evolution of the morphology of right and left bundle branch block (from normal, to partial and advanced BBB).

○ *Third-degree sinoatrial block*. If the third-degree block is at a sinoatrial level, no normal sinus activity is recorded (no P wave is seen in the ECG), and usually AV junctional escape rhythm is initiated (Figure 3.18D).

○ *Third-degree atrial block*. The complete block of the stimulus at a Bachman bundle and a mid-high part of atrial septum initiates a retrograde depolarization of the left atrium, which explains the ± P wave morphology in leads II, III, and VF (Bayés de Luna *et al.*, 1985) (Figure 3.19C). These cases are frequently associated with supraventricular arrhythmias (Bayés de Luna *et al.*, 1988), and therefore constitute an arrhythmological syndrome (Bayes Syndrome) (Conde *et al.*, 2015; Bacharova *et al.*, 2015; Martínez-Sellés *et al.*, 2016) (see Chapter 10, Advanced Interatrial Block with Left Atrial Retrograde Conduction).

○ *Third-degree AV block*. In the case of a third-degree block at AV level, the electrical activity of the atria and ventricles are independent, thus resulting in an AV dissociation (Figure 3.21D). These interfered with the conduction of the atrial rhythm by entering the AV junction and leaving it in refractory period. This

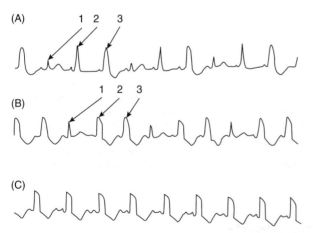

Figure 3.24 Lead I in a patient with different degrees of left bundle branch block. (A) progressive left bundle branch block – Wenckebach type (1–3); (B) intermittent left bundle branch block (2 and 3); (C) fixed left bundle branch block (adapted from Brenes *et al.*, 2006).

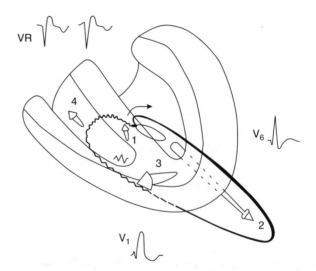

Figure 3.25 Descriptive diagram of the ventricular activation in cases of advanced right bundle branch block (RBBB). The figure shows the vectors that explain the ventricular depolarization and the global QRS loop, as well as the QRS morphology in the three key leads (VR, V1, and V6) (see Figure 6.24).

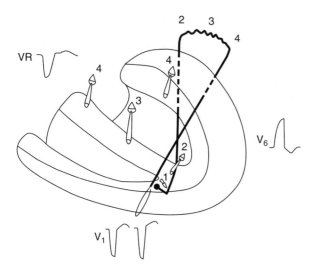

Figure 3.26 Descriptive diagram of the ventricular activation in cases of advanced left bundle branch block (LBBB). The figure shows the vectors that explain the ventricular depolarization and the global QRS loop, as well as the QRS morphology in the three key leads (VR, V1, and V6) (see Figure 6.25).

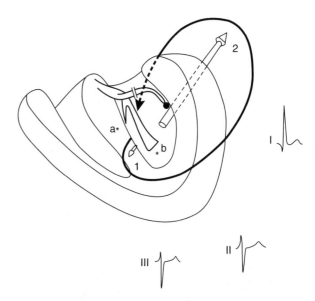

Figure 3.27 Descriptive diagram of ventricular activation in cases of superoanterior hemiblock (SAH). The figure shows the two vectors that explain the ventricular depolarization and the global QRS loop, as well as the QRS morphology in the three key leads (I, II, and III) (see Figure 6.26).

is called AV dissociation with interference. When, in the presence of an AV dissociation, some sinus stimuli may be conducted to the ventricles, a sinus capture is observed (see Figure 5.23). In this case, the AV dissociation is incomplete. A fusion complex is produced when both the sinus and the ventricular stimuli each partially activate the ventricle (Figure 3.30).

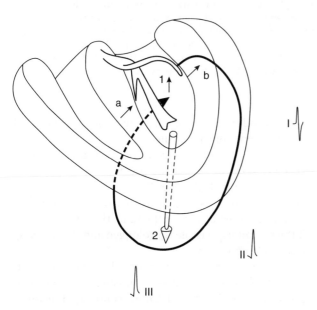

Figure 3.28 Descriptive diagram of the ventricular activation in cases of inferoposterior hemiblock (IPH). The figure shows the two vectors that explain the ventricular depolarization and the global QRS loop, as well as the QRS morphology in the three key derivations (I, II, and III) (see Figure 6.27).

○ *Third-degree intraventricular block.* The third-degree intraventricular block may initiate the typical patterns of the advanced right bundle branch block (RBBB) (Figure 3.25) and left bundle branch block (LBBB) (Figure 3.26), as well as the advanced superoanterior and inferoposterior hemiblocks of the left bundle (Rosenbaum *et al.*, 1968) (Figures 3.27 and 3.28), when the block takes place in these fascicles.

The peripheral block of the right bundle (Cosín *et al.*, 1983; Gras *et al.*, 1981) has also been described. As well, the block of the middle fibers of the left bundle (Uhley, 1973, Pastore *et al.*, 2003;, Perez Riera *et al.*, 2011) must exist, although diagnostic confirmation by surface ECG has not yet been completely confirmed (Bayés de Luna *et al.*, 2012).

Aberrant Conduction

Aberrant conduction is an abnormal and transient distribution of an impulse through the atria, or more frequently through the ventricles, resulting in a change in the P wave (atrial aberrancy) (Chung, 1972; Julia *et al.*, 1978) (Figures 3.22 and 3.23) or in the QRS complex morphology (ventricular aberrancy) (El-Sherif *et al.*, 1974; Rosenbaum *et al.*, 1973; Singer and Ten Eick, 1971) (Figures 3.31–3.34). When a ventricular aberrancy occurs in a healthy heart, given that the right bundle branch usually constitutes the structure of the specific system of ventricular conduction with the longest refractory period, the most frequent ECG pattern found is an advanced right bundle branch block.

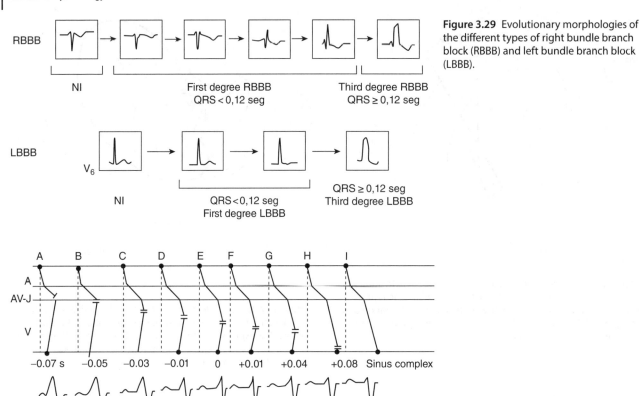

Figure 3.29 Evolutionary morphologies of the different types of right bundle branch block (RBBB) and left bundle branch block (LBBB).

Figure 3.30 Descriptive diagram of the different degrees of ventricular fusion. (A) Ventricular extrasystole in the PR interval. (B)–(D) The fusion complex presents a shorter PR interval compared with the normal PR interval. (B)–(H) Fusion complexes of different degrees. (E)–(H) Fusion complexes with the same PR interval. (I) Normal sinus impulse. Ventricular extrasystoles, regardless of their origin, require at least 0.06 s to reach the His fascicle and depolarize it. Thus, a wide impulse with a PR interval that is shortened >0.06 s (compared with the normal PR interval) may have already depolarized the His fascicle, resulting in no fusion taking place because the descending sinus stimulus will not be able to penetrate the His fascicle already in refractory period. A ventricular extrasystole with a PR interval that is shortened <0.06 s (compared with the normal PR interval) will not have reached the His fascicle at the time the sinus stimulus reaches it, which will result in a minimal ventricular fusion (B). The later the ventricular extrasystole, the less aberrant the fusion complex, as a wider ventricular area will have been depolarized by the sinus impulse. As the sinus QRS complex usually lasts 0.08–0.09 s when a ventricular extrasystole is originated >0.08 s after the time point at which the sinus stimulus penetrates into the ventricle, no fusion takes place. This is explained because the area in which the ectopic ventricular extrasystole is initiated depolarizes thanks to the sinus stimulus before the ventricular ectopic impulse is generated (I).

Phase 3 Aberrancy

The aberrant ventricular conduction pattern is, by definition, a transient pattern (second-degree ventricular block) and is generally related to a shortening of the RR interval (Phase 3 Rosenbaum aberrancy) (Figure 3.31).

o A premature supraventricular complex may or may not have aberrant conduction depending, basically, on the ratio between the preceding diastole length and the coupling interval (Figure 3.32).
o If the coupling interval is not changed, aberrancy occurs when the preceding RR cycle is longer, as it implies that the subsequent TAP is wider (Figures 3.31 and 3.32). Therefore, an impulse with a similar coupling interval (E in Figure 3.32A and D) may fall in the refractory period of the right bundle branch and may not be conducted (D), or it may be normally conducted (A) if the previous RR is shorter.
o In the presence of a shorter coupling interval, aberrancy occurs with the same previous RR (compare E and E′ in Figure 3.32A and B).
o Obviously, there is a greater chance of aberrancy if both phenomena occur at the same time, for example, if the preceding diastole is prolonged and the coupling interval becomes shorter.
o Premature supraventricular impulses in the sinus rhythm follow this rule consistently (prolonged preceding RR interval + short coupling interval = aberrancy; Gouaux and Ashman criteria (Figure 3.33). The subsequent complexes of a supraventricular tachycardia with a preceding short RR interval show an aberrant morphology less frequently, unless the refractory

Figure 3.31 Note how as cycle length (CL) shortens, the transmembrane action potential (TAP) duration (TAD) decreases as well.

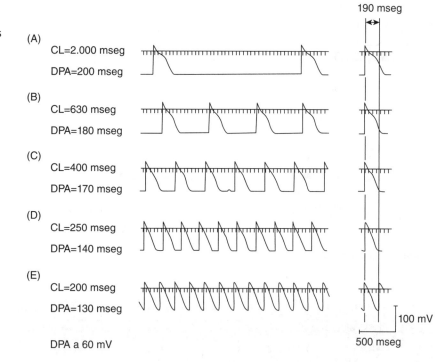

Figure 3.32 (A), (B), (C), and (D) Diagrams showing how the combination of a preceding long diastole and a short coupling interval favor the appearance of aberrancy related to a shortened cycle (Phase 3 aberrancy). Left: Right bundle branch transmembrane action potential (TAP) (top); right bundle branch absolute refractory period (ARP) (bottom, grey); right bundle branch relative RP (bottom, black) (the sum of both equals the total refractory period of the right bundle). Also, the morphology of V₁ in different situations, depending on the preceding RR interval (cycle length) and the coupling interval, is shown. Right: Diagrams (A), (B), (C), and (D) showing whether a more or less premature stimulus falls in or out of the ARP (gray) or RRP (black) left by the preceding RR cycle (distance 1–2). A premature stimulus is not conducted through the right bundle branch if it falls into its ARP (E′ in B and D). If the preceding RR is longer (D), a premature stimulus (E) (which could be conducted when the preceding RR were shorter) (A), may fall in ARP (D), thus not being conducted (rsR′ in V₁) or being slowly conducted showing a partial right bundle branch block (RBBB) morphology (rsr′ in V₁) if it falls in the relative refractory period (C) (E′ in C). A premature stimulus falling out of the total RP (E in A) is normally conducted, although if the preceding RR interval is longer (D), the same premature stimulus may fall into the total refractory period and thus it may not be conducted (compare E in A and D). To summarize, a stimulus falling in the final part of Phase 3 of a TAP of the right bundle (E′ in C, in the relative refractory period of right bundle) is conducted with a partial RBBB morphology, and a stimulus falling in Phase 2 or an initial part of Phase 3 of a TAP of the right bundle (ARP of such branch, E′ in B and D) is conducted with a morphology of advanced RBBB. Rosenbaum called this type of aberrancy "Phase 3 aberrancy," which means that a stimulus that falls in Phase 3 of TAP of the right or left bundle branch is not conducted through such bundle branches, and will present a right or left bundle branch block morphology.

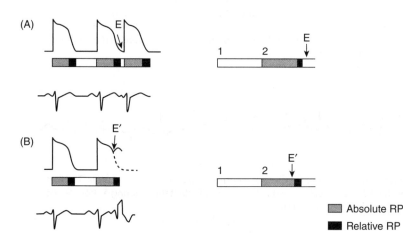

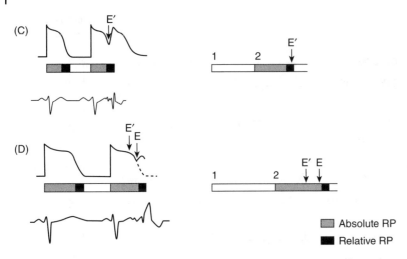

Figure 3.32 (*Continued*)

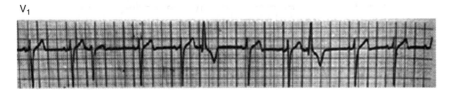

Figure 3.33 The first atrial extrasystole is conducted with minimal aberrancy, even without rsr′ morphology, whereas the following extrasystoles are conducted with a morphology corresponding to an advanced right bundle branch block. By means of the compass it is observed how the Gouaux and Ashman criteria are met. Therefore, the 6th and 9th complexes, clearly aberrant, show a slightly shorter coupling interval and/or a slightly longer preceding diastole than the 3rd complex. This is enough to fall in an absolute (6th and 9th complexes) or relative (3rd complex) refractory period of the right bundle.

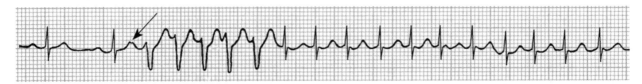

Figure 3.34 Sustained aberrancy during different complexes at the beginning of a supraventricular paroxysmal tachycardia. The first complex of the tachycardia presents classical aberrancy Phase 3, the others occur due to the lack of adaptation, during a short period, of part of the intraventricular conduction system due to sudden change in heart rate.

period of some SCS parts (right or left bundle branch) is pathologically prolonged. Occasionally, aberrancy may persist for several complexes when the refractory period of some SCS parts are not able to adapt to sudden changes in the heart rate (Figure 3.34).

o Exceptions may commonly be observed in premature AF complexes, as, occasionally, complexes that should be aberrant are not, whereas other complexes not following Gouaux and Ashman criteria are aberrant. This may be explained by the different degrees of concealed "f" wave conduction in the AV junction, as well as in the branches (see Figures 4.50 and 4.51). Maintained aberrant morphologies, secondary to concealed retrograde conduction in the branches, may also occur (see Figures 4.46 and 4.47).

o From a clinical viewpoint, it should be noted that in the presence of atrial fibrillation, most wide QRS complexes are ectopic, especially if they do not have the typical RBBB morphology (see Figure 4.45). Therefore, the presence of a typical RBBB morphology in lead V1 (rsR′) favors the occurrence of aberrancy, and not the presence of an R morphology with a notch in the descending limb of the R wave (compare Figures 4.45 and 4.48). In the presence of AF, the irregular ventricular rhythm of fibrillation is also present when there are aberrant QRS complexes (see Figure 4.47). When the QRS complexes present the same morphology but the RR intervals are regular, the atrial fibrillation is considered to have turned into an atrial flutter. If a regular rhythm but a different

QRS morphology exists, the presence of VT should be considered.

Phase 4 Aberrancy

In some cases, the aberrant morphology is associated with a lengthening of the RR cycle (Rosenbaum Phase 4 aberrancy). This may be explained by the presence of a spontaneous diastolic depolarization increasing the right bundle branch TDP up to the level observed in a Phase 3 aberrancy (Figures 3.35B and 3.36).

Aberrancy Without RR Changes

Sometimes different mechanisms result in aberrant QRS complexes without changes in the RR intervals (Figure 3.37).

Concealed Conduction

Sometimes a structure may be partially depolarized by a stimulus that does not cross it completely. This partial depolarization is not directly observed on the surface ECG. However, it may be seen by its effect on the conduction of successive complexes (concealed conduction). An example of this is seen in interpolated premature ventricular complexes. The PR interval of the complex following the premature ventricular impulse is usually longer, as it partially depolarizes the AV junction. As a consequence, the atrial stimulus (P wave) finds the AV junction in relative RP, and thus is conducted more slowly (Figure 3.38).

Concealed conduction explains other phenomena in the field of arrhythmology, including but not limited to:

o The irregular rhythm of the QRS complex in the presence of AF, as a result of the "f" waves, depolarizes the AV junction to a lesser or greater extent, leading to an irregular conduction (Figure 3.39).

o Wide aberrant QRS in AF that do not follow the Gouaux–Ashman rule. Some examples: the presence, in the case of AF with frequent wide QRS complexes of a premature narrow QRS complex after a long-short sequence, is due to an "f" wave being partially conducted through the two branches during the long interval and changing the sequence. This is

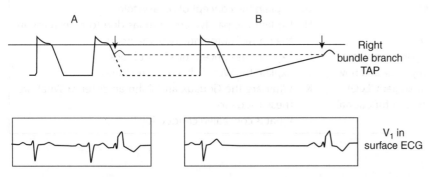

Figure 3.35 Comparison between the aberrancy related with cycle shortening (Phase 3) (A) and that related with cycle lengthening (less frequent) (Phase 4) (B). In this case, due to an important diastolic depolarization during the long cycle, the right bundle gets to a point, as in Phase 3 aberrancy, where it is not excitable, and thus not able to generate a TAP to be conducted (arrow in B at the same level as A). As in Phase 3, in the surface ECG an aberrant QRS complex with right bundle branch block morphology (rsR′) is recorded.

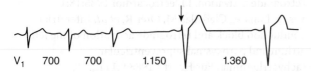

Figure 3.36 Example of a Phase 4 left bundle branch block. Note the left bundle branch block pattern appearing after a significant lengthening of the previous RR cycle. The presence of the same PR interval in all complexes favors Phase 4 aberrancy instead of an idioventricular escape rhythm.

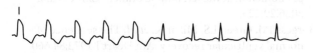

Figure 3.37 Intermittent aberrancy without apparent changes in heart rate.

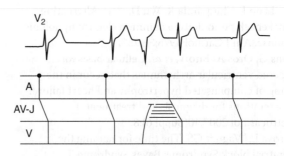

Figure 3.38 Interpolated ventricular extrasystole. The following P wave is conducted with a longer PR due to the concealed conduction of the ventricular extrasystole at the atrioventricular (AV) junction.

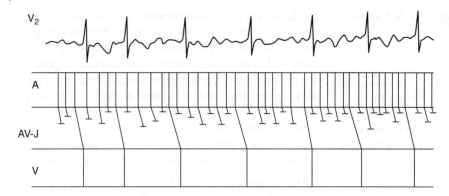

Figure 3.39 V_2 recording showing the different morphologies of "f" waves (atrial fibrillation) and the variability of RR due to different degrees of conduction of the "f" waves in the atrioventricular node (concealed conduction).

shown in Figure 4.51, which shows that complex 3 presents normal conduction and complex 6 a wide QRS, even though complex 3 presents a longer–shorter sequence. This may be explained (see before) by concealed conduction in two branches of an "f" wave that has changed the sequence (see Figure 4.51). On other occasions, some complexes that should not show aberrant conduction because they are late may be conducted with aberrancy if one "f" wave partially depolarizes the right or left branches and changes the sequence as well (see complex 3 in Figure 4.50).

Self Assessment

A. What are the automaticity alterations that may explain some active and passive arrhythmias?

B. What is triggered electrical activity?

C. Explain the classical concept of reentry.

D. Describe the circuits of different types of paroxysmal atrio-ventricular (AV) junctional reentrant tachycardia and how to distinguish them by surface electrocardiogram (ECG).

E. Describe the main types of reentry with a functional basis.

F. What is the gap phenomenon?

G. Explain the concept of parasystole.

H. Explain the passive arrhythmias due to a decrease in the normal automaticity of the heart.

I. Explain the concept of a heart block.

J. Explain the Wenckebach phenomenon.

K. What are the Gouaux and Ashman criteria? What are these used for?

L. What is concealed conduction?

References

Allesie MA, Bonke FI, Schopman FJ. Circus movement in rabbit atrial muscle as a mechanism of tachycardia. III. The "leading circle" concept: a new model of circus movement in cardiac tissue without the involvement of an anatomical obstacle. Circ Res 1977;41:9.

Amat y Leon F, Chuquimia R, Wu D, *et al.* Alternating Wenckebach periodicity: a common electrophysiologic response. Am J Cardiol 1975;36:757.

Antoons G, Oros A, Bito V, *et al.* Cellular basis for triggered ventricular arrhythmias that occur in the setting of compensated hypertrophy and heart failure: considerations for diagnosis and treatment. J Electrocardiol 2007;40(Suppl 6):8.

Bacharova L, Wagner GS. The time for naming the interatrial block Syndrome: Bayes Syndrome. J Electrocardiol 2015;48:133.

Bayés de Luna A. Clinical electrocardiography. John Wiley & Sons Ltd, Chichester, 2011.

Bayés de Luna A, Fort de Ribot R, Trilla E, *et al.* Electrocardiographic and vectorcardiographic study of interatrial conduction disturbances with left atrial retrograde activation. J Electrocardiol 1985;18:1.

Bayés de Luna A, Cladellas M, Oter R, *et al.* Interatrial conduction block and retrograde activation of the left atrium and paroxysmal supraventricular tachyarrhythmia. Eur Heart J 1988;9:1112.

Bayés de Luna A, Pérez Riera A, Baranchuk A, *et al.* Electrocardiographic manifestation of the middle fibers/septal fascicle block: a consensus report. J Electrocardiol 2012;45:454.

Brenes JC, Brenes-Pereira C, Castellanos A. Wenckebach-phenomenon at the left bundle branch. Clin Cardiol 2006;29:226.

Burgess JM, Green LS, Millar K, *et al.* The sequence of normal ventricular recovery. Am Heart J 1972;84:660.

Castellanos A, Lemberg L, Johnson D, *et al.* The Wedensky effect in the human heart. Br Heart J 1966;28:276.

Childers RW. Supernormality: recent developments. PACE 1984;7:1115.

Chung EK. Aberrant atrial conduction. Unrecognized electrocardiographic entity. Br Heart J 1972;34:341.

Conde D, Baranchuk A, Bayés de Luna A. Advanced interatrial block as a substrate of supraventricular tachyarrytymias: a well recognized syndrome. J Electrocardiol 2015;48:135.

Cosín J, Gimeno JV, Bayés de Luna A, *et al*. Estudio experimental de los bloqueos parcelares de la rama derecha. Rev Esp Cardiol 1983;36:125.

Coumel P, Fidelle J, Attuel P, *et al*. Les tachycardies réciproques à évolution prolongée chez l'enfant. Arch Mal Cœur 1974;1:23.

El-Sherif N, Scherlag BJ, Lazzara R, *et al*. Pathophysiology of tachycardia and bradycardia dependent block in the canine proximal H-P system after acute myocardial ischemia. Am J Cardiol 1974;33:529.

El-Sherif N, Chinushi M, Caref EB, Restivo M. Electrophysiological mechanisms of the characteristic electrocardiographic morphology of *torsade de pointes* tachyarrhythmias in the long QT syndrome-detailed analysis of ventricular tridimensional activation patterns. Circulation 1997;96:4392.

Franz MR, Bargheer K, Rafflenbeul W, *et al*. Monophasic action potential mapping in human subjects with normal electrocardiograms: direct evidence for the genesis of the T wave. Circulation 1987;75:379.

Gallagher JJ, Damato AN, Caracta AR, *et al*. Gap in the A-V conduction in man; types I and II. Am Heart J 1973;85:78.

Gras X, Bayés A, Cosín J. Experimental and clinical study of right periphereic block in the subpulmonar anterior zone. Adv Cardiol 1981;28:242.

Gussak I, Antzeleritch Ch (eds). Electrical diseases of the heart. Springer-Verlang, London, 2008.

Haïssaguerre M, Jaïs P, Shah DC, *et al*. Spontaneous initiation of atrial fibrillation by ectopic beats originating in the pulmonary veins. N Engl J Med 1998;339:659.

Haïssaguerre M, Hocini M, Sanders P, *et al*. Catheter ablation of long-lasting persistent atrial fibrillation: clinical outcome and mechanisms of subsequent arrhythmias. J Cardiovasc Electrophysiol 2005;16:1138

Halpern MS, Elizari MV, Rosenbaum MB, *et al*. Wenckebach periods of alternate beats. Clinical and experimental observations. Circulation 1973;48:41.

Jalife J, Berenfeld D, Mansour M. Mother rotors and fibrillation conduction: a mechanism of atrial fibrillation. Circ Research 2000;54:204.

Julia J, Bayés de Luna A, Candell J. Auricular aberration: apropos of 21 cases. Rev Esp Cardiol 1978;31:207.

Katritsis D, Becker A. The AV nodal re-entrant circuit. A proposal. Heart Rhythm 2007;4:1354.

Koulizakis NG, Kappos KG, Toutouzas PK. Parasystolic ventricular tachycardia with exit block. J Electrocardiol 1990;23:89.

Lambiasse PD, Ahmed AK, Ciaccio EJ, *et al*. High-density substrate mapping in Brugada Syndrome. Combined role of conduction and repolarization heterogeneities in arrhythmogenesis. Circulation 2009;12:116.

Martínez-Sellés M, Massó-van Roessel A, Álvarez-Garcia J, *et al*. Interatrial block and atrial arrhythmias in centenarians: prevalence, associations, and clinical implications. Heart Rhythm 2016;13:645.

Moe GM, Méndez C. Physiological basis of reciprocal rhythm. Prog Cardiovasc Dis 1966;8:561.

Morel E, Meyronet D. Identification and distribution of interstitial Cajal cells in the human pulmonary veins. Heart Rhythm 2008;5:1068.

Noble D. The initiation of the heartbeat. Oxford University Press, Oxford, 1979.

Opthof T, Coronel R, Wilms-Schopman FJ, *et al*. Dispersion of repolarization in canine ventricle and the ECG T wave: T interval does not reflect transmural dispersion. Heart Rhythm 2007;4:341.

Oreto G, Satullo G, Luzza F, *et al*. Irregular ventricular parasystole: The influence of sinus rhythm on a parasystolic focus. Am Heart J 1988;115:121.

Perez-Riera A, Ferreira C, Ferreira Filho C, *et al*. Electrovectrocardiographic diagnosis of left septal fascicular block: anatomic and clinical considerations. Ann Noninvasive Electrocardiol 2011;16:196.

Pastore CA, *et al*. Guidelines for interpreting rest electrocardiogram. Arq Bras Cardiol 2003;80:1.

Qu Z, Gurfinkel A. Nonlinear dynamics of excitation and propagation in cardiac muscle. In: Zipes D, Jalife J (eds), Cardiac electrophysiology. From cell to bedside. 4th edn. Saunders, Philadelphia, PA, 2004, p. 327.

Rosenbaum MB, Elizari M, Lazzari JO. Los hemibloqueos. Edit. Paidos, Buenos Aires, 1968.

Rosenbaum MB, Elizari M, Lazzari JO, *et al*. The mechanism of intermittent bundle branch block. Relationship to prolonged recovery, hypopolarization and spontaneous diastolic depolarization. Chest 1973;63:666.

Singer D, Ten Eick, R. Aberrancy: Electrophysiological aspects. Am J Cardiol 1971;28:381.

Takenaka K, Ai T, Shimizu W, *et al*. Exercise stress test amplifies genotype-phenotype correlation in the LQT1 and LQT2 forms of the long-QT syndrome. Circulation 2003;107:838.

Uhley H. The quadrifascicular nature of the peripheral conduction system. In: Dreyfus L, Likoff W (eds), Cardiac arrhythmias. Grune-Stratton, New York, 1973.

Vaquero M, Calvo D, Jalife J. Cardiac fibrillation: from ion channels to rotors in the human heart. Heart Rhythm 2008;5:872.

Voss F, Opthof T, Marker J, *et al*. There is no transmural heterogeneity in an index of action potential duration in the canine left ventricle. Heart Rhythm 2009;6:1028.

Watanabe N, Kobayashi Y, Tanno K, *et al*. Transmural dispersion of repolarization and ventricular tachyarrhythmias. J Electrocardiol 2004;37:191.

Wit AL, Boyden PA. Triggered activity and atrial fibrillation. Heart Rhythm 2007;4(3 Suppl):S17.

Wu D, Yeh S. Double loop figure of eight reentry as a mechanism of multiple AV reentry. Am Heart J 1994;127:83.

Yamabe H, Tanaka Y, Morihisa K, *et al*. Electrophysiologic delineation of the tachycardia circuit in the slow-slow form of atrioventricular nodal reentrant tachycardia. Heart Rhythm 2007;4:713.

Yamaguchi M, Shimizu M, Ino H, *et al*. T wave peak-to-end interval and QT dispersion in acquired long QT syndrome: a new index for arrhythmogenicity. Clin Sci 2003;105:671.

Yan GX, Anzelevitch C. Cellular basis for the normal T wave and the electrocardiographic manifestations of the long-QT syndrome. Circulation 1998;98:1928.

Zipes DP. Mechanisms of clinical arrhythmias. J Cardiovasc Electrophysiol 2003;14:902.

Part II

Diagnosis, Prognosis and Treatment of Arrhythmias

4

Active Supraventricular Arrhythmias

This chapter describes premature supraventricular complexes (PSVC) and supraventricular tachyarrhythmias. This last term refers to the different types of supraventricular tachycardias, atrial fibrillation, and flutter (Table 4.1). Table 4.2 shows the classification of supraventricular tachyarrhythmias, depending on whether the RR is regular or irregular.

Premature Supraventricular Complexes

Premature supraventricular complexes are actually "electrical impulses" that cause "contractions" of the heart, which can be detected as "heart beats" by auscultation or palpation, or recorded on the electrocardiogram (ECG) as "complexes". As the diagnosis is performed by ECG we will use the term "complexes".

Concept and Mechanisms

Premature supraventricular complexes are premature complexes of supraventricular origin. These include those of atrial (A-PSVC) and atrioventricular (AV) junctional origin (J-PSVC). Clinical, prognostic, and therapeutic approaches differ according to the origin of the beats, the hemodynamic consequences, and symptoms (see later).

Most PSVC have a fixed or nearly fixed coupling interval (distance from the beginning of the previous sinus P wave to the beginning of the premature ectopic P′), because their origin is dependent on the baseline heart rhythm. They are commonly called extrasystoles. The most frequent mechanism causing PSVC is micro-reentry in the atrial muscle, although sometimes the circuit is macro-reentrant (see Chapter 3, Reentry). Supraventricular premature complexes can also be caused by an increase in the automaticity or triggered by electric activity (post-potentials). In the AV junction the origin may be in an ectopic focus or an aborted reentrant AV junctional tachycardia (reciprocal beat or complex, see Figure 1.18 B).

Premature supraventricular complexes that have an extremely variable coupling interval are called parasystoles, and originate in an automatic focus. The automatic focus is protected to be depolarized from the basic rhythm, and is therefore independent of it (see Chapter 3, Active Arrhythmias with Variable Coupling Interval: the Parasystole). Occasionally, the ectopic focus can be modulated either by the sinus rhythm or by the autonomic nervous system; these are called "modulated parasystolic beats".

Electrocardiographic Findings

Morphology

In the ECG, a premature ectopic P (P′) wave is observed, which is followed, if not blocked in the AV junction, by a QRS complex, which is also premature. The P′ wave usually has a different morphology from the sinus P wave, although it is frequently hidden in the previous T wave, which is usually modified by the P′ wave, resulting in a masked P′ morphology (Figure 4.1).

The A-PSVC may originate in different regions of the atrium. If an atrial monomorphic tachycardia is initiated, then every complex will have the same morphology. The morphology of P′ has a good correlation with the place of origin (see Figure 4.15).

If the origin of PSVC is the AV junction (J-PSVC), then the premature P wave is always negative in II, III, and VF with a short PR interval (<120 ms). In atrial PSVC that originates in the low atria, the P′ is also negative in II, III, and VF, but usually the PR interval is ≥120 ms. If the conduction of junctional PSVC to the atria is slow, the P′ may be hidden within the QRS, or may occur just after the QRS.

Premature supraventricular complexes may be isolated or occur in runs. If the runs last at least 30 seconds, they are considered runs of supraventricular tachycardia (Figure 4.2). They may present with fixed sequences, trigeminy, and so on. (Figure 4.3A). The coupling interval is fixed or nearly fixed.

Premature supraventricular complexes occasionally may comply with the following ECG criteria for atrial

Clinical Arrhythmology, Second Edition. Antoni Bayés de Luna and Adrian Baranchuk.
© 2017 John Wiley & Sons Ltd. Published 2017 by John Wiley & Sons Ltd.

Table 4.1 Supraventricular active rhythms.

Premature supraventricular complexes

Supraventricular tachyarrhythmias
- Sinus tachycardia
- Monomorphic atrial tachycardia (MAT)
- Atrioventricular (AV) junctional reentrant tachycardia (AVNRT and AVRT)
- AV junctional tachycardia due to an ectopic focus (JT-EF)
- Chaotic or multimorphic atrial tachycardia
- Atrial fibrillation
- Atrial flutter

Table 4.2 Classification of supraventricular tachyarrhythmias according to RR (regular or irregular).

Regular RR (Figure 4.70)

- Sinus tachycardia with fixed atrioventricular (AV) ratio (almost always 1:1) (including sinus node-dependent reentry) (Figures 4.7–4.10)
- Monomorphic atrial tachycardia due to an ectopic focus (MAT-EF), with fixed AV ratio (generally 1 × 1) (Figures 4.11 and 4.12) or to macroreentry (MAT-NR) (p. 98)
- Junctional reentrant tachycardia (JRT) (AVNRT and AVRT) (Figures 4.16–4.29 and 4.21)
- Junctional tachycardia due to an ectopic focus, with fixed AV conduction to ventricles (JT-EF) (Figure 4.27)
- Atrial flutter with fixed AV conduction, generally 2 × 1 (Figure 4.60)

Irregular RR (Figure 4.71)

- Atrial fibrillation (Figure 4.37)
- Atrial flutter with variable AV conduction (Figure 4.63A)
- Multimorphic or chaotic atrial tachycardia (Figure 4.31)
- Monomorphic atrial tachycardia with variable AV conduction (Figure 4.14)
- Junctional tachycardia due to an ectopic focus, with AV variable conduction to the ventricles (Figure 7.6H)

parasystole (see Chapter 3: Parasystole): (i) variable coupling interval of the P′, (ii) interectopic intervals of P′ being multiples, and (iii) possible atrial fusion complexes will be found, if there is a long recording (Figure 4.4).

Conduction of the PSVC to the Ventricles

This may occur in three different ways (Figure 4.1): normal conduction, morphology of aberrant conduction (generally right bundle branch block), or blocking in the AV junction, leading to a pause (nonconducted beats). In the latter, the diagnosis is based on the fact that the concealed atrial premature complex slightly modifies the preceding T wave, and also because the pause is similar to the distance between two QRS complexes when there is an atrial premature complex in between (AB = CD) (Figure 4.3A). This sequence may be observed in the

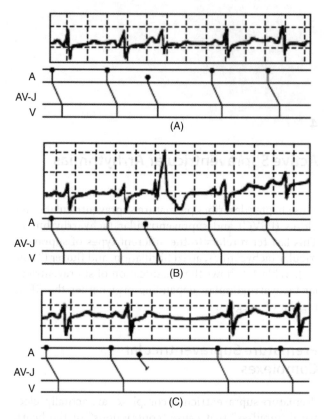

Figure 4.1 A patient in sinus rhythm with paroxysmal atrial fibrillation (AF) episodes and frequent premature supraventricular complexes (PSVC). (A) A PSVC is conducted normally. (B) A PSVC is conducted with aberrancy because it occurs earlier. (C) A PSVC is blocked (arrow), because it occurs even earlier and the preceding diastole is a little longer. The pause is due to an active, not to a passive, arrhythmia.

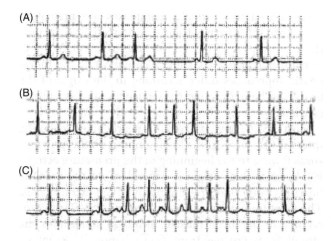

Figure 4.2 Examples of supraventricular premature complexes: (A) isolated; (B) in pairs; (C) in runs.

same patient if the premature complexes become more and more premature (Figures 4.1 and 4.3A).

When supraventricular tachyarrhythmias runs occur, sometimes the first complexes of the runs show a sus-

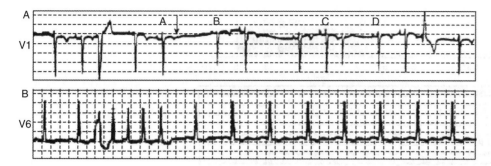

Figure 4.3 (A) A healthy 8-year-old girl with atrial trigeminy, at times normally conducted and at other times blocked (see change in T wave morphology in the A–B pause, arrow (compare AB = CD)). Sometimes it was conducted with right bundle branch (RBB) or left bundle branch (LBB) morphology. (B) A short run of supraventricular tachycardia. Only the first complex of the run is aberrant due to the Gouax–Ashman phenomenon.

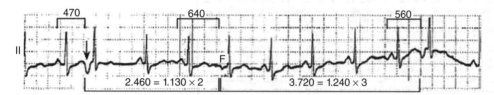

Figure 4.4 Example of atrial parasystole. Note the different coupling intervals (470, 640, and 560 ms), the interectopic intervals that are multiples (2.460 = 1.130 × 2 and 3.720 = 1.240 × 3) and the presence of fused atrial complexes (F).

tained aberrant morphology (see Figure 3.34) due to the refractory periods of some part of the specific conduction system (SCS) not adapting to the sudden changes in heart rate. However, it is usually only the first complex of the run that is aberrant, which is a result of the Gouaux–Ashman phenomenon (see Chapter 3, Aberrant Conduction) (Figure 4.3B).

The differential diagnosis between aberrant PSVC and ventricular complexes is shown in Table 4.3.

Clinical, prognostic, and therapeutic implications

Atrial PSVC may be the origin of any type of atrial tachycardias and also of junctional reentrant tachycardias more often than the PSVC of the AV junction. The latter may trigger the junctional tachycardia mainly due to ectopic focuses (Figures 4.11 and 4.18).

From a clinical point of view, PSVC are generally benign. It is important to determine: (a) their frequency; (b) if they are associated with paroxysmal arrhythmias; (c) if they disappear with exercise; (d) their impact on the left ventricular ejection fraction; and (e) any etiological factors.

Premature supraventricular complexes may be associated with heart disease (i.e., ischemic heart disease (IHD), cor pulmonale, thyroid dysfunction, pericardial diseases, psychologic factors, drugs, digitalis intoxication, etc.) or may be due to functional disturbances. In healthy individuals, they are usually related to digestive problems (aerophagia, etc.), coffee consumption, alcohol, and stress.

Table 4.3 Electrocardiographic evidence indicative of the presence of ectopy or aberrancy, when early wide isolated QRS complexes are observed, in the presence of sinus rhythm[a].

Indicative of ectopy: ventricular extrasystoles

- Wide QRS complex not preceded by a P′ wave (premature ectopic P) (it should be confirmed it is not concealed within the previous T wave)
- RS morphology in V1: and QRS morphology in V6:
- Presence of complete compensatory pause.

Indicative of aberrancy: supraventricular extrasystoles

- P′ wave preceding a wide QRS complex (slight changes in the previous T wave should be identified)
- QRS morphology in V1: , particularly if QRS morphology in V6 is
- In the presence of wide and narrow premature QRS complexes, it should be checked that only wide QRS complexes meet Gouaux–Ashman criteria (see Chapter 3, Aberrant Conduction).

a) Specificity ≥90%.

If atrial PSVC are very frequent and premature, and especially if they occur in runs, they may be predictive of paroxysmal atrial fibrillation (AF) (PSVC arising in the pulmonary vein area in particular) (Figure 4.5, and see Figures 4.34 and 4.35). On some occasions they may trigger different types of atrial or AV junctional tachycardias. Treatment should be individualized and based on the presence of symptoms, left ventricular ejection fraction

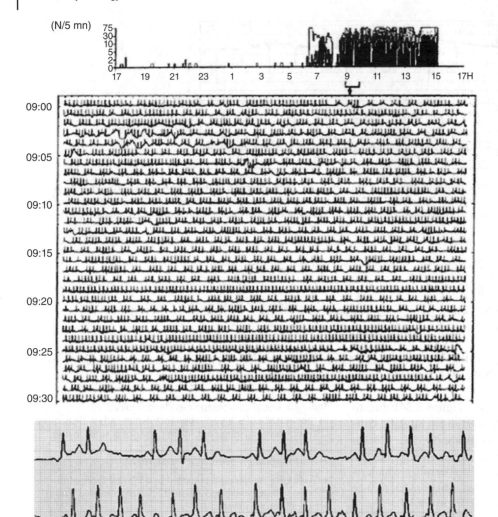

Figure 4.5 Taken from a 60-year-old woman with frequent clinical episodes of long-lasting supraventricular tachyarrhythmias (several hours) (see above). Holter tracings depicting incessant runs of atrial fibrillation.

deterioration or progression to sustained form of arrhythmias (i.e., paroxysmal atrial fibrillation). In the absence of heart failure or post-myocardial infarction, one approach may be if PSVC appear frequently and/or in runs, or are very symptomatic, to prescribe the "pill-in-the-pocket" approach (see Appendix A-5, The Current Role and Future of Antiarrhythmic Agents).

In cases of heart disease, patients with PSVC may receive treatment, if the PSVC occurs frequently and especially if the P-wave presents ± (biphasic) pattern in leads II, III and aVF (advanced interatrial block) (Figure 4.6). However, in addition to pharmacologic treatment; reversible triggering factors should be resolved (toxins like alcohol, coffee, etc.) and certain diseases

(hyperthyroidism) should be compensated first, reassuring the patient about the usually benign condition of PSVC. If there are signs suggesting that these are clearly related to sympathetic overdrive activity (exercise or emotions), β-blockers may be prescribed. In patients with advanced heart disease class I drugs have to be avoided.

Sinus Tachycardia

Concept

Sinus tachycardia is defined as sinus rhythm with a rate greater than 100 bpm at rest (in adults).

Figure 4.6 (A) Example of advanced interatrial block with left atrium retrograde conduction (P± in II, III, and aVF). (B) Associated atypical flutter. The association of advanced interatrial block with supraventricular arrhythmias (specifically AF and atypical atrial flutter; is known now as "Bayes' syndrome" (see later).

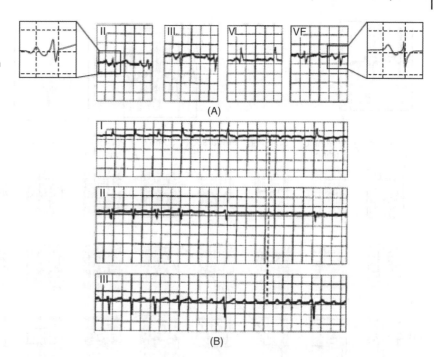

(A)

(B)

Mechanisms

Most of the cases of sinus tachycardia are due to an increase of sinus automaticity as a response to **different physiologic sympathetic stimuli** (exercise, emotions, etc.) (Figures 4.7 and 4.8), or other specific causes such as fever, hyperthyroidism, sympatomimetic drugs, pulmonary embolism, acute myocardial infarction (MI), heart failure (HF), and so on.

Occasionally, **orthostatism** leads to an exaggerated sinus tachycardia (postural orthostatic tachycardia syndrome (POTS)), which had been considered, due to an alteration of the autonomic nervous system (ANS), as probably related to a partial sympathetic denervation of the lower limbs (Jacob *et al.*, 2000; Karas *et al.*, 2000; Carew *et al.*, 2009). However, more recently it has been postulated (Fu *et al.*, 2010) that autonomic function is intact in POTS and that marked tachycardia during orthostatism was attributable to a small heart coupled with reduced blood volume.

In a limited number of cases, sinus tachycardia is present without an evident underlying cause. These cases are caused by an **inappropriate increase of sinus automaticity,** probably due to a lack of autonomic modulation of the sinus node or a **sinoatrial reentrant tachycardia** (Figure 4.9) (Gomes *et al.*, 1985).

Inappropriate sinus tachycardia is a condition characterized by persistent tachycardia above 100 bpm during the day and night. Its mechanism is not completely understood. However, a lack of autonomic modulation of the sinus node has been postulated as the most plausible mechanism. Usually the diagnosis requires Holter monitoring and ruling out extrinsic causes for sinus tachycardia as well as POTS. Available treatment includes beta and calcium blockers, a new drug called Ivabradine, and, in extreme cases, modification of the sinus node using intracardiac catheters (Femenia *et al.*, 2012).

Also, atrial tachycardia originating very close to the sinus node (parasinus origin) may present a P′, identical to sinus P wave.

Clinical Presentation

From a clinical point of view, sinus tachycardia is often asymptomatic. However, it sometimes causes palpitations that may be badly tolerated by patients. Very occasionally may trigger or exacerbate heart failure or be the mechanism for left ventricular dilation (tachycardiomiopathy) (Yusuf *et al*, 2005)

Generally, sinus tachycardia (see Differential Diagnosis) is the normal physiologic response to exercise, emotions, and stress. In patients with predisposition to a sympathetic overdrive (autonomic nervous system imbalance), an exaggerated response of the heart rate (up to 200 bmp in young people) to a specific level of exercise might be observed. It is sometimes related to the underlying condition (i.e., fever, hyperthyroidism, HF, acute MI, pulmonary embolism, sympathic drugs or drinks, etc.).

Cases of tachycardia during orthostatism are much more frequent in females (smaller heart) (see previously) (Fu *et al.*, 2010).

Rare cases of sinus tachycardia due to sinoatrial reentry generally occur as paroxysmal tachycardias (without heart rate warming up or progressive acceleration), and

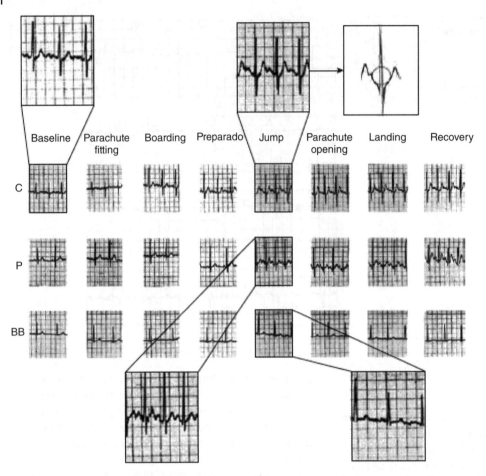

Figure 4.7 Sinus tachycardia in a 32-year-old man at different moments during a parachute jump: control jump (C), with placebo (P), and after taking a β-blocker (BB). β-Blocker (propranolol) administration leads to a less accelerated heart rate. During the control and placebo jumps, a typical electrocardiogram sympathetic overdrive pattern is observed (140 bpm), where PR and ST are part of an arch circumference (drawing).

may be initiated and terminated by programmed electrical stimulation or atrial premature beat. In both cases, the P wave has the same or very similar morphology as baseline sinus P-waves (Gomes *et al.*, 1985).

Electrocardiographic Findings

In the ECG, sinus tachycardia presents an increase in heart rate that occurs progressively in the majority of cases and persists over a certain length of time, with certain changes, until the triggering stimulus resolves. Heart rate during exercise, especially in young people with sympathetic overdrive, may reach 180–200 bpm. Frequently, a change in the morphology of the P-wave (more peaked) is observed, but it always preserves a sinus polarity (upright in leads II, III, and aVF) and shows a PR<RP pattern. If the P wave falls in the refractory period of AV junction and conducts with a long PR interval, this rule may not be applicable, resulting in a PR>RP. In this situation, the P wave falls into the T wave, hindering its

identification, although it may be correctly visualized with the slight changes of heart rate occurring with respiration (Figure 4.10). In such cases, in order to better visualize the P wave, an amplifying technique, a filtering T wave technique, or special leads (Lewis leads) are useful (see Appendix A-3, Other Surface Techniques to Register Electrical Cardiac Activity).

In patients with sinus tachycardia due to physiologic sympathetic overdrive (exercise, emotions, etc.), it is frequently observed that the PR and ST segments are part of a circumference, as the PR segment descends whereas the ST segment ascends (Figure 4.7 drawing).

Differential Diagnosis

The differential diagnosis between orthostatic sinus tachycardia and an inappropriate sinus tachycardia (IST) is based on the presence of tachycardia during orthostatism, as well as on the presence of signs of ANS imbalance during IST, such as in the intrinsic heart rate or in

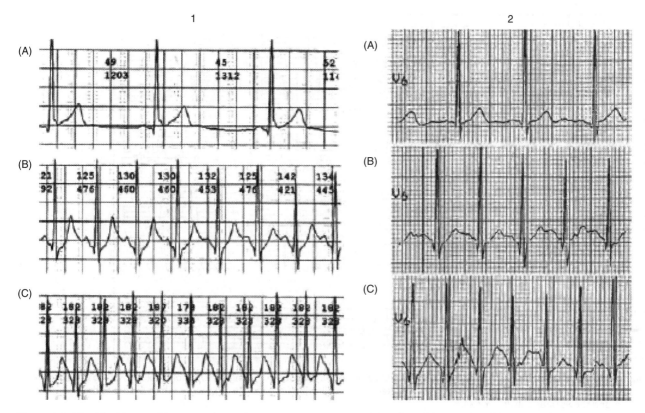

Figure 4.8 A healthy 38-year-old patient who underwent an exercise testing (2) and a Holter recording (1). (A) Recording at rest. (B) and (C) Note the different degrees of sinus tachycardia in both situations with a pattern similar to that in Figure 4.7.

Figure 4.9 Sudden onset of supraventricular tachycardia at a rate of 110 bpm with P wave identical to the sinus wave. This may correspond to reentrant sinoatrial tachycardia.

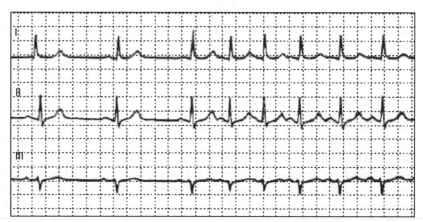

the total peripheral resistance (Morillo *et al.*, 1994; Brady *et al.*, 2005; Femenia *et al.*, 2012).

It is very difficult to differentiate by the ECG once sinus tachycardia is established, between: (i) a physiologic sinus tachycardia; (ii) an inappropriate sinus tachycardia; (iii) a sinoatrial reentrant tachycardia; or (iv) a focal micro-reentrant atrial tachycardia initiated in the upper part of the crista terminalis–parasinus origin. (Lesh and Rohithger, 2000). Each tachycardia present very similar electrocardiographic P wave morphologies. However, at the onset of tachycardia due to a sinoatrial

reentry, we can see more sudden changes of heart rate that are more abrupt than those caused by an inappropriate increase of sinus automaticity; even the increase in heart rate caused by physiologic sinus tachycardia is still less abrupt.

Table 4.2 shows classification of supraventricular tachyarrhythmias based on whether the QRS complexes are regular or irregular. In Table 4.4 the electrocardiographic diagnostic keys of atrial activity in different types of supraventricular arrhythmias are shown, whereas in Table 4.5 the electrocardiographic characteristics of the

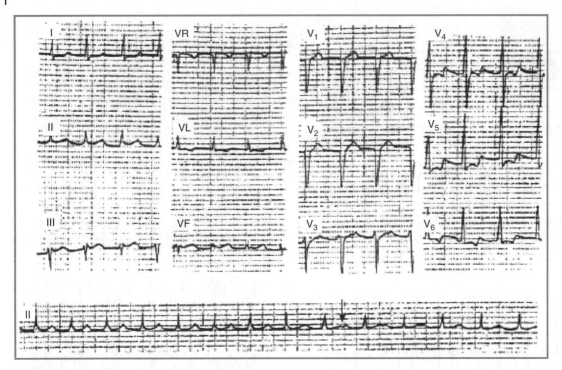

Figure 4.10 Top: tachycardia at 110 bpm with barely visible atrial activity (a notch following the QRS complex is observed in V3). Bottom; breathing results (II, continuous trace) in a slowed down tachycardia, allowing us to see the atrial wave, which is close to the end of the T wave, and shows sinus polarity (arrow).

most frequent types of regular paroxysmal supraventricular tachycardias with narrow QRS are established. Additionally, in Table 1.5 sinus tachycardia response to the carotid sinus massage, including reentrant sinus tachycardia, is shown.

Prognostic and Therapeutic Implications

Classic sinus tachycardia generally subsides when the triggering physiologic stimulus (exercise, emotions) or cause (stimulant drugs intake, fever, etc.) resolves. Nevertheless, in patients with significant sympathetic overdrive, sinus tachycardia occasionally persists for long time. It should be noted that sinus tachycardia caused by a great sympathetic overdrive decreases at night or at rest because of vagal prevalence. This helps to distinguish it from sinus tachycardia due to pathologic causes such as pulmonary embolism, hyperthyroidism, or HF, in which sinus tachycardia is more persistent. Holter recordings are very useful for recording the circadian changes of heart rate.

The prognosis of sinus tachycardia associated with different pathologic processes or heart diseases varies depending on the clinical setting and the heart rate. In patients with acute MI or HF, as well as in post-MI patients, the presence of sinus tachycardia is a marker of poor prognosis (see Chapter 11). A heart rate at rest ≥70 bpm in patients with chronic IHD is associated, in a 5-year follow-up, with a 40% increased risk of all-cause mortality and doubled risk of HF hospitalization (Ho *et al.*, 2010). Also (Bohm *et al.*, 2010), the SHIFT trial demonstrated that in patients with HF treated with ivabradine, heart rate decreasing below 70 bpm reduced mortality and hospitalizations by 25%.

Treatment for sinus tachycardia consists of suppression of the underlying triggering cause, if feasible (i.e., stimulant intake). Physiologic tachycardia disappears when the triggering factor is removed, as previously discussed. The treatment of a sinus tachycardia that accompanies certain pathologic processes basically implies treating the underlying disease. In patients with HF, IHD, and hyperthyroidism, β-blockers may be useful (Class I C). The efficacy of ivabradine, a specific and selective "If" current inhibitor, has also been demonstrated (Di Francesco and Camm, 2004)

Sinus tachycardia due to orthostatism (POTS) may improve with nonpharmacologic measures (salt, water intake, exercise) or pharmacologic treatment (flurocortisone, β-blockers, ivabradine, etc.) (Carew *et al.*, 2009). It has been shown that a low dose of propranolol (20 mg) provides a great clinical benefit to these patients (Raj *et al.*, 2009), and that exercise training alone (Fu *et al.*, 2010) improves or even cures this syndrome in most patients.

Table 4.4 Characteristics of atrial activity in supraventricular tachycardias[a].

Electrocardiographic diagnosis	Atrial activation	Morphology (II, III, VF)	Morphology V1	Atrial activity rate	AV delay
1. Sinus tachycardia (Figures 4.7–4.10)	Sinus	Generally, positive or ± in III. Rarely may be ± in II, III and VF	Positive or ±	100–180 bpm. Sometimes, it may be >200 bpm	Rarely present, even in the fastest types
2. Atrial tachycardia (Figures 4.11 and 4.12)	Focal origin (AT-EF) or due to an atrial macro-reentry* (AT-MR)	Depends on the focus location in cases of ectopic origin (Figure 4.15) Macro-reentrant tachyarrhythmias may feature different morphologies	Depends on the focus location (Figure 4.15) Macro-reentrant tachyarrhythmias may feature different morphologies	From 100 bpm till 200-220 bpm. Especially may be high in macroreentrant AT.	Sometimes, in the fastest types
3. Cavo-tricuspid typical atrial flutter (Figure 4.56)	Counter clockwise activation. This explains the lack of isoelectric baseline in the inferior leads.	Saw-tooth F predominantly negative waves in II, III, VF. No isoelectric baseline	Generally positive and not wide F waves, except in the presence of significant atrial disease	200–300 bpm	Generally present
4. Cavo-tricuspid reverse atrial flutter (Figure 4.60)	Clockwise activation. Generally permanent	Positive F waves in II, III, and VF, generally without isoelectric baseline	F waves generally wide and negative in V1, with no isoelectric baseline	200–300 bpm	Generally present
5. Atypical flutter[b] (Figure 4.61)	Probably a left atrial macro-reentry	Generally positive waves in II, III, and VF. Frequently a slight undulation is observed	Usually positive	220–280 bpm	Very frequently
6. Junctional reentrant tachycardia (JRT) (Figures 4.16–4.18)	Retrograde, either in the AV junction or in an accessory pathway	Concealed in the QRS complex or immediately after the QRS complex (AVNRT) or following the QRS complex (AVRT)	If the circuit exclusively comprises the AV junction, it frequently simulates an r′	Generally 130–200 bpm	In AVNRT rarely a block above or below the His can occur (i.e., 2:1 AVNRT). This cannot happen in AVRT as the ventricle is part of the circuit.
7. Junctional tachycardia due to an ectopic focus (JT-EF) (Figure 4.27)	Retrograde, except in the case of AV dissociation	Negative if retrograde activation is observed	Variable	100–200 bpm	AV dissociation due to interference is frequently observed (Figure 4.27)

a) Atrial tachycardias generated in the areas surrounding a post-surgical scar in patients operated on for congenital heart disease or subjected to atrial ablation procedures (atrial macro-reentry) (MAT-MR) may feature different electrocardiographic morphologies: the most characteristic ones are identical to those observed in the cavo-tricuspid atypical atrial flutter, although sometimes they may show the same morphology as the common or atypical flutter, or even AT-EF.

b) It is usually considered that its morphology cannot be distinguished from that of fast macro reentrant atrial tachycardias (AT-MR), and that both mechanisms are the same (generally left atrial macro-reentry).

Table 4.5 Electrocardiographic characteristics of the different types of paroxysmal supraventricular tachyarrhythmias with regular RR and narrow QRS complexes[a]

	Junctional reentrant tachycardia (JRT)[a]		AVRT[c]	Sinus tachycardia	Atrial tachycardia (AT)[d]	Junctional tachycardia due to an ectopic focus (JT-EF)
	Atrial flutter	AVNRT[b]				
Beginning of tachycardia	Usually initiated with a premature supraventricular impulse	P' wave initiating the tachycardia shows a different morphology, compared with the subsequent P' waves	P' initiating the tachycardia is also different to subsequent P' waves	Progressive P wave does not feature significant changes	Initial P' wave is identical to the subsequent P' waves	Initiation and termination usually abrupt may be gradual. Initial P' wave is identical to the following P' waves
Status of the atrial activity wave (P, P' or F) during tachyarrhythmia I	Flutter waves, generally two waves for QRS complex. Almost never 1 × 1	P' within the QRS complex = 65%. P' after but very close QRS = 30%	P' following the QRS complex in 100% of the cases, but with RP'<P'R	P preceding the QRS complex shows a sinus polarity. Almost always P-QRS<QRS-P	P' wave usually precedes the QRS complex, with P'-QRS<QRS-P'	It is generally concealed in the QRS complex or, more frequently, an AV dissociation is observed
Presence of ventricular block	Depends on the underlying disease and the heart rate	Rarely seen. Almost always features a RBBB morphology	Sometimes observed	Depends on the underlying disease and the heart rate	Depends on the underlying disease and the heart rate	Depends on the underlying disease and the heart rate
QRS alternant (voltage difference >1 mm)	No	No	20% of the cases	No	No	No
AV dissociation	Usually a 2 × 1 AV block is present	Never, unlike that observed in JT-EF	Never.	Generally not present	2 × 1 AV block may be present	Frequently, in many cases it is observed in heart disease patients.
Mechanism and clinical presentation	Atrial macro-reentry, usually in heart disease patients.	Reentry exclusively in the AV junction. Almost always paroxysmal	Reentry through an accessory pathway. Almost always paroxysmal	Generally, it is due to a physiologic increase of automatism.	It may be due to EF (paroxysmal or incessant) or to macro-reentry (MR).	Incessant types may be observed

a) Basal ECG with or without WPW-type pre-excitation.
b) JRT with circuit exclusively involving the AV junction (AVNRT).
c) JRT with a circuit also involving an accessory pathway (AVRT).
d) AT may be due to an ectopic focus (AT-EF) or an atrial macro-reentry (AT-MR).

Sinus tachycardia due to an inappropriate increase of sinus automaticity is the result of an intrinsic increase in sympathetic activity (Bauernfeind *et al.*, 1979). It occurs more frequently in young women who present palpitations, and, as episodes are frequent, they are often badly tolerated. Palpitations are due to abrupt increase of heart rate, for example, with emotions or light exercise. The diagnosis is made from both a clinical and electrocardiographic approach and it is done after ruling out other etiologies. Once established, the differential diagnosis by surface ECG with other types of sinus tachycardias (see before) is impossible. β-blockers (Class I C recommendation) and ivabradine are useful treatments.

The clinical significance and prognosis of cases due to inappropriate increase of automaticity and sinoatrial reentrant tachycardia are dependent on several factors: the number of episodes, the presence of heart disease, heart rate during the episodes, and the duration of the episodes.

In rare cases of inappropriately increased sinus automaticity or sinoatrial reentry (but not in cases of orthostatic sinus tachycardia), tachycardia control has been achieved by modulating the sinus node during electrophysiologic study (Lesh and Rohithger, 2000; Femenia *et al.*, 2012). In selected, very refractory and – in our opinion – exceptional cases, sinus node ablation and pacemaker implantation may be necessary, although the results are not very encouraging (Class II B).

Atrial Tachycardia

Concept

Atrial tachycardia includes all types of atrial tachycardias that present nonsinus monomorphic P waves (P′) on the surface ECG. Both the initial P′ waves, which initiate the tachycardia, and the subsequent waves have the same morphology (Figures 4.11 and 4.12; Tables 4.3 and 4.4). High atrial tachycardias originated close to the sinus node – parasinus origin – usually present a P′ wave that may be identical to a sinus P wave.

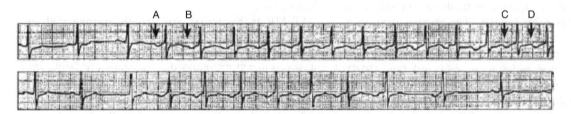

Figure 4.11 Upper tracing: a 20-year-old patient with dilated cardiomyopathy and incessant atrial tachycardia due to an ectopic focus. Note the warming-up of the ectopic focus (AB = 0.64 s and CD = 0.52 s). Lower tracing: after amiodarone administration, the focus activity is slowed down, with a progressive reduction of rate discharge. All of this suggests that the cause is increased automaticity (see Table 4.6).

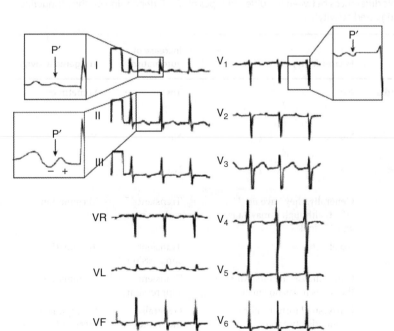

Figure 4.12 The P wave polarity is clearly indicative of its ectopic origin in the low right atrium around the tricuspid ring (negative P′ wave in V1, III, VF, and −/+ in II). Therefore, this is a clear case of monomorphic atrial tachycardia at a low rate (110 bpm) misdiagnosed as sinus tachycardia by the computerized interpretation as a result of the erroneous assessment of the polarity in lead II (−/+), which cannot be a sinus polarity. A stress test showed that the tachycardia disappeared when the sinus rhythm accelerated to a higher rate.

Mechanisms

There are two well-defined types of monomorphic atrial tachycardia (MAT):

o **Tachycardia originating in a small localized zone (ectopic focus)** from which it expands in a centrifugal direction (AT-EF). This may be due to an increased automaticity, triggered activity or micro-reentry. Its clinical presentation could be paroxysmal or incessant forms. Generally, the different mechanisms cannot be differentiated with a conventional surface ECG, especially when the tachycardia is already established. There are certain differences in the way they are initiated and terminated, and in their responses to different maneuvers and drugs, which may be indicative of the different types of tachycardia. The most important and useful differences, from a clinical point of view, are shown in Table 4.6 (Chen *et al.*, 1994; Wharton, 1995).

o **Tachycardia due to an atrial macro-reentry (AT-MR).** This is usually paroxysmal and is observed in patients with atrial post-surgical incisions, generally operated on for congenital heart disease or subjected to atrial ablation procedures. The reentry location is usually around a scar, either in the right or left atrium. This may constitute the most frequent organized tachycardia after pulmonary vein isolation (PVI). Tachycardia due to an atrial macro-reentry may present morphologies of different types of flutter, and even of AT-EF, by surface ECG (see later). Using electrophysiologic studies (EPS), it usually presents characteristics of macro-reentry, like atrial flutter (Saoudi *et al.*, 2001; Waldo and Touboul, 1996), but the location of the macrocircuit is related to the place (scar) at which the tachycardia originates.

Clinical Presentation

AT-EF may occur in all age groups and are seen particularly in valvular heart disease, IHD, and dilated cardiomyopathy (CM). In one study (Bazán *et al.*, 2010), patients with AT-EF from the pulmonary veins (PV) and the right atrium (RA) presented a lower incidence of heart disease (10–20%) when compared with AT-EF from other location (50%). **AT-EF may be paroxysmal or incessant** (Table 4.6). Tolerability to arrhythmia depends on the heart rate and eventual underlying heart disease. Incessant tachycardias are often associated with lower heart rate and frequently are well tolerated. On some occasions, especially when tachycardias are fast and long-lasting they may be poorly tolerated. This can lead to hemodynamic overload and left ventricle dysfunction.

AT-MR tachycardias are usually paroxysmal, and are frequently related to atrial post-surgical incisions or post-ablation procedures (see before). Similar to that observed in AT-EF, their tolerance depends on the clinical context as well as the duration of the tachycardia and the associated heart rate. As the heart rate is frequently high, the tachycardia is usually not well tolerated.

Table 4.6 Clinical, electrophysiologic and pharmacologic differences between the different types of AT-EF, depending on their triggering mechanism (micro-reentry, increase of automatism or triggered activity).

	Micro-reentry	Increase of automatism	Triggered activity
• Progressive acceleration and deceleration of tachycardia, both at the beginning (warming-up) and at the end (cooling-down)	No	Yes	Sometimes
• Initiation due to premature systole or programmed stimulation (PS)	Yes	No	Yes
• Termination due to premature systole or programmed stimulation	Yes	No	No
• Vagal maneuvers (sinus carotid massage)	Generally, they have no effect, although it may cause an AV block	Transient suppression	Termination
• β-blockers	No effect	Transient suppression	Termination
• Adenosine	Contradictory results. Most of the times it has no effect	Transient suppression	Termination
• Clinical presentation	Paroxysmal form is more frequently observed	Generally incessant	Paroxysmal or incessant

Electrocardiographic Findings

Atrial Tachycardia due to an Ectopic Focus (AT-EF)

P Wave Morphology in Sinus Rhythm

The P wave usually shows, in the case of AT-EF of the left atrium, the majority originating from the pulmonary veins, a prolongation of P wave that often notched.

The ECG During the Tachycardia

- **The heart rate and rhythm**
  - It is organized fairly regularly, although rarely the rate may be irregular especially in cases of digitalis intoxication (see Figure 11.13). The heart rate is usually not greater than 180 bpm. Typically, the AT-EF initiated in the RA presents a lower heart rate (usually ≤150 bpm), lower than the AT-EF from the left atrium (LA), especially those originating in the pulmonary veins (Bazán *et al.*, 2010). The latter may even present an atrial rate of over 200 bpm. In particular, in the case of incessant tachycardias the rate is not very high (100–130 bpm) (Figures 4.11 and 4.12).
  - Occasionally in the AT-EF, the heart rate accelerates at the beginning of the tachycardia (warm-up) slowing down prior to resolution (cool-down). This is not usually observed in the paroxysmal AT-EF caused by micro-reentry or triggered activity, although it typically occurs in incessant AT-EF caused by increased automaticity (Figure 4.11, Table 4.6). On the other hand, in those cases where the tachycardia is caused by micro-reentry, the onset is usually abrupt. Once the tachycardia is established the heart rate is generally fixed, and if it is caused by increased automaticity in particular, especially in the presence of digitalis intoxication, it may show some variations from one complex to another. At other times, the heart rate increases with exercises and decreases during sleep and under the effects of different drugs.

  - In cases where the tachycardia heart rate is not very fast, these can be mistaken for sinus tachycardia, especially when it is difficult to correctly visualize the atrial P wave morphology. Frequently, the atrial wave morphology, even if well seen, is not correctly identified in all the leads. Figure 4.12 shows a case misdiagnosed as sinus tachycardia not only by computerized interpretation but also by expert cardiologists. However, looking carefully at lead II we can identify an atrial wave in lead II with −+ morphology that is clearly of nonsinus origin. Therefore, relatively often it is difficult to recognize the morphology of atrial P′ because it is hidden in the previous P wave. It is then useful to perform vagal maneuvers or use other methods (see Appendix A-3) to try to visualize the P′ morphology, which is especially difficult in rapid paroxysmal tachycardias. Vagal maneuvers, such as carotid sinus massage, may help in distinguishing AT-EF arising from an area close to the sinus region from sinus tachycardia. While in sinus tachycardia the increased vagal tone may transiently decrease the tachycardia, in AT-EF there will be no response to vagal maneuvers.

- **The morphology of ectopic atrial wave (P′)**
  - The place or origin of AT-EF explains the morphology of the atrial P′ wave, both in paroxysmal and incessant types (Shenasa *et al.*, 1993; Kistler *et al.*, 2006). As the tachycardia is initiated and maintained in the same atrial area, the P′ wave seen in the first complex does not vary in the remaining complexes (Figure 4.11).
  - In most cases, an isoelectric baseline can be clearly seen in between the P′ waves in all leads, even when the rate is high. The AT-EF is characterized by a P wave, which characteristically is narrow (Figure 4.13), although sometimes may be wide and with notches (see before) (Figures 4.11 and 4.14, and Figure 4.69D). The P′ wave voltage is usually

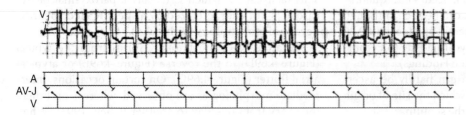

Figure 4.13 A 65-year-old patient with congestive heart failure (HF) and digitalis intoxication. An atrioventricular (AV) dissociation exists, as QRS complexes and P waves show independent discharge rates: regular RR intervals at 120 bpm with a partial right bundle branch block (RBBB) pattern (QRS <120 ms) and regular PP intervals at 85 bpm are observed. The P wave is most probably of an ectopic origin because it is very narrow (0.06 s) and presents the same polarity as the preceding extrasystolic P wave. An ectopic P wave at 85 bpm leads us to think that an exit 2×1 block of the ectopic focus exists, and that the ectopic atrial tachycardia has a rate of 170 bpm. Therefore, this is a case of double tachycardia: atrial and AV junctional ectopic tachycardia (or fascicular ventricular tachycardia) with a 2×1 exit block of the atrial tachycardia and complete AV dissociation. These arrhythmias are very suggestive of digitalis intoxication.

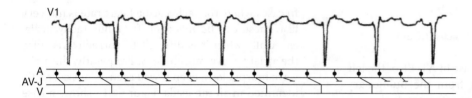

Figure 4.14 A digitalis-intoxicated patient with atrial tachycardia due to an ectopic focus at 175 bpm, with P waves that are different from the preceding sinus waves but not narrow as in Figure 4.13. The atrial waves present some variable cadence and different degrees of AV block.

low and the P′R interval is characteristically shorter than the RP′ interval, except when the P′ wave falls on the AV junctional refractory period and then is conducted with some delay.

- o **If the ectopic P′ wave is well seen, it may be possible to determine the origin of the ectopic beats, according the morphology of the ectopic P-wave, for example:**
  - (iv) **Negative or ± P wave in lead** V1 suggests that the tachycardia originates in the right atrium (100% specificity).
  - (v) **Positive or −/+ in lead V1** suggests a left atrium origin (100% sensitivity). The left atrial origin is even more probable if the P wave is not only monophasic and positive in lead VI but also positive in II, III, and VF.
- o When the focus of tachycardia is located in the upper region of the crista terminalis, the P′ wave morphology is similar to that of the sinus P-wave (see Differential Diagnosis).
  - (i) **The presence of a negative P-wave in I and VL** indicates that the origin is a focus located in the left atrium appendix, with SE, SP, PPV, and NPV >90% (Yamada *et al.*, 2007).
  - (ii) **If the focus is located in a low atrial region, the P′ wave will be negative in leads II, III, and VF.** These cases are very difficult to differentiate from junctional tachycardia due to an ectopic focus, where the retrograde conduction is faster than the anterograde, which occurs infrequently. In both cases, a short P′R can be seen, although in the MAT-EF it is frequently greater than 0.20 s (see AV Junctional Tachycardia Due to Ectopic Focus: Electrocardiographic Findings).
  - (iii) The exact place of origin can hardly be ascertained in the rare cases in which the site of origin of the tachycardia is near the septum.
  - (iv) Kistler (Kistler *et al.*, 2006) published an algorithm using the P-wave morphology to locate the anatomic site of origin of AT-EF (Figure 4.15)
- **The AV conduction**
  The AV conduction is often 1:1. When the rate of the tachycardia is high, sometimes due to the effect of

different drugs (digitalis), various degrees of AV block and even AV dissociation may be seen (Figures 4.13 and 4.14). The P′R usually is less than RP′ (P′R < RP′). (Figures 4.11 and 4.19D). However in cases of first degree AV block may be P′R ≥ RP′. In this case it may be difficult to make the differential diagnosis with other paroxysmal tachycardias, especially AVRT (Tables 4.4 and 4.5) once the tachycardia is established. As previously said, the mechanism of initiation of the tachycardia helps in understanding the mechanism of the whole arrhythmia.

- **The QRS complex**
  The QRS complex is usually equal to the QRS of the baseline rhythm. However, QRS complexes are occasionally wide due to an aberrant ventricular conduction. Sometimes alternating aberrancy is observed (bidirectional supraventricular tachycardia) (see AV Junctional Tachycardia Due to Ectopic Focus: Electrocardiographic Findings).
- **Carotid sinus massage**
  This has a variable effect (Table 4.6). It does not terminate the tachycardia due to reentry in the atrium, although it may provoke transient delay in the AV node. Usually produces a transient slowing down when the tachycardia is due to increased automaticity, but rarely terminates it. It usually terminates the tachycardia due to triggered activity.

Atrial Tachycardia Due to Macro-reentry (AT-MR)

This tachycardia, which is usually a paroxysmal tachycardia, **is not characterized by a specific electrocardiographic morphology (Table 4.4).**

The atrial wave morphology varies from the typical (Figure 4.69D) to the reverse (Figure 4.69E) or atypical atrial flutter (Figure 4.69G). On certain occasions, intermediate morphologies are observed, whereas on others they vary from one day to another (Chen, 1994). When the atrial rate is very high (>200 bpm), arrhythmic is called atypical atrial flutter (Figure 4.69G).

Different degrees of AV node delay are present (Figure 4.69).

AT-MR behavior in an electrophysiology laboratory is more comparable to a flutter than an atrial tachycardia

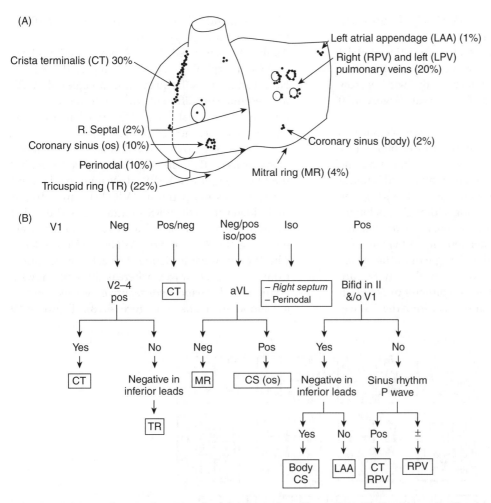

Figure 4.15 (A) Most frequent locations of atrial tachycardias of focal origin. (B) Algorithm to localize the most frequent sites of origin of tachycardias based on P′ wave morphology in V1 (see location inside the figure) (adapted from Kistler *et al.*, 2006).

due to an ectopic focus (AT-EF). Electrophysiologic studies may distinguish the macro-reentrant mechanism, including atrial flutter and AT-MR, from AT-EF. The presence of electrical activity throughout the cycle of the tachycardia and the evidence that an anatomic/functional obstacle exists support the macro-reentrant circuit. Occasionally, more than one mechanism causes the arrhythmia, which explains why the P wave morphology in the ECG may change from one day to another (Saoudi *et al.*, 2001; Waldo and Touboul, 1996).

Differential Diagnosis

Differential diagnosis of AT should be done with other supraventricular tachycardias with narrow QRS complexes (Tables 4.4 and 4.5).

AT-MRs, as previously mentioned, are usually paroxysmal tachycardias and show electrocardiographic and electrophysiologic characteristics more similar to the characteristics of the different forms of flutter than to

those of AT-EF. **Therefore, the ECG differential diagnosis of AT-MR will not be discussed here.**

AT-EF includes both paroxysmal and incessant tachycardias (Table 4.6). Comment will be made on the differential diagnosis in both cases.

- **Paroxysmal atrial tachycardia due to an ectopic focus (P-AT-EF)**
  The algorithm shown in Figure 4.70 and Tables 4.4 and 4.5 comprises the differential characteristics of the most frequent regular paroxysmal tachyarrhythmias with narrow QRS complexes. The specific parameters of atrial activity in the different monomorphic supraventricular tachycardias are provided in Table 4.4, whereas Table 4.6 shows the differences between the types of AT-EF, according to their underlying mechanism. When the atrial activity is visible, the differential diagnosis is quite simple. However, if it is not visible the diagnosis may be very difficult, although the carotid sinus massage as well as other clinical and

electrocardiographic data may be of help (Figures 1.15 and 4.70 and Tables 1.5, 4.4, and 4.5).

We will review some of the characteristics of atrial activity, as this helps to perform the differential diagnosis between all types of tachycardia with narrow QRS complexes and regular RR intervals (Figure 4.70 and Tables 4.4 and 4.5):

○ In the AT-EF, heart rate is usually variable but less than 180 bpm, except in some cases of pulmonary vein–LA tachycardia. The P′ wave initiating the tachycardia is equal to those that follow and is found before the QRS complex (generally, P′R < RP′). The PR interval is not usually long, although it is longer than in the rare cases of junctional tachycardia due to ectopic focus with faster retrograde than anterograde conduction. The site of origin of the tachycardia accounts for the P′ wave morphology (Figure 4.15). However, it is sometimes difficult to ascertain that ectopic P′ exists because it is within the T wave.

More frequently, P′ wave is visible, but it is difficult to see the morphology clearly.

○ As already mentioned, AT-MR may sometimes have an ECG morphology similar to that of the AT-EF. However, the most frequent morphologies of MAT-MR resemble the different types of flutter (common, reverse, and atypical flutter) (see Atrial Tachycardia Due to Macro-reentry (AT-MR).

○ In the case of paroxysmal AV junctional reentrant tachycardias (JRT), the atrial activity is: (i) behind the QRS complex (P′R>RP′) (AV junctional circuit with an accessory pathway-AVRT) (Figure 4.16), or (ii) hidden within the QRS, or attached to the end of it, resembling an "s" or "r′" wave (circuit exclusively involving the AV junction-AVNRT) (Figure 4.17). The P or P′ wave initiating the tachycardia differs from consecutive waves; whereas the first shows a craniocaudal shape, consecutive waves display a caudocranial shape (Figure 4.18). Figure 4.19

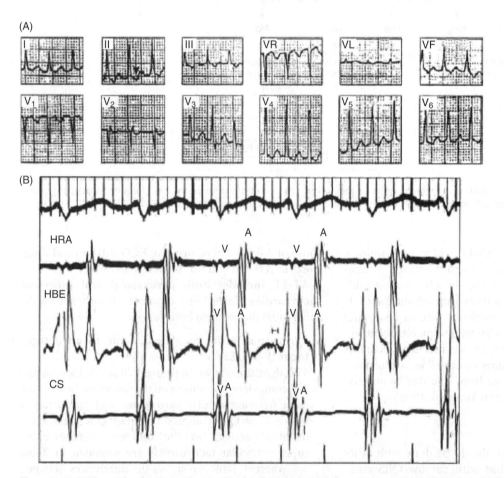

Figure 4.16 (A) Example of junctional paroxysmal tachycardia with left accessory pathway (Kent bundle) in the reentrant circuit. The QRS complex is narrow and the ectopic P is negative in I, II, III, VF, and V6 (arrow), with RP′<P′R. In V3 the QRS complex alternans is presumed (see Figure 4.18(C1)). (B) Electrophysiologic study showing an atrial retrograde activation being the left atrium the area first depolarized. As seen in the CS lead (distal), it is where the retrograde atrial activation (A) is first recorded. This may be suggested by surface ECG because in I and V6 the retrograde p′ is clearly negative (lead I and V6 are facing the tail of atrial activation vector). HRA: high right atrium; HB: his bundle; CS=coronary sinus (see Figure 4.18C).

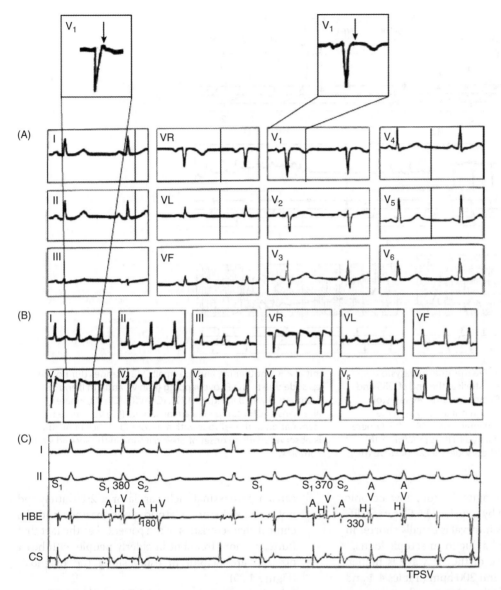

Figure 4.17 (A) ECG of a patient with no heart disease and episodes of paroxysmal supraventricular tachycardia. The tracing is virtually normal. (B) ECG during tachycardia: "s" wave appears in II and VF, whereas a minimal R′ is observed in V1 (pseudo r′-wave). Apart from this, no other modifications are observed in the ECG. (C) The same patient during programmed stimulation ($S_1 S_2$ at 380 ms): a significant AH lengthening is reported (180 ms) but no paroxysmal tachycardia (PT) is initiated. When extrastimulus is coupled at 370 ms, a critical AH lengthening (330 ms) is reached, initiating the junctional reentrant tachycardia with synchronic atrial and ventricular activation (AV junctional exclusive circuit). HB: His Bundle; CS: coronary sinus (see Figure 4.18B).

summarizes the P-QRS relationship in these types of tachycardias.

o In the cases of AV junctional tachycardia due to ectopic focus (Figure 4.27), the sinus P wave, or the ectopic atrial electrical activity (P′, "f" or "F" waves), are often dissociated. If this is not the case and retrograde conduction is observed, the P′ wave is not usually seen because it is hidden within the QRS complex. If the retrograde conduction to the atria is slower than the anterograde conduction, the P′ wave could be identified immediately after the QRS complex. Although this frequently happens in escape rhythms, it is infrequent in cases of AV junctional ectopic focus tachycardia. In these cases, differential diagnosis of junctional tachycardia ectopic focus (JT-EF) should be performed with junctional reentrant tachycardia (JRT) (Padanilam *et al.*, 2008) (see AV Junctional Tachycardia Due to Ectopic Focus: Electrocardiographic Findings) On the other hand, if the retrograde conduction is faster than the anterograde conduction, the P′ could appear before the QRS complex, but with a very short PR. In these

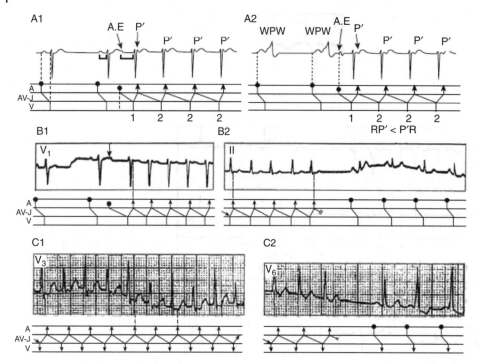

Figure 4.18 (A1) Onset of AVNRT. See the atrial extrasystole leading to a long PR interval, the P′ stuck at the end of QRS and Lewis diagram. (A2) Onset of AVRT. See the atrial extrasystole leading to a long PR interval, although not as long as in the previous case. See also the Lewis diagram, with RP′ < P′R (where P′ is separated from R and not attached to it, as in AVNRT). (B) Onset and termination of a AVNRT episode. We can observe the initial P′R lengthening and the small QRS changes during the episode due to the P′ overlapping (r′ in V1 and s in II and VF (compare A and B in Figure 4.17). (C) AVRT. (C1) V3, where alternans of QRS complexes are observed. (C2) V6, where the termination of the episode with anterograde block in AV junction is observed, with an onset of pre-excitation in the second sinus complex.

cases the differential diagnosis from low ectopic focus atrial tachycardia by a surface ECG is very difficult. However, the P′R interval is usually shorter in the junctional tachycardia due to an ectopic focus.

o In atrial flutter, the rate of the "f" wave is higher, generally between 250 and 300 bpm (Tables 4.4 and 4.5). Sometimes, when the common flutter waves are present with 2×1 conduction, they are assumed to be there, but are not always seen. However, if the ECG is more carefully observed, it can usually be presumed that they are present. The inferior leads frequently have a sawtooth morphology, without an isoelectric baseline in between and with a predominant negative morphology, whereas in V1 they are typically positive and usually have an isoelectric baseline (see Figures 4.56–4.59). On certain occasions, as in paroxysmal junctional reentrant tachycardia with an exclusive junctional circuit (AVNRT), a flutter wave is located at the end of the QRS complex, simulating an "r′" (in V1) or "S" wave (in II, III, and VF) (also known as "pseudo-S or pseudo-r′").

On the other hand, if atrial activity is not evident and the serial ECG during both day and night confirms that the heart rate is fixed, this positively indicates a paroxysmal tachycardia or a 2:1 flutter, and not a sinus rhythm. Carotid sinus massage and the clinical characteristics of the patient (i.e., the fact that flutter is more frequent in elderly people with heart disease) are helpful in establishing the diagnosis (Figure 4.20).

In the case of reverse atrial flutter, the atrial wave (F) is positive in leads II, III, and VF. It is dome-shaped with a wide base and sometimes significant voltage, without an isoelectric baseline between them, and is usually negative in lead V1 (Table 4.4 and see Figure 4.60).

One type of atypical flutter may be observed, in cases of advanced interatrial block with left atrial retrograde conduction, and also after AF ablation (PVI). The morphology of atrial waves is negative in lead 1 and positive in II, III, VF, and VI (Figure 4.61). In fact, there is no real difference between some types of AT-MR and one type atypical flutter (Daubert, 1996). The name atypical flutter may be used when the rate of atrial wave is faster (>220 bpm) (see Electrocardiographic Findings AT-MR) (Figure 4.6, and see Figures 4.61 and 4.69G) and when flutter waves are positive in inferior leads and V1 (Figure 4.61).

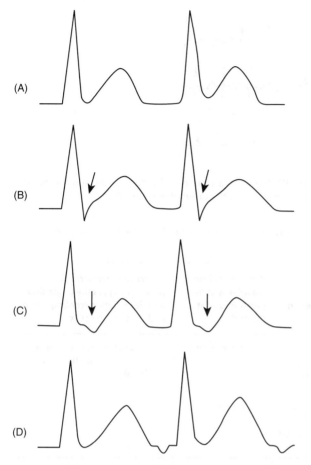

Figure 4.19 Location of P′ waves in paroxysmal supraventricular tachycardias. (A) Nonvisible P′ wave, hidden by the QRS (circuit exclusively involving the AV junction). (B) P′ wave that distorts the end of the QRS (simulating that it ends with an S wave) (circuit exclusively involving the junction as well). (C) P′ wave separated from the QRS, but with RP′ < P′R (reentrant) (circuit involving an accessory pathway). (D) P′ wave preceding the QRS, with P′R <RP′ (atrial circuit or atrial ectopic focus).

o Finally, sinus tachycardia should not be forgotten. If atrial activity is visible and sinus polarity is confirmed, this is probably the correct diagnosis.

However, it should be noted that parasinus atrial focal tachycardias usually feature sinus polarity (see Sinus Tachycardia). Occasionally, the sinus P wave is hidden by the preceding T wave. Careful examination of the ECG and simple maneuvers (such as breathing) (Figure 4.10), as well as determining whether the P wave appears when the heart rate decreases in the case of an exercise test (Figure 4.8), may help to establish the correct diagnosis.

- **Incessant atrial tachycardia due to an ectopic focus (I-AT-EF)**

In this case the heart rate typically varies between 90 and 150 bpm and P′R < RP′. All the aspects related to the morphology of ectopic P′ have been previously explained (see Atrial Tachycardia Due to an Ectopic Focus (AT-EF)). The I-AT-EF occasionally is permanent, except when the sinus rhythm is faster than the rate of the tachycardia.

The main differential diagnosis of I-AT-EF (Figure 4.11) is with incessant junctional reentrant tachycardia (I-JRT), which once established also features a P′R<RP′ interval (Figure 4.21).

The I-AT-EF is characterized by:

o tachycardia onset not associated with a critical shortening of the sinus RR;

o the polarity of subsequent P waves is similar to that of the P or P′ wave that initiates the tachycardia;

o atrial fusion complexes are often observed at the onset or at the end of the tachycardia;

o heart rate acceleration (warm-up) or slowing down (cool-down) is often observed during tachycardia.

In contrast, incessant-junctional reentrant tachycardia (I-JRT) (Coumel *et al.*, 1974) (Figure 4.21) do not show any of these characteristics (Table 4.7).

Prognostic and Therapeutic Implications

The prognosis depends on the heart rate, the underlying pathology, and whether the tachycardias are paroxysmal or incessant. Paroxysmal AT-EF (see Atrial tachycardia: Concept) are more frequently due to micro-reentrant or

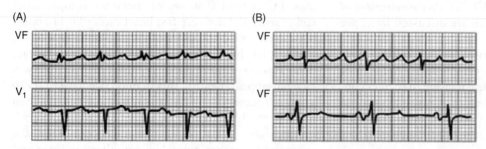

Figure 4.20 (A) VF and V1 in a patient with HF and fixed ventricular rate throughout a 24-h examination. This led us to suspect that the rhythm was not sinus, although a possible sinus P wave around 120 bpm might be inferred in V1. The compression of the carotid sinus blocked the AV node temporarily, which allowed for the identification of "f" waves from an atypical flutter (VF, B top). The cardioversion successfully restored sinus rhythm. Note the P± waves in II, III, and VF corresponding to an advanced interatrial block with retrograde conduction to the left atrium (VF, B bottom).

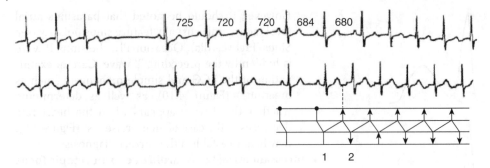

Figure 4.21 Holter continuous recording. Incessant JRT of the fast-slow type JRT. The accessory bundle with slow conduction constitutes the retrograde arm of the circuit (see Figure 3.10). Bottom: Lewis diagram corresponding to the onset of one episode.

Table 4.7 Differential diagnosis between incessant AV junctional reentrant tachycardia and incessant tachycardia due to an atrial ectopic focus

	There is a sinus heart rate increase prior to onset of the tachycardia	Polarity of the P waves following the P-P′ triggering the tachycardia	Presence of fusion complexes at the beginning or at the end	Progressive acceleration (warming-up) at the beginning and deceleration (cooling-down) at the end of the crises
• Incessant tachycardia due to an atrial ectopic focus (Figure 4.11)	Sinus heart rate is not accelerated prior to tachycardia initiation	Polarity of the P′ wave triggering the tachycardia is the same as that from the successive waves	May be present	Yes. Especially in cases due to increase of automaticity (see Table 4.6)
• Incessant AV junctional reentrant tachycardia (I-JRT) (Figure 4.21)	Sinus heart rate is accelerated prior to tachycardia initiation	Polarity of the P or P′ wave triggering the tachycardia is not the same as that from the successive P′ waves	Not present	No

triggered activity mechanisms (Table 4.6). Frequently, and particularly when they are the result of increased automaticity, they are considered incessant tachycardias, at least during certain periods (see Atrial Tachycardia).

Cases with a higher heart rate usually correspond to AT-EF arising from pulmonary veins (Bazán *et al.*, 2010). Some of these cases may also present paroxysmal AF. Although both arrhythmias AT-EF and AF are two different clinical entities, the origin in both cases is due to increased automaticity of one (AT) or several (AF) ectopic focus (Kistler *et al.*, 2006). Other mechanism of AF initiation and maintenance are discussed later; see also Figure 3.14.

The prognosis and treatment of paroxysmal atrial tachycardia either due to an ectopic focus (AT-EF) or AT-MR resulting from a surgical incision to correct congenital heart diseases or post-ablation procedures, or in the setting of different heart disease or other etiologies depend, especially, on the tachycardia rate and the patient's clinical condition.

In the case of a stable patient, a paroxysmal episode may be treated, if vagal maneuvers fail, with adenosine, β-blockers, or amiodarone (Class II aC). However, pharmacologic treatment is often not useful.

If the tachycardia rate is high and is not well tolerated, electrical cardioversion (CV) may be required (Class I B). Later, ablation techniques should be considered to resolve the arrhythmia (Class I A), usually with a high success rate. Detailed location and/or mapping of the ectopic focus or the circuit, which is sometimes complex, is necessary for successful ablation (Lindsay, 2007).

Most incessant AT-EF are well tolerated because heart rate is not usually very high (see Atrial Tachycardia: Concept) (Figures 4.11 and 4.12). In check-up screenings, ECGs with P waves of incessant ectopic atrial tachycardia and not very fast heart rates (90–110 bpm) have been found in 0.33% of cases (Poutiainen *et al.*, 1999). It has been observed that the ectopic focus rate decreases over time and many of these tachycardias will likely disappear. Bearing this in mind, we have to try to avoid permanent drug treatment in these cases. When needed, amiodarone may be an option, or β-blockers if symptomatic. Ablation is currently considered the choice of treatment given low complication rates and high successful results. Sometimes, ablation is indicated even if the patient is asymptomatic, in order to prevent atrial or ventricular dysfunction (tachycardia myopathy).

Junctional Reentrant (Reciprocating) Tachycardia

No consensus has been reached with regard to the most appropriate name for tachycardias due to reentrant mechanisms, whose circuits are exclusively located in the AV junction or involve an accessory pathway (Figure 3.8). However, the most accepted names according to guidelines (see Recommended General Bibliography p. xvii) are junctional AV reentrant (reciprocating) tachycardia with a circuit exclusively involving the AV junction (AV node) (AVNRT) and "junctional reentrant (reciprocating) tachycardia with a circuit involving accessory pathways" (AVRT). We consider that the acronym JRT-E (junctional reentrant tachycardia with a circuit exclusively in the AV junction) and JRT-AP (junctional reentrant tachycardia with a circuit involving accessory pathways) better express the mechanisms of both arrhythmias. We will use both acronyms AVNRT (JRT-E) and AVRT (JRT-AP) because we prefer that the reader chose which he/she considers the best.

Concept

These types of tachycardias include all the reentrant tachycardias involving the AV junction. The reentrant circuit may exclusively involve the AV junction (AVNRT) (JRT-E) or also an accessory pathway (AVRT) (JRT-AP) (Figures 4.16 and 4.17).

Mechanism

The tachycardias may be of the slow-fast type (paroxysmal tachycardias) (Figures 4.16–4.18), which are much more frequent and often have characteristic clinical features (sudden onset, etc.) (Josephson, 1978; Wu *et al.*, 1978; Bar *et al.*, 1984), or fast-slow (incessant or permanent tachycardias) (Figure 4.21), which are much less frequent (Coumel *et al.*, 1974) (see Chapter 3, Reentry). The latter are more frequently observed in children, as a form of incessant tachycardia.

There is evidence to support that fast (β) and slow (α) conduction pathways comprise different anatomic structures and that they are not the expression of a physiologic longitudinal dissociation of the AV node only. It is now known that in JRTs with circuits exclusively in the AV junction, the circuit comprises more than just the AV node (see Figure 2.6). For this reason, we are speaking about AV junctional and not intranodal reentrant tachycardias (see Chapter 2, Anatomy of the Specific Conduction System: Atrioventricular Junction) (Inoue and Becker, 1998; Katritsis and Becker, 2007).

Paroxysmal Tachycardias

In all cases, tachycardia is initiated when there is a unidirectional block (anterograde) in some part of the circuit.

When the circuit exclusively involves the AV junction (see Figure 3.8A), the block takes place in the AV junction where the β pathway is located (see Figure 2.6). The same β pathway is used by the stimulus to reenter. This **slow-fast tachycardia** is thus characterized by a long AH (atrial–His) interval and a short HA interval (His–atrial), as shown in Figure 4.17C. In this figure, it may be observed that when there is a critical lengthening of the AH interval (330 ms), the reentrant tachycardia begins with a short HA conduction (short HA interval) (slow-fast tachycardia) (see Figures 3.8A, 3.9A, 4.18A, and 4.18B). The fact that the atrial retrograde activation does not always take place in the same location (generally in the lower right atrial septal zone, but sometimes in the coronary sinus with a slightly longer HA interval), confirms that the circuit has an anatomic basis and that it is not always exactly the same.

When a Kent bundle-type accessory pathway is involved in the circuit, the anterograde block generally occurs in the accessory pathway and the stimulus reaches the ventricles through the normal AV conduction. The stimulus reenters retrogradely over an accessory pathway. The retrograde atrial activation shows a longer HA interval than when the circuit exclusively involves the AV junction, as the circuit is larger (compare Figures 4.16B and 4.17C). Later, the stimulus reaches the ventricles again (Figure 4.18(A2)). Because the anterograde conduction is through the normal AV junction, paroxysmal tachycardias with the involvement of an accessory pathway have a narrow QRS complex, although very often a pre-excitation delta wave is observed in the ECG without tachycardia (Wolff–Parkinson–White (WPW) syndrome) (see Chapter 8, Table 9.1, and Figure 4.18(A2) and (C2)). Only in very few cases showing anterograde conduction through the accessory pathway can a wide QRS complex be observed during tachycardia (see Figure 5.26) (also known as "antidromic tachycardias").

The onset of paroxysmal junctional reentrant tachycardias (Figure 4.18) is triggered by a premature impulse, which is more often supraventricular than ventricular (see Figure 1.18 B). It is blocked anterogradely in the β pathway (AVNRT) or in an accessory pathway (AVRT), and reenters retrogradely by the same β pathway (AVNRT) or over an accessory pathway (AVRT) (slow-fast type) (see Figure 3.9). The end of the tachycardia occurs as a consequence of a block in some part of the circuit, usually in the AV junction itself (Figure 4.18(B2)).

Paroxysmal junctional reentrant tachycardias may be initiated and terminated by programmed electrical stimulation. The premature stimulus acts as an atrial extrasystole, triggering the tachycardia when it causes a critical lengthening of the AH interval (330 ms in Figure 4.17C). Reentrant atrial or ventricular tachycardias may also be triggered and terminated by a programmed stimulation, unlike the tachycardias caused by increased automatism (Table 4.6).

Incessant Tachycardias

Incessant tachycardias usually start as a result of/a critical shortening of the sinus RR interval (Figure 4.21).

In incessant or permanent tachycardias, the antegrade block takes place in the AV junction (α pathway) (see Figure 3.10). The stimulus reaches the ventricles by the β pathway and reentry was once thought to be through the α pathway (Coumel *et al.*, 1974). However, it is now known that the retrograde conduction takes place over an anomalous bundle with a slow retrograde conduction (Farré *et al.*, 1979; Critelli *et al.*, 1984). This anomalous bundle corresponds more to atypical pre-excitation than to the Kent-type accessory pathway (fast-slow tachycardia) (see Figures 3.10 and 4.21) (see Chapter 3, Reentry).

Clinical Presentation

Paroxysmal Tachycardias

These generally appear in subjects with no apparent heart disease. They characteristically present an abrupt onset, with a fast rate (frequently >150 bpm) and vary in duration, from seconds to hours. The patient often presents not only uncomfortable palpitations but also paroxysmal dyspnea that may require urgent treatment (see later). Long-lasting tachycardias are accompanied by polyuria caused by an abrupt atrial distention.

○ **Some clinical differences exist between the two types of paroxysmal junctional reentrant tachycardias (AVNRT and AVRT)** (González-Torrecilla *et al.*, 2009). AVNRT: (i) are frequently accompanied by a pounding in the neck due to the simultaneous atrial and ventricular contraction, (ii) occur more frequently in women, and (iii) appear at more advanced ages, rarely before the age of 20–30. On the other hand, AVRT: (i) does not usually present pounding in the neck, (ii) is not gender-associated, and (iii) may even occur during childhood.

○ It has been suggested that the AVNRT may be related to a post-inflammatory fibrotic process. This could justify the fact that they appear at a later age (≈20–30 years) when compared with AVRT, which may appear during childhood (Porter *et al.*, 2004). A similar hypothesis may account for some of the non-ischemic right ventricular outflow tract VTs (Kautzner *et al.*, 2003; Marchlinski, 2007).

Incessant Tachycardias

Incessant tachycardias present slower heart rates. The accompanying symptoms depend on the heart rate and especially on the number and duration of episodes (Figure 4.21) (see Chapter 1).

Electrocardiographic Findings

(Josephson, 1978; Wu et al., 1978; Bar et al., 1984; Marchlinski, 2009)

Paroxysmal Junctional Reentrant Tachycardia (Slow-Fast Type Circuit)

Sinus Rhythm

The ECG of patients with AVNRT is usually normal. A bigeminal rhythm with alternance of the PR interval and even sometimes two QRS complexes for each P wave, due to the special characteristics of the α and β pathways may be seen rarely. In nearly 40% of cases, a usually nonischemic ST depression negative and a T wave is present at the end of the episode (Paparella *et al.*, 2000). In AVRT a WPW pattern may be present, except in cases of accessory pathway with retrograde conduction only (concealed pre-excitation) (see Table 8.1).

During the Tachycardia

(Figures 4.16–4.19)

The heart rate generally varies between 130 and 200 bpm. The QRS complex morphology is the same as or very similar (see later) to the baseline rhythm when the circuit exclusively involves the AV junction (Figures 4.17, 4.18A(1) and 4.18B, and 4.19A and 4.19B), or when the accessory pathway only has retrograde conduction (see Table 8.1). If the baseline ECG shows WPW type pre-excitation, this pattern disappears during the tachycardia (narrow QRS complex), because the anterograde block is located in the accessory pathway (Figures 4.16B and 4.18C).

To determine which type of circuit is involved in the paroxysmal junctional reentrant tachycardia, it is essential to determine the relationship between the P′ wave and the QRS complex (Figure 4.19):

○ **If the circuit contains the AV junction exclusively,** then the P′ wave will be within the QRS in 60% of the cases, or will appear immediately afterwards (30–40%). In this case, the P′ wave may be mistakenly believed to be the end of the QRS complex. It simulates an "r′" in lead V1, a slurred "s" in inferior leads, or a notch in VL. Thus, in these latter cases the ECG is slightly different from the basic ECG (see above). All of these small changes are highly specific (≈90%) and show a high PPV (>90%), even though their sensitivity is lower (≈40–50%), because the P′ wave is frequently hidden in the QRS complex. The notch in VL may be considered to be the most useful criterion (Di Toro *et al.*, 2009) (Figure 4.19B).

○ **If an accessory pathway is involved in the circuit** that forms its retrograde arm, the path from the ventricles to the atria is longer, resulting in a P′ wave that is always slightly behind the QRS complex (Figures 4.16, 4.18B, and 4.19C). If the accessory pathway is found on

(A)
(B)

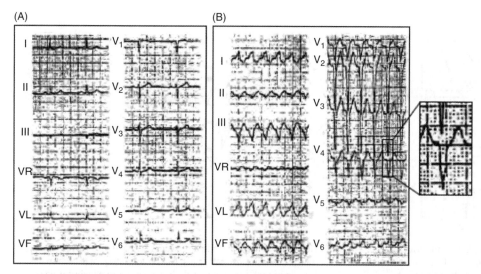

Figure 4.22 A 28-year-old patient without heart disease and a normal electrocardiogram (ECG) (A), who presented episodes of paroxysmal tachycardia with wide QRS (B). This is an antidromic tachycardia through an accessory tract (right atriofascicular pathway) (atypical pre-excitation), (see Chapter 8, Atypical Pre-excitation) that shows a morphology similar to that of an advanced left bundle branch block (LBBB), with wide QRS complexes and an rS morphology in V2–V4, as opposed to the relevant R wave in V3–V4 that is observed in antidromic supraventricular tachycardias over a long right atrio-fascicular tract (Kent bundle) (see Figure 5.26, and Table 8.1). Note there is a delayed transition to RS in precordial leads (R only in V6) compared with supraventricular tachycardia through normal accessory pathway that present a transitory to R already in V3 (see Figure 5.26)

the left side, the P′ wave is frequently negative in lead I, because the atrial activation occurs from left to right (Figure 4.16A).

Relatively often (≅40% cases) during JRT, ST segment depression appears but does not confirm the existence of ischemia (Figure 4.25). In the case of AVRT, the leads with ST depression may predict the location of the accessory pathway (Riva *et al.*, 1996).

If during the tachycardia, the AV conduction is over one accessory pathway (Kent bundle (see Figure 5.26) or a long atriofascicular tract (Figure 4.22)), the QRS is wide (antidromic tachycardia) (see Table 8.1). This type of tachycardia often involves other accessory pathways as a retrograde arm of the circuit (see Chapter 8, WPW-type Pre-excitation: Clinical, Prognostic, and Therapeutic Implications). These types of tachycardias must be included in the differential diagnosis of wide QRS tachycardias, along with supraventricular tachycardias with bundle branch block (aberrancy) and ventricular tachycardias (see Chapter 5, Classic Monomorphic VT).

When a bundle branch block morphology appears during a paroxysmal AV junctional reentrant tachycardia, the RR lengthens if the accessory pathway is on the same side as the blocked branch. This happens because the stimulus descending through SCS will have to cross the septum (a longer distance) to complete reentry (Figure 4.23).

If there is a baseline bundle branch block, the morphology of paroxysmal tachycardia shows obviously a wide QRS complex (see Figure 5.25).

Maneuvers in the EP Lab to distinguish AVNRT from AVRT and AT (pacing 20–30 ms faster than the cycle length of the tachycardia without interruption) allows the sequence of the return cycle to be determined. A V-A-A-V sequence suggests an automatic mechanism (AT) while a V-A-V sequence suggests a reentry mechanism (either AVNRT or AVRT). Subsequently, introducing PVCs during a His-refractory period, will allow differentiating the reentry mechanism. While in AVNRT there will be no change in the A-A interval, if the retrograde conduction occurs over an accessory pathway (AVRT), the A-A will shorten (Knight *et al.*, 2000; Michaud *et al.*, 2001).

ECG Differential Diagnosis

In Tables 4.4 and 4.5 all the electrocardiographic characteristics of paroxysmal supraventricular tachycardias with regular RR and narrow QRS are shown, including junctional reciprocating tachycardia, atrial flutter, sinus tachycardia, monomorphic atrial tachycardia, and AV junctional tachycardia due to an ectopic focus.

Figure 4.70 shows the step-by-step diagnosis of regular tachycardias with narrow QRS complexes. Some of the most interesting aspects of this differential diagnosis were mentioned earlier in this chapter. Some of the most interesting characteristics are now emphasized from a practical point of view.

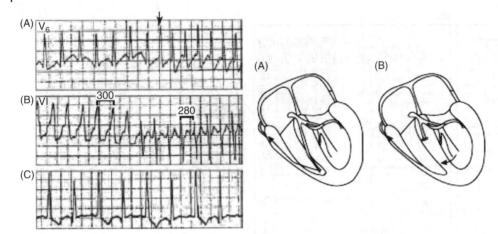

Figure 4.23 (A) In a patient with Type III intermittent Wolff–Parkinson–White syndrome with paroxysmal tachycardia episodes, a very fast tachycardia episode occurred. (B) A transient morphology of the bundle branch block, with an RR interval longer than that recorded before and after the block (300 vs 280 ms), was seen. The episode was terminated by performing cardioversion. In a Holter reading performed afterwards, the patient showed an intermittent pre-excitation (C). The prolongation of RR, when a bundle branch block occurs during a paroxysmal tachycardia of the Wolff– Parkinson–White syndrome, indicates that the accessory pathway is homolateral to the blocked branch, as in this case (B) the path that the stimulus has to cover is longer (drawing).

> Junctional reentrant tachycardias (JRT) usually have a narrow QRS complex, either when the circuit exclusively involves the atrioventricular (AV) junction (Figure 4.17), or when it also involves an accessory pathway (Figure 4.16), because the stimulus usually reaches the ventricles through the AV junction using a normal intraventricular conduction.

To a great extent, the location of the P′ wave contributes to the establishment of a differential diagnosis (Table 4.4 and Figure 4.19). If the P′ is hidden within the QRS complex or simply modifies the last part of it, it corresponds to junctional reentrant tachycardia with a circuit exclusively in the AV junction (Figure 4.19A and 4.19B). If an accessory pathway is involved in the circuit, the P′ is located slightly after the QRS complex, with QRS-P′<P′QRS (Figure 4.19C).

The presence of AV dissociation rules out the junctional reentrant tachycardia with accessory pathway involvement (JRT-AP), because in this tachycardia the stimulus goes from the ventricles to the atrium and back to the ventricles. Additionally, it is very unlikely that it is a tachycardia with an exclusively AV junctional circuit (AVNRT) because, as we mentioned before, at least some part of the atria (see Figure 2.6) is involved in this circuit (Tables 4.4 and 4.5).

The presence of alternating QRS complexes is highly suggestive of AV junctional reentrant tachycardias associated to AVRT (Table 4.5 and Figure 4.18C). This sign is very specific but presents a low sensibility.

The PR interval of the premature impulse that triggers the tachycardia clearly lengthens in comparison with the previous sinus PR interval. This is especially evident when the circuit exclusively involves the AV junction because, in this case, the premature impulse, usually one atrial extrasystole, initiating the tachycardia is completely blocked in the β pathway and travels to the ventricles through the α pathway (Figures 3.9A and 4.18A). However, when an accessory pathway is involved in the circuit, the premature stimulus may advance, although slowly, through the β pathway, which is in relative refractory period (Figures 3.9B and 4.18A).

Once established, junctional tachycardias due to an ectopic focus (JT-EF), with a retrograde conduction to the atria at the same or slower rate as the anterograde conduction, are difficult to discern from JRT with a P′ wave hidden within the QRS complex or immediately after it (Figure 4.19A). Recently, it has been described (Padanilam *et al.*, 2008) that in these cases the application of atrial extrastimuli during the electrophysiologic test may distinguish a focal origin, in which case the tachycardia cycle length does not change from a reentrant origin. In the latter situation the tachycardia is terminated or the following QRS complex moves forwards or backwards.

It should be taken into consideration that atrial flutter with a 2:1 conduction is a very frequent arrhythmia. Therefore, when we find a tachycardia with narrow QRS complexes, atrial flutter should always be ruled out, particularly if the heart rate is around 150 bpm, and especially if the patient is elderly and suffers from heart disease. In these cases we must carefully monitor the atrial activity (check for presence of "F" waves) and perform carotid sinus massage. (Table 1.5 and Figure 4.70).

Incessant Junctional Reentrant Tachycardia (I-JRT) (Fast-Slow Type Of Circuit)
(Coumel et al., 1974)

The ECG characteristics of I-JRT are the following (Figure 4.21):

o The heart rates are usually lower (120–150 x′) than in paroxysmal junctional reentrant tachycardias.

o The P′ wave is located before the QRS complex and, therefore, the RP′ interval is >P′R interval (Figure 4.21)

o The beginning of the tachycardia is associated with a critical shortening of the baseline RR interval. The triggering atrial wave is generally of sinus origin, although it may also be due to an atrial extrasystole or a programmed early atrial stimulation.

o The polarity of the initial atrial wave (usually sinus) is different from the remaining atrial waves (P′), which, as previously discussed, present caudocranial polarity (Figure 4.21).

o Generally, tachycardias occur in runs, which are usually short and separated by a few sinus impulses (incessant) (Figure 4.21). When the tachycardia is always present it is considered a permanent tachycardia.

Differential Diagnosis

It is important to differentiate I-JRT from I-MAT-EF. The most relevant data have already been mentioned (see Incessant monomorphic atrial tachycardia due to an ectopic focus (I-MAT-EF) and Table 4.7).

Prognostic and Therapeutic Implications

1. Generally, paroxysmal AVNRT are not life-threatening, although they can be very troublesome, because of fast heart rate, the duration of the tachycardia, and the underlying illness, if present. Cases with an accessory pathway involved in the circuit (AVRT) (JRT-E) may be potentially dangerous because in rare cases a rapid AF may be triggered (see later).

2. To terminate an episode due to a paroxysmal junctional reentrant tachycardia (P-JRT) immediately after it starts, it is necessary to block the circuit at any level, usually at the AV junction. This may be achieved by:

o Coughing hard five to eight times, or performing some vagal maneuver (oculocardiac reflex, Valsalva maneuver, etc.), may stop the tachycardia in about 50% of the cases

o Performing a carotid sinus massage (CSM), if feasible (see Figures 1.15 and 4.70).

o Administering drugs immediately, if the episode persists, to terminate it as soon as possible. Adenosine is the drug of choice giving its immediate action and rapid degradation (thermolisis). The doses could be started at 6 mg IV and increased to 12 mg IV (ACLS recommendations). Other antiarrhythmic drugs may be useful too (Alboni *et al.*, 2004). These drugs prolong conduction time in the AV node and increase anterograde and retrograde refractoriness in accessory pathways and in the AV node.

o If the crisis does not cease, after some time (from minutes to hours depending on the tolerance) the patient should be hospitalized, and if the tachycardia is of AVNRT type (this diagnosis may be suggested by ECG – nonvisible P′ or a slight change at the end of QRS (Figure 4.24)) intravenous adenosine should be given. The effects of adenosine are quicker (Figure 4.24) but it is not recommended for patients with bronchial asthma (Glatter *et al.*, 1999). Intravenous verapamil, β-blockers, and digitalis (Table A-11) may be administered as well, in case of AVNRT (nonvisible P′ or a slight change at the end of QRS) (Figure 4.24). **However, we do not recommend drugs such as verapamil, digitalis, β-blockers, and adenosine in case of suspicion, by ECG, that the JRT is of accessory pathway type (P′ after QRS), (AVRT)** (Figure 4.18C); because if the tachycardia degenerates to AF, these drugs may block the AV junction more than the accessory pathway (in fact, digoxin decreases the ERP of AP) and can increase the rate of AF, which can be dangerous. One option may be Type 1A and 1C, which block the refractory period of the accessory bundle but for us the best option is amiodarone (see before). The real risk of degeneration into AF is quite slim and blocking the tachycardia may be safe, even if prior pre-excitation has been observed. In the case of significant dyspnea or hemodynamic instability, urgent electrical CV is required (Class I c).

3. In patients with frequent episodes of AVNRT, especially if they do not stop coughing, the problem may be definitively resolved in nearly all cases by radiofrequency ablation techniques (Type I A recommendation) (Figure 4.25). Currently, ablation of the slow pathway is the most used technique, with a success rate of ≈98%, recurrences <2%, and incidence of heart block requiring permanent pacing <1% (Calkins *et al.*, 1999).

Decision making is less clear when episodes are not very frequent or are well tolerated. It is probably necessary to wait until the patient has had more than one episode and especially important to wait until the patient has taken a final decision. If the first episode was accompanied by severe hemodynamic impairment (very high heart rate, etc.) and/or in cases of specific professions (pilots, athletes, divers, etc.) the ablation may already be advisable. If prophylactic drug treatment is chosen, several options may be considered. Beta blockers and class IB antiarrhythmic

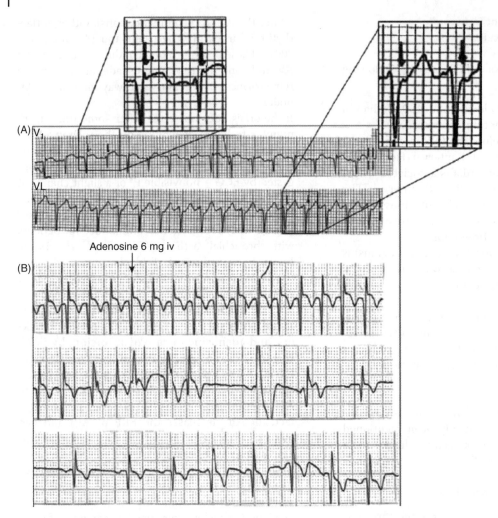

Figure 4.24 Electrocardiogram of a young patient with junctional reentrant tachycardia with a circuit exclusive of the atrioventricular junction (AVNRT) at 200 bpm (A) that ceases a few seconds after the intravenous administration of adenosine (arrow) (B) (continuous tracing). The notch in the end of QRS in V1 and VL strongly suggests the diagnosis of AVNRT.

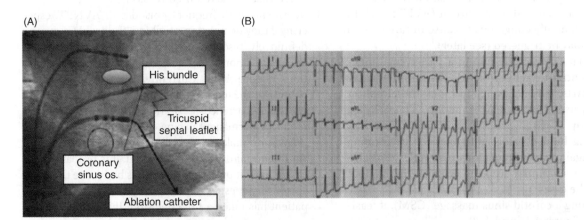

Figure 4.25 Ablation of a junctional reentrant tachycardia with a circuit exclusive of the atrioventricular junction (AVNRT). (A) Position of catheters for the ablation of a slow pathway. The image shows the placement of the catheters in an oblique right anterior projection, as well as the schematic radiologic anatomy. The ablation of the slow pathway is accomplished at the level of the Koch triangle, demarcated by the opening of the coronary sinus, the His, and the septal tricuspid valve. The ablation takes place at approximately 0.5–1 cm below the His bundle, in front of the opening of the coronary sinus. (B) Electrocardiogram during an episode. In V1, r′ is not seen because the P′ is hidden in the QRS (Figure 4.19A).

drugs are the drugs most frequently used by us, when not contraindicated (see Appendix A-5).

4. In the case of AVRT and with a baseline ECG showing a pre-excitation, we recommend ablation (Figure 4.26) (see Chapter 8, WPW-type Pre-excitation). This is because a remote but real danger exists whereby a new crisis of paroxysmal tachycardia triggers AF. This may be dangerous if fast anterograde conduction exists in the accessory pathway. The risk of complications from ablation techniques is very low (see Chapter 8, Arrhythmias and Wolff–Parkinson–White Type Pre-excitation: Wolff–Parkinson–White Syndrome, and Appendix A-4, Catheter Ablation) and when being treated at experienced heart centers there is no more risk in performing these techniques than the risk of AVRT itself.

5. We recommend taking into account the profession of the patient, when there are no episodes of tachycardia but the ECG shows a pre-excitation pattern. For instance, it is especially recommended for airplane pilots. Other factors to consider are age (especially in younger patients who practice high-risk sports) and the results of some tests. One exception for ablation may be when the WPW pattern is intermittent, according to the results of Holter monitoring, and especially when the WPW pattern disappears at a higher rate with exercise testing. However, it has been recently demonstrated that in young patients with an asymptomatic WPW pattern, performing the EPS may provide the best information to stratify risk: the presence of a refractory period over AP <240 ms, and the evidence that there are multiple AP, are the most important risk factors. Ablation was highly recommended if these risk factors were present (Santinelli *et al.*, 2009) (see Chapter 8, WPW-type Pre-excitation).

6. In patients with concealed WPW syndrome in which the accessory pathway conducts only retrogradely, intravenous amiodarone to terminate the tachycardia can be used. It is also probably an option to use drugs that prolong the refractory period of the accessory bundle like type 1A and 1C. On the contrary, is not advisable to use drugs that block AV conduction, such as verapamil, and digoxin to successfully terminate the episode of tachycardia. Usually, if AF appears, it will not be accompanied by rapid heart rate. However, in the presence of catecholamine stimulation, anterograde conduction may occur over an apparently concealed accessory pathway. Because of this, chronic prophylactic therapy with drugs that block AV conduction (verapamil, digitalis) are not recommended because, in these circumstances, in cases of atrial fibrillation, an excessive and rapid anterograde conduction over the accessory pathway can occur.

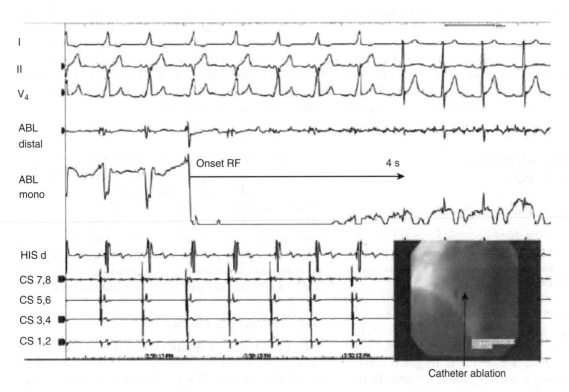

Figure 4.26 Ablation of right inferoseptal accessory pathway. After 4 s of application of radiofrequency energy, the pre-excitation disappeared and the electrocardiogram was normalized.

Therefore, in order to prevent a new episode from occurring, we use antiarrhythmic agents (AAA), such as amiodarone. So then, although a fast atrial fibrillation is very unlikely (as the accessory pathway only has retrograde conduction), ablation is generally recommended when there are frequent episodes. Currently, given high success rate and low complication rate, ablation is the preferred choice if anterograde conduction occurs over an accessory pathway.

> In cases of AVRT, after discussing the situation with the patient, especially in the case of young people practicing sports, we advise ablation in well-experienced centers after examining the results of the exercise testing, Holter monitoring, and electrophysiologic studies. This is based on the infrequent but real risk that the first episode could lead to a fast atrial fibrillation (AF) that, in rare cases, may lead to death.

7. The rare cases of JRT with anterograde conduction over an accessory pathway (wide QRS complex, antidromic tachycardia) should be distinguished from ventricular tachycardias and supraventricular tachycardias with bundle branch block morphology (see Chapter 5, Differential Diagnosis of Wide QRS Complex Tachycardias). Once the diagnosis is made, ablation of the accessory pathway is recommended.
8. In less than 5% of cases, JRT are incessant tachycardias. In these cases the circuit includes a slow anomalous bundle with retrograde conduction (fast-slow reentrant tachycardia). The type of circuit has to be confirmed by EPS. Ablation of the anomalous bundle, if it is demonstrated that it is part of the circuit, will resolve the problem.

> Paroxysmal atrioventricular (AV) junctional reentrant arrhythmias are generally of a slow-fast type. The electrocardiogram (ECG) usually reveals whether the circuit is exclusively of the AV junction or if an accessory pathway is involved. If the reentry occurs with exclusive participation of the AV junction, the P′ wave is hidden within the QRS complex or slightly modifies the end of it (i.e., r′ in lead V1). If the tachycardia occurs with the accessory pathway involved, the P′ wave will be recorded after the QRS but with a RP′<P′R and, in 20% of cases, alternans of QRS complexes may be observed in the ECG (Figures 4.16 to 4.18).
>
> Tables 4.4 and 4.5, and Figure 4.70 show the most important electrocardiographic characteristics of these two types of tachycardias, as well as the differential diagnosis with other types of supraventricular paroxysmal tachycardias with narrow QRS and regular RR. The location of the P′ wave is a key point (Figure 4.19).
>
> In diagnosing paroxysmal junctional reentrant tachycardias (JRTs), these may first be strongly suspected by history taking, especially when the onset and end are sudden, and because polyuria is observed especially in long-lasting episodes. Diagnosis of AVNRT is supported by the presence of pounding in the neck, and is more common in female patients whose first episode appears after childhood.
>
> In the majority of cases, ablation techniques resolve the problem (see Appendix A-4, Percutaneous Transcatheter Ablation). Ablation is the best solution for patients who tolerate JRTs poorly or experience them frequently.

AV Junctional Tachycardia Due to Ectopic Focus

Concept, Mechanism, and Clinical Presentation

Junctional tachycardia due to ectopic focus (JT-EF) is a rare tachycardia, which originates in an ectopic focus of the AV junction, as a result of increased automaticity or triggered activity (Ruder *et al.*, 1986).

From a clinical point of view, heart rate usually varies between 100 and 200 bpm. Generally, these are paroxysmal tachycardias, although there is one type characterized by nonabrupt onset and end (not paroxysmal type) (Pick and Dominguez, 1957), due to triggered activity that usually presents a low rate (100–130 bpm). In rare cases this tachycardia is incessant (see Prognostic and Therapeutic Implications).

JT-EF are observed in adult patients with severe heart disease, for example, acute MI and electrolyte disorders. It is also found in children, and in some cases is considered congenital (McCanta *et al.*, 2010; Dubin *et al.*, 2005). Nonparoxysmal types of JT-EF that present AV dissociation, were frequently seen in cases of digitalis intoxication. Currently, these tachycardias are not very common due to advances in the treatment of acute MI and to a decrease in cases of digitalis intoxication.

Electrocardiographic Findings

This arrhythmia is usually characterized by a fast rhythm (>150 bpm), a sudden onset and end, and often by AV dissociation. The atrial rhythm may be of sinus origin (Figure 4.27), ectopic atrial rhythm (Figure 4.13), atrial fibrillation (Figure 4.28A), or flutter (Figure 4.28B).

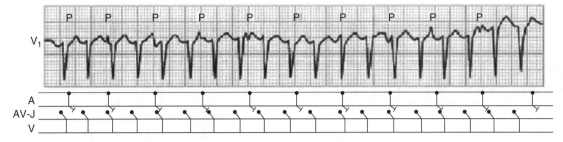

Figure 4.27 Example of a fast junctional ectopic focus tachycardia (180/min) with complete atrioventricular (AV) dissociation. Atrial rhythm is sinus rhythm.

(A)

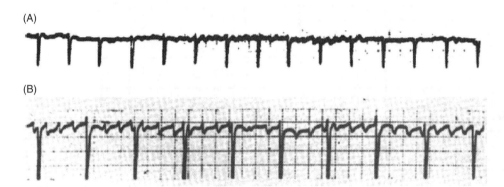

(B)

Figure 4.28 (A) Atrial fibrillation with regular RR. The electrocardiogram (ECG) is from a patient with a junctional tachycardia and digitalis intoxication who showed atrial fibrillation as an atrial rhythm. (B) F flutter waves of variable morphology due to drug effect (digitals) (p. 144) and changing FR intervals coinciding with fixed QRS intervals. This supports the existence of a junctional ectopic focus at a heart rate greater than 85 bpm that may be considered an active rhythm, that is dissociated from the atrial rhythm (atrial flutter).

Conduction into the ventricles is usually fixed (Figures 4.13, 4.27, and 4.28). When a 1:1 conduction exists to the atria and ventricles, the atrial retrograde activation is usually slower than the anterograde conduction. Thus, the P wave usually is located after the QRS, or it may be concealed inside it. In these cases when the AV junction is in refractory period, the application of atrial stimuli during EPS allows us to distinguish between junctional tachycardias of focal origin, where the tachycardia cycle length is not modified, and junctional reentrant tachycardias where the tachycardia is terminated or the next QRS is moved forward or delayed (Padanilam *et al.*, 2008) (see Junctional Reentrant Tachycardia ECG Finding).

The JT-EF that present progressive onset and termination (nonparoxysmal) usually have a slower heart rate (<130 bpm) (Pick and Dominguez, 1957) (see before).

Figure 4.70 shows how we can perform diagnosis of this type of tachycardia in a surface ECG in the setting of a step-by-step diagnosis of supraventricular tachyarrhythmias with regular RR and narrow QRS complexes. Additionally, Tables 4.4 and 4.5 show some of the most important aspects of differential diagnosis.

Bidirectional tachycardias of supraventricular origin are atrial, or more often AV junctional tachycardias due to ectopic focus with alternans ventricular aberrancy (right bundle branch block + superoanterior hemiblock, alternating with right bundle branch block + inferoposterior hemiblock) (see Chapter 5, Other Polymorphic Ventricular Tachycardia).

When the rate is between 50–60 and 70–80 bpm, it is considered an **accelerated AV junctional rhythm**, an arrhythmia that may appear in digitalis intoxication, acute MI, during anesthesia, and also in normal people. It frequently coincides with depression of sinus automaticity. Often, when the sinus rate slows, slightly accelerated AV junctional rhythms (60–70 bpm) are observed. In these cases, there is generally an atrial retrograde conduction, which, if faster than the anterograde conduction, shows on the ECG a negative P' wave in leads II, III, and VF with a very short PR interval. These characteristics are similar to low atrial ectopic rhythm (Figure 4.29). Occasionally, the accelerated idionodal rhythm competes with the sinus rhythm, originating numerous atrial fusion complexes (Figure 4.30). The rhythms of the AV junction that presents heart rates below 50 bpm are called escape rhythms and are studied in Chapter 6.

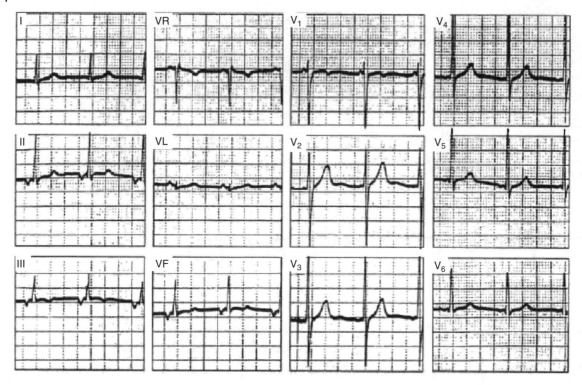

Figure 4.29 Electrocardiogram (ECG) taken from a healthy man with an accelerated junctional atrioventricular (AV) rhythm. Note the negative P wave in II, III, VF, V5, and V6, and positive in V1, indicating that the impulse is generated at the inferior-left-posterior area of the AV junction. The PR interval is short, lasting 0.10–0.11 s, denoting faster conduction to the atria than to the ventricles. Differentiation between junctional and low atrial rhythms is not possible in a surface ECG, although the PR interval in junctional rhythm usually is shorter.

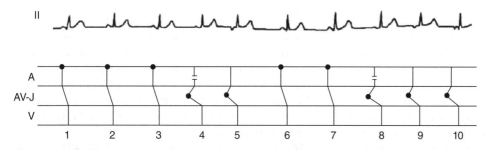

Figure 4.30 The sinus node and AV junction both compete to be the pacemaker at a heart rate around 65 bpm. The heart is at times commanded by the sinus node (Complexes 1, 2, 3, 6, and 7), and sometimes by the junction (5, 9, and 10). On occasion, an intermediate P morphology is observed (4 and 8) (atrial fusion beats). In the fifth and tenth complexes the junctional focus is accelerated, exceeding 60 bpm, showing a discrete increase of atrioventricular (AV) junction automaticity.

Prognostic and Therapeutic Implications

The prognosis depends on the clinical context and the heart rate. If the heart rate is <80–90 bpm (accelerated idionodal rhythm), the prognosis is good and the arrhythmia may disappear during follow-up. If a fast heart rate is observed, the prognosis is worse. Tachycardia that occurs in childhood, especially newborns, may be serious and may need very quick treatment. Sudden death sometimes occurs but it is usually due to congenital advanced AV block (Dubin *et al.*, 2005).

Pharmacologic treatment (especially β-blockers and/ or amiodarone) may be an option (Class II a C recommendation). It may be necessary to perform ablation, although it should be taken into account that there is some risk of causing AV block (Class II C recommendation). In children the incidence of AV block due to ablation procedure, is of 4% in the greatest series published (Collins *et al.*, 2009). In nonparoxysmal types, the first therapeutic measure is to reverse any possible cause of the tachycardia (electrolyte disorders, digitalis intoxication, acute ischemia) (Class I C recommendation).

Chaotic Atrial Tachycardia

Concept, Mechanism, and Clinical Presentation

This is an arrhythmia with a variable heart rate (between 100 and 200 bpm) due to the presence of three or more atrial ectopic focus.

From a clinical point of view, this is an infrequent arrhythmia. It usually occurs in patients with cor pulmonale and is associated with hypoxia episodes. Given the irregularity of the ventricular rhythm, the palpation may lead to incorrect diagnosis of AF. The most frequent symptom is the increase of dyspnea, which is usually present because of an underlying disease, particularly if a fast heart rate is observed.

Electrocardiographic Diagnosis

Electrocardiographic diagnosis may be made (Figure 4.31) when the following electrocardiographic criteria are met:

o Three or more different P wave morphologies.
o Isoelectric baseline lines in between P waves.
o Absence of a dominating atrial pacemaker, which means that there are no more than two consecutive identical P waves.
o Variable PP and PR intervals, which cause an irregular heart rate, sometimes fast and sometimes slow, which makes it difficult to clinically distinguish it from AF. At first glance, an incorrect diagnosis of AF may be made. It is important to avoid confusing different ectopic P waves and atrial "f" waves (see Atrial Fibrillation: ECG Diagnosis).

Prognostic and Therapeutic Implications

The best treatment for this arrhythmia is treating the hypoxic crisis. Calcium antagonists may be useful (Type IV drugs in Vaughan–Williams classification), at least to slow the ventricular rate (Table A-11). Types I or III drugs should not be administered, nor should Type II drugs be given to patients who suffer from cor pulmonale. It is important to perform the correct diagnosis because CV or ablation should not be considered in this arrhythmia.

Atrial Fibrillation

Concept

Atrial fibrillation, the most frequent sustained arrhythmia and truly an epidemic of the twenty-first century, is a rapid (between 500 and 700 bpm), chaotic, and disorganized atrial rhythm that results in loss of effective atrial contraction. Conduction to the ventricles is irregular and the ventricular rate is usually high (120–150 bpm). The clinical presentation may be paroxysmal persistent or permanent (Camm *et al.*, 2012) (see Atrial Fibrillation Types). Although diagnosis is made by ECG (see Electrocardiographic Findings), it may be strongly suspected during history taking and physical examination (sensation of palpitations – irregular and quick beats – and/or palpation or auscultation of a rhythm with these characteristics).

As the diagnosis is based particularly on the presence of rapid and completely irregular rhythm, it is necessary to rule out other arrhythmias that have similar features. This is usually easy with the ECG but often very difficult or even impossible with a physical examination alone. The following arrhythmias must be ruled out: (i) atrial flutter with irregular variable conduction, (ii) chaotic atrial tachycardia, and (iii) sinus rhythm with frequent random atrial extrasystoles (see Electrocardiographic Findings).

Atrial fibrillation has to be considered as a progressive disease, starting usually with episodes that are self-controlled (paroxysmal), and it is difficult to predict when these will repeat, but in at least in 10% of cases there will be recurrences at 1 year. Finally, in the majority of cases, with more or less time (sometimes several decades) the disease becomes persistent (more than 7 days) but with the option to cardiovert to sinus rhythm, or permanent, when all attempts to cardiovert to sinus rhythm have been abandoned, and a rate-control strategy will be pursued (permanent AF) (see later) (Camm *et al.*, 2012; Wyse *et al.*, 2002).

The epidemiology, electrophysiologic mechanisms, and electrocardiographic findings will now be discussed.

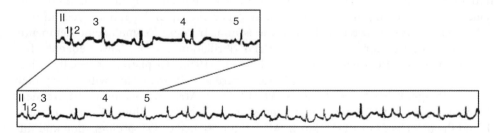

Figure 4.31 A patient with decompensated chronic obstructive pulmonary disease showing all the features of multimorphic or chaotic atrial tachycardia. Note the five different types of P waves in the first five QRS complexes.

The most important prognostic and therapeutic implications of AF will also be discussed.

Epidemiology and Etiology

Atrial fibrillation is the most prevalent tachyarrhythmia in outpatient clinics as well as in hospitals. However, the total burden of AF extends beyond its symptoms because around 30-40% of AF episodes are asymptomatic. These silent episodes may impact quality of life and cardiac function (Savelieva and Camm, 2000). Therefore, in patients at risk, especially those who suffer from valvular heart disease or have had a stroke, it is convenient to use extended monitoring to rule out the possibility of silent AF episodes.

Due to the long life expectancy, AF is now of great importance because of its increasing incidence, and the significant complications (HF, embolism) that may appear during follow-up. These are associated with a shortened life expectancy (see later).

At present, it is presumed that there are about five million people in Europe and more than four million in the United States with AF, and it is expected that in year 2050 there will be more than 7–8 million cases the United States. In Spain, the number of patients with AF is more than 500 000 (Moro Serrano and Hernández-Madrid, 2009). Atrial fibrillation increases the number of hospitalizations, which not only produces a problem for the patient but also increases healthcare costs (Reynolds *et al.*, 2009). The clinical profile of AF patients in Spain has been published (Alegret *et al.*, 2008).

Sporadic paroxysmal episodes of AF may occur in relation to alcohol intake and in patients with different diseases such as acute MI, pericarditis, hyperthyroidism, WPW syndrome, and so on (see Prognostic Implications).

Atrial fibrillation is very infrequent before the age of 20–30 years, including the sporadic appearance of paroxysmal types. Atrial fibrillation occurring in very young people obliges us to consider a genetic origin and leads us to rule out short QT syndrome (see Chapter 9, Short QT Syndrome, and Atrial Fibrillation of Genetic Origin) and other channelopathies. There are cases of paroxysmal AF occurring before the age of 40 that do not turn into persistent AF until more than 20 or 30 years later. Thus, a paroxysmal AF episode in the beginning may represent an isolated finding ("lone AF"). However, these patients may present risk factors (i.e., hypertension) or develop heart diseases that increase the risk of permanent AF years later.

The incidence of AF increases with age. It has been demonstrated (Martínez-Sellés *et al.*, 2016) that 10% of octogenarians suffer from AF, and the prevalence of AF in centenarians is of 25%. Although permanent AF may be an isolated finding, in the majority of cases it occurs in patients with heart disease, especially heart valve disease (mainly mitral stenosis), IHD, hypertensive heart disease, cardiomyopathies, HF, and may be also present in other specific situations.

In mitral stenosis, AF appears very often in the natural course of the disease and is usually accompanied by significant worsening of symptoms. Therefore, patients with advanced mitral stenosis should undergo a surgical procedure, if possible, before AF occurs.

In HF, AF is frequently seen, especially in advanced phases. Globally, it is present in 10–30% of cases and is an indicator of bad prognosis and poor quality of life (Niemwlaat *et al.*, 2009; Martínez-Sellés *et al.*, 2016) (see Chapter 11, Heart Failure).

Arterial hypertension is associated with a higher incidence of AF. It has been reported (Conen *et al.*, 2009; Barrios *et al.*, 2010) that there is a relationship between systolic, more than diastolic, hypertension and AF in middle-aged women.

Atrial fibrillation occurs more frequently in patients with ischemic heart disease. In acute MI, AF occurs transiently in 10% of cases. Its presence is a sign of a more serious prognosis (see Chapter 11, Ischemic Heart Disease).

Atrial fibrillation occurs in 25% of patients undergoing coronary artery bypass grafting (CABG) and some authors (Mathew *et al.*, 2004; Villareal *et al.*, 2004) have found increased risk of mortality, stroke, and congestive HF from AF after CABG (see Therapeutic Approach for Prevention and Treatment of Post-CABG AF). It has been demonstrated (Conen *et al.*, 2010) that higher birth weight is associated with an increased risk of AF during adulthood. Sleep Apnea increases the risk of post-CABG AF (Van Oosten *et al.*, 2014; Qaddoura *et al.*, 2014).

Atrial fibrillation and/or flutter may affect some patients with congenital heart disease, especially patients with atrial septal defect (ASD) over 50 years of age and patients who underwent surgery for some congenital heart defects (see Chapter 11, Congenital Heart Disease).

Atrial fibrillation occurs frequently in inherited heart disease such as cardiomyopathies, especially obstructive CM, and channelopathies (Chapter 9).

It has also been reported (Guglin *et al.*, 2009) that arrhythmias, especially AF and VT, may occur in relation to the administration of some chemotherapeutic drugs. Atrial fibrillation is especially frequent after anthracyclines (2–10%). Cisplatin, especially when used intrapericardially, is associated with a very high rate of AF (12–30%). Atrial fibrillation is also frequent with the use of melpholen, e-fluoracil, and interleukin-2. Also, the presence of QT prolongation and different bradyarrhythmias have been reported (Yeh and Bickford, 2009).

It has been postulated, too, that patients with sinus bradycardia and first-degree AV block present a higher incidence of AF (see Chapter 10, Severe Sinus Bradycardia). It has been demonstrated (Sadiq *et al.*, 2015; Enriquez *et al.*, 2014, 2015a) that the presence of interatrial block (P ≥120ms) is a marker of AF during close follow-up.

Persistent and permanent AF is more frequent in patients with alcoholism (Mäki *et al.*, 1998), obesity, metabolic syndrome, diabetes, renal impairment (Iguchi *et al.*, 2008), and chronic obstructive pulmonary disease (COPD) in people who practice competitive sports (Mont *et al.*, 2002), and in people with sleep disorders (Monahan *et al.*, 2009; Baranchuk, 2012).

However, relatively often AF appears as an isolated finding, especially in the elderly, or perhaps only in the presence of some risk factors. In cases of lone atrial fibrillation it seems clear that there is some genetic predisposition (Roberts and Gollob, 2010). In this case, if the heart rate is controlled, the patient may be asymptomatic and the prognosis may be good but needs to be treated following all the recommendations for stroke prevention (see Therapeutic approach).

Triggering and Perpetuating Mechanisms

In recent years significant advances have been made in the understanding of different mechanisms of AF. We may summarize saying that the process of triggering and maintenance of AF usually occurs (Figure 4.32) because in the presence of the atria "at risk" some trigger factors induce and maintain an electrophysiologic and ultrastructural remodeling of the atria, especially in the left atrium. Some premature atrial complexes, originating from different mechanisms, may then precipitate AF. This immediately starts the process that perpetuates AF and that may be summarized with the sentence "**atrial fibrillation begets atrial fibrillation**" (Wijffels and Allesie, 1995). To restore sinus rhythm as soon as possible, it is very important to try to start a reverse remodeling process, or at least try to avoid a deterioration of the remodelling process. Figure 4.32 summarizes the following concepts:

- **Atria "at risk"**
  The following factors contribute to the atria being "at risk" of developing AF:
  o In general, the presence of structural heart disease is an important factor, especially in cases of future persistent AF.
  o **Autonomic nervous system** involvement is crucial to modulate the arrhythmia onset. The reduction of the relative atrial refractory period, modulated by vagal stimulation, is very important for triggering atrial fibrillation (see later). A short refractory period favors the occurrence of AF, especially if it is nonhomogeneous through the atria, particularly in the case of coexisting atrial pathology. On the other

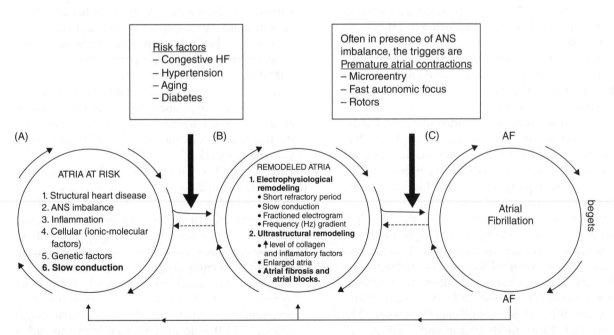

Figure 4.32 Summary of the pathophysiologic mechanisms involved in the initiation and perpetuation of atrial fibrillation. In the presence of atria at risk (see Triggering and Perpetuating Mechanisms: New Concepts) some risk factors maintain electrophysiologic and structural remodeling of the atria. At a certain point some premature atrial contractions, usually in the presence of autonomic nervous system (ANS) imbalance, may trigger atrial fibrillation. If the sinus rhythm is not restored soon, the arrhythmia is maintained by itself (atrial fibrillation begets atrial fibrillation) and becomes permanent.

hand, fast atrial activation of the AF leads to a shortening of the ARP, perpetuating the arrhythmia.

o Numerous studies have demonstrated that **inflammation** plays also an important role in preparing the atria for triggering and perpetuating AF (see later) (Issac *et al.*, 2007).

o There are some **cellular mechanisms** (ionic and molecular) involved in the development of AF, although they are not well known (Workman *et al.*, 2008). These include: (i) an increase in K currents (IKi, Ikr and Iks) favoring the shortening of the atrial refractory period and (ii) altered Ca handling, responsible for the TAP plateau, as well as Ito, which favors the TAP change observed during AF (triangulated TAP) (Drobev and Nattel, 2008). All these mechanisms work together with ANS imbalance to trigger the activity that initiates and perpetuates AF.

o The **genetic origin** of AF has been described in rare cases of familiar AF in young subjects and in lone atrial fibrillation (Roberts *et al.*, 2010). Similarly, new factors (ionic channels and sarcomere proteins defects, and SCN5A gene mutations) have been brought to light that may explain the AF occurrence in genetically determined cardiomyopathies and in channelopathies (Maron *et al.*, 2006; Otway *et al.*, 2007). Other genetic factors involved in the AF occurrence by decreasing atrial TAP, as well as the gain in potassium channels (see before), have been recently described (Tsai *et al.*, 2008). Finally, the importance of genetic factors has been shown in cases of nonfamiliar atrial fibrillation (Gudbjartsson *et al.*, 2007).

o Finally, has been demonstrated that in these cases there usually exists very clearly **slow conduction of the stimulus in the atria**.

- **Remodeling of the atria**

There are risk factors, such as congestive heart failure, hypertension, aging, and diabetes (Figure 4.32), that, when the atria is "at risk", contribute to the initiation and maintenance of the remodeling process of the atria. The most important aspects of this process are:

o **There is ultrastructural remodeling** usually in the presence of enlarged atria, especially the left, although the remodeling of the right atrium is important for the susceptibility to AF (Ishida *et al.*, 2010). This is expressed with specific characteristic changes such as clear LA dilation, atrial fibrosis increased levels of collagen and inflammation markers, and different degrees of interatrial block. The interatrial blocks are divided in partial (P-IAB) (P wave duration ≥120 ms) and advanced (A-IAB) (P wave duration ≥120 ms plus biphasic ± pattern in II, III, VF) (Bayés de Luna *et al.*, 1985, 1988, 1989, 2012). Figure 4.33 shows which are the patients with

A-IAB that are at higher risk to present AF and the pathophysiological mechanisms that favor, in patients with A-IAB, the appearance of AF.

Finally, the structural remodeling of the atria has been confirmed recently by contrast enhanced cardiac magnetic resonance (CE-CMR). Oakes (Oakes *et al.*, 2009) demonstrated that the presence of atrial fibrosis by CE-CMR is a very important marker to decide electrical CV and possibility of ablation. **Fibrosis (fibrotic atrial cardiomyopathy)** (Hirsh *et al.*, 2015; Kottkamp, 2013) **is a key factor for ultrastructural remodelling**.

o **There is also evidence of electrophysiologic remodeling**. This is explained by the electrophysiologic changes that occur in the atria, such as shortening of the atria refractory period, conduction velocity, alterations of the atrial impulse, sinus node dysfunction, and also the presence of complex fractioned atrial electrograms (CFAE). These are two or more deflections with continuous electrical activity distributed randomly chaotically that may trigger and perpetuate AF. Because they are difficult to visualize, special algorithms are required for this purpose. Changes of maximal frequency gradients between LA and RA reflect the existence of high-frequency (Hz) areas in the LA, whereas the RA is passively activated during AF. The sites of high-frequency activity identified by spectral analysis play a crucial role in the maintenance of electrophysiologic remodeling in AF (Sanders *et al.*, 2005). It has also been proven that in paroxysmal AF the pulmonary vein area is the place with dominant frequency differences (Arenal *et al.*, 2009). Furthermore, Stiles *et al.* (2009) have demonstrated that patients with lone paroxysmal AF also present an abnormal atrial electrophysiologic and anatomic "substrate" (longer atrial volumes, longer refractory periods and conduction times, more fractioned ECGs, and abnormal sinus node function).

- **Atrial fibrillation: initiation and maintenance (Figures 4.32 and 3.14)**

o In the presence of atrial "at risk" and "remodeled atria", especially the left atrium, some triggers will precipitate atrial fibrillation. The initiation of AF may be explained not only by the classical concept of a **micro-reentry** (Figure 3.14A) but also by fast depolarization atrial extrasystoles (automaticity increase) that lead to a fibrillatory conduction, perpetuating the arrhythmia. This **automatic focus** (Figure 3.14B) is located preferably in the carina region of the pulmonary veins. It may also be located in other parts of the LA (coronary sinus) and even in some parts of the RA (zone of superior cava vein). It is the initial mechanism responsible

(A)

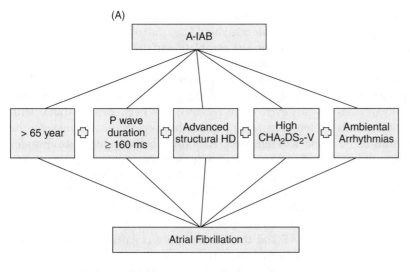

Figure 4.33 (A) Patients with A.IAB that are older than 65 years, with P-wave duration longer than 160 ms, advanced structural HD (and high CHA_2DS_2-Vasc), and ambiental arrhythmias are at high risk of AF in less than 2–3 years. (B) Pathophysiological mechanism that favor, in patients with A-IAB, the appearance of AF.

(B)

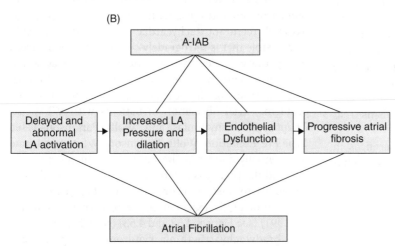

for the majority of cases of paroxysmal AF without apparent heart disease (Haïssaguerre *et al.*, 1998) (see later Figure 4.34). These frequent atrial extrasystoles present in cases of paroxysmal AF very short coupling intervals. When one of them falls in the atrial vulnerable period (VP), it may trigger an episode of paroxysmal AF.

o The premature automatic atrial complexes may also be the origin of persistent AF in patients with structural heart disease, in which case some other factors may be involved. It has been shown that AF may also originate from a unique **high-rate rotor** (see Figure 3.14C), which perpetuates arrhythmia by the successive reexcitation of a spiral wave (rotors) also leading to a fibrillatory conduction (Jalife, 2003) (see Figure 3.144C). An interplay between rotors and automatic stimuli has been observed, and these tend to terminate and perpetuate each other. In both

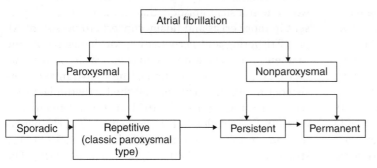

Figure 4.34 Types of atrial fibrillation according to clinical presentation.

cases, the initial 1:1 high rate excitation is converted into fibrillatory conduction because the neighboring tissues are not able to depolarize fast enough. It has been demonstrated in animal experiments (Wijffels, 1995) that once AF is established, the longer it is maintained the more difficult it will be to restore sinus rhythm, either spontaneously or even with the support of drug therapy or other methods (CV or ablation). Returning to sinus rhythm seems to be a "temporal" phenomenon. The longer the AF, the less the chance of returning to sinus rhythm, in other words, "atrial fibrillation begets atrial fibrillation" (Wijffels, 1995) (Figure 4.32).

Miscellaneous Aspects

Although in many aspects they are different arrhythmias (see Atrial Flutter: Electrophysiologic Mechanisms), there is a correlation and connection between AF and atrial flutter. Atrial flutter may be directly converted into atrial fibrillation or facilitate its appearance, and also may be a transient arrhythmia in the conversion of AF to sinus rhythm and vice versa (Yang *et al.*, 2003).

In cases of WPW and bradycardia-tachycardia syndromes, there are some particular mechanisms that cause AF (see later, and Chapters 8 and 10).

Atrial and ventricular similarities and differences in the initiation and maintenance of the fibrillatory mechanism will be discussed later (see Figure 5.45).

Clinical Presentation

Symptoms

Patients with AF may present troublesome symptoms, such as palpitations or decreased physical capacity. Dyspnea may be present if heart rate increases more than usual with exercise. However, the symptoms of patients with AF are quite variable. Sometimes AF may go unnoticed (asymptomatic AF), not only in cases of short crisis detected by Holter monitoring, but also in patients with chronic heart disease and a relatively high ventricular rate. On the other hand, repetitive episodes of paroxysmal AF may be poorly tolerated by healthy patients.

When AF is associated with a fast ventricular rate ($\geq$150 bpm), this may induce hemodynamic angina or paroxysmal dyspnea and, in heart disease patients, particularly those suffering from mitral stenosis, AF may lead to pulmonary edema. In patients with poor ventricular function, especially those with high ventricular rate, AF may lead, not only to left ventricular failure or hemodynamic angina episodes, but even to congestive HF (tachycardiomyopathy). Therefore, every effort should be made to revert it to sinus rhythm, either with drugs, electrical CV, or ablation, whichever is considered

feasible. If none of these options is possible, the patient's ventricular rate should be controlled in order to prevent HF. In some cases, ablation of the AV node and pacing is the only solution.

In the past, it was considered that stroke or embolism can occur during shifting from AF to sinus or vice versa. However, more recently, has been demonstrated with long recording implantable devices (or pacemakers) the lack of temporal relationship between high rate episodes of AF, and ischemic strokes (Glotzer *et al.*, 2009; Hohnoloser *et al.*, 2006; Martín *et al.*, 2015; Healey *et al.*, 2005). Therefore, AF it is not the final cause of stroke but clearly an important risk factor of it. Sometimes the cerebral embolism is asymptomatic. Lastly, the association of AF and the risk of future cognitive impairment has also been demonstrated (Savelieva and Camm, 2000).

Patients with WPW pre-excitation syndrome may present paroxysmal AF episodes that may be triggered by paroxysmal reentrant tachycardia or by one ventricular extrasystole that is retrogradely conducted over an accessory pathway. When the retrograde atrial activation falls in the atrial vulnerable period, it precipitates AF. In these cases, ablation of the accessory pathway will solve the problem. Atrial fibrillation in patients with WPW (see Chapter 8, Arrhythmias and Wolff–Parkinson–White Type Pre-excitation: Wolff–Parkinson–White Syndrome) is potentially dangerous because of the high ventricular rate and the potential risk of sudden death, as well as the possibility to mistake it for ventricular tachycardia (VT) due to broad QRS (Klein *et al.*, 1979; Torner-Montoya *et al.*, 1991) (see Figures 4.52 and 4.53) (see Chapter 8).

In bradytachyarrhythmia syndrome, the paroxysmal tachyarrhythmia episodes (generally AF) are favored by the dispersion of the atrial refractory period that occurs during bradycardia. Also, at the end of the episode, a potentially dangerous pause is frequently observed (see Figure 4.42). For this reason, the insertion of a pacemaker may be required, not only to prevent pauses and the occurrence of frequent arrhythmias but also to prevent long pauses after the arrhythmia episode (see Figure 4.43 and Chapter 10).

Atrial Fibrillation Types

Atrial fibrillation is a progressive disease that often starts with one transient episode, that in many cases will present in more crisis and finally converts to persistent AF (see Triggering and Perpetuating Mechanisms). At the moment of presentation, AF may appear in paroxysmal (abrupt onset and termination of the arrhythmia) or persistent (more than 7 days) (established arrhythmia) forms (Figure 4.34) (Camm *et al.*, 2012). Factors related to progression are included in the acronym HAT_2CH_2 (hypertension, age >75 years, transient ischemic attack (TIA) or stroke ($\times$2), COPD and HF ($\times$2) (De Vos *et al.*, 2010). The higher the score, the more the AF progresses. A score of 0 represents an incidence of progression of only 5% yearly, but a score of >5 represents more than 50% yearly incidence of progression. To predict progression other parameters may be used, such as the presence in the ECG of advanced interatrial block pattern (see later, therapeutic approach).

Sporadic paroxysmal AF may be related to alcohol consumption, hyperthyroidism, pericarditis, acute MI, or post-cardiac surgery. It may constitute the first stage of **repetitive paroxysmal AF (true paroxysmal AF)**, and also of future persistent AF. Sometimes it occurs only sporadically, with no triggering cause. When it is observed in very young people, a genetic origin should be considered (see Chapter 9, Genetic Atrial Fibrillation).

Repetitive paroxysmal AF (R-PAF) (Figure 4.35) consists of nonsustained repetitive AF episodes, frequently triggered by a vagal initiating stimulus (occurring at night or while resting and favored by alcohol consumption after big meals, and aerophagia). Rarely, these episodes are triggered by sympathetic overdrive (with exercise or stress). Traditionally, it was believed that patients with R-PAF episodes did not present heart disease that may play an important role in the triggering of arrhythmia. However, it has already been demonstrated (Tanigawa *et al.*, 1991), and more recently reinforced (Stiles *et al.*, 2009) that there is not only a clear imbalance of ANS, especially with a predominant vagal overdrive, but also different electrophysiologic changes and ultrastructural abnormalities that are the first

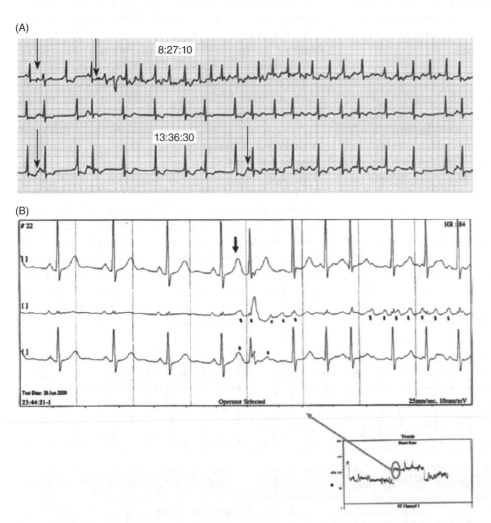

Figure 4.35 (A) Three strips of an electrocardiogram (ECG) taken from a 45-year-old patient with repeated palpitation episodes that sometimes lasted several hours and were being self-limited (paroxysmal). Note the short (few seconds) runs of atrial fibrillation with many premature atrial extrasystoles in the rest of the tracing. This is a typical Holter morphology of paroxysmal atrial fibrillation with a focal origin. Sinus rate is slow, often with escape complexes. (B) A 37-year-old patient who showed frequent paroxysmal atrial fibrillation (AF) episodes despite drug therapy and who was a good candidate for ablation. We see the onset of an episode of paroxysmal AF after a very premature atrial systole that distorts the preceding T wave and is conducted with an aberrant QRS (arrow). Bottom: Onset and end of the episode in the heart rate trend of a Holter recording.

manifestation of atrial remodeling. In addition, atrial extrasystoles may be seen, sometimes in the form of repetitive runs, and the baseline sinus rhythm in most cases is slow (vagal stimulation) (Figure 4.34). Usually, patients suffer from episodes for many years. As time passes, chances are higher that paroxysmal AF evolves into persistent AF (Figure 4.34).

AF may be persistent, in which case it is necessary to administer drugs or electrical CV to restore sinus rhythm. In other cases it may be **permanent**. In such cases, despite drugs or electrical CV, the sinus rhythm is not reestablished. Persistent AF is more frequent in patients with rheumatic valvular heart disease, cardiomyopathy, IHD, and hypertension, and particularly in the presence of HF (Maisel and Stevenson, 2003). It may also be seen as isolated arrhythmia in elderly patients. Obviously, persistent and sometimes permanent AF is often the final event that appears after some years of self-limited paroxysmal AF (see before).

ECG Findings

Diagnosis of AF, although it may be suspected during history taking and physical examination, is confirmed by the ECG. It is based on observation of the fibrillation "f" waves and the ventricular response, which is completely irregular. It is also desirable, if possible, to check the ECG morphology at onset and at the end of the episode (see later).

During Sinus Rhythm

The ECG in cases of paroxysmal (P) AF may be normal, although relatively often the P wave presents notches and even clear signs of partial interatrial block.

In sinus rhythm there are some ECG changes in the P wave that have been considered "premonitory markers" for future AF/atrial flutter. It has been demonstrated that

in a global population older than 65 years, the presence of atrial premature beats in basal surface ECG, and the duration of P-wave and the presence of ECG criteria of left atrial enlargement and partial or advanced interatrial block, are markers of risk of AF in the follow-up. In the cohort ARIC has been demonstrated that the presence of A-IAB multiplies by four the incidence of AF in one-year follow-up (3% vs 0.7%). As long ago as 1988 it was published that in cases of very advanced heart disease with ECG criteria of advanced interatrial block the occurrence of paroxysmal supraventricular arrhythmias (AF and/or atrial flutter) is very frequent (≈50%) at one-year follow-up (Bayés de Luna *et al.*, 1988) (Figures 10.4–10.7). The presence of partial interatrial block is also a marker, but less so, of AF in the future (Bayés de Luna *et al.*, 1988; Holmqvist *et al.*, 2009, 2010). It has also been demonstrated (Ishida *et al.*, 2010) that the presence of LA enlargement (P± V1 with duration ≥120 ms) and signs of RA overload (tall initial part of P wave in V1) may be critical for susceptibility to AF.

The rest of the ECG is usually normal in P-AF and presents different ECG signs according to the underlying heart disease in case of persistent AF.

Atrial Waves: "f" Waves
(Figures 4.36 and 4.37)

The ECG shows small waves (named "f") with a rate between 400 and 700 pm. Figure 4.38 shows different shapes and voltages of the "f" waves in lead V1. This is generally the most appropriate lead for observing the fibrillation waves. Even in this lead they are occasionally barely visible. The fibrillatory waves measuring ≥1 mm (coarse "f" waves), are usually present in patients with left atrial enlargement, or elevated left atrial pressure and often the "f" waves become smaller after treatment (Thurmann and Janney, 1962).

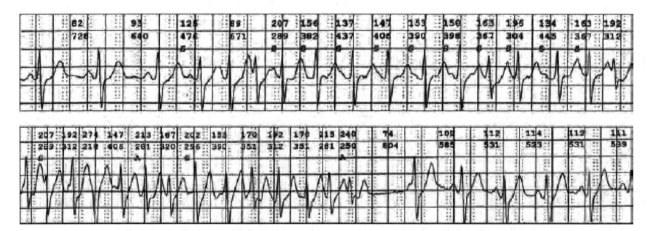

Figure 4.36 An episode of atrial fibrillation in a patient with a fast baseline sinus rhythm. After onset the ventricular response is very rapid, and it is followed by a sinus rhythm above 100 bpm, at the end of the episode. All these features are indicative of a sympathetic overdrive to trigger the episode.

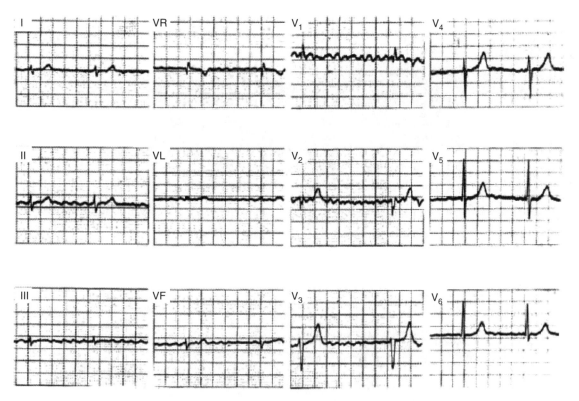

Figure 4.37 A 45-year-old patient with a tight mitral stenosis and mild aortic regurgitation. Note the typical atrial fibrillation (AF) medium-sized waves, which are especially visible in V1.

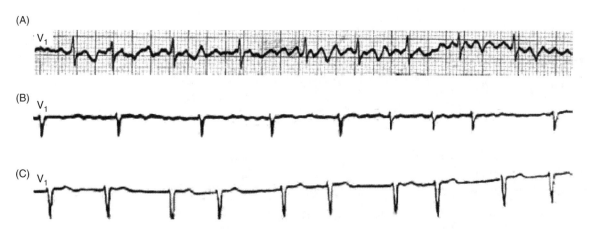

Figure 4.38 (A) Atrial fibrillation (AF) with "f" waves with prominent voltage. (B) and (C)"f" waves with lower voltage, almost not visible in (C).

To visualize the "f" waves sometimes it is necessary to amplify the waves by external methods (Figure 4.39) or, in very rare cases, to perform an intracavitary ECG (Figure 4.40). When in doubt, the hisiogram allows determination of whether the QRS complexes are supraventricular or ventricular. In supraventricular QRS complexes, the interval between the His and the ventricular deflections (HV) is normal, whereas in ventricular QRS complexes the HV interval is shorter (fascicular premature ventricular complexes), or the H deflection is hidden in the V deflection, or can be seen right after it (Figure 4.40).

On some occasions, if the sinus P waves are not particularly visible and there are frequent premature atrial contractions, AF may be misdiagnosed (Figure 4.41) (see later).

The majority of "f" waves are blocked somewhere in the AV junction with different degrees of concealed conduction, originating an irregular ventricular response (Figure 4.38) (see later).

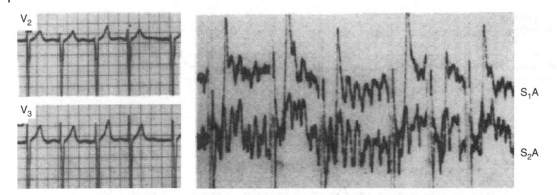

Figure 4.39 Left: V2 and V3 with nonvisible "f" waves. They are easily seen on the right, where they are taken with external voltage amplification.

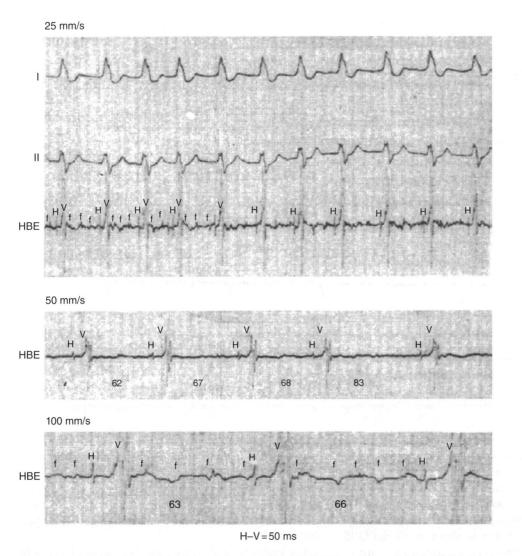

Figure 4.40 Atrial fibrillation with left bundle branch block (LBBB)-QRS complexes in leads I and II. Simultaneous recording of His bundle electrocardiogram (HBE) show the "f" waves, which are nonvisible on surface electrocardiogram (ECG), and demonstrates that the H deflection precedes the ventricular complexes, with a normal H-V interval of 50 ms. Tracings taken at higher speeds show better the oscillations in the duration of RR intervals (50 and 100 mm/s).

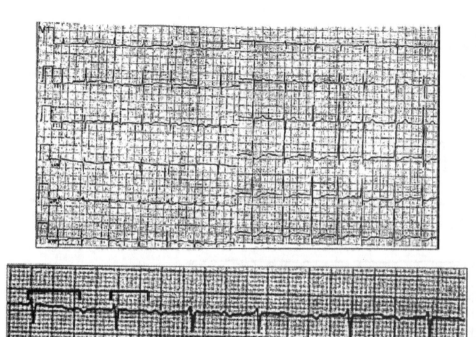

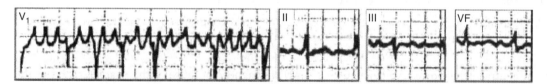

Sinus P   Ectopic   Ectopic   Sinus P   Sinus P

Figure 4.41 Example of the complexity involved in an accurate diagnosis of an arrhythmia, when the atrial wave is not clearly visible and the QRS are irregular. A sinus rhythm with atrial extrasystoles has to be ruled out, as in this case (see V1 = second and third P waves where atrial premature complexes show a distinct morphology, bimodal P, and are more premature).

Figure 4.42 Sometimes the atrial waves show a fairly regular, slightly faster rate in V1 (as in the flutter), a little faster, and do not show a sawtooth morphology in II, III, or VF (as in AF). This case represents AF and could easily be confused with atrial flutter. These cases have been called fibrilo-flutter.

On some rare occasions the shape of the waves in some leads is typical of fibrillation (variable morphology and voltage), whereas in others they may look like flutter waves (regular and monomorphic) (Figure 4.42). This phenomenon is related to the distance between the rotor and the ECG electrode. The closer to the rotor, the more disorganized the waves are, the farther from the rotor the more organized the waves are. This is comparable to dropping a coin in a lake (in the center, the waves are disorganized, however; as they expanded from the epicenter, the waves get more organized.

Onset and End of Episodes

Repetitive paroxysmal AF is initiated by early premature atrial contractions (short coupling interval) falling in the atrial vulnerable period (AVP) and often with repeated short runs of supraventricular tachyarrhythmias, before triggering more prolonged (paroxysmal) episodes (Figure 4.35).

The end of the episode is usually followed by a short pause. However, often the pause is more or less prolonged (Figure 4.43), sometimes interrupted by the spike of the pacemaker (Figure 4.44). When the pause is very long it may be indicative of bradycardiatachycardia syndrome due to concomitant sinus node dysfunction (see Figures 10.2 and 10.3, and Chapter 10, Severe Sinus Bradycardia)

Ventricular Response and QRS Complex Morphology

The spontaneous ventricular response is completely irregular due to the different degrees of concealed conduction of the "f" waves (Figure 4.38). In normal conditions it is usually fast (from 130 to 160 bpm). Higher rates are seen in hyperthyroidism and in cases with an

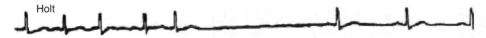

Figure 4.43 A long pause frequently occurs after an episode in tachy-bradyarrhythmia syndrome, which in this case finishes with a sinus P wave.

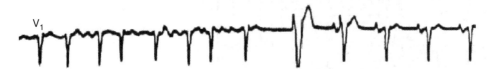

Figure 4.44 Note how, in this case, the pause at the end of the atrial fibrillation (AF) episode is finished by a pacemaker rhythm followed by a sinus P wave and QRS fusion complex with the pacemaker. This provides an appropriate treatment for AF patients with fast rates during the day and slow rates during the night.

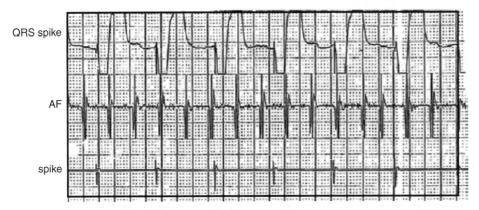

Figure 4.45 The prevailing pacemaker rhythm in a patient with atrial fibrillation (AF) (atrial recording) and advanced atrioventricular (AV) block.

accessory pathway; in contrast, the slowest ventricular rates occur in cases of spontaneous depressed AV conduction or as a consequence of drug administration.

In the presence of AF, a regular and slow ventricular rhythm is explained by the presence of an escape rhythm of the AV junction (narrow QRS complex), or ventricular (wide QRS complex) or pacemaker rhythm (Figure 4.45 and see Figure 6.2). If the ventricular rhythm is regular and fast, it is due to an AV junctional tachycardia with narrow QRS (Figure 4.28A) or wide QRS in the case of aberrant conduction, or due to ventricular tachycardia (wide nonaberrant QRS morphology). In both situations no "f" wave passes through the AV junction to the ventricles, and therefore there is a complete AV dissociation due to interference of the high ectopic rhythm (JT-EF) (Figure 4.28A), or AV block, if the ventricular rate is slow (see Figure 6.2). If the QRS is wide and the heart rate is fast, the "f" waves are often difficult to recognize (Figure 4.40).

Differential Diagnosis

- **With other irregular tachyarrhythmias**. Diagnosis of AF is electrocardiographic. As stated in general, it is easy to diagnose because of the characteristics of the "f" waves and the irregularity of the ventricular rhythm. However, it can be confused with the following irregular rhythms:
  - o **Chaotic atrial tachycardia**. The characteristics of this infrequent tachyarrhythmia, which usually appears in patients with cor pulmonale and disappears with hypoxia treatment, may be seen in the section on Chaotic Atrial Tachycardia (Figure 4.31).
  - o **Atrial flutter with variable AV conduction**. The "F" waves of flutter are almost always monomorphic, although different types may exist (see Figure 4.69). The monomorphic morphology of "F" waves rarely changes. It occurs usually due to drug effect (Figure 4.28). The treatment in terms of anticoagulation is in general similar to the treatment for AF (see Atrial Flutter).
  - o **Sinus rhythm with low voltage P waves and frequent and irregularly located atrial extrasystoles** (Figure 4.41). It is important not to confuse these rhythms because the treatment may be different. In this case, we have to prevent, not treat, AF (see Atrial Fibrillation: Treatment: Prevention of the

First Episode). It may be useful to amplify the ECGs (Figure 4.39), and to use T wave filtering if it is incorporated to commercial devices (see Appendix A-3, Other Surface Techniques to Register Electrical Cardiac Activity).

Differential Diagnosis Between Aberrancy and Ectopy in Wide QRS Complexes

- This differential diagnosis is not only of academic interest, but also has prognostic and therapeutic implications. The following must be taken into account:

  o It has been demonstrated that when in the presence of AF, the majority (90%) of wide QRS complexes are ectopic complexes (Gulamhusein *et al.*, 1985).

  o However, the presence of runs with a typical right bundle branch block (RBBB) morphology (rsR′ in V1 and/or qRs in V6) favors aberrancy (Figure 4.46), mainly if the irregularity of the rhythm during the runs with the RBBB pattern is similar to that observed in the basic rhythm with narrow QRS (Figures 4.47 and 4.48). The maintained aberrancy with RBBB morphology may be explained by

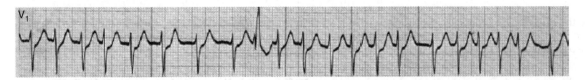

Figure 4.46 Atrial fibrillation (AF) patient with one wide premature QRS complex with a distinct morphology in V1. In general, the Gouaux–Ashman criteria in the presence of wide QRS complexes during AF are not as useful to distinguish between aberrancy and ectopy as in sinus rhythm. Nevertheless, the rsR′ morphology in V1, as seen in this case, suggests that aberrancy is more probable.

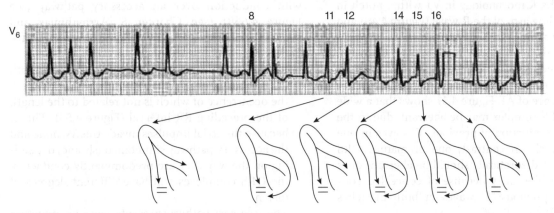

Figure 4.47 Sustained aberrancy. Several wide complexes with right bundle branch block (RBBB) morphology (wide S) are shown in the V6 lead. The 8th wide complex is probably aberrant and may be explained by a Phase 3 mechanism (long preceding diastole-short coupling interval). Afterwards, there is a couple (complexes 11 and 12), as well as a run (complexes 14, 15, and 16), of aberrant complexes. Complexes 11 and 14 may be aberrant

because of the aforementioned classical mechanism (short coupling interval, relatively long preceding diastole). In contrast, the aberrant complexes 12, 15, and 16 without these characteristics may be explained because the preceding ones (11, 14 and 15) may initiate a concealed retrograde conduction over the RBB, preventing the subsequent stimuli 12, 15, and 16 from crossing this branch in an anterograde fashion (* millivolt).

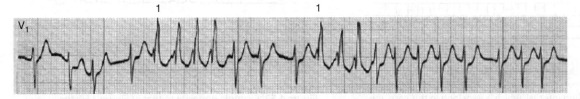

Figure 4.48 Taken from the same patient as in Figure 4.45, two runs of QRS with sustained aberrancy are shown. The first complex in each run (1) would be explained by Phase 3 aberrancy but not the others. The first aberrant complex of each run, and also the 2nd and 3rd of first run, and the 2nd of second run probably retrogradely invades the right bundle branch (RBB) and the

subsequent QRS is aberrant because it cannot be conducted over the RBB as it is in its refractory period due to concealed conduction in the right branch of the preceding QRS complex (see diagram in Figure 4.46). The typical right bundle branch block (RBBB) morphology (rsR′ in V1), and also the irregular RR cadence, similar to narrow subsequent QRS, strongly suggests aberrancy.

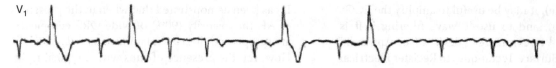

Figure 4.49 A patient with atrial fibrillation (AF) showing wide QRS complexes with a single R in V1. The notch in the descending arm of the QRS and the fixed coupling interval definitely point to an ectopic origin, ruling out aberrant conduction.

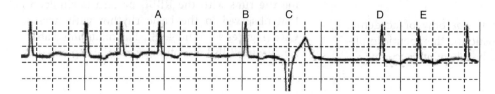

Figure 4.50 In this case, the QS morphology of the wide complex in V6 definitely indicates an ectopic origin despite the previous diastole being very long (AB). Note that even with a longer preceding diastole (CD), the following QRS (E) shows a normal morphology, probably because of the concealed conduction of some "f" waves in the branches (see Figure 4.51).

retrograde concealed conduction in the right bundle (Figures 4.47 and 4.48).

o The rest of the morphologies are observed to a greater extent when the complexes are ectopic, including the R morphology in V1 with a notch in the descending arm of the R wave (Figure 4.49) and the QS morphology in V6 (Figure 4.50).

o It has already been mentioned that the Gouaux–Ashman phenomenon (see Chapter 3, Aberrant Conduction) is not useful for diagnosing aberrancy in the presence of AF. Figure 4.51 shows that a wide and late QRS complex may be aberrant, due to the concealed conduction of previous "f" waves in one bundle branch. In contrast, one premature QRS complex that theoretically should be aberrant does not present aberrancy because of concealed conduction of previous "f" waves in both branches (Figure 4.52).

o The irregularity of the RR intervals generally allows us to distinguish a rapid AF with aberrant complexes due to a bundle branch block morphology from a VT.

- **Differential diagnosis between AF in WPW syndrome and VT.** We will comment on this differential diagnosis (Figure 4.53), which is even more difficult to perform in cases of atrial flutter in WPW syndrome with conduction over an accessory pathway (see Figure 4.66B) (see Chapter 8, Arrhythmias and Wolff–Parkinson–White Type Pre-excitation: Wolff–Parkinson–White Syndrome).

o In WPW syndrome with AF, QRS complexes with different degrees of pre-excitation may be observed, the occurrence of which is not related to the length of the preceding RR interval (Figure 4.53). This is because the atrial impulses invade the AV node and the accessory pathway simultaneously and, depending on the way they are predominantly conducted, the QRS complexes will have different degrees of fusion.

o The accessory pathway presents a faster conduction than the SCS, and therefore AF in the presence of WPW syndrome frequently shows QRS complex morphology with significant pre-excitation and fast

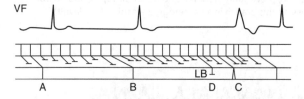

Figure 4.51 Taken from an atrial fibrillation (AF) patient with generally narrow QRS and eventual wide QRS complexes with a variable coupling interval, which is very long in this case. It is probably not a ventricular escape because it is identical to other previous wide QRSs with shorter coupling intervals; it may be explained by the concealed conduction of a previous "f" wave in the left bundle branch (LBB) that has changed its sequence from AB-BC, which should not show left bundle branch block (LBBB) aberrancy, to BD-DC, which may show this aberrancy.

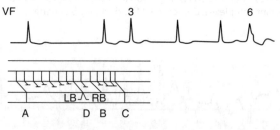

Figure 4.52 Example opposite to that of Figure 4.50: the premature QRS complex (number 3) does not show aberrancy, whereas other less premature complexes with a shorter preceding diastole show aberrancy (6). An explanation for this may be that an "f" wave located in the preceding diastole has penetrated into both branches, changing the sequence from AB-BC (aberrant) to DB-BC (not to be aberrant).

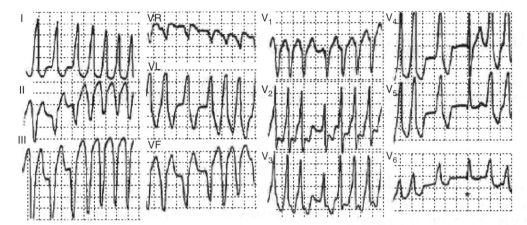

Figure 4.53 Twelve-lead electrocardiogram (ECG) of a Wolff–Parkinson–White syndrome in atrial fibrillation. Note the great degree of aberrancy of the complexes, complicating the differential diagnosis with ventricular tachycardia, especially in the presence of a regular ventricular conduction (atrial flutter) (see Figure 4.66). This arrhythmia should always be taken into account, because it may easily be mistaken for a very serious ventricular tachycardia. In this case the diagnosis of Wolff–Parkinson–White syndrome with atrial fibrillation is supported by: (i) the presence of d waves in some leads (V2, V3) and the presence of different morphologies of QRS, with more or less degrees of aberrancy, as the expression of different degrees of conduction over the accessory pathway; (ii) irregular RR; (iii) narrow QRS, which may or may not be premature (see asterisk and Figure 4.66). In VT, narrow QRS complexes are always premature (captures); and (iv) awareness of this arrhythmia existing.

heart rate. However, as the refractory period is longer, sometimes an early stimulus is blocked, which is the key to explaining how the wideness of QRS may change from one complex to another, as well as how an atrial premature beat blocked in the accessory pathway may trigger a AVRT (JRT-AP) (see Figure 3.9B).

o In AF in the presence of pre-excitation it is necessary to make the differential diagnosis with fast VT runs. The following criteria are indicative of AF in the presence of WPW syndrome (Figure 4.53):

- The presence of QRS complexes with different degrees of pre-excitation, sometimes with evident δ waves not related to the length of the preceding cycle (see before).

- The irregularity of the RR intervals is another criterion that helps to distinguish a fast AF with wide QRS complexes from a VT.

- In VT the presence of narrow QRS complexes, if they exist, are sinus captures (premature complexes), whereas in AF with WPW syndrome, the narrow QRS complexes are usually characterized by random occurrence and may be early or late (Figure 4.52).

Prognostic Implications

Mortality for any reason in patients with AF **is higher than the mortality observed in patients with similar clinical status in sinus rhythm**. Isolated AF has a better prognosis. In the rest of the cases it depends on the underlying disease. It has been demonstrated that AF is associated with an increased risk of complications in several pathologies (hypertension, ischemic cardiomyopathy, HF, etc.) (Benjamin *et al.*, 1998; Dries *et al.*, 1998; Fuster *et al.*, 2006). It has also been demonstrated that in HF patients, AF not only has an impact on prognosis but also aggravates the symptoms (dyspnea and exercise capacity). Patients with diastolic HF, perhaps because they are elderly patients, present a poorer prognosis (Fung *et al.*, 2007).

We have shown that patients with grade II–III HF, and AF + advanced LBBB have a poorer prognosis than patients with none or just one of these two electrocardiographic abnormalities (see Chapter 11, Heart failure) (Vazquez *et al.*, 2009).

Furthermore, in patients with acute MI, the occurrence of AF is relatively frequent (≈10%) and is associated with a worse prognosis, increased mortality, and cerebrovascular embolism (Saczynski *et al.*, 2009) (see Chapter 11, Ischemic Heart Disease). The presence of previous AF was even associated with greater mortality over a long-term follow-up (Lau *et al.*, 2009).

In general, **the main problems associated with AF are: (i) fast ventricular rates** that are difficult to control with drugs – this may lead to hemodynamic deterioration, LV dysfunction, and even to HF (tachycardio-myopathy), especially in cases with previous heart disease; additionally, in rare cases, WPW syndrome may induce serious ventricular arrhythmias, including ventricular fibrillation (Figure 4.54) (see before) – and **(ii) being an important risk factor**, although not the final cause, of developing systemic embolism, especially cerebral embolism.

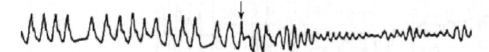

Figure 4.54 A patient with Wolff–Parkinson–White syndrome and a very fast atrial fibrillation. Some RRs are at times shorter than 200 ms and QRS complexes are aberrant. A very premature QRS complex (arrow) falls into the atrial vulnerable period, triggering a ventricular fibrillation that was reverted with electrical cardioversion.

Therapeutic Approach

The treatment comprises four objectives: (i) prevention of the first episode, (ii) conversion to a sinus rhythm and maintenance of sinus rhythm (rhythm- control strategy), (iii) if neither of these are possible, control of ventricular rate (rate-control strategy), and (iv) prevention of thromboembolism (Fuster *et al.*, 2006; Kirchhof and Breithardt, 2009; Camm, 2010; Wyse *et al.*, 2002). We will comment on the role of the different therapeutic approaches: antiarrhythmic agents (AAA), anticoagulants, cardioversion (CV), and ablation. Because AF is a progressive disease, we show in Figure 4.55 at what stages these different approaches should be used.

Prevention of the First Episode

The best general approach for AF prevention is to prevent and treat risk factors and heart diseases in which AF is more prevalent (IHD, HF, arterial hypertension, obesity, sleep disorders, etc.), with angiotensin converting enzyme inhibitors (ACE-I), angiotensin receptor blockers, aldosterone antagonists, and statins. From an epidemiologic point of view, fish consumption has been associated with reduced risk of AF. Long chain n-3 PUFAS in fish are thought to account for this beneficial effect (Virtanen *et al.*, 2009). However, at present more evidence is needed to recommend the global use of PUFAs for primary or secondary prevention of AF (Camm, 2010) The use of C-PAP in patients with obstructive sleep apnea contribute to induce reversed atrial electrical remodeling, thus reducing AF (Baranchuk *et al.*, 2012).

From a practical point of view it is necessary to take different measures with patients that have a high risk for AF (patients with valvular heart disease, especially those with advanced mitral stenosis and patients suffering from HF, and also patients with IHD, hypertension, hyperthyroidism, etc.). In these cases we recommend detection and treatment of PSVC, if frequent, and especially runs of supraventricular tachycardia. Furthermore, we advise:

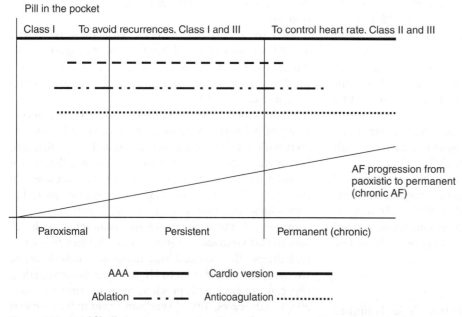

Figure 4.55 Atrial fibrillation is a progressive disease from paroxysmal to persistent and permanent (chronic). The figure shows the time schedule of prescription of different treatments given during the follow-up for this disease. Note that anticoagulation may already have been started if paroxysmal crises are frequent and must be taken during the entire follow-up if there are no contraindications. Antiarrhythmic agents (AAA) may be used already in paroxystic crisis (pill in the pocket approach) and to avoid recurrences and control heart rate.

o Immediate surgery, if the criteria for surgery are met, in patients with valvular heart disease.

o Limiting coffee, tea, alcohol, any energetic drink, and carbonated drink intake, especially at night, due to the importance of vagal influence.

o Remembering that the presence of an interatrial block, especially advanced interatrial block (P± in II, III, VF), is a marker for important supraventricular tachyarrhythmias in a follow-up, especially in patients with advanced heart disease and/or CHA_2DS_2-Vascular ≥3 (see Chapter 10, Advanced Interatrial Block with Left Atrial Retrograde Conduction).

o Preventing post-CABG-AF (see Atrial Fibrillation: Epidemiology). β-blockers may be useful (recommendation Class I) (Fuster *et al.*, 2006). Amiodarone has also been proven to reduce the risk of post-CABG-AF (Budeus *et al.*, 2006).

o In an apparently isolated AF (lone AF) consider some diseases such as hyperthyroidism, sleep disorders, and so on, in order to rule them out or choose the appropriate treatment for them.

Conversion to Sinus Rhythm and Prevention of Recurrences

Drugs or Electrical CV

We have to consider the following situations:

- **Sporadic paroxysmal** AF is often resolved with the treatment of the underlying disease, or removing the triggering causes (see atrial fibrillation types).
- **Recurrent paroxysmal** AF episodes in patients without advanced heart disease, usually reverts within a few hours, sometimes in a few minutes. We recommend urging the patient to cough hard immediately (six to eight times) once the episode is perceived, and if so increases could be terminated by a strategy called "pill-in-the-pocket" approach, usually taking a dose of an antiarrhythmic agent (AAA), Type IC drug (we use preferably propafenone), if HF or advanced ultrastructural heart disease is not present (Class II a recommendation) (Alboni *et al.*, 2004) (Appendix A-5.3, Antiarrhythmic Agents, and Tables A-7 and A-11). In combining these measures, the episode frequently reverts.
- **If AF persists despite the abovementioned measures** and the patient is stable and without rapid ventricular rate we may start an oral treatment with amiodarone and digoxin or betablockers (in the absence of pre-excitation or other contraindications) to block the AV node and try to revert AF. Often, however, if the arrhythmia is poorly tolerated, the patient is admitted to the emergency room and intravenous pharmacologic treatment is administered to revert AF to sinus rhythm, provided that the patient is hemodynamically stable. Our first option is intravenous amiodarone (5 mg/kg in 1 h) (Class II a recommendation) or recently a new atrial selective antiarrhythmic drug called vernalakant, which proved to be safe and effective in converting paroxysmal AF into normal sinus rhythm. Vernakalant is available in some countries in Europe and a few countries in South America (Conde and Baranchuk, 2014) (see Appendix A-5, Antiarrhythmic Agents and Table A-11). If it is necessary to block more of the AV junction (in cases of very rapid ventricular response) then other drugs should be added. When selecting drugs for rate control, especially in cases of lone paroxysmal AF, clinicians should evaluate not only their efficacy to depress AV nodal conduction but also their effects on the atrial muscle itself. Thus, in the absence of pre-excitation, β-blockers may be considered the drug of choice in rate control of AF. Other drugs, such as verapamil, may also control heart rate, but there is some evidence that may favor the appearance of new high-rate sources in the atria that may lead to new crises (Raatikanen, 2010). If HF is clinically present, digitalis associated to amiodarone may be the best drug to control heart rate. When drug treatment fails, or the patients as hemodinamically unstable electrical CV should be performed (Class I B). Electrical CV may be performed within the first 24–48 h without previous anticoagulation therapy, only prescribing heparin.

- **If sinus rhythm is not recovered with drug treatment**, or in the case that we see the patient for the first time, and they are in a stable situation, and the AF lasts for more than 48 h or is unknown, and it is decided to perform a programmed non-urgent electrical CV, we may follow two paths:

(i) A transoesophageal-guided echo (TEE) strategy to check if thrombi are present in the left atrium appendage (LAA), and act according to the results. If there are thrombi, we prescribe three months of anticoagulation and later on perform a new TEE before cardioversion. If, after this, there are still LAA thrombi, the most convenient therapy is to control the heart rate and long-term oral anticoagulation is indicated (usually Warfarin is preferred over the new oral anticoagulants, in this case).

(ii) In clinical practice we usually perform the following before an elective CV: anticoagulation over a 3–4-week period in order to achieve an international normalized ratio (INR) ≥2, and drug treatment (amiodarone and ACE inhibitors or angiotensin II receptor antagonists (ARA II)) (Madrid *et al.*, 2002). Alternatively, three weeks of Rivaroxaban (Cappato *et al.*, 2014) is also safe and efficient. This will lead to a more successful electrical CV and also help to prevent an embolism. With this pre-treatment, the electrical CV is more successful (>70% of selected patients). Furthermore, some patients return spontaneously to sinus rhythm during the pre-treatment period.

It is advisable to perform TEE before electrical CV, especially in patients at risk of embolism (previous stroke, frequent recurrences, advanced heart diseases, etc.) to be sure that there are no thrombi in LAA. If found, although they may be endotheliazed, CV is not recommended. However, there is no clear recommendation in the guidelines about the need of a TEE in these patients. We consider that this decision has to be taken, in any case, after careful evaluation, and if necessary discussing with the patient. In our experience, in patients of low/moderate risk, the incidence of cerebral embolism is very small.

- **In persistent AF** it is important to know: (i) which cases are more difficult to revert to sinus rhythm, (ii) in which cases the CV is probably not necessary, and (iii) the probability of recurrences.
  - ○ **Eligibility for CV**. In persistent AF, electrical CV is not usually effective if: the duration of the AF is more than one year; the left atrium is very large (>50 mm); heart disease is very advanced; the ECG shows advanced interatrial block and the patient is very old. As these factors increase in number, the results worsen proportionally.
  - ○ On the other hand, electrical **CV may be not so necessary**, especially in the elderly, if: the mean ventricular rate is under control; there are only few symptoms; and it is not associated with significant heart disease (Wyse *et al.*, 2002).
  - ○ **Recurrences**. If CV was successful, the most common prognostic indicators of recurrence are the following:
    - ○ Clinical parameters, such as: age (>70 years), duration of the AF (more than 1–2 years), presence of hypertension, HF, impairment of renal function, mitral valve disease, hypertrophic cardiomyopathy, previous TIA or stroke, sleep disorders, COPD, advanced interatrial block frequent, atrial extrasystoles (Holter), and history of paroxysmal AF. These include all parameters of the HAT_2CH_2 score–risk factors of progression (see Atrial Fibrillation) and some others.
    - ○ Imaging techniques: presence of spontaneous echo contrast and a large left atrium by echocardiography (>50 mm). The importance of the degree of atrial fibrosis, which can be detected by CE-CMR, has been reported (Oakes *et al.*, 2009). However, in clinical practice with "conventional" CMR it is difficult to detect atrial fibrosis. The presence of advanced interatrial block in the ECG, probably, reflects a high degree of atrial fibrosis.
    - ○ Blood test: serological parameters related to matrix remodeling, fibrosis, atrial stretching, and chemotaxis, such as transforming growth factor (TGF-β) and stromal cell derived factor (SDF-1α), can predict failure or recurrence of AF after electrical CV (Kim *et al.*, 2009). However, these tests are not easy to perform on a routine basis. Elevated levels of C-reactive protein as a marker of inflammatory disease are a significant prognostic factor of success and recurrence (Mazza *et al.*, 2009). The role of the hs-CRP has also been suggested (Lin *et al.*, 2010) (see later).

All these parameters should be taken into account at the time of deciding the therapeutic approach.

- **Treatment after recovery of sinus rhythm.** In cases where the sinus rhythm is recovered after the CV, it is necessary to continue administering treatment, at least for several months, and often forever in order to prevent recurrences, which are frequent when untreated (50–70%/year) (Top-Pedersen *et al.*, 2010). Usually the scientific society guidelines (AHA/ESC) recommend the administration of different drugs according the associated disease. If the first line drug fails we may try others. After the initial enthusiasm with the use of Dronaderone to control paroxysmal AF without the inconvenient of amiodarone (Hohnoloser *et al.*, 2009); several patients were switched from amiodarone to dronaderone (Connolly *et al.*, 2009b; Cook *et al.*, 2010). The same group of investigators decided to expand the use of dronaderone, to sicker patients with persistent AF (Connolly *et al.*, 2011). Unfortunately, this study needed to be discontinued early due to increase mortality in the treatment group in comparison to placebo. The fact that AF is a progressive disease, motivated several groups to practically abandon the use of dronaderone, given the fact that is impossible to predict who would evolve from paroxysmal to persistent AF (Davy *et al.*, 2008; Køber *et al.*, 2008; Piccini *et al.*, 2009; Zimetbaum, 2009; Singh *et al.*, 2010; Mohajer *et al.*, 2013). Therefore, amiodarone remains the first-choice drug only in patients with HF although compared with placebo in patients with grade II-III NYHA HF does not reduce total mortality (Bardy *et al.*, 2005). With all this information in mind, now (January 2016) we recommend the following to maintain sinus rhythm in our patients:
  - ○ The decision to prescribe amiodarone depends not only on the possible side effects of the drug, but also on the risk of recurrences, the frequency of them, and the importance of heart disease, especially the grade of HF. To avoid the most frequent side effect,

the thyroid dysfunction it is necessary to control carefully the levels of TSH and chest X-ray to rule out pulmonary fibrosis.

o Type I drugs alone can also be administered to prevent recurrences. We use more propafenone, although other authors recommend also flecainide (Capucci *et al.*, 1999). No Class I drugs are recommended when there is evident structural heart disease, especially in the presence of HF, given their proarrhythmic and negative inotropic effects. However, in spite of these limitations, Class I drugs may be administered in selected cases, always with a close follow-up (Andersen *et al.*, 2009) (see Appendix A-5).

o Beta-blockers may be useful to prevent recurrences in rare cases of adrenergic mediated AF.

o Sotalol is the second drug of choice if no QT prolongation at two weeks of initiating the drug. Women with coronary artery disease should not receive Sotalol (Verma *et al.*, 2014)

o Even though certain discrepancies exist regarding benefits of the use of statins, ACE inhibitors, and/ or ARA II (Disertori *et al.*, 2009; Smit and Van Gelder, 2009), we usually administer them several months after CV. Some discordant results have been published. A meta-analysis has been published (Schneider *et al.*, 2010) that demonstrates substantial benefits from renin–angiotensin system (RAS) inhibition in the primary and secondary prevention of AF, especially when patients also received amiodarone.

o **To prevent recurrences**, it is also in our opinion extremely important to **remove any triggering** factors (i.e., alcohol, aerophagia) that may be different for different people, and to remember that many patients present the crisis by night.

Chronic Treatment for Rhythm Control

To avoid triggering factors:
- Amiodarone: useful in all cases, if no contraindications.
- Class I AAA: useful in cases of normal heart.
- β-blockers: useful in some cases, Sotalol may be an option.
- Other drugs: uncertain usefulness of statins, ACE-I, and ARA II.
- Useful to avoid alcohol, aerophagia, etc.

- **Treatment of AF in WPW syndrome**. A good pharmacologic option for decreasing ventricular rate is intravenous amiodarone, which may even resolve the episode, or intravenous procainamide, especially if the QRS complex is wide (see Table A-11). The drugs that block the AV node more than the accessory pathway, such as adenosine, digitalis, ß-blockers, calcium antagonists, and lidocaine, *cannot be administered* because they may improve the conduction over the accessory pathway and, therefore, increase ventricular rate, creating a dangerous scenario (see Chapter 8, Arrhythmias and Wolff–Parkinson–White Type Pre-excitation: Wolff–Parkinson–White Syndrome). However, as the ventricular rate is usually very high (>150 bpm), the most convenient measure is to perform an urgent electrical CV. Once the episode is over it is necessary to perform an ablation of the accessory pathway.

- Very few trials have studied how to best treat **post-CABG-AF**. There are no trials that compare a rhythm versus rate control strategy. The AHA/ACC/ESC guidelines (Fuster *et al.*, 2006) consider "both treatments reasonable". However, it seems that rhythm control is more frequently used (Al-Khatib *et al.*, 2009). Amiodarone is most likely a good choice. Sleep disorders should be treated energically in order to reduce post-CABG-AF (Qaddoura *et al.*, 2014).

- AF in patients with acute MI is usually transient but may need early treatment at least to decrease heart rate (see Chapter 11, Ischemic Heart Disease, and Table 11.1).

Ablation Techniques

Discussed here are the most practical aspects of this important treatment for AF that radically try "to resolve and cure" AF. The state-of-the-art ablation techniques for AF are (see Appendix A-4.4):

- **Circumferential pulmonary vein ablation** has already shown very good results in paroxysmal AF (PAF) (success rate >70–80%) (Haïssaguerre *et al.*, 2000a, 2000b; Pappone and Santinelli, 2006) (Figure 4.56). This corresponds to **trigger-based strategy**. Currently in cases of P-AF, additional left atrial linear ablation should not be advised as an initial ablation approach. There is evidence that there is no added benefit, and even that an increased risk of left atrial flutter exists (Sawhney *et al.*, 2010).

- Currently in many cases of **persistent AF**, acceptable results are obtained using a trigger-based strategy (circumferential pulmonary vein ablation). However, in order to improve the results, other techniques have been developed to eliminate the substrate (**substrate-based strategy**). The stepwise approach may include: (i) the use of left atrial lines (Valles *et al.*, 2008) (the importance of a circular mapping catheter (CMC), graded technique for detection and closing the gaps within the LA ablation lines has been reported (Eitel *et al.*, 2010)); (ii) inclusion of zones with maximal high-frequency drivers and with CFAEs, in the ablation area. Furthermore, as AF is frequently associated

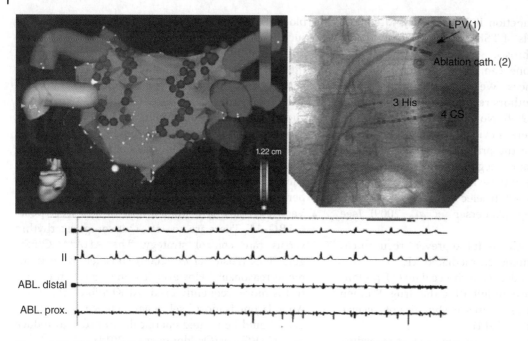

Figure 4.56 Ablation of atrial fibrillation. Currently, ablation of atrial fibrillation consists of circular perimetral isolation of pulmonary veins. Generally, electroanatomic navigation–reconstruction systems are used (left), which allow the anatomic reconstruction of the left atrium, as well as the performance of the ablation lines. The right panel shows the placement of catheters through X-rays during the procedure. A circular catheter may be seen inside the upper left pulmonary vein (1), as well as a mapping-ablation catheter to perform punctual ablations around the ostium (2). Another catheter has been placed by the His bundle (3), and an additional multipolar catheter in the coronary sinus (4). The bottom panel shows how after isolation the pulmonary vein remains in AF without transmitting it to the atria, which remain in sinus rhythm.

with atrial flutter it is also recommended to perform flutter ablation (this may be also done in cases of paroxysmal atrial fibrillation (P-AF)). It is convenient to perform ablation after sinus rhythm has been restored by electrical CV. With this stepwise approach and with the use of new generation of catheters, very acceptable results have been obtained even in patients with enlarged atria (>5 cm) and long-lasting AF (over >1–2 years) (60–80% of success, and even more in some subgroups) (Khaykin *et al.*, 2009; Nair *et al.*, 2009; Scharf *et al.*, 2009; Lin *et al.*, 2010). A multicentric trial of ablation favoring the combined trigger + substrate strategy approach versus trigger strategy or substrate strategy alone in patients with permanent AF has been published (Verma *et al.*, 2010).

If these promising results could be confirmed in a larger series, and especially if the recurrences are low in a long follow-up, indications for ablation could be expanded in future. We have to remember, however, that there are some complications associated with AF ablation, and that to restore and maintain sinus rhythm may be impossible in advanced cases (see later).

After ablation AA agents, especially amiodarone, may be prescribed to prevent recurrences. In spite of this, the incidence of recurrences is still relatively high.

Koyama *et al.* (2010) has demonstrated that transient use of corticosteroids shortly after AF ablation may be effective and safe for preventing AF recurrences during the mid-term follow-up period after PVI ablation, however; they are not systematically used.

- In cases of AF in **WPW syndrome**, curative treatment includes the ablation of the accessory pathway.It has been suggested that some **AF cases of sympathetic origin** may be resolved by the ablation of the Marshall ligament, a neuromuscular bundle richly innervated with sympathetic fibers, located in the left atrium (Katritsis and Ioannidis, 2001).

- One of the problems related to ablation is that we do not know **which patients will not respond to this treatment** and which responding patients will maintain the sinus rhythm (Lubitz *et al.*, 2008). In general, the prognostic markers of recurrence in performing an electrical CV are also valid (see before). We will now look at some aspects of this problem in more detail.

  ○ It has been described (Matsuo *et al.*, 2009) that, in general, if the duration of AF is less than two years, the success of ablation and the maintenance of sinus rhythm is high. If the duration is longer than two years, or unknown, it might be necessary to include CFAE in targetting of ablation areas (see before).

o New hope has been raised by demonstrating, using contrast enhanced CV magnetic resonance (CE-CMR) (Oakes *et al.*, 2009), that the quantification of atrial fibrosis and atrial scars, indicative of irreversible atrial remodeling, may identify candidates for ablation (see before).

o It has also been shown (Lin *et al.*, 2010) that high levels of hs-CRP are associated with an abnormal left atrium substrate, high incidence of pulmonary vein AF sources, and less successful ablation and higher rate of recurrence (see before). In patients with long-lasting AF, the level of hs-CRP decreases if AF recurrences do not occur after three months of ablation (Rotter *et al.*, 2006).

o Caldwell *et al.* (2014) demonstrated that longer P-wave duration (>140 ms) is associated with higher recurrence rate, despite same (or lower) number of pulmonary veins reconnection (indicating that P-wave duration may be an easier way to demonstrate abnormal substrate and fibrosis).

o The first three months after a pulmonary vein isolation are considered a "time window", where recurrences may not necessary imply long-term recurrence. If AF does not resolve, it should be treated as any other recurrence, until this "time window" expires. Recurrences after the first three months are considered "true" recurrences and patients should be considered for re-do procedures, where re-isolation for the pulmonary veins is the more frequent strategy.

• Few severe **complications** associated with AF ablation can be seen. Some serious (<1%) and even fatal complications (<1%) have been described. Frequently between 5% and 30% of patients (it depends very much in different series) who have undergone a pulmonary vein ablation show recurrences of AF or new atrial tachycardias (AT) in the follow-up, which present different ECG characteristics according to the place of ablation (Gerstenfeld *et al.*, 2007; Matsuo *et al.*, 2010). There may be focal (easily amenable to ablation) and macro-reentrant tachycardias (which are usually more difficult to ablate). The noninducibility of atrial tachycardias (AT) after circumferential pulmonary vein isolation may be very helpful in recognizing the patients not prone to recurrences of AF (Chang and Chen, 2010). Therefore, it is necessary to explain to patients not only the advantages of the procedure but also the improbable, but possible, severe complications and the real success of the procedure. We have to note the possible need for a second ablation in cases of recurrences in order to increase the success rate of the procedure.

• It appears that ablation techniques have practically replaced **surgical procedures** aimed at resolving AF (the Maze procedure) (Cox *et al.*, 1991). Nevertheless, new minimally invasive surgical approaches have been developed, which, in select cases and sometimes combined with ablation (hybrid treatment), allow the isolation of autonomic ganglia that actively trigger AF. At the same time, surgery is useful for the isolation ablation of the left appendage, which is the main location for thrombus formation (Lee *et al.*, 2009). If patients are surgical candidates, for example, to mitral valve replacement, MAZE IV technique to treat AF should be also considered (Tinetti *et al.*, 2010, 2012).

• We also have to stress that **anticoagulation** is recommended for all patients for at least three months after ablation. It is advisable to continue anticoagulation, even in all patients with CHADS$_2$ ≥1 score, until new clinical trials can help recommend the best therapy for these patients (Cakulev and Waldo, 2010).

• **With all this information in mind, we consider that the application of this technique is currently advised:**

o For many cases of repetitive paroxysmal AF, especially when they are frequent and troublesome; or when antiarrhythmic drugs failed to control the arrhythmia.

o It is also advisable in selected cases of chronic AF, when recovering sinus rhythm, it is considered a feasible and convenient method for improving quality of life and the general clinical condition of the patient (for instance, selected cases of hypertrophic cardiomyopathy and HF). It has been published (Khan *et al.*, 2008, PABA trial) that in patients with AF+HF+QRS duration <120 ms, pulmonary vein ablation (PV-A) was superior to biventricular pacing + AV node ablation in terms of exercise capacity and increase of ejection fraction (EF). This study shows that rhythm control if possible, is better than the most perfect rate control (biventricular pacing + AV ablation). However, in cases with very advanced HF + AF and QRS >120 ms not available for ablation, several studies demonstrated that cardiac resynchronization therapy (CRT) was effective not only in sinus rhythm but also in AF. In one study (Gasparini *et al.*, 2006), this was effective particularly when AV node ablation was also performed, but in another (Khadjooi *et al.*, 2008) it occurred even without AV node ablation.

• However, it should be noted that the **real value of ablation is still not completely known,** especially in the long term, in elderly people and in patients with advanced heart disease. Our feeling is that in the future it will be performed much earlier during the evolution of the disease (Katritsis *et al.*, 2009). At present, we have to consider that not all centers, even in developed countries, are equipped with the appropriate technology and logistics to perform this procedure safely.

Current developments in ablation robotic techniques, in catheter technology, and in the applied energy for ablation, as well as the possibility to perform ablation beyond pulmonary veins in the most appropriate areas where frequency gradients arise, and fractioned electrograms exist, have already reduced ablation time and radiation, and increased its success rate.

The goal is to continue making significant progress in this field with the hope that this technique will become cheaper and expand throughout the world. This would be very beneficial to patients.

Rate-Control Strategy

If reversion to sinus rhythm is not feasible, ventricular rate should be controlled.

- *Drugs should be administered to slow the ventricular rate*

  This is true in cases of permanent AF that are not resolved with pharmacologic treatment or electrical CV, and also in patients who do not respond to or are not clear candidates for ablation techniques.

  This is usually achieved by administering oral digoxin, and/or diltiazem or ß-blockers (Class II aB). Obviously, these are cases without pre-excitation. In the presence of evident HF, β-blockers, associated with calcium antagonists, have to be used with caution, and in some situations they may not be prescribed, for example, in cases of bronchial asthma. β-blockers are especially useful in cases where heart rate increases significantly with exercise, and in the presence of IHD. Long-term treatment with amiodarone need to be very well controlled for avoiding side effects especially thyroid dysfunction

- *Rhythm control versus rate control*

  Some studies have demonstrated that heart rate control is as efficient as sinus rhythm control, especially in elderly patients (AFFIRM trial, Wyse *et al.*, 2002; RACE trial Van Gelder *et al.*, 2002). To properly control the ventricular rate, the following are required: (i) ventricular rate at rest should be between 60 and 80 bpm, (ii) ventricular rate should not be >110 bpm after the 6-min walk test, and (iii) the average rate in a 24-h Holter study should be <100 bpm, whereas the maximum rate should be <110% of the age-adjusted maximum rate in sinus rhythm. However, one study shows that a not-so-strict rate control may also be effective (Van Gelder *et al.*, 2010). In spite, however, of the demonstrated noninferiority of rate control, in practice many patients remain symptomatic despite adequate control of ventricular rate (Mazzini and Monahan, 2008). It is in these cases that rhythm control becomes first-line therapy.

  These studies (rhythm vs rate control) have raised a great deal of controversy (Wyse *et al.*, 2002; Van Gelder *et al.*, 2002). There is no definitive study demonstrating the superiority of rhythm control over rate control for either end point. It was believed that rhythm control was not better than rate control (Steinberg *et al.*, 2004), probably due to the side effects associated with AAA (Roy *et al.*, 2008). The increased risk of proarrhythmic effects is observed mostly in patients with an EF <40% (Kaufman *et al.*, 2004). On the other hand, the lack of differences observed between the treatment groups may be explained because the electroanatomic remodeling of the atria starts from the time AF is initiated. For many authors this may lead to a conclusion of irreversible AF. Finally, several studies (Shelton *et al.*, 2009; Kong *et al.*, 2010) resulted in the appearance of a trend toward better survival in patients with AF and HF managed with rhythm control. However, large randomized clinical trials are needed to verify this hypothesis in this group of patients.

Our opinion regarding this matter is as follows: on the one hand, in some cases heart rate control is a good option, such as in asymptomatic or mildly symptomatic elderly patients with permanent AF (duration greater than 1–2 years), a large left atrium, and a well-controlled ventricular rate. On the other hand, CV should be attempted in those patients who are expected to maintain sinus rhythm (relatively recent AF, left atrium not too large), as well as in those patients whose prognosis and symptoms you expect will improve after sinus rhythm is restored. This includes some patients with valvular heart disease, HF, cardiomyopathies, and so forth. It should to be noted (Shelton *et al.*, 2009) that in patients with AF and HF, restoration of sinus rhythm improves the left ventricular EF significantly and decreases NT-proBNP levels. For this reason, one or two electrical CV may be performed on many patients with HF. Ablation, should be considered if maintenance of sinus rhythm is not achievable with AAA (see before). If sinus rhythm is restored, it is important to maintain it especially with amiodarone, or sometimes with Class I drugs. In patients with no heart disease, propafenone may be administered in monotherapy or in combination. If sinus rhythm cannot be restored, rate control may be sufficient. However, bearing in mind the clinical situation of the patient and the experience of the medical center, one should decide if a new CV or catheter ablation with new techniques may be performed (see before).

Prevention of Thromboembolism

- *Risk of embolism*

  Studies performed with transesophageal echocardiography (TEE) have shown that thrombi are more frequently in the left than in the right atrium. This is in part related to the increased platelet reactivity found in the left atrium. Cerebral embolism is unfortunately the most frequent and dangerous complication. In permanent AF, the risk of cerebral embolism is set to increase fivefold (Lubitz *et al.*, 2008). In some cases, such as mitral stenosis, the risk without treatment is around 20–25% per year. In nonvalvular AF with previous embolism the risk is also high ($\cong$10%/year). We had the feeling that thromboembolism may occur at the moment of the first AF episode or in patients with paroxysmal repetitive crises of AF (see Atrial Fibrillation Types). Therefore, anticoagulant treatment if indicated, according to the CHADS$_2$ score, has to be prescribed as soon as AF was detected to reduce the risk of stroke (Friberg *et al.*, 2010).

However, studies using long recording systems (implantable loop reorders or storage capabilities of pacemakers and ICDs) (Glotzer *et al.*, 2009; Martin *et al.*, 2015) have demonstrated that AF is not the direct cause of stroke, because there is no temporal relation between the appearance of stroke and the presence of AF. This fact leads us to speculate whether anticoagulation may need to be started even before the first episode of AF is demonstrated, especially in old patients with enlarged LA, interatrial block and fibrotic atrial cardiomyopathy, because all these situations especially together favor the presence of thrombosis in the LA (see before).,

- ### *Preventive treatment*

Prevention of thromboembolism with anticoagulants is paramount to reduce the risk of stroke. A 70% decrease of cerebral embolism, and a 25% decrease of mortality, with very low incidence of complications (bleeding) can be expected. Such treatment should be done knowing the bleeding risk of each patient (see HAS-BLED* score from ESC guidelines for AF (Camm, 2010)), and according to the risk stratification for cerebrovascular events in every patient following the CHADS$_2$** score (Gage *et al.*, 2001; Fuster *et al.*, 2006; Niemwlaat *et al.*, 2009). In 2016, the newest risk score for stroke is the well-established CHA$_2$DS$_2$-Vasc (Lip, 2014).

This treatment should be indefinitely administered with very strict control with except in specific cases where anticoagulants are completely contraindicated

(INR between 2 and 3, closer to 3 in patients with valvular prostheses if Warfarin is used), to patients with (i) previous cerebral embolism, (ii) HF, (iii) hypertrophic cardiomyopathy, (iv) mitral valve disease, (v) implanted mechanical valve prosthesis and (vi) evident heart failure.

Anticoagulation is also recommended in patients with ≥1 point (one or more risk factors taken from CHADS$_2$ score), including: (i) elderly patients, (ii) patients with hypertension, or (iii) patients with diabetes, (iv) heart failure or (v) prior TIA or stroke. The guidelines of the ESC on AF (Camm, 2010) emphasize more in this group of patients with 1 point and consider important some modification of CHADS$_2$ score, including as a risk factors patients between 65 and 75 years old, female gender, and those who present vascular diseases (score CHA$_2$DS$_2$-VAsc). According to this score, anticoagulants are not necessary only in the small number of nonelderly patients (<65 years for women and <75 for men) with isolated AF to whom aspirin should be administered. In patients with 1 point the decision has to be taken at individual level, but usually anticoagulation is preferably to aspirin. Patients over 80 years of age (Gage *et al.*, 2001), in particular, may benefit from anticoagulant treatment but should be closely followed-up. The results of a prospective BAFTA trial (Mant *et al.*, 2007) demonstrated that in elderly patients with AF warfarin is more effective than aspirin at preventing stroke (annual risk of stroke 1.8% with warfarin compared to 3.8% with aspirin). Finally, the Canadian guidelines have simplified the decision flow even more: age >65-years-old and AF is enough to start full anticoagulation (Verma *et al.*, 2014).

In patients with several of the previously mentioned factors (i.e., elderly patients with HF and hypertension), the yearly incidence of cerebral embolism when no anticoagulants are administered may be over 15%.

The addition of aspirin or clopidogrel to the anticoagulant treatment does not decrease the risk of embolism but increases the risk of bleeding (Lip and Lane, 2009). On the other hand, it has been shown that the combination of acenocumarol with the antiplatelet agent trifusal is more effective than anticoagulant monotherapy, with an even lower rate of hemorrhagic complication (Pérez Gómez *et al.*, 2004). Currently, double antiplatelet therapy or adding one platelet agent is discouraged due to increased risk of bleeding with no incremental benefit on stroke prevention. However, this association may be mandatory in some cases as we will see now.

Patients with AF receiving chronic anticoagulant treatment who have presented an acute coronary syndrome (ACS) requiring stent implantation represent a

---

* HAS-BLED in an acronym (H, hypertension; A, abnormal liver or renal function; S, previous stroke; B, bleeding (cerebral); L, labil INR; E, elderly; D, drug intake including alcohol and aspirin or equivalents). Each factor has 1 point. The risk of embolism increases with the number of factors.
** CHA$_2$DS$_2$-Vascular is an acronym (C, congestive heart failure; H, hypertension; A, aging>75 years for men, more than 65 years for women with double risk at 75 years; D, diabetes; S, stroke). All factors have 1 point (S2 = 2 points).

real clinical dilemma. These patients also require anti-platelet treatment. The decisions should be taken on an individual basis. Experts on anticoagulation may be consulted and, after considering the pros and cons of each case, a decision should be taken with regard to the best combination and dosage, bearing in mind that the risk of bleeding or embolism is high (Halbfass *et al.*, 2009). The wiser option is probably to follow the recommendations published by the experts committee (Rubboli *et al.*, 2008, 2009). Patients with mechanical valves, AF, and repetitive emboli represent also a similar difficult dilemma.

It should be pointed out that cerebral embolisms are frequently asymptomatic, as demonstrated by magnetic resonance imaging. However, they may lead to a significant cognitive deficit (Vermeer *et al.*, 2003). That is the reason why Holter recordings (or extended monitoring using implantable loop recorders) should be performed in patients at risk for developing AF (i.e., patients with valvular heart disease or sleep apnea), or in patients who have suffered cerebral embolism (Gladstone *et al.*, 2014; Sanna *et al.*, 2014), including transient ischemic attack, to assess whether they have experienced asymptomatic AF episodes. In cases where the presence of asymptomatic embolism is detected by CMR, and/or the presence of asymptomatic episodes of AF is detected by Holter, it is necessary to start anticoagulant treatment (Brambatti *et al.*, 2014).

If reversion to sinus rhythm is achieved, administration of anticoagulants should continue even forever depending on the clinical situation of each case patient (frequent recurrences, presence of HF, results of Holter monitoring, etc.).

Anticoagulant treatment leads to a significant decrease in the incidence of systemic embolism, including cerebral embolism, with a very low risk of bleeding if proper monitoring is performed. The advantages of the new oral anticoagulants over Warfarin include: no need to monitoring, higher adherence, fewer drug–drug or drug–food interactions, easier pre- and post-operative management, and probably lower risk of intracranial hemorrhage. The disadvantages are that they are much more expensive, which could be a problem for many people in many countries, and (see later) there is not currently, except for dabigatran, an antidote in case of bleeding (see later).

• *New oral anticoagulants (NOACS)*

Considerable research has been done in an attempt to prevent thromboembolism without the necessity for performing the frequent controls needed with current anticoagulation drugs like coumadin or warfarin (Eriksson *et al.*, 2009). A summary of these trials include: Xa factor inhibitors such as rivaroxaban (Halperin *et al.*, 2014) – ROCKET AF trial, which demonstrated that it is equally efficacious as warfarin and with less complications such as intracranial bleeding and general bleeding; apixaban (Keating, 2013) – the ARISTOTELE and AVERROES trials, which have demonstrated that apixaban is superior to warfarin to prevent embolism and with less serious bleeding; edoxaban (Kato *et al.*, 2016, ENGAGE-AF-TIMI 48), which showed that the new drug is not inferior to warfarin, or **direct thrombin inhibitors** (Factor IIa) such as ximelagatran, which is no longer used due to its hepatotoxic potential, or, currently, dabigatran. The RE-LY study (Connolly *et al.*, 2009a) demonstrates that dabigatran, at both 150 mg or at 110 mg (twice daily) doses, was found to be a useful alternative to warfarin in the prevention of embolism in AF patients with no valvular heart disease and at least one risk factor for cerebrovascular events. The higher dose provides a better protection than warfarin with similar risk of bleeding, whereas the lower dose provides the same degree of protection but is associated with a lower risk of bleeding. In all current anticoagulation guidelines, NOACs are preferred over warfarin. In 2016, there are no "head-to-head" comparisons between NOACs. However, all guidelines recommend NOACs over warfarin (Verma *et al.*, 2014) in nonvalvular AF. However, in valvular patients or in patients with severe renal disease (eGFR <30), warfarin still is recommended over NOACs. Despite in clinical practice, anticoagulation reversal is not a serious or frequent challenge, patients have been misinformed and several of them will feel reluctant to use NOACs due to the absence of a reversal agent. The first anticoagulation reversal for Dabigatran, the drug Idurixizumab is now available in Europe and the USA (FDA) and has helped physicians to re-assure patients about the potential risk of requiring their anticoagulation to be reversed (Enriquez *et al.*, 2016).

• *Devices for LA occlusion*

A new therapeutic option, which in some cases may be an alternative to drug therapy (if contraindicated), is the placement of a device (Watchman) in the left atrial appendage, the most important origin of thrombus. This seems to significantly reduce the combined risk of cardiovascular death and vascular embolic and hemorrhagic episodes (Sick *et al.*, 2007; Holmes, 2009). This would provide a great advantage to many patients with AF, especially those who are not able to receive anticoagulation treatment (Holmes *et al.*, 2014).

Atrial fibrillation

1. Atrial fibrillation (AF) is a very frequent arrhythmia that can be paroxysmal (sporadic or repetitive), persistent (more than 7 days) or permanent (no intention to return to sinus rhythm). It is usually initiated by atrial extrasystoles and maintained by repetitive micro-reentries, rotors, or simply by fibrillatory conduction.

2. From an electrocardiogram (ECG) point of view, the diagnosis is easy and is based on evidence of the presence of "f" fibrillation waves (variable voltage and morphology and high rate (>500 bpm)) with an irregular ventricular rhythm (QRS with RR intervals completely variable). The following should be taken into account:
   a) If the ventricular rhythm is regular this indicates that there is an AV dissociation (Figure 4.27).
   b) If there are wide QRS complexes, these may be ventricular ectopic or conducted with aberrancy. Therefore, it is necessary to make the correct differential diagnosis (Figures 4.44–4.48).
   c) The AF associated to Wolff–Parkinson–White (WPW) syndrome can be mistaken with ventricular tachycardia (VT). The key for the differential diagnosis is shown in Figure 4.52.

3. Serious complications are associated with AF, such as systemic embolism (mostly cerebral), hemodynamic impairment, and heart failure (HF). These complications should be prevented and treated if they appear.

4. Currently, pharmacologic treatments and electrical cardioversion (CV) used to revert the AF into sinus rhythm, and the administration of drugs to avoid recurrences, are often useful. If it is not possible to restore sinus rhythm with drugs or cardioversion, ablation is offered to dissociate the pulmonary veins.

5. Finally, in some cases, the control of the ventricular rate may be the most convenient therapeutic approach.

6. To prevent embolism, it is necessary to prescribe anticoagulant therapy to patients who are at risk for stroke according to the CHA2DS2 –Vascular score.

7. Finally, NOACs to prevent embolism that do not need monthly control are available, (see above). New devices for blocking the left atrial appendage, the most important origin of thrombus, are another interesting alternative to anticoagulant drug therapy (Di Biase *et al.*, 2010).

Atrial Flutter
(Figures 4.57–4.71)

Concept

This is a fast atrial rhythm (240–300 bpm). The cases with a slower rate even ≈200 bpm are explained by the effect of pharmacologic therapy and/or the presence of important conduction delay in the atria. The rhythm is organized and regular, and initiates atrial waves that do not have, at least in some leads, especially the inferior leads, an isoelectric baseline between them (flutter "F" waves).

Electrophysiologic mechanism

Although atrial flutter (AFl) has aspects very similar to AF, it is really a very different arrhythmia, at least because the maintenance mechanism is different. Atrial flutter is predominantly a RA arrhythmia; the maintenance mechanism relies on a macro-reentry using the cavo-tricuspid isthmus. However, the triggering and modulating factors (PSVC, ANS imbalance, interatrial block, inflammatory markers, etc.) are similar to AF.

It is possible that all types of flutter start with a very premature atrial extrasystole, which, when it finds some zone of the atria with unidirectional block, initiates a circular movement (reentry). The slower the conduction of the stimulus or the longer the circuit, the easier it is to perpetuate the arrhythmia (Figure 3.6C and D). There is evidence suggesting that in the typical or common flutter, the reentry circuit is located in the RA and that there is an area with slow conduction in the lower RA. The combination of valvular and venous orifices and the obstacle of the crista terminalis due to its anatomic structure make the RA an ideal place for reentry. In the past, it was believed that it was necessary to have an anatomic obstacle (cava or pulmonary veins), around which the circular movement was perpetuated. However, it is now known that an anatomic obstacle is not required for a flutter to perpetuate.

The depolarization in **common (typical) flutter** is counterclockwise, going down through the anterior and lateral walls of the RA and up through the septum and the posterior wall of the RA, with a zone of slow conduction in the lower RA. Thus, when depolarization reaches the lower part of the septum, another "F" wave is already in development (Figures 3.7A and 4.57). This explains the lack of isoelectric baseline between "F" waves, and why "F" waves are predominantly negative in leads II, III, and VF. From leads such as VF, the positive (craniocaudal) part of the wave lasts longer and is smoother (less visible) than the negative part (caudocranial) (Figures 4.57–4.59). Because of this, in II, III, and VF, the negative morphology part predominates over the positive one, especially in the absence of large atria.

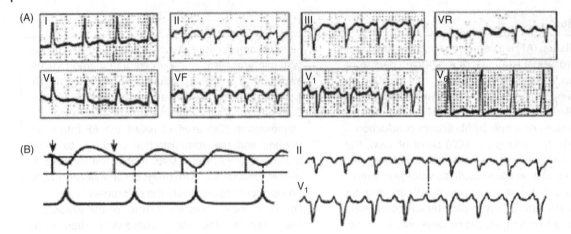

Figure 4.57 (A). Morphologies of the common 2:1 flutter waves in the six frontal leads, V1 and V6. Note one "f" wave visible at the end of the QRS in V1, which may simulate a partial right bundle branch block (RBBB) morphology. (B) Morphology correlation between II and V1 in a common 2:1 flutter, with an eventual 3:1 conduction.

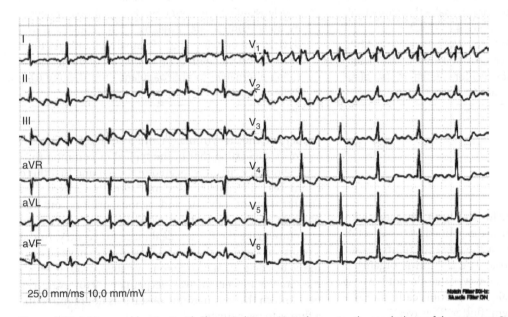

25,0 mm/ms 10,0 mm/mV

Figure 4.58 A 15-year-old patient with Ebstein's disease. Note the sawtooth morphology of the common 3×1 flutter waves, which show a voltage greater than usual because of the large size of the atria.

In a small number of cases, flutter activation uses the same circuit but follows a clockwise rotation, ascending through the anterior and lateral wall and descending through the posterior and septal wall, so that the circuit is the same, but the rotation is different (**inverse or reverse flutter**) (Figure 3.7B). Usually, the ECG shows a different morphology (wide positive waves in leads II, III, and VF, and wide negative in V1) (Figure 4.60).

It is also possible to find other morphologies that require EPS to identify the circuit. On such occasions rapid atrial waves that are usually narrow and positive appear (>220 bpm), often with a certain undulation. They are probably related to a reentry in the LA, and

correspond to an uncommon type of flutter (**atypical flutter**) (Figure 4.61). These cases are equivalent to macro-reentrant atrial tachycardia but with a higher rate (>200–220 bpm) (see Atrial Tachycardia Due to Macro-reentry (AT-MR)).

○ The rapid atrial rhythms related to atrial incisions, and sometimes to the placing of patches, especially in the right atrium (Mustard, Fontan, Senning operations, etc.), or to ablation techniques (macro-reentry circuit surrounding the ablated area) do not have a unique electrocardiographic morphology. They can show a morphology similar to the monomorphic atrial tachycardia from an ectopic focus, but also different electrocardiographic patterns (reverse flutter, common flutter, or atypical flutter) (see Monomorphic Atrial Tachycardia Due to Macro-reentry (AT-MR).).

- ○ Lastly, different types of atrial circuits activating different parts of the atria can occasionally coexist (atrial dissociation). They can only be confirmed by intracavitary techniques. These cases can explain the morphologies called fibrilloflutter (Figure 4.41).

In the classification of all supraventricular tachyarrhythmias that we make at the end of this chapter (see Supraventricular Tachyarrhythmias and Atrial-Wave Morphology), we pay more attention to the ECG morphology than to the electrophysiologic mechanism of the arrhythmia. According to this classification, we have: (i) sinus P wave (Figure 4.69A), (ii) and (iii) the P' wave of the monomorphic atrial tachycardia of ectopic focus (Figure 4.69B and C), (iv) the "F" waves of common flutter (Figure 4.69D), (v) the "F" waves of inverse flutter

(Figure 4.69E), (vi) the P' behind the QRS complex in cases of paroxysmal junctional reentrant tachycardia through an accessory pathway (Figure 4.69F), and (vii) the atrial wave from the so-called atypical flutter (Figure 4.69G). We have also already mentioned that atrial tachycardias by macro-reentry can have different ECG morphologies (see before, Atrial Tachycardia Due to Macro-reentry (AT-MR), and Table 4.4).

For some authors (Saoudi *et al.*, 2001), all of the atrial tachyarrhythmias due to macro-reentrant circuits with fixed or functional obstacles that can be entrained during the electrophysiologic study could be classified under the category of **macro-reentrant atrial tachyarrhythmia**. This term would include typical flutter, reverse flutter, atypical flutter, due to a macro-reentry in the LA, and all other types of fast atrial rhythms associated with postsurgical incisions that have an atrial macro-reentry mechanism (macro-reentrant atrial tachycardia). Atypical flutter presents the same monomorphic atrial wave as

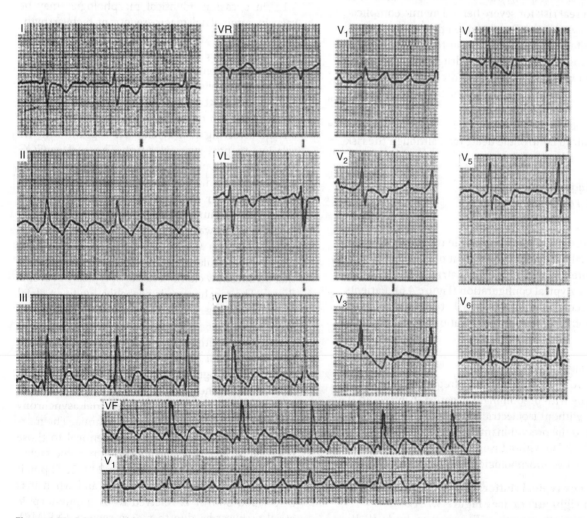

Figure 4.59 A 30-year-old patient who underwent surgery because of a complete transposition of the great vessels (Fontan procedure). Note the typical common flutter morphology (3×1) with unusually high voltages (negative F in II, III, and VF, and positive with an isoelectric line in V1), which is caused by macro-reentry around the atrial scar.

MAT-MR but we refer to atypical flutter if the rate is >200–220 bpm and MAT-MR if the atrial rate is lower. They are, in fact, the same arrhythmia with two different names.

Clinical Manifestations

From a clinical point of view, the etiological characteristics, clinical presentation, and prognosis of atrial flutter are similar to those of AF. Therefore, it may present paroxysmal (sporadic and repetitive) and chronic (persistent and or permanent) forms. On some occasions, runs of flutter waves or alternating flutter and fibrillation waves can be seen, showing characteristics of incessant forms. Very often the same patient presents recurrences with separate and alternant episodes of AF and atrial flutter.

As with all tachyarrhythmias, symptoms depend mainly on the heart rate, associated heart disease, and the duration of arrhythmia (see Chapter 1).

1:1 Flutter is infrequent but very badly tolerated, and represents a real risk for severe hemodynamic complications and may trigger VF and sudden death (SD), unless it is self-limited (Figure 4.65). 1:1 Flutter may be seen in patients taking some cardioactive drugs, in Ebstein disease, in pre-excitation, in some children with congenital heart disease, and in the presence of a hyperconductive AV node (i.e., hyperthyroidism).

With respect to AF in patients with atrial flutter, it is more difficult to control the heart rate, although the risk of embolism is lower.

Electrocardiographic Diagnosis
(Figures 4.58–4.67)

Sinus Rhythm
The same considerations discussed in the AF section, are valid for atrial flutter. Remember that often patients with advanced interatrial block presents atrial flutter that frequently is of atypical configuration (Figure 4.6). Patients with advanced IAB and paroxysmal atrial flutter, have a higher incidence of post-flutter ablation AF (Enriquez *et al.*, 2015b).

Flutter "F" Waves
There are two morphologies more frequently found: the common type with predominant negative "f" waves in II, III, and VF, without isoelectric baselines (sawtooth morphology), and the predominantly positive morphology in II, III, and VF, also without isoelectric baselines. We will analyze these two morphologies in more detail:

- **Common or typical flutter: counter clockwise activation in right atrium (see Figure 3.7 A)**
  - Predominantly negative "F" waves in leads II, III, and VF. These are "F" waves with a small voltage, in the absence of large atria, and are without an isoelectric baseline (Figures 4.56–4.59), giving them a sawtooth morphology. They are predominantly negative in leads II, III, and VF, and positive in V1, where the "F" wave is usually narrow and often presents an isoelectric baseline.
  - Occasionally, in the presence of large atria, especially in congenital defects, the voltage of the "F" waves is larger but generally has the typical sawtooth morphology (Figures 4.58 and 4.59). Although the typical rate is 300 bpm, it can be even lower than 200 bpm when antiarrhythmic drugs are taken and/or there are atrial conduction defects.

- **Noncommon flutter**
  - **Reverse or inverse flutter**: clockwise activation in the right atrium (Figure 3.7B). Generally, it initiates wide and positive "F" waves in leads II, III, and VF, without isoelectric baselines between them and with predominantly negative and wide waves in lead V1. On occasion, identical morphologies may be seen in some atrial macro-reentrant tachyarrhythmia due to a surgical incision or post-ablation (Figure 4.60) (see Monomorphic Atrial Tachycardia Due to Macro-reentry (MAT-MR), and later).

- **Other types of atrial morphology**
  - **Left septal flutter** (Marrouche *et al.*, 2004). This infrequent form of flutter is produced by a reentry circuit involving mainly the left septum with no relation to post-surgical scars. The surface ECG shows high and peaked "F" waves in V1 and flat "F" waves in the remaining leads (Anselme, 2008).
  - **Atypical flutter**. Possibly macro-reentrant circuit in the left atrium (see Figure 3.7C). This term includes atrial wave positive in II, III, VF and V1, with high rates (>200–220 bpm) and sometimes with some undulating waves in at least some leads that do not show characteristics of typical or reverse flutter. The mechanism is probably due to an atrial macro-reentry, generally in the left atrium (Bayés de Luna *et al.*, 1996; Daubert, 1996). Very often, tachyarrhythmias with these characteristics are recorded in patients that present an advanced interatrial block with retrograde left atrial conduction (Figures 4.6 and 4.61). The presence of inhomogeneous activation of the LA and major interatrial asynchrony favors the appearance of this arrhythmia. The morphology of these waves may be identical to those observed in macro-reentrant monomorphic tachycardia. When the atrial rate is over 200–220 bpm, it is referred to it as atypical flutter, and when it is below 200 bpm it is referred to as monomorphic atrial tachycardia due to macro-reentry (AT-MR). In fact, these are the same arrhythmia with different

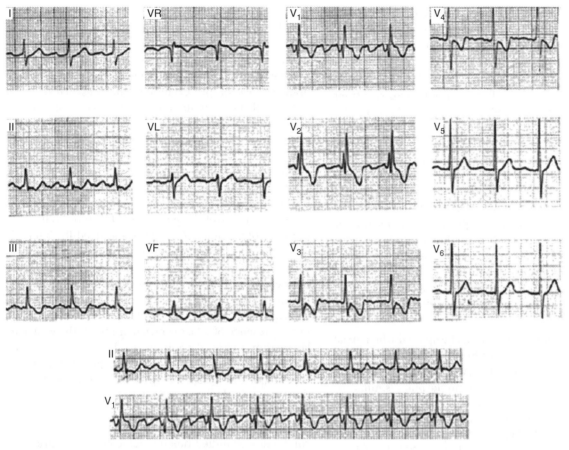

Figure 4.60 Example of reverse atrial flutter ("F" waves + I, II, III, and VF, and wide negative in V1) that appeared after surgery for anomalous drainage of pulmonary veins.

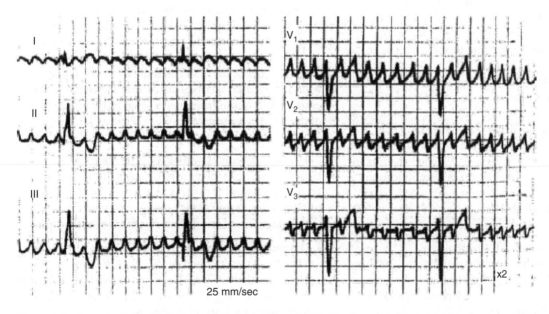

25 mm/sec

Figure 4.61 Example of atypical flutter with fast atrial waves (≈280 x′) and predominantly negative waves in I and positive waves in II, III, VF, and V1.This type of flutter is very often recorded in patients with advanced interatrial block with retrograde activation of the left atrium (see Figure 4.6).

rates. When the atrial rate is on the border (200–220 bpm), this may be called "atrial tachysystole" (see Monomorphic Atrial Tachycardia Due to Macro-reentry (AT-MR)).

Atrial tachyarrhythmias that have been generated around a scar after cardiac surgery (macro-reentrant atrial tachycardia) has no specific morphology and can appear with an electrocardiographic morphology identical to reverse flutter (Figure 4.60), a focal atrial tachycardia (Figure 4.69C) and also typical flutter (Figure 4.56), although the "F" waves clearly have a higher voltage. A new very frequently form of atypical flutter seen in clinical practice, is the post-PVI atrial flutter, usually involving the prior lines of ablation or the mitral isthmus. These arrhythmias can be difficult to re-ablate and require well-trained EP services. Noncontact mapping is useful in helping the ablator to locate the circuit of these flutters. Anterior lines from the mitral isthmus to the right superior pulmonary vein are usually needed.

○ The term **fibrilloflutter** has be applied when atrial waves are highly visible in some leads in the same ECG, especially in lead V1, when the waves are quite regular and relatively monomorphic, similar to those in atrial flutter although with a higher rate, but with irregular waves on other leads, especially II, III, and VF (Figure 4.41). Endocavitary studies performed many years ago (Puech, 1956) have demonstrated that in certain areas of the atria flutter waves exist, whereas fibrillation waves exist in others. These can be considered varieties of atrial dissociation. However, as we have said, currently it is considered that these changes of morphology are due to the recording process (distance between the rotor and the surface of atria).

○ **The morphology of the flutter wave may vary** suddenly along the recording (Figure 4.28B) on some rare occasions, especially when patients are taking cardioactive drugs (i.e., digitalis).

○ The **flutter "F" waves may not be visible** or only barely visible on the surface ECG when there is significant atrial fibrosis. External amplification or intracavitary techniques may be needed to make them visible (Bayés de Luna *et al.*, 1978) (Figure 4.62).

Ventricular Response and QRS Morphology

In typical flutter, with a rate between 250 and 300 bpm, one of every two "F" waves is blocked in the AV junction, as a rule, and therefore the ventricular response is between 125 and 150 bpm (Figure 4.56). The FR interval, starting from the beginning of the negative "F" wave, has a duration ≥0.20 s (Figure 4.63B). However, a higher degree block (3:1 (rare), 4:1, 6:1, or more) (Figure 4.63) are found, especially with certain drugs that have depressor effects on the AV conduction. Sometimes, in the same patient the degree of conduction is variable and can be inclusively 1:1 in the same patient (Figure 4.64). If the basal QRS complex is wide because of a bundle branch block or pre-excitation, the presence of atrial flutter with 1×1 conduction mimics a ventricular flutter aspect (Figure 4.65). Flutter 1:1 is very badly tolerated and represents a real risk of SD due to its high ventricular rate that is usually >220 bpm (see before, Clinical Manifestations).

Normally, the common flutter wave (F), starting from the beginning of the negative component, conducts with a fixed and relatively long FR interval (Figure 4.63B). The presence of variable FR intervals and fixed RR intervals means that AV dissociation exists. If the ventricular rate is fast (>80–90 bpm), there is an AV dissociation by interference with AV ectopic junctional tachycardia with narrow QRS complexes (Figure 4.28B). If the QRS is wide it would be very difficult to identify the atrial waves in the presence of a fast ventricular rate. If the ventricular rhythm is slow, there is an AV dissociation by block with atrial flutter dissociated from junctional escape rhythm (narrow QRS) (see Figure 6.4). If the QRS is wide, the escape rhythm is ventricular or due to an AV junction with aberrancy.

The wide QRS morphology may be due to aberrant conduction (bundle branch block pattern) (Figure 4.65) or conduction along an anomalous pathway (Figure 4.66B). In cases of 2:1 flutter and primarily 1:1 conduction, an accessory pathway must be considered when the aberrant QRS complex morphology does not correspond with a bundle branch block pattern and especially if a delta wave is suspected. If the flutter is 1:1, the morphology can look like ventricular flutter (compare Figures 4.65B and 5.40). In these cases the differential diagnosis with ventricular tachycardia is more difficult than in cases of WPW syndrome with atrial fibrillation because of the regular ventricular rhythm (Figures 4.52 and 4.66).

Diagnostic Difficulties and Differential Diagnosis

Usually, the ECG diagnosis of atrial flutter is simple. However, in several cases it may present different kinds of difficulties that make it necessary to perform a differential diagnosis of atrial flutter with other arrhythmias.

● **Diagnostic Difficulties Due to "F" Wave Morphology**
The "F" waves may present many of the different morphologies that we have just mentioned. Naturally, it is important to be familiar with all of these possibilities to perform the correct diagnosis:
– Common flutter (Figure 4.57).
– Reverse flutter (Figure 4.60).
– Atypical flutter (Figure 4.61).

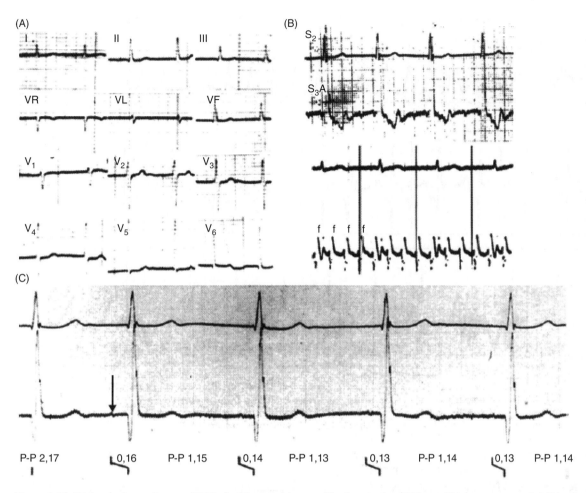

Figure 4.62 (A) An electrocardiogram (ECG) of a 66-year-old man with a heart rate of 55 bpm. Atrial waves are not visible, simulating a junctional escape rhythm. (B) With the use of external wave amplification and intracavitary ECG, the concealed flutter waves were exposed. (C) A successful cardioversion was performed, showing afterwards, thanks to external amplification of waves ($S_{III}A$), that it was a small but visible sinus P wave (see arrow) (C).

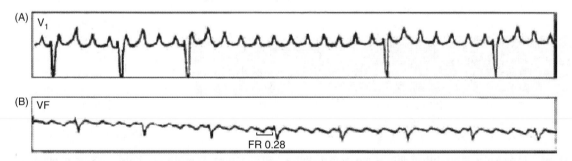

Figure 4.63 (A) Atrial flutter ("F" waves in V1 at 280 bpm) with a significant atrioventricular (AV) block. (B) Typical flutter with a fixed 4×1 AV conduction. Note the fixed and long FR interval.

– Flutter with a changing morphology (Figure 4.28).
– Concealed flutter (Figure 4.62).
– Fibrilloflutter (Figure 4.42).

• **Diagnostic difficulties due to the "F" wave rate**
When the "F" waves are slow (around 200 bpm) the diagnostic difficulties are especially important. They can be confused with a MAT-MR (see before, Monomorphic Atrial Tachycardia Due to Macro-reentry (MAT-MR)) if conduction is 1:1 and 2:1 they can be confused with a sinus rhythm (Figure 4.20). When the AV conduction is 1:1 and the QRS complex is wide, it can be mistaken for ventricular flutter (Figure 4.65B).

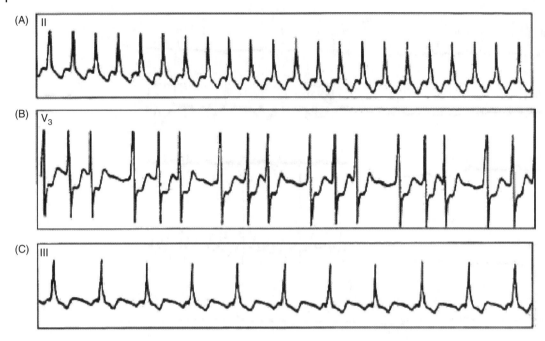

Figure 4.64 (A) A patient with tight mitral stenosis taking antiarrhythmic agents who presented a 1×1 flutter that turned into a Wenckebach-type 4×3 conduction (B) and finally a 2×1 flutter (C).

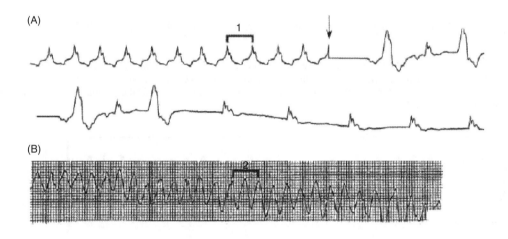

Figure 4.65 (A) 52-year-old patient with an Ebstein disease and rapid rhythm at 160 bpm suggestive of a 2×1 flutter (QRS morphology similar to sinus rhythm), which ceased after cardioversion (arrow), turning into a slow escape rhythm with retrograde conduction toward the atria. (B) Afterwards, this patient showed a short (monitor strip) run of tachycardia with a heart rate doubled from previous (~320 bpm) (1 = 2), which was very badly tolerated, probably indicating a 1:1 flutter, which fortunately ceased spontaneously after a few seconds. This tracing, seen isolated, may be taken as a ventricular flutter/fibrillation.

- **Diagnostic difficulties due to the width of the QRS complex**

Cases of flutter with 2×1 with bundle branch block morphology, or conduction along an accessory pathway (Figures 4.65 and 4.66B) can be mistaken for a ventricular tachycardia or flutter (see before). Knowledge of the patient's clinical details, having access to a previous ECG, and thinking about the

(A)

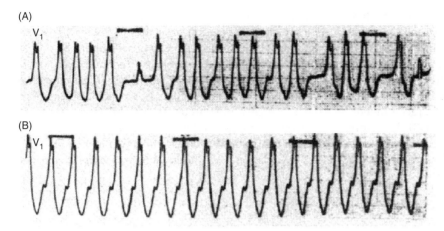

(B)

Figure 4.66 A 50-year-old patient with type IV Wolff–Parkinson–White atrial fibrillation (top) and atrial flutter (bottom) episodes simulating a ventricular tachycardia. (A) The isolated, wide R morphology, with a notch in the descending arm does not correspond to a right bundle branch block (RBBB)-type conduction aberrancy type RBBB. The following facts are in favor of a Wolff–Parkinson–White syndrome with atrial fibrillation (in addition to other clinical features and the prior awareness of the Wolff–Parkinson–White syndrome diagnosis): (i) the wide complexes show a very irregular rate and morphology (varying wideness) because of the presence of different degrees of pre-excitation, and (ii) the narrow complexes, 6 and the last ones in A, are one late and the other premature, respectively. In sustained ventricular tachycardia, QRSs are more regular and if captures occur (narrow complexes), they are always premature (see Figures 4.52 and 5.23). (B) In the Wolff–Parkinson–White syndrome with atrial flutter, (in this case 2:1, 150 bpm) the differential diagnosis with sustained ventricular tachycardia through the electrocardiogram is even more difficult.

different pathologies that could be responsible for these patterns (WPW syndrome, Ebstein disease, etc.) are very useful in making the correct diagnosis.

- **Diagnostic difficulties due to artifacts**

It is also very important to know that, on occasion, artifacts simulating atrial waves may occur. This has been seen with diaphragm contractions (hiccups) and also as a result of recording problems, for example, when a patient is trembling (Parkinson's tremor disease). In this last case the artifact is seen only in certain leads (Figure 4.67). It is necessary to remember that these artifacts disappear if the electrodes are placed at the root of the extremities.

Prognostic and Therapeutic Implications

In comparison to AF, in atrial flutter it is more difficult to control the heart rate, but the risk of embolism seems to be lower. However, AF frequently alternates with flutter episodes in the same patient (see Clinical Manifestations). Thus, the prognosis is similar to AF.

There are different options (drugs, electrical CV, atrial pacing, and ablation) for treatment of rapid atrial flutter episodes in hospital. The aim of treatment is to restore the sinus rhythm. Amiodarone may be used as first-choice drug. Remember that digitalis, β-blockers, and verapamil are not recommended in the presence of pre-excitation, as happens with AF (see before, Conversion to Sinus Rhythm and Prevention of Recurrences). Usually, control of heart rate is more difficult than in cases of AF (see before). Electrical CV is recommended (Class I C) to treat episodes of rapid poorly tolerated flutter as a first choice (i.e., 1:1 atrial flutter), or if the sinus rhythm is not restored with drugs.

Electrical CV (Class I C), or atrial pacing (Class I A), may also be performed in case of chronic stable atrial flutter, and is helpful for restoring the sinus rhythm.

Digitalis, diltiazem, or β-blockers are recommended for rate control if restoration of sinus rhythm is not possible, but with the same limitations (pre-excitation, HF) as in AF (see before Conversion to Sinus Rhythm and Prevention of Recurrences). However, as in AF, we may use also

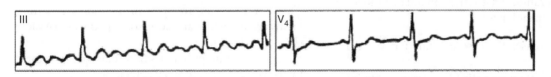

Figure 4.67 A patient with Parkinson's disease who simulates an atrial flutter in some leads (III), although the P wave is clearly visible in other leads (V4).

amiodarone if not contraindicated. In atrial flutter we have the advantage that ablation is more feasible and successful.

In common flutter, and also currently in reverse flutter, radiofrequency ablation in the zone of the cavum-tricuspid isthmus allows us to treat atrial flutter with a success rate of more than 90% and a very small number of complications (<0.5%) and no deaths (Class I B recommendation) (Figure 4.68) (García Cosío *et al.*, 1993). Therefore, the ablation procedure is strongly recommended in many cases of atrial flutter. Nevertheless, recurrence of flutter, and/or AF are frequently observed in the same

patient during the long-term follow-up, which may require another ablation procedure. This is why is recommended to perform AF and atrial flutter ablation at the same time (see before Ablation Techniques). In other types of flutter nonresponders to drug treatment, we advise catheter ablation, after the correct localization of the macro-reentrant circuit, to avoid recurrences.

In very rare cases of flutter with a ventricular response poorly controlled by drugs and not manageable with flutter ablation, AV node ablation with pacemaker implantation may be performed.

Atrial flutter

1. Atrial flutter is a frequent arrhythmia that is often a "transient step" between sinus rhythm and atrial fibrillation, or vice versa. It is generated by an organized and regular rhythm that originates in an atrial macro-circuit by a reentry mechanism.
2. From the electrocardiographic point of view, it is characterized by the presence of "F" waves that in their most typical form (common flutter) do not have an isoelectric baseline between them, especially in leads II, III, and VF, and are positive in lead V1 (Figure 4.56).
3. The reverse form also does not show an isoelectric baseline in leads II, III, and VF, and in lead V1 it is usually negative (Figure 4.60).
4. The common and reverse form may be "cured" in a high percentage of cases by ablation techniques.
5. The following must be taken into account:
   a) If the conduction is fixed 2:1 and the flutter waves are slow (≈200 bpm), it can be mistaken for sinus rhythm when taking the patient pulse and even in

the electrocardiogram (ECG) (Figure 4.20). The behavior of the heart rate during exercise, over a 24-h period, and/or with carotid sinus massage allows for a differential diagnosis (see Figure 1.15 and Table 1.5).
   b) The presence of 1:1 flutter is a real emergency. The ventricular rate is usually higher than 230 bpm.
   c) If the AV conduction is fixed in the ECG, the RR intervals and the FR intervals are regular. The conducted "F" wave has an FR interval of ≥0.20 s. (Figure 4.63B)
   d) In Figure 4.69 different types of monomorphic atrial waves of supraventricular tachycardias can be seen.
   e) In Tables 4.4 and 4.5, the most important electrocardiographic characteristics for the differential diagnosis of paroxysmal supraventricular tachycardias with a regular RR interval and narrow QRS complex are shown.

Supraventricular Tachyarrhythmias and Atrial Wave Morphology: Monomorphic and Polymorphic Morphology

Monomorphic Atrial Morphology
(Figure 4.69)

Monomorphic atrial morphology can be caused by craniocaudal or caudocranial activation.

The cases with craniocaudal activation include the following types of morphologies:

o Sinus P-wave in cases the case of sinus tachycardia. (Figure 4.69A).
o P′ wave of the atrial tachycardia (AT) (Figure 4.69C).

o "F" waves of common flutter (counterclockwise activation) (Figure 4.69D).
o "F" waves of reverse flutter (clockwise activation) (Figure 4.69E)
o Atrial waves of atypical atrial flutter can also be found (Figure 4.69G).

If there is some degree of AV block, the RR intervals may sometimes be irregular (Figure 4.69D and 4.69G)

Cases of caudocranial atrial activation correspond to:

1. The P′ waves that are seen in junctional reentrant tachycardias with an accessory pathway (AVRT) (JRT-AP) (Figure 4.69F).
2. Some cases of junctional tachycardias due to ectopic focus with retrograde atrial activation.

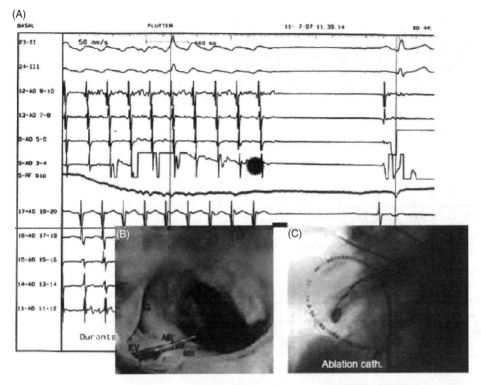

Figure 4.68 Ablation of a typical atrial flutter. (A) The tracings II and III indicate the presence of a typical atrial flutter that ceases and turns into sinus rhythm after the ablation of the cavum-tricuspid isthmus. (B) Anatomic scheme of the cavum-tricuspid isthmus, where the ablation of the typical flutter is performed between the opening of the tricuspid valve and the inferior vena cava. (C) An oblique left anterior projection shows the intracavitary catheters. The multipolar catheter (20 poles) surrounds the right atrium and records all electrical activity. The mapping-ablation catheter is placed in the cavum-tricuspid isthmus to perform a "linear" ablation.

3. Cases of monomorphic atrial tachycardias that originate in the lower part of the atria (Figure 4.69B).

Polymorphic Atrial Morphology

Rapid supraventricular rhythms with polymorphic atrial wave include:

- Chaotic atrial tachycardia (Figure 4.31).
- Atrial fibrillation (Figures 4.36 and 4.37).
- On some rare occasions, atrial flutter "F" waves can suddenly change the morphology (Figure 4.28B), or show waves in some leads that look like atrial flutter and sometimes like atrial fibrillation (fibrilloflutter) (Figure 4.41).

Differential Diagnosis of Supraventricular Tachyarrhythmias with Regular RR Intervals and Narrow QRS

Paroxysmal Tachycardias

In Tables 4.4 and 4.5, the electrocardiographic characteristics of the different paroxysmal supraventricular tachycardias with narrow QRS complexes are explained. Figure 4.69 shows examples of the different atrial activation waves seen in these tachycardias. We will comment on some of the characteristics of atrial activation activity used to make the differential diagnosis shown in Table 4.4.

- **In the junctional reentrant tachycardia with an accessory pathway (AVRT),** the atrial activity is behind the QRS complex with a relation of P'-QRS complex > QRS complex-P'. In **AVNRT** the P' is hidden within the QRS complex, or stuck to the end of the QRS, simulating an S or r' wave. The P' wave that initiates the tachycardia (craniocaudal) is different in both types from the caudocranial types described below (Figures 4.16–4.18).
- **In junctional tachycardia due to ectopic focus (JT-EF),** the P' wave is frequently dissociated (Figure 4.27). If the atrial rhythm is flutter, the AV dissociation is manifested by regular RR intervals and different FR intervals (Figure 4.28B), and if the atrial rhythm is fibrillation, the "f" waves are accompanied by regular RR intervals (Figure 4.28A).

Meanwhile, if the P' is not dissociated, it is frequently not seen because it is hidden in the QRS complex.

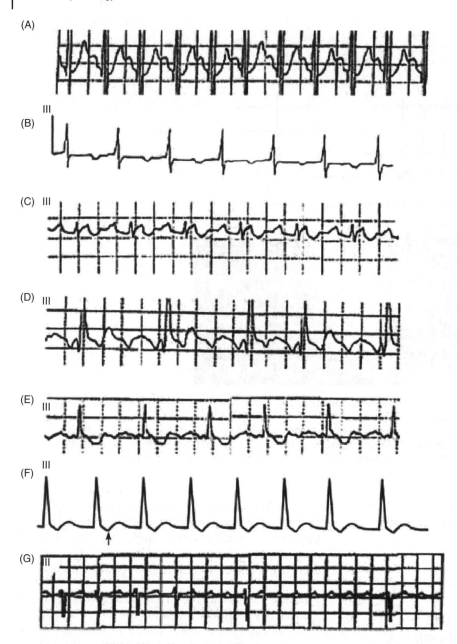

Figure 4.69 Different morphologies of monomorphic atrial waves. (A) Sinus P wave. (B) Monomorphic atrial tachycardia due to ectopic focus (MAT-EF) with 1×1 conduction. (C) MAT-EF with 2×1 atrioventricular (AV) conduction. (D) "F" waves of common flutter with variable AV conduction. (E) "F" waves of reverse flutter with a 3×1 conduction. F: Retrograde P' in case of AVRT (junctional reciprocating tachycardia-accessory pathway). (G) Atypical flutter waves with variable conduction.

However, if the retrograde conduction is faster or slower than the anterograde conduction, the P' wave will be seen before the QRS complex, but with a very short P'R, or just after the QRS complex. In any case, the P' wave has a caudocranial polarity (negative in II, III, and VF) and the first atrial depolarization, first P', has the same morphology as the others.

- **In atrial tachycardia (AT)** due to atrial macro-reentry or to an ectopic focus, the P' wave that starts the tachycardia is the same as the following waves and appears before the QRS complex, usually with P'-QRS < QRS-P'. The P' R interval is often short (Figures 4.12 and 4.19D). Sometimes there is a second- or third-degree AV block (Figures 4.13–4.14). If the AV block is first degree P'QRS may be > QRSP'. If the P' is negative in II, III, and VF, the P'R is not usually as short as in JT-EF.

- **In atrial flutter** with a regular ventricular rate, some flutter waves tend to be presumed rather than seen. If the ECG is carefully observed, in cases of 2×1 flutter in lead V1, one of each of the two "F" waves (Figures 4.56

and 4.57), can simulate r′. The same thing occurs in the case of AVNRT (Figure 4.17). In slow flutter with 2×1 block, one P wave may be hidden in the QRS or at the end of QRS, and the other mistaken for a sinus P wave (Figure 4.20).

• Finally, **sinus tachycardia** must not be forgotten, although its presentation is not usually paroxysmal and the heart rate is not very high except during exercise or emotions (Figures 4.7 and 4.8) (see Sinus Tachycardia: Clinical Presentation). If atrial activity can be seen, verifying that it has sinus polarity, this will strongly support the diagnosis. Sometimes the sinus P wave is hidden in the preceding T wave. The diagnosis may be made with careful observation of the ECG and the performance of simple maneuvers (i.e., breathing) (Figure 4.10). Sometimes it is necessary to amplify the waves or to filter the T wave, which allows us to see the P wave hidden in the T wave (Figure A-13), or to use leads such as the Lewis lead (see Appendix A-3, Other Surface Techniques to Register Electrical Cardiac Activity).

Incessant Tachycardias

The differential diagnosis of incessant supraventricular tachycardias must be made mainly between the incessant monomorphic atrial tachycardia due to ectopic focus (MAT-EF) and the incessant junctional reentrant tachycardia (I-JRT). Both show a P′R < RP′(Figures 4.11 and 4.21). The factors that help to make the differential diagnosis are (Table 4.7):

o In incessant JRT, initiation of the tachycardia is related to a critical shortening of the sinus RR. Therefore, tachycardia is initiated by a premature sinus P wave. This does not happen in MAT-ET (Figures 4.11 and 4.21).

o In incessant JRT, the sinus P-wave that initiates the tachycardia shows a different polarity from the following P-waves that presents a caudocranial polarity (Figure 4.21). This does not happen in incessant MAT-EF, where the polarity is the same (Figure 4.11).

o Incessant JRTs do not show progressive acceleration and slowing down of the heart rate (warming-up and cooling-down), something that may occur in MAT-EF (Figures 4.11 and 4.21).

o Incessant JRT does not present fusion complexes at the beginning or at the end of the episode, whereas in IMAT-EF they may appear.

Electrocardiographic Diagnosis of the Paroxysmal Supraventricular Tachycardias: a Sequential Approach

We will examine supraventricular tachycardias, according to whether the RR is regular or irregular, and whether the atrial activity is visible or not in the surface ECG. Here, we will refer to paroxysmal tachyarrhythmias. The differential diagnosis between the two most frequent types of incessant tachycardias (junctional reentrant tachycardia, and monomorphic atrial tachycardia due to ectopic focus) has been previously commented on previously (see previous section).

Supraventricular Tachycardias with Regular RR Intervals
(Tables 4.2, 4.4 and 4.5, and Figure 4.70)

Here, we will look at those intervals with a narrow QRS complex. The differential diagnosis of tachyarrhythmias with wide QRS complexes (supraventricular with intraventricular aberrant conduction or an accessory pathway) has been analyzed in Chapter 5 (see Table 5.5 and Figure 5.28).

Visible Atrial Activity

From an electrocardiographic point of view, the following types of atrial electrical activity are found in patients with supraventricular tachyarrhythmia and regular RR (Tables 4.4 and 4.5):

Situations in which the Atrioventricular Relationship is 1×1

• **Tachycardias with the P or P′ waves before the QRS complex**
  o **Sinus tachycardia** (Figure 4.8), including reentrant sinus tachycardia (sinus node-dependent) (Figure 4.9). The atrial activity is compatible with sinus P wave. The atrial rate is fast, but generally lower than 200 bpm. The AV relation is usually fixed 1×1, and therefore the RR intervals are regular, although they modify over time, with the changes in heart rate (Figure 4.8). The conducted P wave is nearer to the following QRS complex than the preceding one (RP′ > P′R), except in some cases with a first-degree AV block exist.
  o **Monomorphic atrial tachycardia** (Figure 4.12). Atrial activity can be very **high**, but is usually below 180 bpm and has a different morphology from the sinus P wave, except in the rare cases in which the atrial focus is very close to sinus node (parasinus). In the majority of cases, the distance RP′ > P′R (Figures 4.12 and 4.69B), although, as already mentioned in sinus tachycardia, there can be exceptions if the P′ wave falls into the AV junctional relative refractory period.
  o **Exceptionally in cases of junctional tachycardia due to ectopic focus (JT-EF)** (see later) (Fig. 4.29).
• **Tachycardias with the P′ wave after the QRS complex (RP′ < P′R)**
  o **Paroxysmal** junctional reentrant tachycardias (P-JRT) (Figures 4.16–4.19). In this case, the rate of

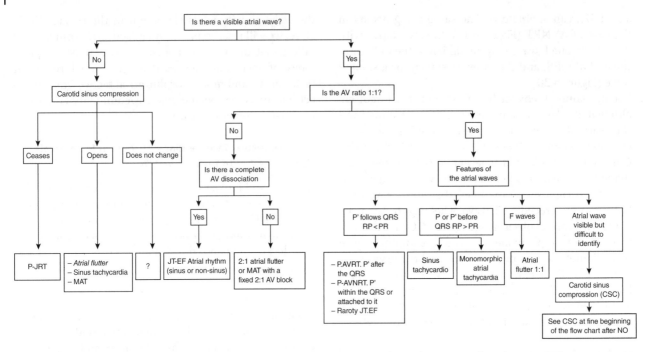

Figure 4.70 Algorithm for the diagnosis of active supraventricular arrhythmias with regular RR intervals and narrow QRS.

retrograde atrial activity is fast but usually less than 200 bpm, and its polarity is caudocranial (slow-fast type circuit). If the circuit is exclusively in the AV junction, the P′ wave can be within the QRS complex or just after it (Figures 4.17, 4.18A and 4.18B, and 4.19A and 4.19B). If an accessory pathway is involved in the circuit, the P′ wave is slightly separated from the QRS complex, but has a relation of P′R>RP′ (Figures 4.16, 4.18A and 4.18C, and 4.19C).

o **In junctional tachycardia due to ectopic focus (JT-EF)**, the conduction to the atria may be 1:1 on some occasions. In these situations, and also in the accelerated idiojunctional rhythms, the P′ wave may be: (i) after the QRS complex, if the retrograde conduction is slower than the anterograde, (ii) hidden within the QRS complex, or (iii) situated before the QRS complex. This occurs more frequently in the slow or mildly accelerated AV junctional rhythms due to ectopic focus (Figure 4.29).

- **Atrial flutter with 1:1 atrioventricular conduction**
  o When the flutter waves have a 1:1 AV conduction, the flutter rate is usually slow, reaching around 200–240 bpm. This occurs when the "F" waves are slowed down because of drugs or associated heart disease. Sometimes the same patient can show different types of AV conduction (Figure 4.64). Usually, it is very difficult to distinguish from other types of paroxysmal tachycardia with only one ECG. We have already mentioned that the slow flutter (≈200 bpm) and the atrial tachycardia (AT) with a similar rate

are impossible to distinguish with a surface ECG. In fact, atypical flutter and MAT-MR may be considered the same arrhythmia.

To make the differential diagnosis between 1×1 flutter with a rate around 200 bpm and very fast paroxysmal AV junctional reentrant tachycardia, it is very useful to perform a CSM or other similar maneuvers. In cases of atrial flutter, the CSM can slow the AV conduction and induce AV block, whereas in paroxysmal reentrant junctional tachycardia, the CSM can suppress the tachycardia or have no effect (Table 1.4 and Figure 1.16).

It must be taken into account that atrial flutter generally appears in elderly people or in young patients with heart disease, especially after surgery for congenital defects. In contrast, paroxysmal junctional reentrant tachycardias are habitually seen in young people without heart disease.

Situations in which the Atrioventricular Relation is not 1:1

- With complete AV dissociation
  o Junctional tachycardia due to ectopic focus (JT-EF) with complete AV dissociation (regular RR intervals dissociated from the atrial activity).

The rate of the QRS complexes can be relatively fast (150–180 bpm), but the sinus or nonsinus atrial activity is dissociated from the JT-EF (QRS complex conducted from the AV junction) (AV dissociation) (Figures 4.13, and 4.27, 4.28).

- Without complete AV dissociation

o Atrial flutter with fixed AV relation that is not 1×1, but frequently 2×1 and sometimes also 3:1 or 4:1, but not usually more. The average ventricular rate depends on the degree of AV block. The atrial activity and "F" waves are fast, between 200 and 300 bpm, without an isoelectric line between "F" waves in leads II, III, and VF (Figures 4.57–4.61).

o If the atrial activity is slower than 200 bpm, it is probably a monomorphic atrial tachycardia with an AV block (Figure 4.69C).

Nonvisible Atrial Activity

Relatively often, it is difficult to determine where the atrial activity is in the surface ECG, either because it is hidden in the QRS complex (Figure 4.19A) or the T wave (Figure 4.10). Sometimes atrial activity is not visible (unapparent voltage) because of atrial fibrosis (concealed sinus rhythm or atrial flutter) (Bayés de Luna *et al.*, 1978). The concealed rhythm may be also seen in patients with irregular heart rate (atrial flutter or fibrillation) (see later). Often, the atrial activity is generally seen during the longer pauses, at least in some leads, although there may be exceptions (Figure 4.62).

In the presence of rapid regular supraventricular rhythms (tachycardia or flutter with fixed AV conduction) without apparent atrial activity, the following must be considered:

o The P′ wave of junctional reentrant tachycardia of AVNRT (JRT-E) type or one of two "F" waves of a 2×1 flutter can simulate the last part of the QRS complex and create a morphology similar to a partial RBBB (Figures 4.17 and 4.57). Obviously, in the case of 2×1 atrial flutter, the other "F" wave will be clearly seen, and this will help to make the diagnosis (Figure 4.57).

o It is necessary to make sure that the P′ wave is not masked in the T wave, modifying it in a very subtle manner. This can happen frequently in all types of regular tachycardias that have been mentioned, including sinus tachycardia. Sometimes, with simple maneuvers, such as deep breathing, the rate of the tachycardia is modified and the atrial activity is clearly seen (Figure 4.10). The fact that the tachycardia rate is clearly modified with breathing makes it quite possible that it is of sinus origin (check the morphology). However, this can also happen in monomorphic atrial tachycardias due to ectopic focus, but not in reentrant tachycardias from any origin, which follow the rule of all or nothing: either they cease, for example, with compression of the carotid sinus, or nothing happens (Figures 1.16 and 4.70, and Table 1.4). This difficulty may be overcome when ECG devices include P wave amplification and also T wave filtering, which will allow us to see the P, P′, or "F" waves

hidden in the T wave (www.medicalproductguide.com), or with the use of special recording leads (Lewis lead) (see Appendix A-3, Analysis of Late Potentials Using a Signal Averaging Electrocardiogram (SAEG)).

o The response to vagal stimulation maneuvers such as CSM is very useful for differentiating types of tachyarrhythmias. When no atrial activity is recorded in the presence of regular RR intervals, the compression of the carotid sinus can help establish the correct diagnosis. If the tachycardia ceases, it is a paroxysmal junctional reentrant tachycardia. If it does not cease, and a transient AV block is generated, the atrial waves may be seen (see Table 1.4, Figures 1.16 and 4.70).

o Nevertheless, in some cases the problem is not resolved with CSM because there is not any change. In this situation, previous clinical and electrocardiographic data can help determine the diagnosis. Here are some examples:

• A relatively slow heart rate (between 130 and 150 bpm) is in favor of flutter 2:1, whereas a rate higher than160 bpm is in favor of AV junctional reentrant tachycardias or atrial tachycardias.

• It is very difficult to distinguish slow flutter with common flutter waves from 1×1 AV conduction and fast monomorphic atrial tachycardia. Observing heart rate may help. If the rate is faster than 220 bpm, it is considered atrial flutter; if it is slower than 180 bpm, atrial tachycardia. The borderline cases (180–220 bpm) may be referred to as "tachysystole" (see Flutter "F" Waves).

• On the other hand, slow flutter (i.e., at 220 bpm) with 2:1 conduction, the most frequent situation, can be mistaken for sinus tachycardia at 110 bpm. It is useful to observe the changes of heart rate during exercise or over a period of 24 h. If there is a gradual increase in heart rate with exercise, or it changes over time but never abruptly, the rhythm is sinus. If the rate is fixed during 24 h or changes abruptly with exercise, it is most likely ectopic (flutter) (Figure 4.20).

Supraventricular Tachycardias with Irregular RR Intervals
(Table 4.2 and Figure 4.71)

Generally, QRS complexes are narrow, although sometimes isolated or repetitive wide QRS complexes may be seen. This leads us to make a differential diagnosis between aberrancy and ectopy of the wide QRS complexes (see Atrial Fibrillation, ECG Diagnosis). If they are repetitive with irregular RR intervals, the most probable cause of wide QRS is aberrancy. It is compulsory to make the differential diagnosis between AF of WPW syndrome and ventricular tachycardia (see before, Differential Diagnosis Between Aberrancy and Ectopy in Wide QRS

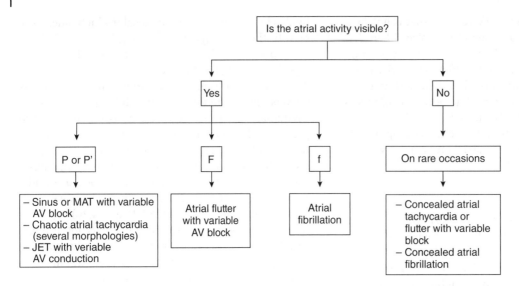

Figure 4.71 Algorithm for the diagnosis of active supraventricular arrhythmias with irregular RR intervals and narrow QRS.

Complexes, and Figure 4.52). We will comment on this situation and discuss whether the atrial activity can be visible or not.

Visible Atrial Activity

The following arrhythmias may be considered:

o Atrial fibrillation (Figures 4.37- 4.39). The atrial activity is fast (400–700 bpm) with irregular and changing wave morphologies ("f" waves), and variable AV conduction.

o **Flutter with variable AV conduction**. Usually, regular flutter "F" waves can be seen (Figures 4.63A and 4.69D).

o **Chaotic atrial tachycardi**a (Figure 4.31). Atrial rate is usually high but variable (100–200 bpm) and atrial waves have different morphologies and change continuously (not more than two identical P waves in a row), although they are easily identifiable (P or P′ waves), with isoelectric baselines in between them and variable AV conduction. It is impossible to distinguish from atrial fibrillation using palpitation.

o **Sinus tachycardia or monomorphic atrial tachycardia with variable AV block.** Monomorphic P or P′ waves are seen with variable AV block (Figure 4.14). In addition, the presence of premature beats (atrial or ventricular extrasystoles) may explain the irregular RR in sinus tachycardia or other types of tachycardia.

o **Atrioventricular junctional tachycardia due to ectopic focus with variable AV conduction, or the presence of premature beats.**

Atrial Activity Not Clearly Visible

On certain rare occasions, when RR intervals are irregular, the atrial activity cannot be seen. When this occurs, there is often atrial fibrosis that explains low-voltage atrial waves (P, P′, f or F) or even invisible waves. In these cases, atrial flutter with variable AV conduction or AF is usually the most common cause. Generally, in lead V1 F or f, waves can be seen with a very low voltage, especially if the recordings are made using equipment provided with a wave amplifier system (Figure 4.39) without having to proceed to intracavitary recordings (Fig. 4.40).

Self Assessment

A. What are the key concepts of premature supraventricular complexes (PSVC)?

B. Explain how PSVC conduction to the ventricles can happen in different ways.

C. What are the factors that favor the appearance of PSVC?

D. Comment on the different types of sinus tachycardia and their prognostic and therapeutic implications.

E. Explain the concept of monomorphic atrial tachycardias (MAT).

F. How many types of MAT are there?

G. How does the place of origin of the MAT-EF influence the shape of the P wave?

H. How do you make a differential diagnosis of paroxysmal MAT due to ectopic focus?

I. How do you make a differential diagnosis of incessant MAT due to ectopic focus?

J. What tachycardias are included in the concept atrioventricular (AV) junctional reentrant tachycardia (JRT)?

K. How can a paroxysmal junctional reentrant tachycardia with a circuit that is exclusive to the AV junction be distinguished from one with a circuit that also involves an accessory pathway?

L. What are the electrocardiographic characteristics of incessant JRT?

M. Should ablation always be done to cure paroxysmal JRT?

N. What are the electrocardiographic characteristics of the junctional tachycardia due to ectopic focus (AVNRTF)?

O. What are the ECG characteristics of chaotic atrial tachycardia?

P. Describe the initiation and perpetuation mechanisms of atrial fibrillation (AF).

Q. What are the characteristics of AF waves?

R. What is the morphology of QRS and the ventricular response in AF?

S. How is the differential diagnosis between AF with Wolff–Parkinson–White (WPW) syndrome and ventricular tachycardia made?

T. What is the prognosis of patients with AF?

U. What are the objectives of treatment?

V. Comment on the definition and mechanism of atrial flutter.

W. What are the morphologies that atrial flutter waves may present?

X. What are the clinical, prognostic, and therapeutic implications of atrial flutter?

Y. Discuss the different types of monomorphic and polymorphic atrial waves observed in supraventricular tachyarrhythmias.

Z. How is the differential diagnosis of supraventricular tachycardias with regular RR intervals made?

AA. Describe how to carry out the sequential ECG diagnosis of regular and irregular paroxysmal supraventricular tachyarrhythmias is made.

References

Alboni P, Botto GL, Baldi N, *et al*. Outpatient treatment of recent-onset atrial fibrillation with the "pill-in-the-pocket" approach. N Engl J Med 2004;351:2384.

Alegret JM, Viñolas X, Sagristá J, *et al*; on behalf of REVERSE study investigators. Clinical characteristics of patients with persistent atrial fibrillation referred for cardioversion: Spanish Cardioversion Registry (REVERSE). Rev Esp Cardiol 2008;61:630.

Al-Khatib SM, Hafley G, Harrington RA, *et al*. Patterns of management of atrial fibrillation complicating coronary artery bypass grafting: Results from the PRoject of Ex-vivo Vein graft Engineering via Transfection IV (PREVENT-IV) Trial. Am Heart J 2009;158:792.

Andersen SS, Hansen ML, Gislason GH, *et al*. Antiarrhythmic therapy and risk of death in patients with atrial fibrillation: a nationwide study. Europace 2009;11:886.

Anselme F. Macroreentrant atrial tachycardia: pathophysiological concepts. Heart Rhythm 2008;5(6 Suppl):S18.

Arenal A, Datino T, Atea L *et al*. Dominant frequency differences in atrial fibrillation patients with and without left ventricular systolic dysfunction. Europace 2009;11:450.

Bar FW, Brugada P, Dassen WR, *et al*. Differential diagnosis of tachycardia with narrow QRS complex (shorter than 0.12 second). Am J Cardiol 1984;54: 555.

Baranchuk A. Sleep apnea, cardiac arrhythmias and conduction disorders. J Electrocardiol 2012;45:508.

Baranchuk A, Pang H, Seaborn GEJ, *et al*. Reverse atrial electrical remodeling induced by continuous positive airway pressure in patients with severe obstructive sleep apnea. J Interventional Card Electrophysiol 2013;36(3):247.

Bardy GH, Lee KL, Mark DB, *et al*. Amiodarone or an implantable cardioverter-defibrillator for congestive heart failure. N Engl J Med 2005;352(3):225.

Barrios V, Escobar C, Echarri R. Letter by Barrios *et al.* regarding article "Influence of systolic and diastolic blood pressure on the risk of incident atrial fibrillation in women". Circulation 2010;121:e29.

Bauernfeind RA, Amat-y-Leon F, Dhingra RC, *et al.* Chronic nonparoxysmal sinus tachycardia in otherwise healthy persons. Ann Intern Med 1979;91:702.

Bayés de Luna A, Boada FX, Casellas A, *et al*. Concealed atrial electrical activity. J Electrocardiol 1978;11:301.

Bayés de Luna A, Fort de Ribot R, Trilla E, *et al*. Electrocardiographic and vectorcardiographic study of interatrial conduction disturbances with left atrial retrograde activation. J Electrocardiology 1985;18:1.

Bayés de Luna A, Cladellas M, Oter R, *et al*. Interatrial conduction block and retrograde activation of the left atrium and paroxysmal supraventricular arrhythmias. Eur Heart J 1988;9:1112.

Bayés de Luna A, Cladellas M, Oter R, *et al*. Interatrial conduction block with retrograde activation of the left atrium and paroxysmal supraventricular tachyarrhythmias: influence of preventive antiarrhythmic treatment. Int J Cardiol 1989;22:147.

Bayés de Luna A, Viñolas X, Guindo J, *et al.* Frontiers of atrial flutter. In: Waldo A, Touboul P (eds) Atrial flutter: Advances in mechanisms and management. Futura Publishing Company, New York, 1996, p. 321.

Bayés de Luna A, Platonov P, Cosio FG, *et al.* Interatrial blocks. A separate entity from left atrial enlargement: a consensus report. J Electrocardiol 2012;45(5):445.

Bazán V, Rodríguez-Font E, Viñolas X, *et al.* Atrial tachycardia originating from the pulmonary vein: clinical, electrocardiographic, and differential electrophysiologic characteristics. Rev Esp Cardiol. 2010;63:149.

Benjamin EJ, Wolf PA, D'Agostino RB, *et al.* Impact of atrial fibrillation on the risk of death: the Framingham Heart Study. Circulation 1998;98:946.

Böhm M, Swedberg K, Komajda M, *et al.* Heart rate as a risk factor in chronic heart failure (SHIFT): the association between heart rate and outcomes in a randomized placebo-controlled trial. Lancet 2010;376:847.

Brady PA, Low PA, Shen WK. Inappropriate sinus tachycardia, postural orthostatic tachycardia syndrome, and overlapping syndromes. Pacing Clin Electrophysiol 2005;28:1112.

Brambatti M, Connolly SJ, Gold MR, *et al.* Temporal relationship between subclinical atrial fibrillation and embolic events. Circulation 2014;129(21):2094.

Budeus M, Hennersdorf M, Perings S, *et al.* Amiodarone prophylaxis for atrial fibrillation of high-risk patients after coronary bypass grafting: a prospective, doubleblinded, placebo-controlled, randomized study. Eur Heart J 2006;27:1584.

Cakulev I, Waldo AL. Do not stop the warfarin until … J Am Coll Cardiol 2010;55:744.

Caldwell J, Koppikar S, Barake W, *et al.* Prolonged P wave duration is associated with atrial fibrillation recurrence after successful pulmonary vein isolation for paroxysmal atrial fibrillation. J Interv Card Electrophysiol 2014;39(2):131.

Calkins H, Yong P, Miller JM, *et al.* Catheter ablation of accessory pathways, atrioventricular nodal reentrant tachycardia, and the atrioventricular junction: Final results of a prospective, multicenter clinical trial. Circulation 1999;99:262.

Camm AJ. Chairman. Guidelines for the management of atrial fibrillation. European Society of Cardiology 2010 (www.escardio.org/guidelines).

Camm AJ, Lip GY, De Caterina R, *et al.* 2012 focused update of the ESC Guidelines for the management of atrial fibrillation: an update of the 2010 ESC Guidelines for the management of atrial fibrillation – developed with the special contribution of the European Heart Rhythm Association. Europace 2012;14(10):1385.

Capucci A, Villani GQ, Piepoli, MF *et al.* The role of oral 1C antiarrhythmic drugs in terminating atrial fibrillation. Curr Opin Cardiol 1999;14:4.

Carew S, Connor MO, Cooke, J *et al.* A review of postural orthostatic tachycardia syndrome. Europace 2009;11:18.

Cappato R, Exokowitz MD, Klein GJ, *et al.* Rivaroxaban vs. vitamin K antagonists for cardioversion in atrial fibrillation. Eur Heart J. 2014;35(47):3346.

Chan PS, Nallamothu BK, Oral H. Amiodarone or dronedarone for atrial fibrillation: too early to know the winner? J Am Coll Cardiol 2009;54:1089.

Chang S, Chen S. From a chaotic to organized tachyarrhythmia. Heart Rhythm 2010;7:673.

Chen SA, Chiang CE, Yang CJ, *et al.* Sustained atrial tachycardia in adult patients. Electrophysiological characteristics, pharmacological response, possible mechanisms, and effects of radiofrequency ablation. Circulation 1994;90:1262.

Collins K, Van Hare G, Kertesz N, *et al.* Pediatric non-postoperative junctional ectopic tachycardia. J Am Coll Cardiol 2009;53:690.

Conde D, Baranchuk A. Vernakalant for the conversion of atrial fibrillation: the new kid in the block? Ann Noninv Electrocardiol 2014;19(4):299.

Conen D, Tedrow UB, Koplan BA, *et al.* Influence of systolic and diastolic blood pressure on the risk of incident atrial fibrillation in women. Circulation 2009;119:2146.

Conen D, Tedrow UB, Cook NR, *et al.* Birth weight is a significant risk factor for incident atrial fibrillation. Circulation 2010;122:759.

Connolly SJ, Ezekowitz MD, Yusuf S, *et al.* Dabigatran versus Warfarin in patients with atrial fibrillation. N Engl J Med 2009a:361:1139.

Connolly SJ, Crijns H, Torp-Pedersen Ch., *et al* Analysis of stroke in ATHENA: a placebo-controlled, double-blind, parallel-arm trial to assess the efficacy of dronedarone 400 mg BID for the prevention of cardiovascular hospitalization or death from any cause in patients with atrial fibrillation/atrial flutter. Circulation 2009b;120:1174.

Connolly SJ, Camm AJ, Halperin JL, *et al.* Dronedarone in high-risk permanent atrial fibrillation. N Engl J Med 2011; 365 (24): 2268.

Cook GE, Sasich LD, Sukkari SR. Atrial fibrillation. DIONYSOS study comparing dronedarone with amiodarone. Br Med J 2010;340:c285

Coumel Ph, Fidelle J, Cloup M, *et al.* Les tachycardies réciproques à évolution prolongée chez l'enfant. Arch Mal Coeur 1974;67:23.

Cox JL, Schuessler RB, D'Agostino HJ Jr, *et al.* The surgical treatment of atrial fibrillation. III. Development of a definitive surgical procedure. J Thorac Cardiovasc Surg 1991;101:569.

Critelli G, Gallagher JJ, Monda V, *et al.* Anatomic and electrophysiologic substrate of the permanent form of junctional reciprocating tachycardia. J Am Coll Cardiol 1984;4:601.

Daubert J-C. Atrial flutter and interatrial conduction block. In: Waldo A, Touboul P (eds) Atrial flutter: advances in mechanisms and management. Futura Publishing Company, New York, 1996, p. 331.

Davy JM, Herold M, Hoglund C, *et al.* Dronedarone for the control of ventricular rate in permanent atrial fibrillation: the efficacy and safety of dronedarone for the control of ventricular rate during atrial fibrillation (ERATO) study. Am Heart J 2008;156:527.

De Vos CB, Pisters R, Nieuwlaat R, *et al.* Progression from paroxysmal to persistent atrial fibrillation clinical correlates and prognosis. J Am Coll Cardiol 2010;55:725.

Di Biase L, Burkhardt J, Mohenty P, *et al.* Left atrial appendage: an under recognized trigger site of atrial fibrillation. Circulation 2010;122:109.

Di Francesco D, Camm JA. Heart rate lowering by specific and selective I(f)current inhibition with ivabradine: a new therapeutic perspective in cardiovascular disease. Drugs 2004;64:1757.

Di Toro D, Hadid C, López C *et al.* Utility of the aVL lead in the electrocardiographic diagnosis of atrioventricular node re-entrant tachycardia. Europace 2009;11:944.

Disertori M, Latini R, Barlera S, *et al.* GISSI-AF Investigators Valsartan for prevention of recurrent atrial fibrillation. N Engl J Med. 2009 16;360:1606.

Dobrev V, Nattel S. Calcium handling abnormalities in AF. J Cardio Pharmacol 2008;52:293.

Dries DL, Exner DV, Gersh BJ. Atrial fibrillation is associated with an increased risk for mortality and heart failure progression in patients with asymptomatic and symptomatic left ventricular systolic dysfunction: a retrospective analysis of the SOLVD trials. Studies of Left Ventricular Dysfunction. J Am Coll Cardiol 1998;32:695.

Dubin A, Cuneo B, Strasburger J, *et al.* Congenital junctional ectopic tachycardia and congenital AV block: A shared etiology? Heart Rhythm 2005;2:313.

Eitel C, Hindricks G, Sommer P, *et al.* Circumferential pulmonary vein isolation and linear left atrial ablation as a single-catheter technique to achieve bidirectional conduction block: the pace-and-ablate approach. Heart Rhythm 2010;7:157.

Enriquez A, Conde D, Hopman W, *et al.* Advanced interatrial block is associated with recurrence of atrial fibrillation post pharmacological cardioversion. Cardiovas Ther 2014;32(2):52.

Enriquez A, Conde D, Redfearn DP, Baranchuk A. Progressive interatrial block and supraventricular arrhythmias. Ann Noninvasive Electrocardiol 2015a;20(4):394

Enriquez A, Sarrias A, Villuendas R, *et al.* New-onset atrial fibrillation after cavotricuspid isthmus ablation: identification of advanced interatrial block is key. Europace 2015b;17(8):1289.

Enriquez A, Lip GYH, Baranchuk A. Anticoagulation reversal in the era of the non-vitamin K oral anticoagulants (NOACs). Europace 2016;18(7):955.

Eriksson B, Quinlan D, Weitz J. Comparative pharmacodynamy and pharmacokinetics of oral thrombin and factor Xa inhibitors in development. Clin Pharmacokinet 2009;48:1.

Farré J, Ross D, Wiener I, *et al.* Reciprocal tachycardias using accessory pathways with long conduction times. Am J Cardiol 1979;44:1099.

Femenia F, Baranchuk A, Morillo CA. Inappropiate sinus tachycardia: current therapeutic options. Cardiol Rev 2012;20(1):8.

Friberg L, Hammar N, Rosenqvist M. Stroke in paroxysmal atrial fibrillation: report from the Stockholm Cohort of Atrial Fibrillation. Eur Heart J 2010;31(8):967.

Fu Q, Van Guyindy T, Galbreath M, *et al.* Cardiac origin of the postural tachycardia orthostatic syndrome. J Am Coll Cardiol 2010;55:2858.

Fung JW, Sanderson JE, Yip GW, *et al.* Impact of atrial fibrillation in heart failure with normal ejection fraction: a clinical and echocardiographic study. J Card Fail 2007;13:649.

Fuster V, Rydén LE, Cannom DS *et al.* Cardiology/ American Heart Association Task Force on Practice Guidelines; European Society of Cardiology Committee for Practice Guidelines; European Heart Rhythm Association; Heart Rhythm Society. ACC/ AHA/ESC 2006 Guidelines for the Management of Patients with Atrial Fibrillation: a report of the American College of Cardiology/American Heart Association Task Force on Practice Guidelines and the European Society of Cardiology Committee for Practice Guidelines (Writing Committee to Revise the 2001 Guidelines for the Management of Patients With Atrial Fibrillation): developed in collaboration with the European Heart Rhythm Association and the Heart Rhythm Society. Circulation 2006 15;114:e257.

Gage B, Waterman AD, Shannon W, *et al.* Validation of clinical classification schemes for predicting stroke: results for the national registry of atrial fibrillation. JAMA 2001;285:2864.

García Cosio F, López-Gil M, Goicolea A, *et al.* Radiofrequency ablation in of the inferior vena cava-tricuspid valve isthmus in common atrial flutter. Am J Cardiol 1993;71:705.

Gasparini M, Auricchio A, Regoli F, *et al.* Four-year efficacy of cardiac resynchronization therapy on exercise tolerance and disease progression: the importance of performing atrioventricular junction ablation in patients with atrial fibrillation. J Am Coll Cardiol 2006;48:734.

Gerstenfeld EP, Dixit S, Bala R, *et al.* Surface electrocardiogram characteristics of atrial tachycardias occurring after pulmonary vein isolation. Heart Rhythm 2007;4:1136.

Gladstone DJ, Spring M, Dorian P, *et al.* Atrial fibrillation in patients with cryptogenic stroke. N Engl J Med 2014; 370(26):2467.

Glatter K, Cheng J, Dorostkar P, *et al.* Electrophysiologic effects of adenosine in supraventricular tachycardias. Circulation 1999;99:1034.

Glotzer TV, Daoud EG, Wyse DG, *et al.* The relationship between daily atrial tahyarrhythmiaa burden from implantable device diagnostics and stroke risk. The TRENDS Study. Circ Arrhythmia Electophysiol 2009;2:474.

Gomes JA, Hariman RJ, Kang PS, *et al.* Sustained symptomatic sinus node reentrant tachycardia: Incidence, clinical significance, electrophysiologic observations and the effects of antiarrhythmic agents. J Am Coll Cardiol 1985;5:45.

González-Torrecilla E, Almendral J, Arenal A, *et al.* Combined evaluation of bedside clinical variables and the electrocardiogram for the differential diagnosis of paroxysmal atrioventricular reciprocating tachycardias in patients without pre-excitation. J Am Coll Cardiol 2009;53:2353.

Gudbjartsson DF, Arnar DO, Helgadottir A, *et al.* Variants conferring risk of atrial fibrillation on chromosome 4q25. Nature 2007;448:353.

Guglin M, Aljayeh M, Saiyad S *et al.* Introducing a new entity: chemotherapy-induced arrhythmia. Europace 2009;11:1579.

Gulamhusein S, Yee R, Ko PT, *et al.* ECG criteria for differentiating aberrancy and ventricular premature systole in chronic atrial fibrillation: Validation by intracardiac recordings. J Electrocardiol 1985;18:41.

Haïssaguerre M, Jaïs P, Shah DC, *et al.* Spontaneous initiation of atrial fibrillation by ectopic beats originating in the pulmonary veins. N Engl J Med 1998;339:659.

Haïssaguerre M, Jais P, Shah DC, *et al.* Electrophysiological end point for catheter ablation of atrial fibrillation initiated from multiple pulmonary veins foci. Circulation 2000a;101:1409.

Haïssaguerre M, Jaïs P, Shah DC, *et al.* Catheter ablation of chronic atrial fibrillation targeting the reinitiating triggers. J Cardiovasc Electrophysiol 2000b;11:2.

Halbfass P, Janko S, Dorwarth U, *et al.* Dilemma of antithrombotic therapy in anticoagulated atrial fibrillation patients squeezed between thrombosis and bleeding events: a single-centre experience. Europace 2009;11:957.

Halperin JL, Hankey GJ, Wojdyla DM, *et al.* Efficacy and safety of rivaroxaban compared with warfarin among elderly patients with nonvalvular atrial fibrillation in the Rivaroxaban Once Daily, Oral, Direct Factor Xa Inhibition compared with vitamin K antagonism for prevention of stroke and embolism Trial in Atrial Fibrillation (ROCKET AF). Circulation 2014;130(2):138.

Healey J, Baranchuk A, Crystal E, *et al.* Prevention of atrial fibrillation with angiotensin converting enzyme inhibitors and angiotensin receptor blockers: a meta-analysis. J Am Coll Cardiol 2005;45:1832.

Hirsh BJ, Copeland-Halperin RS, Halperin JL. Fibrotic atrial cardiomyopathy, atrial fibrillation, and thromboembolism: mechanistic links and clinical inferences. J Am Coll Cardiol 2015;65:2239.

Ho J, Bitner V, De Micco D, *et al.* Usefulness of heart rate as a predictor of mortality and HF (TNT trial). Am J Card 2010;105:905.

Hohnoloser SH, Capucci A, Fain E, *et al.* ASSERT Investigators and Committees. Asymptomatic atrial fibrillation and stroke evaluation in pacemaker patients and the atrial fibrillation reduction atrial pacing Trial (ASSERT). Am Heart J 2006;152:442.

Hohnloser SH, Crijns HJ, van Eickels M, *et al.* ATHENA Investigators. Effect of dronedarone on cardiovascular events in atrial fibrillation. N Engl J Med 2009;360:668.

Holmes DR Jr, Kar S, Price MJ, *et al.* Prospective randomized evaluation of the Watchman left atrial appendage closure device in patients with atrial fibrillation versus long-term warfarin therapy: the PREVAIL trial. J Am Coll Cardiol 2014;64(1):1.

Holmqvist F, Platonov PG, Carlson J, *et al.* Altered interatrial conduction detected in MADIT II patients bound to develop atrial fibrillation. Ann Noninvasive Electrocardiol 2009;14:268.

Holmqvist F, Platonov P, Nitt S, *et al.* Abnormal P wave morphology is a predictor of AF development and cardiac death in MADIT II patients. ANE 2010;15:63.

Iguchi Y, Kimura K, Aoki J, *et al.* Prevalence of atrial fibrillation in community-dwelling Japanese aged 40 years or older in Japan: analysis of 41,436 non-employee residents in Kurashiki-city. Circ J 2008;72:909.

Inoue S, Becker A. Posterior extension of human AV node. Circulation 1998;97:188.

Ishida K, Hayushi H, Miyamoto A, *et al.* P wave and the development of atrial fibrillation. Heart Rhythm 2010;7:289.

Issac TT, Dokainish H, Lakkis NM. Role of inflammation in initiation and perpetuation of atrial fibrillation: a systematic review of the published data. J Am Coll Cardiol 2007;20(50):2021.

Jacob G, Costa F, Shannon JR, *et al.* The neuropathic postural tachycardia syndrome. N Engl J Med 2000;343:1008.

Jalife J. Rotors and spiral waves in atrial fibrillation. J Cardiovasc Electrophysiol 2003;14:776.

Josephson ME. Paroxysmal supraventricular tachycardia: An electrophysiological approach. Am J Cardiol 1978;41:1123.

Karas B, Grubb BP, Boehm K, *et al*. The postural orthostatic tachycardia syndrome: A potentially treatable cause of chronic fatigue, exercise intolerance, and cognitive impairment in adolescents. PACE 2000;23:344.

Kato ET, Giugliano RP, Ruff CT, *et al*. Efficacy and safety of edoxaban in elderly patients with atrial fibrillation in the ENGAGE AF-TIMI 48 Trial. J Am Heart Assoc 2016;5(5).

Katritsis D, Becker A. The AV nodal re-entrant circuit. A proposal. Heart Rhythm 2007;4:1354.

Katritsis D, Ioannidis JP, Anagnostopoulos CE, *et al*. Identification and catheter ablation of extracardiac and intracardiac components of ligament of Marshall tissue for treatment of paroxysmal atrial fibrillation. J Cardiovasc Electrophysiol 2001;12:750.

Katritsis D, Giazitzoglou E, Sougiannis D, *et al*. Complex fractionated atrial electrograms at anatomic sites of ganglionated plexi in atrial fibrillation. Europace 2009;11:308.

Kaufman ES, Zimmermann PA, Wang T, *et al*. Atrial Fibrillation Follow-up Investigation of Rhythm Management investigators. Risk of proarrhythmic events in the Atrial Fibrillation Follow-up Investigation of Rhythm Management (AFFIRM) study: a multivariate analysis. J Am Coll Cardiol 2004;44:1276.

Kautzner J, Cihák R, Vancura V, *et al*. Coincidence of idiopathic ventricular outflow tract tachycardia and atrioventricular nodal re-entrant tachycardia. Europace 2003;5:215.

Keating GM. Apixaban: a review of its use for reducing the risk of stroke and systemic embolism in patients with nonvalvular atrial fibrillation. Drugs 2013;73(8):825.

Khadjooi K, Foley PW, Chalil S, *et al*. Long-term effects of cardiac resynchronisation therapy in patients with atrial fibrillation. Heart 2008;94:879.

Khan MN, Jaïs P, Cummings J, *et al*. PABA-CHF Investigators. Pulmonary-vein isolation for atrial fibrillation in patients with heart failure. N Engl J Med 2008;359:1778.

Khaykin Y, Skanes A, Champagne J, *et al*. A randomized controlled trial of the efficacy and safety of electroanatomic circumferential pulmonary vein ablation supplemented by ablation of complex fractionated atrial electrograms versus potential-guided pulmonary vein antrum isolation guided by intracardiac ultrasound. Circ Arrhythm Electrophysiol 2009;2:481.

Kim SK, Pak HN, Park JH, *et al*. Clinical and serological predictors for the recurrence of atrial fibrillation after electrical cardioversion. Europace 2009;11:1632.

Kirchhof P, Breithardt G. (LAFNET/EHRA consensus conference on AF). Early and comprehensive management of atrial fibrillation. Europace 2009;11:860.

Kistler PM, Roberts-Thomson KC, Haqqani HM, *et al*. P-wave morphology in focal atrial tachycardia: development of an algorithm to predict the anatomic site of origin. J Am Coll Cardiol 2006;48:1010.

Klein GJ, Bashore TM, Sellers TD. Ventricular fibrillation in the Wolff–Parkinson–White syndrome. N Engl J Med 1979;1111:300.

Knight BP, Ebinger M, Oral H, *et al*. Diagnostic value of tachycardia features and pacing maneuvers during paroxysmal supraventricular tachycardia. J Am Coll Cardiol 2000;36:574.

Køber L, Torp-Pedersen C, McMurray JJ, *et al*. Increased mortality after dronadorone therapy for severe heart failure. N Engl J Med 2008;358:2678.

Kong M, Shaw L, O'Connor C. Is rhythm-control superior to rate-control in patients with AF and diastolic heart failure. Ann Noninvasive Electrocardiol 2010;15:209.

Kottkamp H. Humal atrial fibrillation substrate: towards a specific fibrotic atrial cardiomyopathy. Eur Heart J 2013;34:2731.

Koyama T, Tada H, Segikuchi Y, *et al*. Prevention of AP recurrence with corticosteroids after radiofrequency catheter ablation. J Am Coll Cardiol 2010;56:1463.

Lau DH, Huynh LT, Chew DP, *et al*. Prognostic impact of types of atrial fibrillation in acute coronary syndromes. Am J Cardiol 2009;104:1317.

Lee R, Kruse J, McCarthy PM. Surgery for atrial fibrillation. Nat Rev Cardiol 2009;6:505.

Lesh M, Rohithger F. Atrial tachycardia. Future Publishing Company, New York, 2000.

Lin YJ, Tsao HM, Chang SL, *et al*. Prognostic implications of the high-sensitive C-reactive protein in the catheter ablation of atrial fibrillation. Am J Cardiol 2010;105:495.

Lindsay BD. Focal and macroreentrant atrial tachycardia: from bench to bedside and back to the bench again. Heart Rhythm 2007;4:1361.

Lip GY. Atrial fibrillation and stroke prevention: brief observations on the last decade. Expert Rev Cardiovasc Ther 2014;12(4):403.

Lip GY, Lane DA. Combination anticoagulant and antiplatelet therapy in atrial fibrillation patients. Rev Esp Cardiol 2009;62(9):972.

Lubitz SA, Fischer A, Fuster V. Catheter ablation for atrial fibrillation. Br Med J 2008;336:819.

Madrid AH, Bueno MG, Rebollo JM, *et al*. Use of irbesartan to maintain sinus rhythm in patients with long-lasting persistent atrial fibrillation: a prospective and randomized study. Circulation 2002;106:331.

Maisel WH, Stevenson LW. Atrial fibrillation in heart failure: epidemiology, pathophysiology, and rationale for therapy. Am J Cardiol 2003;20(91):2D.

Mäki T, Toivonen L, Koskinen P, *et al.* Effect of ethanol drinking, hangover, and exercise on adrenergic activity and heart rate variability in patients with a history of alcohol-induced atrial fibrillation. Am J Cardiol 1998;82:317.

Mant J, Hobbs R, Fletcher K, *et al.* on behalf of the BAFT Investigators and the Midland Research Practices Network. Warfarin versus aspirin for stroke prevention in an elderly community population with atrial fibrillation (the Birmingham Atrial Fibrillation Treatment of the Aged Study, BAFT): a randomised controlled trial. Lancet 2007;370:493.

Marchlinski FE. Perivalvular fibrosis and monomorphic ventricular tachycardia: toward a unifying hypothesis in nonischemic cardiomyopathy. Circulation 2007; 116:1998.

Marchlinski FE. Diagnosing the mechanism of supraventricular tachycardia: restoring the luster of a fading art. J Am Coll Cardiol 2009;53:2359.

Maron BJ, Towbin JA, Thiene G, *et al.* Contemporary definitions and classification of the cardiomyopathies: an American Heart Association Scientific Statement from the Council on Clinical Cardiology, Heart Failure and Transplantation Committee; Quality of Care and Outcomes Research and Functional Genomics and Translational Biology Interdisciplinary Working Groups; and Council on Epidemiology and Prevention. Circulation 2006;113:1807.

Marrouche NF, Natale A, Wazni OM, *et al.* Left septal atrial flutter: electrophysiology, anatomy, and results of ablation. Circulation 2004;109:2440.

Martin DT, Bersohn MM, Waldo AL, *et al.* Randomized trial of atrial arrhythmias monitoring to guide anticoagulation in patiens with implanted defibrillator and cardiac resynchronization devices. Eur Heart J 2015;36(26):1660.

Martínez-Sellés M, Massó-van Roessel A, Álvarez-Garcia J, *et al.* Interatrial block and atrial arrhythmias in centenarians: prevalence, associations, and clinical implications. Heart Rhythm 2016;13:645.

Mathew JP, Fontes ML, Tudor IC, *et al.* Investigators of the Ischemia Research and Education Foundation; Multicenter Study of Perioperative Ischemia Research Group. A multicenter risk index for atrial fibrillation after cardiac surgery. JAMA 2004;291:1720.

Matsuo S, Lellouche N, Wright M, *et al.* Clinical predictors of termination and clinical outcome of catheter ablation for persistent atrial fibrillation. J Am Coll Cardiol 2009;54:788.

Matsuo S, Wright M, Knecht S, *et al.* Peri-mital atrial flutter in patients with atrial fibrillation ablation. Heart Rhythm 2010;7(1):2.

Mazza A, Bendini MG, Cristofori M, *et al.* Baseline apnoea/hypopnoea index and high-sensitivity C-reactive protein for the risk of recurrence of atrial fibrillation after successful electrical cardioversion: a predictive model based upon the multiple effects of significant variables. Europace 2009;11:902.

Mazzini MJ, Monahan KM. Pharmacotherapy for atrial arrhythmias: present and future. Heart Rhythm 2008;5(6 Suppl):S26.

McCanta AC, Collins KK, Schaffer MS. Incidental dual atrioventricular nodal physiology in children and adolescents: clinical follow-up and implications. Pacing Clin Electrophysiol 2010;33(12):1528.

Michaud GF, Tada H, Chough S, *et al.* Differentiation of atypical atrioventricular node re-entrant tachycardia from orthodromic reciprocating tachycardia using a septal accessory pathway by the response to ventricular pacing. J Am Coll Cardiol 2001;38:1163.

Mohajer K, Fregeau B, Garg V, *et al.* Management of atrial fibrillation by Canadian Electrophysiologists after early termination of the PALLAS study. Can J Cardiol 2013;29(1):131.e1-2. doi: 10.1016/j.cjca.2012.07.848.

Monahan K, Storfer-Isser A, Mehra R, *et al.* Triggering of nocturnal arrhythmias by sleep-disordered breathing events. J Am Coll Cardiol 2009;54:1797.

Mont L, Sambola A, Brugada J, *et al.* Long-lasting sport practice and lone atrial fibrillation. Eur Heart J 2002;23:477.

Morillo CA, Klein GJ, Jones DL, *et al.* Time and frequency domain analyses of heart rate variability during orthostatic stress in patients with neurally mediated syncope. Am J Cardiol 1994;74:1258.

Moro Serrano C, Hernández-Madrid A. Atrial fibrillation: are we faced with an epidemic? Rev Esp Cardiol 2009;62:10.

Nair M, Nayyar S, Rajagopal S, *et al.* Results of radiofrequency ablation of permanent atrial fibrillation of >2 years duration and left atrial size >5 cm using 2-mm irrigated tip ablation catheter and targeting areas of complex fractionated atrial electrograms. Am J Cardiol 2009;104:683.

Niemwlaat R, Eurlings LW, Cleland JG, *et al.* Atrial fibrillation and heart failure in cardiology practice: reciprocal impact and combined management from the perspective of atrial fibrillation: results of the Euro Heart Survey on atrial fibrillation. J Am Coll Cardiol 2009;53:1690.

Oakes RS, Badger TJ, Kholmovski G, *et al.* Detection and quantification of left atrial structural remodeling with delayed-enhancement magnetic resonance imaging in patients with atrial fibrillation. Circulation 2009; 119:1758.

Otway R, Vandenberg JI, Fatkin D. Atrial fibrillation—a new cardiac channelopathy. Heart Lung Circ 2007;16:356.

Padanilam BJ, Manfredi JA, Steinberg LA, *et al.* Differentiating junctional tachycardia and atrioventricular node re-entry tachycardia based on response to atrial extrastimulus pacing. J Am Coll Cardiol 2008;52:1711.

Paparella N, Ouyang F, Fucă G, *et al.* Significance of newly acquired negative T waves after interruption of paroxysmal reentrant supraventricular tachycardia with narrow QRS complex. Am J Cardiol 2000;85:261.

Pappone C, Santinelli V. Ablation of atrial fibrillation. Curr Cardiol Rep 2006;8:343.

Pérez Gómez F, Alegría E, Berjón J, *et al.* Comparative effects of antiplatelet, anticoagulant, or combined therapy in patients with valvular and nonvalvular atrial fibrillation: A randomized multicenter study. J Am Coll Cardiol 2004;44:1557.

Piccini JP, Hasselblad V, Peterson ED, *et al.* Comparative efficacy of dronedarone and amiodarone for the maintenance of sinus rhythm in atrial fibrillation. J Am Coll Cardiol 2009;54:1089.

Pick, A, Dominguez P. Non-paroxysmal AV nodal tachycardia. Circulation 1957;16:1022.

Porter MJ, Morton JB, Denman R, *et al.* Influence of age and gender on the mechanism of supraventricular tachycardia. Heart Rhythm 2004;1:393.

Poutiainen AM, Koistinen MJ, Airaksinen KE, *et al.* Prevalence and natural course of ectopic atrial tachycardia. Eur Heart J 1999;20:694.

Puech P. L'activité électrique auriculaire. Normale et pathologique. Masson&Editeurs, Paris, 1956.

Qaddoura A, Kabali C, Drew D, *et al.* Obstructive sleep apnea as a predictor of post coronary artery bypass graft atrial fibrillation: a systematic review and meta-analysis. Can J Cardiol 2014;30(12):1516.

Raatikanen M. Verapamil a double-edged sword in the rate control of paroxysmal AF. Heart Rhythm 2010;7:584.

Raj S, Black B, Biaggioni I, *et al.* Propranolol decreases tachycardia and improves symptoms in postural tachycardia syndrome. Circulation 2009;120:725.

Reynolds MR, Zimetbaum P, Josephson ME, *et al.* Costeffectiveness of radiofrequency catheter ablation compared with antiarrhythmic drug therapy for paroxysmal atrial fibrillation. Circ Arrhythm Electrophysiol 2009;2:362

Riva SI, Della Bella P, Fassini G, *et al.* Value of analysis of ST segment changes during tachycardia in determining type of narrow QRS complex tachycardia. J Am Coll Cardiol 1996;27:1480.

Roberts J., Gollob M. Impact of genetic discoveries on the classification of lone atrial fibrillation. J Am Coll Cardiol 2010;55:705.

Rotter M, Jaïs P, Vergnes MC, *et al.* Decline in C-reactive protein after successful ablation of long-lasting persistent atrial fibrillation. J Am Coll Cardiol 2006 21;47:1231.

Roy D, Talajic M, Nattel S, *et al.* Rhythm control versus rate control for atrial fibrillation and heart failure. N Engl J Med 2008;358(25):2667.

Rubboli A, Halperin JL, Airaksinen KE, *et al.* Antithrombotic therapy in patients treated with anticoagulation undergoing coronary stenting. Ann Med 2008;40:428.

Rubboli A, Bolognese L, Di Pasquale G, *et al.* A prospective multicentre observational study on the management of patients on oral anticoagulation undergoing coronary artery stenting: rationale and design of the ongoing warfarin and coronary stenting (WAR-STENT) registry. J Cardiovasc Med 2009;10:200.

Ruder MA, Davis JC, Eldar M, *et al.* Clinical and electrophysiologic characterization of automatic junctional tachycardia in adults. Circulation 1986;73:930.

Saczynski JS, McManus D, Zhou Z, *et al.* Trends in atrial fibrillation complicating acute myocardial infarction. Am J Cardiol 2009;104:169.

Sadiq Ali F, Enriquez A, Conde D, *et al.* Advanced interatrial block predicts new onset atrial fibrillation in patients with severe heart failure and cardiac resynchronization therapy. Ann Noninvasive Electrocardiol 2015;20:586.

Sanders P, Berenfeld O, Hocini M, *et al.* Spectral analysis identifies sites of high-frequency activity maintaining atrial fibrillation in humans. Circulation 2005;112:789.

Sanna T, Diener HC, Passman RS, *et al.* Cryptogenic stroke and underlying atrial fibrillation. N Engl J Med 2014;370(26):2478.

Santinelli V, Radinovic A, Manguso F, *et al.* Asymptomatic ventricular preexcitation: a long-term prospective follow-up study of 293 adult patients. Circ Arrhythm Electrophysiol 2009;2:102.

Saoudi N, Cosio F, Waldo A, *et al.* Classification of atrial flutter and regular atrial tachycardia according to electrophysiologic mechanism and anatomic bases: A statement from a joint expert group from the Working Group of Arrhythmias of the European Society of Cardiology and the North American Society of Pacing and Electrophysiology. J Cardiovasc Electrophysiol 2001;12:852.

Savelieva I, Camm AJ. Clinical relevance of silent atrial fibrillation: prevalence, prognosis, quality of life, and management. J Interv Card Electrophysiol 2000;4:369.

Sawhney N, Anoushed R, Chen W, *et al.* Circumferential pulmonary vein ablation with additional linear ablation results in an increased left atrial flutter incidence. Circ Arrhyth Electro 2010;3:243.

Scharf C, Boersma L, Davies W, *et al.* Ablation of persistent atrial fibrillation using multielectrode catheters and duty-cycled radiofrequency energy. J Am Coll Cardiol 2009;54:1450.

Schneider M, Hua T, Böhm M, *et al.* Prevention of atrial fibrillation by RAS inhibition. J Am Coll Cardiol 2010;55:2999.

Shelton RJ, Clark AL, Goode K, *et al.* A randomised, controlled study of rate versus rhythm control in patients with chronic atrial fibrillation and heart failure: (CAFE-II Study) Heart 2009;95:924.

Shenasa H, Merrill JJ, Hamer ME, *et al.* Distribution of ectopic atrial tachycardias along the crista terminalis: An atrial ring of fire? Circulation 1993;88:1.

Sick PB, Schuler G, Hauptmann KE, *et al.* Initial worldwide experience with the Watchman left atrial appendage system for stroke prevention in atrial fibrillation. J Am Coll Cardiol 2007;49:1490.

Singh D,Cingolani E, Diamond GA, *et al.* Dronedarone for atrial fibrillation have we expanded the antiarrhythmic armamentarium?. J Am Coll Cardiol 2010;55:1577.

Smit MD, Van Gelder IC. Valsartan and recurrent atrial fibrillation. N Engl J Med 2009;361:532.

Steinberg JS, Sadaniantz A, Kron J, *et al.* Analysis of causespecific mortality in the Atrial Fibrillation Follow-up Investigation of Rhythm Management (AFFIRM) study. Circulation 2004;109:1973.

Stiles MK, John B, Wong CX, *et al.* Paroxysmal lone atrial fibrillation is associated with an abnormal atrial substrate: characterizing the "second factor". J Am Coll Cardiol 2009;53:1182.

Tanigawa M, Fukatani M, Konoe A, *et al.* Prolonged and fractionated right atrial electrograms during sinus rhythm in patients with paroxysmal atrial fibrillation and sick sinus node syndrome. J Am Coll Cardiol 1991;17:403.

Thurmann M, Janney G. The diagnostic importance of fibrillatory wave size. Circulation 1962;24:991.

Tinetti M, Costello R, Piazza A, *et al.* Rheumatic disease and atrial fibrillation duration are predictors of inability to recover atrial contractility after MAZE IV surgery. Circulation 2010;122:A14718.

Tinetti M, Costello R, Cardenas C, *et al.* Persistent atrial fibrillation is associated with inability to recover atrial contractility after MAZE IV surgery in rheumatic disease. Pacing Clin Electrophysiol 2012;35(8):999.

Top-Pedersen C, Pedersen OD, Kober L. Antirrhythmic drugs: safety first. J Am Coll Cardiol 2010;55:1577.

Torner-Montoya P, Brugada P, Smeets J, *et al.* Ventricular fibrillation in the Wolff–Parkinson–White syndrome. Eur Heart J 1991;12:144.

Tsai ChT, Lai LP, Hwang JJ, *et al.* Molecular genetics of atrial fibrillation. J Am Coll Cardiol 2008;52:241.

Valles E, Fan R, Roux JF, *et al.* Localization of atrial fibrillation triggers in patients undergoing pulmonary vein isolation. Importance of the Carina Region. J Am Coll Cardiol 2008;52:1413.

Van Gelder IC, Hagens VE, Bosker HA, *et al.* Rate Control versus Electrical Cardioversion for Persistent Atrial Fibrillation Study Group. A comparison of rate control and rhythm control in patients with recurrent persistent atrial fibrillation. N Engl J Med 2002;347:1834.

Van Gelder IC, Groenveld H, Crijns H, *et al.* Lenient versus strict rate control in patients with atrial fibrillation. N Engl J Med. 2010;362:1363.

Van Oosten EN, Hamilton A, Petsikas D, *et al.* Effect of pre-operative obstructive sleep apnea on the frequency of atrial fibrillation after coronary artery bypass grafting. Am J Cardiol 2014;113(6):919.

Vazquez R, Bayés-Genis A, Cygankiewicz I, *et al.* The MUSIC Risk score: a simple method for predicting mortality in ambulatory patients with chronic heart failure. Eur Heart J 2009;30:1088.

Verma A, Mantovan R, Macle L, *et al.* Substrate and Trigger Ablation for Reduction of Atrial Fibrillation (STAR AF): a randomized, multicentre, international trial. Eur Heart J 2010;31:1344.

Verma A, Cairns JA, Mitchell LB, *et al.* 2014 focused update of the Canadian Cardiovascular Society Guidelines for the management of atrial fibrillation. Can J Cardiol 2014;30(10):1114.

Vermeer SE, Prins ND, den Heijer T, *et al.* Silent brain infarcts and the risk of dementia and cognitive decline. N Engl J Med 2003;348:1215.

Villareal RP, Hariharan R, Liu BC, *et al.* Postoperative atrial fibrillation and mortality after coronary artery bypass surgery. J Am Coll Cardiol 2004;43:742.

Virtanen JK, Mursu J, Voutilainen S, *et al.* Serum longchain n-3 polyunsaturated fatty acids and risk of hospital diagnosis of atrial fibrillation in men. Circulation 2009;120:2315.

Waldo A, Touboul P, eds. Atrial flutter: advances in mechanisms and management. Futura Publishing Company, New York, 1996, p. 321.

Wharton, M. Atrial tachycardia: Advances in diagnosis and treatment. Cardiol Rev 1995;3:332.

Wijffels M, Allesie M. Atrial fibrillation begets atrial fibrillation. Circulation 1995;92:1954.

Workman AJ, Kane KA, Rankin AC. Cellular bases for human atrial fibrillation. Heart Rhythm 2008;5:S1.

Wu D, Denes P, Amat-y-Leon F, *et al.* Clinical, electrocardiographic and electrophysiologic observations in patients with paroxysmal supraventricular tachycardia. Am J Cardiol 1978;41:1045.

Wyse DG, Waldo AL, DiMarco JP, *et al.* A comparison of rate control and rhythm control in patients with atrial fibrillation. N Engl J Med 2002;347:1825.

Yamada T, Murakami Y, Yoshida Y, *et al*. Electrophysiologic and electrocardiographic characteristics and radiofrequency catheter ablation of focal atrial tachycardia originating from the left atrial appendage. Heart Rhythm 2007;4:1284.

Yang Y, Mangat I, Glatter KA, *et al*. Mechanism of conversion of atypical right atrial flutter to atrial fibrillation. Am J Cardiol 2003;91:46.

Yeh ET, Bickford CL. Cardiovascular complications of cancer therapy: incidence, pathogenesis, diagnosis, and management. J Am Coll Cardiol 2009;53:2231

Yusuf S, Camm AJ. Deciphering the sinus tachycardias. Clin Cardiol 2005;28(6):267.

Zimetbaum PJ. Dronedarone for atrial fibrillation – an odyssey. N Engl J Med 2009;360:1811.

5

Active Ventricular Arrhythmias

Discussed in this chapter are premature ventricular complexes (PVC), both isolated and in runs, and the different types of ventricular tachycardia (VT), as well as ventricular fibrillation and ventricular flutter (Chapter 1, Table 1.1).

Premature Ventricular Complexes

Concept

Premature ventricular complexes (PVC) are premature impulses (complexes) that originate in the ventricles. Therefore, they present a different morphology from that of the baseline rhythm.

If the PVC are repetitive, they form pairs (two consecutive PVC) or VT runs (≥3) (Figures 5.1B and 5.3). Conventionally, a VT is considered to be sustained when it lasts for more than 30 seconds. Infrequent short runs of nonsustained monomorphic VT are included in this section. They correspond to Type 4B of Lown's classification (Lown and Wolf, 1971) (Figure 5.3 and Table 5.1).

In this section, runs of VT have not been included when they occur very frequently (repeated monomorphic nonsustained VT) (Figure 5.4), as they present clinical, hemodynamic, and therapeutic features that are more similar to sustained VT than to isolated PVC (Figure 5.3) (see Other Monomorphic Ventricular Tachycardias). Torsades de Pointes-type VTs (Dessertene, 1966) are not be included either; although they occur in runs, they are considered polymorphic VT and have quite different prognostic and therapeutic implications compared to isolated PVC or the short runs of classical monomorphic VT (Figure 5.5).

Mechanisms

The PVC may be caused by extrasystolic or parasystolic mechanisms (Figures 5.1 and 5.2):

- Extrasystoles, which are much more frequent, are induced by a mechanism related to the preceding QRS complex. For this reason, they feature a fixed or nearly fixed coupling interval (Figure 5.1). This is generally a reentrant mechanism (usually micro-reentry, but also branch-to-branch, or around a necrotic or fibrotic area) (see Figure 3.6). They may also be induced by post-potentials (triggered activity) (see Figure 3.5) or, in some exceptions, may be due to supernormal excitability and conduction. In the latter case, there should be some factor at a particular point of the cycle that turns the subthreshold stimulus into a suprathreshold stimulus, which triggers the premature impulse. This may happen when the stimulus falls in the supernormal excitability zone (see Figure 3.15).

- Parasystoles are much less frequent. They are impulses that are independent of the baseline rhythm. The electrophysiologic mechanism is an ectopic focus protected from depolarization by the impulses of the baseline rhythm. In general, this is due to the presence of a unidirectional entrance block in the parasystolic focus (see Figure 3.17). On the other hand, there usually exists a certain degree of exit block in the parasystolic focus (generally 2:1, 3:1, or Wenckebach-type), accounting for the slow and often irregular parasystolic rhythm. The total or partial disappearance of this block would lead to a more rapid conduction and the occurrence of parasystolic VT (see Other Monomorphic Ventricular Tachycardias). Parasystolic impulses can only activate the ventricular myocardium and originate a QRS complex if the myocardium is not in the absolute refractory period (ARP). Consequently, not all the impulses originating in the parasystolic focus may be detected in the electrocardiogram (ECG) tracing (Figure 5.2). The fact that the parasystolic focus is independent from the baseline rhythm explains the two principal electrocardiographic characteristics of parasystole: (i) the coupling intervals are variable and (ii) the interectopic intervals are multiples of each other, although there are some exceptions (see electrocardiographic diagnosis). Other complicated mechanisms could be responsible for some types of infrequent parasystoles, which do not fulfill these

Clinical Arrhythmology, Second Edition. Antoni Bayés de Luna and Adrian Baranchuk.
© 2017 John Wiley & Sons Ltd. Published 2017 by John Wiley & Sons Ltd.

Table 5.1 Lown's classification of premature ventricular complexes (PVC) (Lown and Wolf, 1971), according to prognostic significance (Holter electrocardiogram).

Grade 0: No PVC

Grade 1: <30/h

Grade 2: ≥30/h

Grade 3: Polymorphic PVC

Grade 4: 4a On pairs 4b Runs of monomorphic ventricular tachycardia

Grade 5: R/T Phenomenon (PVC falls on the preceding T wave)

criteria (modulated parasystole) (Oreto *et al.*, 1988). One easy to understand mechanism occurs when the discharge rate of the baseline rhythm is a multiple of the rate of parasystolic focus (for instance, sinus rhythm at 90 bpm, and parasystolic focus at 30 bpm). In such cases, the ECG would show a ventricular trigeminy with a fixed coupling interval.

Etiological and Clinical Presentation

Premature ventricular complexes, both of extrasystolic and parasystolic origin, may be observed both in healthy

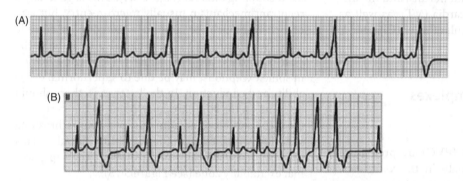

Figure 5.1 (A) A typical example of ventricular extrasystoles in the form of trigeminy. (B) Another example of ventricular extrasystoles, first bigeminal, then one run of nonsustained ventricular tachycardia (VT) (four complexes).

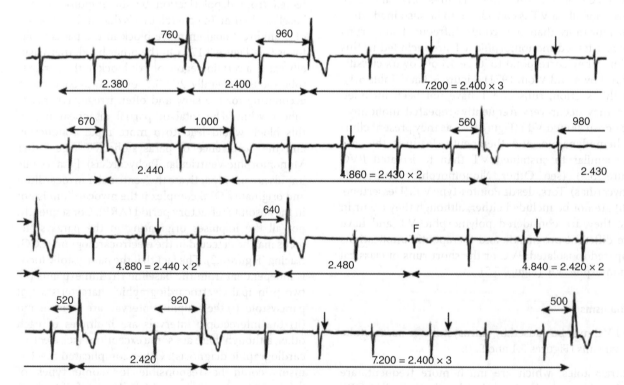

Figure 5.2 An example of parasystole. Note the variable coupling intervals, 760 ms, etc., the interectopic intervals that are multiples 2380, 2400, 2400 × 3, etc. and the presence of a fusion complex (F).

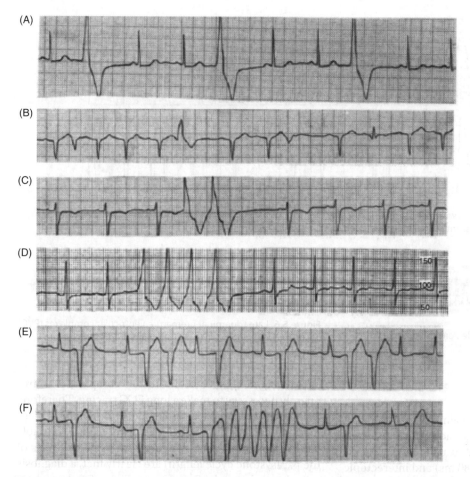

(A)

(B)

(C)

(D)

(E)

(F)

Figure 5.3 Different types of premature ventricular complexes (PVC) according to Lown's classification. (A) Frequent PVC. (B) Polymorphic PVC. (C) A pair of PVC. (D) Run of ventricular tachycardia (VT). (E and F) Examples of R/T phenomenon with a pair and one run.

subjects and in heart disease patients. Premature ventricular complexes are more troublesome while resting, particularly when the patient is lying in bed. When frequent, they can cause significant psychologic disturbances. The incidence increases with age and is more frequent in asymptomatic men after the age of 50 (Hinkle *et al.*, 1969). At times healthy people present with PVC as a result of consuming foods that cause flatulence, in addition to wine, coffee, ginseng, gassy foods and drinks, and some energy drinks. Emotions, stress, and exercise can also cause PVC.

Patients with PVC may be unaware of their presence, or may present palpitations, momentary "pressure or discomfort" in the chest, or the "transient absence of the pulse", often with what is perceived as a long postectopic pause. The patient may also describe a feeling of "the heart turning over", or "the heart stopping", or "a catch in the throat". Often, PVC lead to greater discomfort in healthy subjects, as the feeling of the heart "missing a beat" is mostly due to the post-extrasystolic potentiation of contraction, which is more evident in healthy individuals. The characteristic auscultation finding is

interruption of the normal rhythm by a premature beat or beats followed by a pause. If they are very frequent (many thousands in 24 h), and especially if they appear in runs, they may end up affecting the left ventricular function, even in patients without previous heart disease (tachycardiomyopathy). Nevertheless, in healthy subjects the prognosis is generally excellent (see Prognosis). When runs of PVC are frequent, however, and/or rapid, and/or long, they may not only produce hemodynamic disturbances and ventricular dysfunction, but also trigger a sustained VT. This type of VT (repeated monomorphic nonsustained VT) (Figure 5.4) (see Other Monomorphic Ventricular Tachycardias) jointly with runs of Torsades de Pointes VT (Figure 5.5) (Dessertene, 1966), isdiscussed further later (see Torsades de Pointes Polymorphic Ventricular Tachycardia).

Electrocardiographic Diagnosis

In the ECG, the PVC are represented as premature wide QRS complexes with a different morphology from that of the basal QRS.

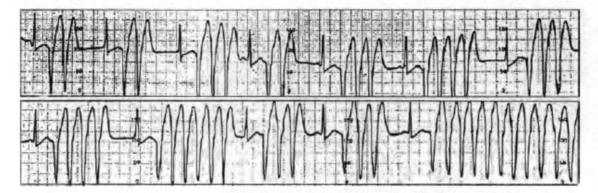

Figure 5.4 Taken from a 66-year-old man with ischemic heart disease. The tracings are successive. Self-limited runs of ventricular tachycardia (VT) with fast rate and incessant rates can be observed, until a sustained VT is initiated.

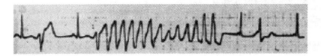

Figure 5.5 A run of a typical Torsades de Pointes ventricular tachycardia (VT).

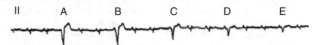

Figure 5.6 Late trigeminal premature ventricular complexes (PVC) occurring in the interval PR, and showing progressive fusion degrees from C to E (see Figure 3.30).

Extrasystole Compared to Parasystole PVC
(Figures 5.1 and 5.2)

Extrasystolic PVC show a fixed or almost fixed coupling interval. Parasystolic complexes, according to their mechanism (previously discussed) usually show a markedly variable coupling interval (>80 ms) and interectopic intervals, which are multiples of the parasystolic cycle length. Certain differences are permitted, as the discharge rate of the parasystolic focus may show fluctuations of up to 200 ms, and, contrary to this, as already explained, the coupling interval in some infrequent circumstances may be fixed (see Mechanisms). Furthermore, the lack of a mathematical relationship between interectopic intervals can be due to either incomplete protection of the parasystolic pacemaker (Cohen *et al.*, 1973) or to electronic modulation of the parasystolic rhythm (Oreto *et al.*, 1988). The hypothesis postulated by Kinoshita (1977) that parasystole may be explained by a reentry mechanism lacks any electrophysiologic and experimental demonstration (Oreto, 2010).

On the other hand, when complexes that originated in the two foci (baseline and parasystolic foci) coincide, they both activate the ventricles and a fusion complex occurs at a certain point in time (Figure 5.2). Figure 3.30 shows how the fusion complex is originated. It should be remembered that fusion complexes may occur during parasystole, and may also have an extrasystolic origin when ventricular extrasystoles occur very late (Figure 5.6). They may also occur in the presence of accelerated idioventricular rhythm (AIVR) (see Figure 5.33) or VT (see Figure 5.23).

To observe a parasystolic fusion complex, it is frequently necessary to make a long ECG tracing. Therefore, a single fusion complex is not enough for making a diagnosis of parasystole. If the other two criteria (variable coupling interval and interectopic intervals multiples of the parasystolic cycle length) are clearly met, a diagnosis may already be made. For instance, Figure 5.2 shows how a diagnosis may already be apparent before the end of the second ECG strip, and the fusion complex appear in the third. When we talk about PVC, we assume that their origins are extrasystolic, and we usually refer to them as simply ventricular extrasystoles. If they have a parasystolic origin, we call them parasystolic PVC.

Parasystolic PVC are very infrequent. They usually occur as isolated complexes (Figure 5.2). Rarely, there might be VT runs (see Figure 5.35) with a generally slow and often irregular rate, which facilitates the presence of capture and fusion beats (see Figure 5.35). In very infrequent cases, parasystolic PVC may trigger sustained VT, and in very exceptional cases a parasystolic PVC with R/T phenomenon may trigger ventricular flutter/fibrillation and sudden death (SD) (see Figure 5.43A).

Electrocardiographic Forms of Presentation

Premature ventricular complexes usually show a complete compensatory pause (the distance between the QRS complex preceding the PVC and the following QRS complex double the sinus cadence) (Figure 5.7A, BC = 2AB). This happens because the PVC usually fails to discharge the sinus node. In consequence, the distance BC

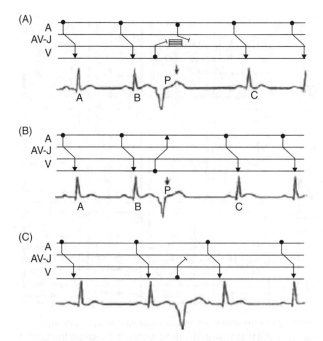

Figure 5.7 (A) Premature ventricular complexes (PVC) with concealed junctional conduction, which hinders the conduction of the following P wave to the ventricles. (B) PVC with retrograde activation to the atria with depolarization of sinus node. A change starts in the sinus cadence. (C) PVC with partial atrioventricular (AV) junctional conduction that permits the conduction of the following sinus P wave to the ventricles, albeit with longer PR.

is doubles the distance AB, represented as two sinus cycles.

If the PVC discharges the sinus node, a noncomplete compensatory pause may be observed (BC < 2AB) (Figure 5.7B).

In contrast, when the sinus heart rate is slow, a PVC, although it may enter the atrioventricular (AV) junction, leaving it in refractory period (RP), will not prevent the following sinus stimulus from being conducted toward the ventricles, although usually with a longer PR interval. This is due to the concealed PVC conduction in the AV junction, leaving it in the relative refractory period (RRP) that slows, but does not prevent, the conduction of the following P wave. Thus, the PVC occurs between two sinus-conducted P waves and does not feature a compensatory pause (Figure 5.7C). This type of PVC is known as **interpolated** PVC (Figures 3.38 and 5.7C).

The isolated PVC may occur sporadically or with a specific cadence. In this case, they may originate a bigeminy (a sinus QRS complex and an extrasystolic QRS complex) (Figure 5.1B), or a trigeminy (two normal QRS complexes and one extrasystolic QRS) (Figure 5.1A). As already noted, they may also occur in a repetitive form (Figures 5.1B and 5.3D). Short and isolated runs of classical monomorphic VT with a rather slow rate (Figures 5.1B and 5.3) are considered repetitive

forms of PVCs and will be dealt with in this section. This is not the case when the runs are very frequent (Figure 5.4) (see before and Other Monomorphic Ventricular Tachycardias). Lown has classified the PVC into different types, according to the characteristics shown in Table 5.1 and Figure 5.3 (Lown and Wolf, 1971). Ventricular tachycardia runs correspond to Class 4b in Lown's classification (Figure 5.3). This classification is hierarchical and has prognostic implications (see later).

Characteristics of QRS Complexes

Width of the QRS complex: most PVCs originate in the Purkinje network or in the ventricular muscle. They usually present a QRS complex ≥0.12 s. Occasionally, if they start in one of the two main branches of the bundle of His or in one of the two divisions of the left bundle branch (LBB), the QRS is <0.12 s (narrow fascicular PVC), and the morphology, although variable, resembles an intraventricular conduction block with a QRS <0.12 s. Some of these are parasystolic impulses.

QRS **morphology** varies according to its site of origin (Figure 5.8). If the QRS complex starts in the right ventricle (RV) it is similar to that of a left bundle branch block (LBBB) (Figure 5.8B). Those originating in the left ventricle (LV) show a variable morphology: when QRS complexes arise mainly from the lateral or inferobasal walls of the heart, they appear positive in all precordial leads (Figure 5.8A); when QRS complexes originate next to the inferoposterior or superoanterior division of left bundle, they resemble a prominent R wave, sometimes with notches in the descending limb of the R wave, but usually without the rsR morphology that is typical of right bundle branch block (RBBB) in lead V1. The ÂQRS may be extremely deviated to the right or the left, depending on their origin in the inferoposterior or superoanterior division, and so on. The presence of QR morphology suggests associated necrosis (see Classic monomorphic VT).

Generally, all QRS of VT show similar morphologic characteristics to the initial PVC. This is because they usually have the same origin and are caused by the same mechanism. Additionally, the intraventricular conduction of the stimulus is usually the same. However, the morphology of QRS complexes may change during a VT episode (pleomorphism) (see Polymorphic VT), or a PVC with a given morphology does not originate a monomorphic but a polymorphic VT as is often the case in Brugada's syndrome (see Chapter 9, Brugada's Syndrome).

In individuals with no evidence of heart disease, PVCs usually show high voltage and unnotched QRS complexes. It is possible for them to present a QS morphology but rarely a notched QR morphology. Repolarization shows an ST segment depression when

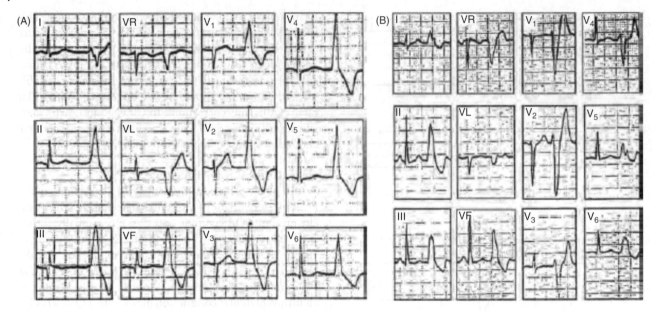

Figure 5.8 (A) Premature ventricular complexes (PVC) that arise in the lateral wall of the heart (QRS always positive from V1 to V6 and negative in I and VL). These are frequently observed in heart disease patients. (B) PVCs that arise in the right ventricle. These are frequently observed in healthy individuals, although they may also occur in heart disease patients.

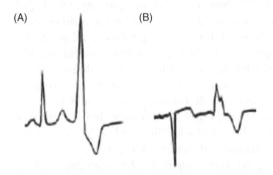

Figure 5.9 Typical electrocardiographic morphologies of premature ventricular complexes (PVC) in healthy individuals (A) and in patients with advanced heart disease (B). Note that the PVC of A may be seen also in patients with advanced heart disease, and much less frequently the PVC of B may be recorded in healthy people.

the QRS is positive, and vice versa, whereas the T wave has asymmetrical branches (Figure 5.9A). This type of PVC may also be observed in heart disease patients. A large proportion of PVCs in individuals with no structural heart disease will be originated in the right ventricular outflow tract (RVOT). These PVCs can be asymptomatic, however: if the density is high (probably more than 10 000/24 h); they can trigger ventricular dysfunction and in this case they may require treatment including ablation. Its morphology is easy to recognize: they present with LBBB-like morphology in lead V1 and with superior to inferior axis (positive QRS complexes in leads II, III and VF (Lamba *et al.*, 2014) (see later).

However, **the PVC of patients with significant myocardial impairment** shows frequently symmetrical T waves, more often than healthy subjects, because of the presence of an additional primary disturbance of repolarization. Also, the QRS complexes present notches and

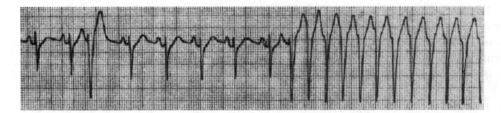

Figure 5.10 Taken from a 51-year-old woman who showed frequent paroxysmal tachycardia episodes. Note how the second and seventh T waves prior to arrhythmia onset are much sharper than the remaining waves, because an atrial extrasystole causes, respectively, an isolated or repetitive aberrant conduction.

slurrings, often with a low voltage pattern and qR morphology (Moulton *et al.*, 1990) (Figure 5.9B).

Differential Diagnosis

Table 4.3 shows the most relevant data indicative of aberrancy or ectopy in cases of premature complexes with wide QRS. It is very important to determine if a P wave preceding a wide premature QRS complex is clearly present or may change the morphology of previous T wave, because this is crucial for the diagnosis of aberrancy (Figure 5.10). It is also essential to thoroughly observe the PVC morphology, as the presence of patterns consistent with the typical bundle branch block is very much in favor of aberrancy, although we have already stated that fascicular PVC may mimic the pattern of an intraventricular conduction disorder with QRS complexes <0.12 s.

Prognosis

As already discussed (see Etiological and Clinical Presentation), PVC may be observed both in healthy subjects and in heart disease patients. Premature ventricular complexes that originate in the RV (LBBB morphology) are considered to be benign. However, arrhythmogenic right ventricular cardiomyopathy (ARVC) should be ruled out, particularly if frequent; any other ECG signs suggestive of ARVC should be closely observed (Figure 5.11). Remember that PVCs with notched wide QRS complexes occur much more often in subjects with myocardial impairment. In addition, PVC

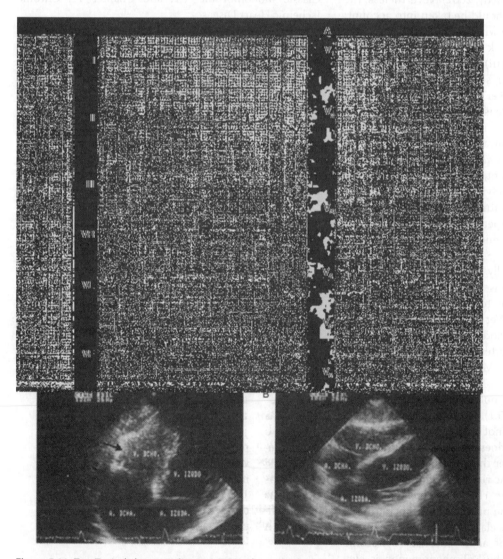

Figure 5.11 Top: Typical electrocardiogram (ECG) of an arrhythmogenic right ventricle (RV) dysplasia/cardiomyopathy. Note the negative and symmetric T wave in V1–V3 and the frequent premature ventricular complexes arising from the RV (left bundle branch block morphology). Bottom: The echocardiogram shows evidences of the impairment of RV wall contractility (arrow) (see Chapter 9).

that trigger ventricular fibrillation (VF) in patients with early repolarization patterns in inferior leads may originate in the inferior wall (left AQRS) (Haïssaguerre *et al.*, 2008) (see Chapter 10, Early Repolarization Pattern). It has been suggested (Moulton *et al.*, 1990) that PVC with QRS complexes <160 ms, and unnotched QRS complexes or notched QRS complexes of less than 40 ms, generally show a normal or nearly normal left ventricular function, although there are exceptions (Figure 5.9). However, a clear impairment of left ventricular function usually occurs when there are notched QRS complexes with a notch separation >40 ms (see Chapter 10, The Presence of Ventricular Arrhythmias in Chronic Heart Disease Patients).

The long-term prognosis of healthy subjects with ventricular premature extrasystoles is generally good (Kennedy *et al.*, 1985; Kennedy, 2002) Nevertheless, the following considerations should be taken into account: (i) if PVC clearly increase with exercise, this indicates an increased long-term risk for cardiovascular problems (Jouven *et al.*, 2000); (ii) it has been reported that during a stress test, the ST segment depression in the PVC may be a better marker for ischemia than the ST segment depression in the baseline rhythm (Rasouli and Ellestad, 2001) (see Figure 10.16); (iii) very frequent PVC (>10–20 000/day) (Niwano *et al.*, 2009), or a PVC burden of >24% (Baman *et al.*, 2010) may lead to ventricular function impairment, in which case ablation of the ectopic focus may be advisable (Bogun *et al.*, 2008; Lamba *et al* 2014 (see Treatment)). Nevertheless, during the five-year follow-up period reported in this study, no one case of SD or death due to heart failure (HF) was observed.

Parasystolic PVCs usually have a good prognosis. Occasionally, they may cause VT, which usually has a slow and irregular rate due to different degrees of exit block (see Figure 5.35). Very rarely, they fall in the vulnerable ventricular period (R/T phenomenon) and may trigger ventricular flutter/fibrillation (Figure 5.43) (see before and Other Monomorphic Ventricular Tachycardias).

In addition, it should be noted that Lown's classification is hierarchical (Table 5.1). For example, if grade 4/5 PVC are present, it does not matter whether they are polymorphic or not, nor does the reported number of QRS complexes. The higher the grade, according to this classification, the higher the risk of triggering malignant arrhythmias. However, the risk also depends on the number of PVC and on the patient's clinical condition. Thus, the usefulness of this classification has been questioned, except in cases of acute coronary syndrome (Myerburg *et al.*, 1984). The R/T phenomenon is currently considered to be dangerous especially in the presence of acute ischemia.

During acute ischemia, especially in acute myocardial infarction (MI), the presence of PVC may be a harbinger, especially in cases of PVC with R/T phenomenon, of VF and SD. Today, with the new efficient treatments for acute MI, the incidence of PVC and the danger of VF/SD decreases if the patient starts the treatment early (see Chapter 11, PVC and SD in acute Myocardial Infarction (AMI)).

It has been demonstrated (Moss, 1983; Bigger *et al.*, 1984) that in chronic ischemic heart disease (IHD) patients, especially post-infarction patients, risk increases after one PVC/h, especially when complex PVC morphologies and/or HF are present (Figures 5.12 and 5.13). It has also been demonstrated (Haqqani *et al.*, 2009) that the characteristics of MI scar are more important than the number of PVCs in the triggering of sustained VT (see Classic monomorphic VT, and Chapter 11: Chronic Ischemic Heart Disease).

In hypertrophic cardiomyopathy, the presence of frequent PVC, and especially the presence of VT runs, during a Holter ECG recording is an indicator of risk for SD (McKenna and Behr, 2002; Zhang *et al.*, 2014) (see Chapter 9, Hypertrophic Cardiomyopathy).

Premature ventricular complexes are also frequent in many other heart diseases: valvular heart diseases, especially aortic valve disease and mitral valve prolapse, cor pulmonale, hypertension, some congenital heart diseases, post-surgery in Fallot's tetralogy and others (see Chapter 11).

In any case, the severity of PVC increases in patients with depressed ventricular function and especially in the presence of evident HF (see Chapter 11, Heart Failure).

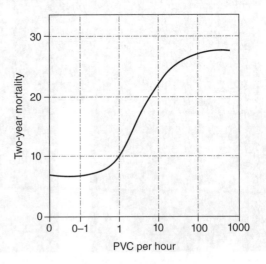

Figure 5.12 Note the increase of mortality among post-infarction patients when the frequency of premature ventricular complexes increases from one to ten per h (Bigger *et al.*, 1984).

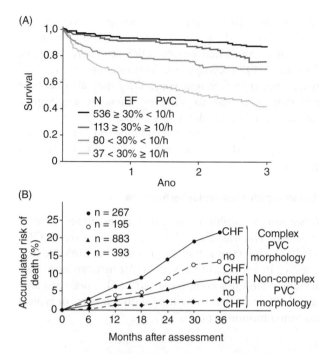

Figure 5.13 (A) A post-infarction survival related to left ventricular function (ejection fraction) and the number of premature ventricular complexes (PVC) (Bigger *et al.*, 1984). (B) Relationship between the presence of PVC with complex morphology (grade II or higher in Lown's classification), and noncomplex morphology, with or without heart failure, and mortality risk in post-infarction patients (Moss, 1983).

Treatment

The treatment of PVC, both in heart disease patients and healthy subjects, should include some general measures, such as: (i) decreasing, or even ceasing, consumption of wine, coffee, tea, and stimulating energetic drinks, as well as avoiding intake of parapharmaceutic products containing stimulants (i.e., ginseng) if a cause–effect relationship is observed; (ii) preventing aerophagia by avoiding soda and foods that cause flatulence and eating too much too quickly; and (iii) avoiding stress as much as possible.

In heart disease patients, pharmacologic treatment is based on the symptoms and the clinical condition of the patient, as well as the number and type of PVC:

- If symptoms are related to sympathetic overdrive, β-blockers should be prescribed.
- Amiodarone may also be prescribed, especially when PVCs are very frequent, or runs of PVC are observed, because they are considered to be markers for a poor prognosis. In IHD patients, the beneficial effects of amiodarone, in terms of prevention of SD, are controversial. In fact, this has been considered in cases with the concomitant administration of β-blockers (Janse *et al.*, 1998). The main disadvantages of amiodarone

treatment are its extracardiac side effects, especially thyroid dysfunction. Periodical monitoring of the thyroid function is recommended if this drug is prescribed.

- Type 1 antiarrhythmic agents, such as quinidine, flecainide, mexiletine, and so forth, should not be administered to post-infarction patients or patients with other types of heart disease, especially in cases of depressed ventricular function, due to their arrhythmogenic potential, as demonstrated in the CAST trial (Echt *et al.*, 1991). In patients with well-preserved ventricular function in whom β-blockers are not effective or amiodarone is contraindicated, low doses of propafenone may be a useful alternative, when PVC are frequent and symptomatic and are suppressed by the drug (acute drug test) (Bayés de Luna *et al.*, 1987). However, this treatment should not be administered to patients with important structural heart disease and LV dysfunction, especially when HF exists.

In the case of patients who are free from heart disease, apart from the general measures already mentioned the patient should be reassured that PVC are likely to disappear at any time, especially if the previously discussed measures are taken. If necessary (i.e., if PVC are symptomatic or occur more frequently with exercise or emotions), β-blockers may be prescribed. As in patients with heart disease, it is also very important to advise patients that PVC are much more likely to stop if they avoid wine, stress, and gassy foods.

Ablation of the right ventricular focus may be recommended in the absence of heart disease in cases with persistent, very frequent (>5–10 000 in 24 h) and symptomatic PVCs (including athletes), and in heart disease patients in whom frequent PVCs may lead to a decreased ejection fraction (tachycardiomyopathy), or if there is evidence that they have triggered a VT of the same origin (Lamba *et al.*, 2014). It has been demonstrated (Bogun *et al.*, 2008) that ablation may suppress PVC in 80% of cases, normalizing the ejection fraction if it has deteriorated due to the arrhythmia. Zhang *et al.* (2009) describe an algorithm that helps to localize the PVC origin in the surface ECG, thereby optimizing ablation.

Also, it has been demonstrated (Sarrazin *et al.*. 2009) that in post-infarction patients with frequent PVC (>5% of the total QRS complex in 24 h, Holter) ablation of the ectopic focus located around the MI scar may improve the ejection fraction so that the patient no longer meets the ejection fraction criteria for an implantable cardioverter defibrillator (ICD) implementation.

Ablation of left ventricular outflow tract (LVOT) PVCs should also be performed if the criteria to ablate (very symptomatic, deteriorating LV function or high density) are met. This usually requires noncontact mapping support and sometimes a concomitant angiogram to determine the anatomic location of the ostia of the coronary arteries.

Premature Ventricular Complexes (PVC)

- Most PVC present wide QRS around 120 ms and show a different morphology from the baseline rhythm.
- Most PVC feature a fixed coupling interval (extrasystoles) and are generally caused by a reentrant ventricular mechanism.
- In few cases do PVCs meet the criteria of parasystole (variable coupling interval, multiple interectopic intervals, and, if a long ECG tracing is taken, the presence of fusion complexes).
- PVC morphology usually allows us to differentiate them from the supraventricular aberrant complexes.
- Treatment and prognosis of PVC largely depends on the clinical condition of the patient.

Ventricular Tachycardias

Ventricular tachycardias may be sustained or appear as runs. They are considered sustained when they last for more than 30 seconds. Based on their morphology, VTs are classified as either **monomorphic or polymorphic** (Table 5.2). The initial complexes sometimes show certain polymorphisms and often may feature some irregularities of the rhythm. Therefore, this classification should be made when the VT is established. **Both monomorphic and polymorphic VTs may be sustained or nonsustained** (runs). Isolated or infrequent monomorphic VT runs have been traditionally studied along with PVC and are now classified as Type IV B in Lown's classification (Table 5.1, Figure 5.3). The clinical, prognostic, and therapeutic aspects of monomorphic frequent VT runs, particularly if they are incessant, may easily trigger a sustained VT in heart disease patients and have a significant hemodynamic impact. They are discussed in

Table 5.2 Ventricular tachycardias (VT).

Monomorphic	Polymorphic
Classical (QRS ≥0.12 s)	Torsades de Pointes
Narrow QRS	Bidirectional
Accelerated idioventricular rhythm	Pleomorphism
Nonsustained monomorphic	Catecholaminergic polymorphic
Parasystolic	Other VT with variable morphology

this section (see Other Monomorphic Ventricular Tachycardias, and Figure 5.4). Tachycardia is considered to be incessant when ectopic QRS are more frequent than sinus QRS complexes. Torsades de Pointes VT usually occur in frequent runs. They may also become incessant and lead to VF (see Torsades de Pointes Polymorphic Ventricular Tachycardia).

All VTs, except for those originating in the upper part of the septum (fascicles), present wide QRS complexes ≥0.12 s.

Monomorphic Ventricular Tachycardia

When monomorphic VT originate in the upper septum/bundle of His branches, they may have a narrow QRS (<0.12 s). However, if they originate in the Purkinje network, or in any area of the ventricular myocardium, they present wide QRS complexes (≥0.12 s). These are sustained VT and occur more frequently (classical or typical sustained monomorphic VT).

Classical Ventricular Tachycardia (QRS ≥ 0.12 s)
Concept
By definition, sustained VT are those lasting longer than 30 seconds. From a clinical point of view, most sustained VT are long enough to develop specific symptoms that may require hospitalization. This is more likely to occur when the tachycardia is fast and long-lasting, particularly in heart disease patients. Most VT are triggered by extrasystolic PVC. Thus, the initial complex, when there are several episodes, presents the same coupling interval. Parasystolic VT are very rare and frequently occur at a slow rate. They are generally nonsustained VT appearing in runs and arise from a protected automatic focus, which explains the variable coupling interval (see Figure 5.35, and Other Monomorphic Ventricular Tachycardias).

The typical monomorphic ventricular tachycardia (VT) is a sustained VT with QRS interval ≥0.12 s, whereas the typical polymorphic VT is a Torsades de Pointes VT.

Electrophysiologic Mechanisms
We will now deal with the most interesting aspects of the electrophysiologic mechanisms that trigger and perpetuate extrasystolic VT in different heart diseases as well as in healthy individuals.

In subjects with heart disease
In acute MI in patients without previous MI scars, sustained VT are relatively rare and sudden death (SD) generally occurs due to a VF triggered by one PVC (see Figures 5.42 and 5.44).

However, when VT occurs in the acute phase of MI, it may be triggered by a combination of factors, including: (i) the presence of fibrotic zones (previous scars) facilitating the anisotropic and intermittent conduction of stimuli; (ii) an increased focal automatic activity in the peripheral part of the ischemic zone; (iii) evident disturbances in the autonomic nervous system (ANS) that may be indirectly assessed by the presence of sinus tachycardia, abnormal heart rate variability, heart rate turbulence, and so on; (iv) a dispersion of repolarization with unidirectional block of the stimulus, which facilitates reentry; and (v) genetic factors probably in relation to Ito current activity in different parts of the heart (more in RV) and in men (see Chapter 11, Acute Ischemic Heart Diseases).

Post-infarction VT are usually triggered by alterations in the ANS assessed by different parameters (see previously) in the presence of frequent PVCs (Bigger *et al.*, 1984; Moss, 1983). It has been demonstrated (Haqqani *et al.*, 2009) that the characteristics of the scar are more relevant to trigger VT in chronic IHD patients without residual ischemia than the presence of PVC (see Chapter 11, Chronic Ischemic Heart Disease).

- The risk factors explained in Chapter 11 (see Figure 11.4), that are considered more important to trigger SD (electrical instability, depressed LV function, and residual ischemia) may interact and trigger a VT in the presence of PVC. The VT may be perpetuated in post-infarction patients by a reentry mechanism in the area surrounding the infarction scar. This reentry may be explained by the classical concept of anatomic obstacle or by the functional reentry (rotors) (see Figures 3.6B and 3.11D). The reentrant VT may be initiated and terminated by programmed stimulation. This is not the case when the mechanism of VT is an increased automatism or a triggered electrical activity.
- The theory of the spiral wave breakdown (rotors) (see Chapter 3, Reentry) explains the conversion of a stable VT into a polymorphic VT, and later to VF (Qu and Garfinkel, 2004).

Ventricular tachycardias observed in other heart diseases, including cases of heart failure (HF), are often due to a reentry mechanism in the area surrounding a fibrotic zone. Different ANS disturbances (assessed by heart rate variability, heart rate turbulence, QT/RR slope, etc.) (Cygankiewicz *et al.*, 2008, 2009) and disorders of K^+ currents resulting in prolonged repolarization (Shah and Hondeghem, 2005), may trigger and/or modulate VT, which may lead to VF and SD (see Figure 1.3).

In some cases, particularly in patients with dilated or ischemic cardiomyopathy, VTs are produced by a reentry where both branches of the specific conduction system (SCS) are involved. This type of VT, also called bundle branch reentry, accounts for 5% of all sustained VT

(Touboul *et al.*, 1983) (see Figure 3.6B). In this case, the VT is initiated by a right bundle PVC that ascends through the left bundle branch and descends over the right bundle branch, thus depolarizing the left ventricle from right to left and showing the typical morphology of the LBBB. In this case it is difficult to diagnose as a VT with a surface ECG (see Figure 5.27, and later ECG findings). The presence of AV dissociation may help to reach the correct diagnosis. In some exceptions this reentrant circuit may be reversed and the VT morphology will be that of a RBBB, which is quite easy to induce (Mizusawa *et al.*, 2009). Ventricular tachycardias originating in an interfascicular reentry circuit have also been described.

In arrhythmogenic right ventricular cardiomyopathy (see Chapter 9, Arrhythmogenic Right Ventricular Dysplasia Cardiomyopathy (ARVC), and Figure 9.7B), VT is related to the anatamopathologic changes caused by the underlying disease, especially when muscle tissue has been replaced by adipose tissue and triggers the development of reentrant VT.

On the other hand, in hypertrophic cardiomyopathy (see Chapter 9, Arrhythmogenic Right Ventricular Dysplasia Cardiomyopathy (ARVC)), VT are produced by the presence of fiber disarray and fibrotic areas, which trigger the development of reentrant VT (Zhang *et al.*, 2014).

Heterogeneous dispersion of repolarization at an intramural (Yan and Antzelevitch, 1998) or global (Opthof *et al.*, 2007) level results in a voltage gradient (see Figure 3.11E), which facilitates reentry during transmembrane action potential (TAP) Phase 2. This explains VT in the long QT syndrome and other channelopathies (see Chapter 3, Reentry, and Figure 3.11E).

In all the cases previously described, especially in heart disease with a depressed left ventricular function and inherited heart disease, the greatest challenge is to recognize why a sustained VT may lead to VF and SD (Chapters 9 and 11).

In subjects with no evidence of heart disease

The most frequent electrophysiologic mechanisms are (Lerman *et al.*, 1995; Lerman, 2007):

- **A micro-reentry**, usually in the region of the inferoposterior fascicle of the left bundle branch, although it may also occur in the superoanterior fascicle (fascicular VTs). These fascicular VTs are sensitive to verapamil. Ventricular tachycardias originating in the papillary muscles have characteristics similar to those of the fascicular VT.
- **Triggered electrical activity**. These VT are sensitive to adenosine.
- **Increased automatism**. These VT are sensitive to propranolol.
- Table 5.3 shows the differences between these three types of idiopathic VTs.

Table 5.3 Ventricular tachycardias in patients with no apparent heart disease.

Mechanism	Triggered activity (late post-potentials) (adenosine sensitive)	Fascicular reentry (verapamil sensitive)	Automatic focus (propranolol sensitive)
Origin	RVOT in 90% of the cases LVOT in 10% of the cases	Inferoposterior fascicle of the LBB in 90–95% of the cases. Rest of the cases in superoanterior fascicle	Different areas of the RV or LV
Incidence	~70% of VT with no apparent heart disease	Rare	Very rare
Induced by	Programmed stimulation	Programmed stimulation	Catecholamine excess
ECG morphology	• RVOT: LBBB with right ÂQRS (Figure 5.17) • LVOT: Atypical LBBB (see Figure 5.15-4)	• RBBB with generally left ÂQRS (Figure 5.16) • QRS: sometimes narrow (even <120 ms (Figure 5.32))	• RBBB • LBBB • Polymorphic morphology
Type and triggering factor	Exercise-induced. catecholamines Incessant (Figure 5.17)	Disappear with exercise if the heart rate exceeds the VT rate (Figure 5.16)	• Exercise-induced Incessant
Treatment	• Possibly terminated with adenosine or verapamil • In 25–50% of cases verapamil or β blockers may prevent new episodes • Resolved by ablation when necessary • Symptoms, CMR anomalies, etc.	• Although VT are terminated when verapamil is administered, this drug does not always prevent new episodes • Ablation constitutes a definitive treatment	• It may respond to β blockers • Polymorphic types are potentially serious • ICD implantation may be required

CMR, cardiovascular magnetic resonance; ICD, implantable cardioverter defibrillator; LBB, left bundle branch; LBBB, left bundle branch block; LV, left ventricle; LVOT, left ventricular outflow tract; RBBB, right bundle branch block; RV, right ventricle; RVOT, right ventricular outflow tract; VT, ventricular tachycardia.

Clinical Presentation

From an etiological point of view, sustained VT are more frequently observed in heart disease patients, especially in the presence of HF or in inherited HD. In the latter, the VT that trigger VF are usually polymorphic, but are not always Torsades de Pointes type (see Polymorphic Ventricular Tachycardia). Different factors, such as electrolyte imbalance and the administration of different drugs, especially digitalis, may trigger different types of ventricular arrhythmia, including VT. It has been reported (Guglin *et al.*, 2009) that several chemotherapy drugs may induce arrhythmias (see Chapter 4, AF: Epidemiology), especially AF and VT. The drugs that induce the most ventricular arrhythmias are interleukin-2, cisplatin, and, especially, e-fluoracil. The last has the potential to induce arrhythmias in the context of a coronary spasm.

From a clinical point of view, symptoms include generally poorly tolerated palpitations, paroxysmal dyspnea, angina, dizziness, or even syncope, and sometimes pulmonary edema, and may lead to VF and SD.

The significance of the symptoms depends on the ventricular rate, the arrhythmia duration, and the presence and type of heart disease. The most dangerous types of VT are sustained and rapid VT associated with acute ischemia and those occurring in patients with depressed ventricular function, particularly if associated with HF and in patients with inherited HD. In some cases, especially in the presence of some triggers (new crises of ischemia, electrolyte imbalance, worsening of heart failure), the crises of VT are recurrent and often lead to VF. If the VT/VF recurrences occur frequently (more than 3 in 24 h), this constitutes the clinical setting named "electrical storm". This clinical setting is seen in 10% of patients with an implanted ICD in a follow-up of five months (Credner, 1998). Usually, patients without heart disease have a better tolerance for VT, a much better prognosis, and require a different treatment (see Treatment). Currently, management of "electrical storm" in patients with ICDs requires a multifactorial treatment: (i) Optimization of antiarrhythmic treatment and (ii) ablation of the VT, either the circuit (critical isthmus) or the anatomical substrate. Recent studies have shown an improvement in survival when VT ablation is added to ICD and optimized antiarrhythmic treatment (Reddy *et al.*, 2007; Sapp *et al.*, 2016).

Electrocardiographic Findings

- **ECG recording in sinus rhythm** If previous ECGs are available, it is useful to compare their morphologies with that of a wide QRS complex tachycardia. For

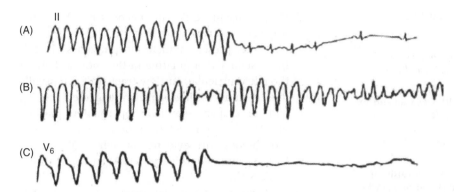

Figure 5.14 Three modes of termination of a sustained ventricular tachycardia (VT). (A) Reverting into sinus rhythm. (B) Initiating a ventricular fibrillation (VF). (C) Turning into asystole (rare).

instance, in the case of a tachycardia with a wide QRS complex ≥0.12 s, the presence of an even wider QRS complex in sinus rhythm due to an advanced LBBB strongly supports the diagnosis of a VT. Meanwhile also, the presence of an AV block during sinus rhythm favors a wide QRS complex being a VT.

- **Onset and end**
- Different triggering or modulating factors are involved in the onset of VT. These mechanisms, when acting on a vulnerable myocardium (post-infarction scar, fibrosis, HF, disarray in hypertrophic heart disease), may trigger the final step: VF and SD (see Figures 1.3 and 5.46). Sustained VT usually starts with a PVC with a morphology similar to the other QRS of the tachycardia, with a relatively short and fixed coupling interval but frequently without R/T phenomena, especially in sustained VT not related to acute ischemia. Sometimes, prior to the establishment of a sustained VT, the number of PVC and runs increases significantly. Sustained VT may trigger VF. This is often the final event in ambulatory patients dying suddenly while wearing a Holter device (Bayés de Luna *et al.*, 1989). Tachycardization of sinus rhythm characteristically occurs prior to the sustained VT, which leads to VF and SD (see Figure 1.4). Other mechanisms have also been proposed as pro-arrhythmogenic: short–long sequences produce a dispersion of the repolarization, increasing the probability of developing VT. This mechanism is highly prevalent in nonischemic cardiomyopathies, and Chagas' disease (Rabinovich *et al.*, 2008).

    The end of a VT may be followed by a short pause and then by a sinus rhythm. In the worst cases it will be followed by VF, sometimes with an intermediate ventricular flutter. Exceptionally, VT leads directly to cardiac arrest (Figure 5.14). It has been described that bidirectional VT can be the mechanism of termination of some ischemic sustained VTs (Siegal *et al.*, 2009)

- **Heart rate**

    Heart rate usually ranges from 130 to 200 bpm. RR intervals occasionally show some irregularities, especially at tachycardia onset and termination. Once the tachycardia has been established, RR intervals are usually fixed or nearly fixed (variability is <0.04 s). Using Holter ECGs, we have demonstrated (Bayés de Luna *et al.*, 1989) that VTs leading to VF are usually fast and show a wide QRS complex. We have seen in cases of VF preceded by VT that VT rate typically increases before VT turns into VF (see Figure 1.4).

- **QRS morphology**
  - By definition, **QRS complexes are monomorphic.** QRS complex patterns depend on the site of origin, the VT pathways, and the presence of heart disease. If the heart rate is very rapid and the QRS complex is very wide, the ventricular repolarization is hard to detect in some leads. In this case it would be difficult, and sometimes impossible, to differentiate VT from ventricular flutter (see Ventricular Flutter).
  - **Subjects with no evidence of heart disease** (Shimoike *et al.*, 2000; Marrouche *et al.*, 2001; Cole *et al.*, 2002; Nogami, 2002).
  a) Usually, the QRS morphology does not have many notches and the T wave is clearly asymmetric. In general terms, the morphology is similar to that of a LBBB or RBBB. However, the bundle branch block pattern is usually atypical.
  b) Table 5.4 describes **the different types of idiopathic VT** according to ECG morphology: RBBB-type with evidence of left or right ÂQRS deviation, or LBBB-type with left or right ÂQRS deviation.
  c) Figures 5.15A and 5.15B show the electrocardiographic characteristics of idiopathic VT, depending on their site of origin (Figures 5.16–5.19). All idiopathic VT with RBBB morphology originate in the LV, whereas most VT with LBBB morphology initiate in the RV. However, there are some idiopathic left VT, which originate in or near the high portion of the septum and/or the aortic valve leaflets. These may have a LBBB morphology, even though a QS type morphology is not usually present in V1 (Figures 5.15 and 5.18). Also, VT

Table 5.4 Idiopathic ventricular tachycardia with QRS ≥120 ms: electrocardiogram morphology[*].

A. Idiopathic VT with LBBB morphology (generally with "r" in V1). May originate in both ventricles (although usually originates in the RV)[†]	
Superior (left) ÂQRS	– **VT originates in the RV free wall and/or near the tricuspid ring.** R in I and QS or rS in V1–V2 and late R transition in precordials. ARVC should be ruled out (Figure 9.7B and 5.15-(1)).
Inferior (right) ÂQRS	– **VT originated in RVOT endocardium.** Features a relatively late R transition (V3–V4); R/S in V3<I) and an isolated unnotched R in V6 (Figure 5.17). 50% of **VT of ARVC show similar morphologies**.
	– **VT originated near the aortic valve.** Features an early R transition (R/S V3>I) and an isolated notched R in V6 (Figure 5.18). With regard to origin (Figure 5.15): (i) if QRS morphology in I is rS or QS (Figure 5.18), the zone close to the left coronary leaflet is involved. (ii) if rs(RS) with notched "r" is observed in V1, the VT originates near the non-coronary leaflet; and (iii) if qrS pattern is present in V1–V3, the VT originates between the right and left coronary leaflet.
	– **If the VT originates in the area surrounding the mitral ring,** usually a rsr' or RS pattern morphology is observed in V1. a qrS pattern morphology is observed in V1.
B. Idiopathic VT with RBBB morphology (generally, R in V1 and "s" in V6; from Rs to rS). Always originates in the LV	
Superior (left) ÂQRS	– Inferior-posterior fascicular VT: activation similar to RBBB + SAH (Figure 5.16)
Inferior (right) ÂQRS	Anterior-superior fascicular VT (Figure 5.19B))
	VT originated in LVOT endocardium near anterior-superior fascicle (Figure 5.19A — Activation similar to the RBBB + IPH

[*] Idiopathic VT with duration <120 ms (narrow QRS) present partial RBBB or LBBB morphologies (see Other Monomorphic Ventricular Tachycardias).
[†] Ouyeng *et al.*, 2002; O'Donnell *et al.*, 2003; Yamada *et al.*, 2008.

IPH, inferior-posterior hemiblock; LBBB, left bundle branch block; LV, left ventricle; LVOT, left ventricular outflow tract; RBBB, right bundle branch block; RV, right ventricle; RVOT, right ventricular outflow tract; SAH, superior-anterior hemiblock; VT, ventricular tachycardia.

originating near the mitral valve feature an atypical LBBB morphology, even with an RS type morphology usually of low voltage in lead V1 (Figure 5.15-(5)). In contrast, high left fascicular VT usually show a typical or atypical RBBB morphology, although usually with a QRS complex <0.12 s (see Other Monomorphic Ventricular Tachycardias, and Figure 5.32).

d) Despite having different mechanisms, VT often originate in areas very close to each other and, therefore, present similar morphologies. This is the case in VT originating in the endocardium of the left ventricular outflow tract (LVOT), usually due to an adenosine- sensitive triggered activity, and the verapamil-sensitive superoanterior fascicular VT. (Nogami, 2002). In both cases, an RBBB morphology with evidence of right ÂQRS deviation is observed (Figure 5.19A and 5.19B, and Table 5.4B).

e) Ventricular tachycardias originating in the left papillary muscles are similar to fascicular VTs; however, they show a wider QRS complex and there is no Q wave in the frontal plane.

o **Heart disease patients** (Josephson *et al.*, 1979; Griffith *et al.*, 1991, 1992; Wellens, 1978, 2001; O'Donnell *et al.*, 2003). The most important characteristics are:

- **The QRS pattern** in heart disease patients with VT compared with the QRS pattern in healthy subjects with VT is usually wider (≥0.16 s), with more notches, slower beginning of the QRS until the point of first change of polarity, and a more symmetrical T wave (Figures 5.20–5.22).

- **Ventricular tachycardias originated in the LV free wall present wider QRS complexes,** whereas narrower QRS complexes are indicative of VT originating in the high septum. The QRS complexes may even be narrower than those in sinus rhythm if the patient presents an advanced bundle branch block. The QRS complex width is also conditioned by several factors, such as ventricular hypertrophy, post-infarction scars, and so on.

- **VT in heart disease patients may show the following QRS morphologies:**
  o A prominent R wave in lead V1 and an "s" wave in lead V6 (**RBBB morphology**) (Figure 5.21).
  o An rS in lead V1 with evident R in V6 (**LBBB morphology**) (Figure 5.22).
  o **Concordance of the QRS complex** patterns in precordial leads (all positive or all negative) (Figure 5.20).
  o Presence of a **QR morphology, usually seen in post-infarction VT** (Wellens, 1978). This morphology sometimes allows for the localization of the MI site, if it is not possible during baseline sinus rhythm due to the presence of a LBBB.
  o Presence in **lead II of R wave peak time** (distance from the beginning of QRS deflection to the **point of first change in polarity,** independent of whether the QRS is positive or negative) ≥ 50 ms (Pava *et al.*, 2010).

(A)

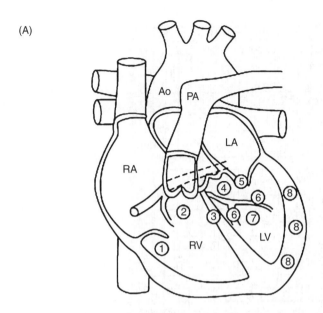

(B)

	Place of origin and incidence	ECG patent	AQRS	QRS in the frontal plane	Morphologies in V1 (depends of AQRS)	RS transition in precordial leads
R **V**	(1) Tricuspid ring 5–10%	LBBB	Never right-handed Between +60° and +30°	R in I and VL	QS or rS	Beyond V3
	(2 and 3) RV outflow tract, pulmonary valve and high septum 60–60%	LBBB	Right	R in II, III and VF	QS or rS	Generally beyond V3
L **V**	(4) Below the aortic valve ≈ 5%	LBBB	Right	R in II, III and VF	– qrS – RS (R < S) – rS – qS	In V2-V3
	(5) Mitral ring	Atypical LBBB	Right	R in II, III and VF	⋀, ⋁	Generally in V1
	(6) Fascicular. Generally inferoposterior 10–20%	RBBB	Left (Fig 5.16) If right handed (Fig 5.19), the origin is in the superoanterior fascicle	It depends Left, in case of inferoposterior fascicle. Right, superoanterior	qR, R	qR, R in VI

Figure 5.15 (A) Place of origin of idiopathic ventricular tachycardia (VT) (see correlation number-location in B). Some, such as the bundle branch (7) and the subepicardial (8) can be observed more in heart disease cases. (B) Electrocardiographic features of the most common of these VTs. RV = right ventricle, RBBB = right bundle branch block, LBBB = left bundle branch block. RV, Right Ventricle, LV, Left Ventricle.

- **Ventricular tachycardias arising from the apex** usually show more negative voltages in precordial leads with evidence of extreme left ÂQRS (Figure 5.20). **Those rising from the basal area** generally have more positive voltages in precordial leads with evidence of right ÂQRS (Figure 5.8A).
- In post-infarction patients or in advanced heart disease patients, morphology depends not only on the site of origin of the VT but also on the

intraventricular distribution of the electric stimulus. It should be noted that sometimes the morphology may change in the same VT episode (**pleomorphism**) (Josephson *et al.*, 1979) (see Polymorphic VT).
- **The bundle branch reentrant VT** (Figure 5.27) (Touboul *et al.*, 1983) accounts for 5–10% of all cases of sustained VT. Both branches of the SCS are usually involved in the reentry circuit. This

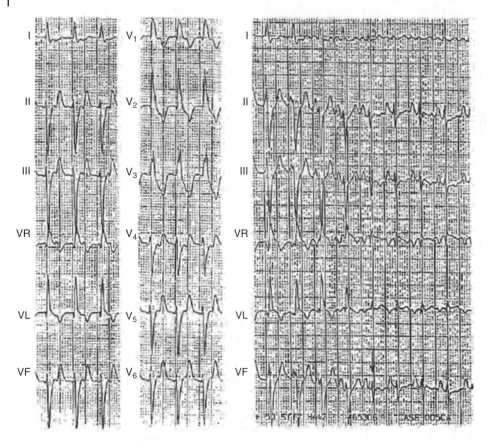

Figure 5.16 An example of verapamil-sensitive ventricular tachycardia (VT) with origin in the infero-posterior zone (infero-posterior fascicular). Note the morphology of right bundle branch block + superoanterior hemiblock (RBBB + SAH), but with qR morphology in V1. In the right panel it can be appreciated how the sinus tachycardia exceeds the VT rate during exercise testing.

VT usually occurs in patients with IHD or dilated cardiomyopathy. It is rarely seen in patients who show no evidence of heart disease. The bundle branch reentrant VT is generally associated with an advanced LBBB morphology (see Chapter 3, Reentry) and is caused by an initial right PVC originating near the right bundle branch. It is blocked in this branch, then retrogradely enters the left bundle branch before descending anterogradely over the right bundle branch. From an electrophysiologic point of view, the H-V interval of the bundle branch reentrant complex equals or exceeds the H-V interval of the normally spontaneous conducted QRS complex. Less frequently, the direction of the reentry circuit is reversed (Mizusawa *et al.*, 2009). In these cases, the depolarization impulses descend through the LBB and ascend over the RBB (bundle branch reentrant VT with RBBB morphology). It is important to point out that the morphology during VT is often similar to that observed during sinus rhythm if the bundle branch block is present in the baseline rhythm. In fact, bundle branch reentrant VT

presents an ECG pattern of LBBB that may be easily diagnosed as aberrant tachycardia (see Figure 5.27). On the other hand, RBB or LBB catheter ablation blocks the circuit and solves the problem definitively.

- Despite the fact that most **VT originating in the RV** (left bundle branch block morphology with superior or inferior ÂQRS deviation) **are idiopathic, the presence of ARVC should always be ruled out** (Table 5.4). Clinical, electrocardiographic, and especially electrophysiologic and imaging data, allow us to differentiate idiopathic right ventricular outflow tract (RVOT) VT from VT due to ARVC (O'Donnell *et al.*, 2003).

- **Ventricular tachycardias** generally originate in the **subendocardial area**. However, in a few cases VT originate in the **subepicardial area**, generally in heart disease patients. In this scenario the impulse conduction is slower because less Purkinje fibers are involved. This results in (i) a pseudo-δ wave, (ii) time of intrinsic deflection >85 ms, and (iii) distance from the onset of the R wave to the nadir of the S wave >120 ms (Brugada

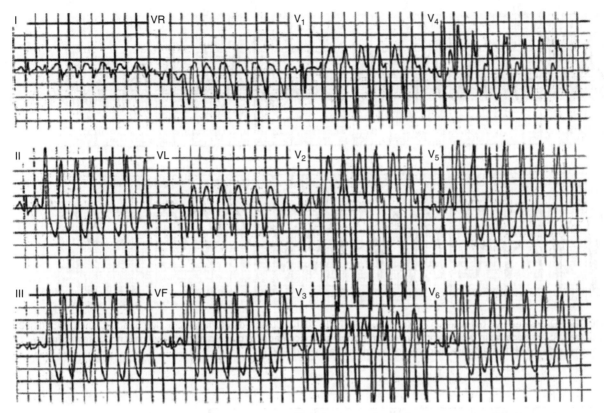

Figure 5.17 An example of left bundle branch block (LBBB)-type ventricular tachycardia (VT) with rightwards QRS occurring as repetitive runs during exercise testing in an individual without heart disease. Example of VT originated in RVOT. See how in V3 the R < S. In case of VT of RVOT (Figure 5.18) the R/S appear before V3.

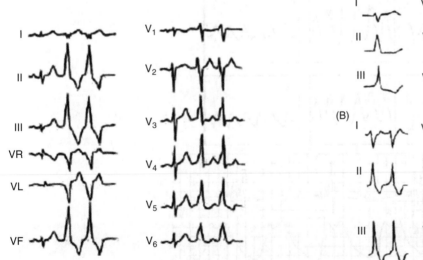

Figure 5.18 Example of runs of a left ventricular tachycardia (VT) arising from septal epicardial zones close to the leaflets of the aortic valve (Type 4 Figure 5.15). The morphology of V1 may present different pattern, see Figure 5.15-(3), and in V3 R>S. Because of the QS morphology in I, the leaflet of the aortic valve closest to the epicardial zone that gives rise to the VT is probably the left coronary one. See in Figure 5.15 the characteristic of RVOT-VT.

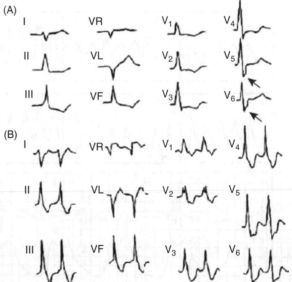

Figure 5.19 Examples of two VT in normal structural heart that present similar morphology (RBBB + right QRS) and are originated in two close zones (A in LVOT and B in zone of antero-superior fascicle) but are originated by different mechanisms the VT of A are generally caused by triggered activity (adenosine-sensitive), whereas those of B are due to reentry (verapamil-sensitive) (adapted from Nogami, 2002).

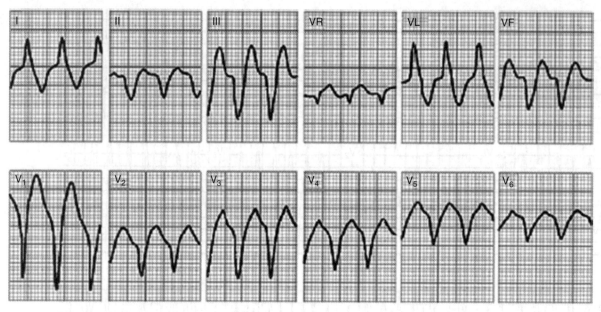

Figure 5.20 The ÂQRS is deviated to the left in the frontal plane, similar to that observed in some cases of left bundle branch block (LBBB). However, all the QRS are negative in the horizontal plane (morphologic concordance in precordial leads), which is not observed in any type of branch bundle block; this supports diagnosis of ventricular tachycardia (VT).

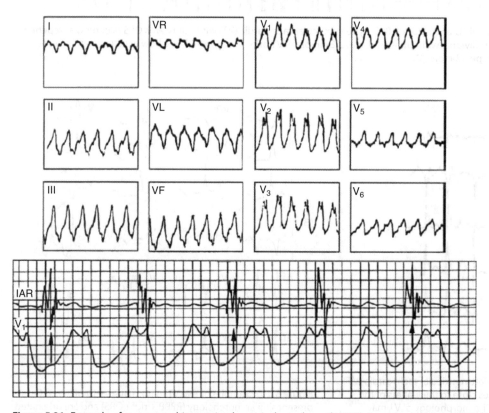

Figure 5.21 Example of monomorphic sustained ventricular tachycardia (VT). An atrioventricular (AV) dissociation is evidenced with the use of a right intra-atrial lead (IAL) and the higher speed of electrocardiogram (ECG) recording, allowing us to better see the presence of small changes of QRS that correspond to atrial activity (arrow). The morphologies of V1 (R) and V6 (rS) also support the ventricular origin.

(A)

(B)

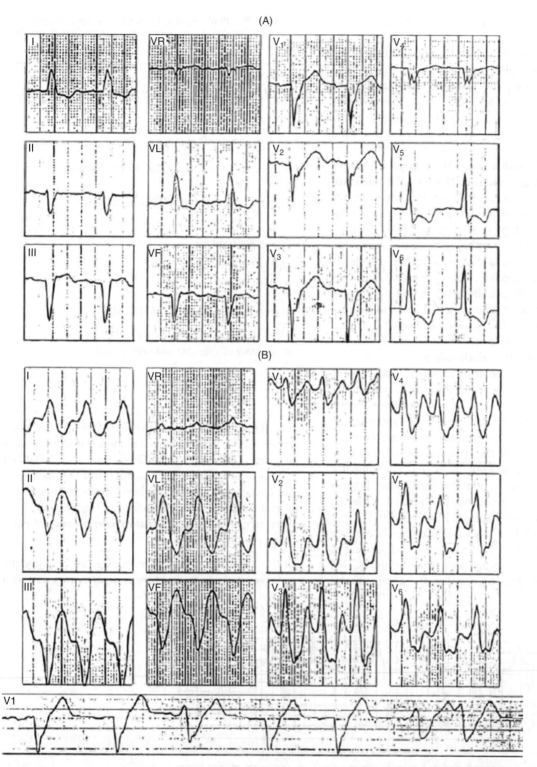

V1

Figure 5.22 A 75-year-old patient with ischemic heart disease. The baseline electrocardiogram (ECG) (A) shows an advanced left bundle branch block (LBBB), with an extremely leftwards ÂQRS and poor progression of R wave from V1 to V4, with a notch in the ascending limb of the S wave, suggestive of an associated myocardial infarction. The patient suffered an episode of paroxysmal tachycardia at 135 bpm, with advanced LBBB morphology (B). Despite the fact that the ECG pattern is of LBBB type and the patient presented baseline LBBB, we diagnose ventricular tachycardia (VT) because: (i) the R wave in V1 was, during the tachycardia, clearly higher than the R wave in V1 during sinus rhythm – additionally, the bottom panel shows that, in the presence of sinus rhythm, the patient showed premature ventricular complexes (PVC) with the same morphology as those present during the tachycardia; the first and second PVC are late (in the PR), and, after the second, a repetitive form is observed – and (ii) according to the Brugada algorithm (Figure 5.28), in some precordial leads featuring an RS morphology, this interval, measured from the initiation of the R wave to S wave nadir, is >100 ms.

et al., 2003; Bazan *et al.*, 2007; Berruezo *et al.*, 2004) (Figure 5.22).

- **The presence of capture and fusion beats** may modify the QRS complex morphology and cadence. If they are frequent, tachycardia may mimic a polymorphic tachycardia. The presence of capture and fusion beats strongly suggests that a tachycardia associated with wide QRS complexes is of ventricular origin (see later) (Figure 5.23).

- **When a VT with a wide QRS complex features a morphology similar to that of a RBB or LBB,** it is necessary to check the morphologies in different leads to determine whether we are in the presence of ectopy or aberrancy. Table 5.5 shows the most typical morphologies that help in making this differential diagnosis in four key leads (V1, V6, VR, and VF). The differential diagnosis between ectopy and aberrancy in wide QRS complex tachycardias is discussed in detail in the section Differential Diagnosis of Wide QRS Complex Tachycardias (see later).

- **P wave–QRS complex relationship**

There is an **AV dissociation in more than 60% of cases**. This means that ventricles and atria are independently activated (there is no relationship between the P wave and the QRS complexes). In the remainder of cases, we can observe variable retrograde conduction (2×1, 1×1, etc.) to the atrium, although 1×1 conduction is more frequently reported. Occasionally, atrial activity (with or without AV dissociation, Figures 5.21 and 5.1B, respectively) may be observed as a notch in the repolarization of isolated PVC or VT.

The presence of AV dissociation is critical in order to make a diagnosis of wide QRS complex tachycardias of ventricular origin. It may be useful to record the ECG at higher speed in order to visualize the atrial impulse

Table 5.5 Differential diagnosis between ventricular tachycardia and wide QRS aberrant supraventricular tachycardia with regular RR intervals (morphologic criteria).

In favor of ectopy

V₁ ∧ ∧ ∿ ∧

V₁ ∿ ∿ especially if in V₆ ∿ ∿

VR ∿ ∿ ∿ ∿ ∿

VF: i) In the presence of wide QRS and RBBB pattern

∨ ∨ ∿

ii) In the presence of wide QRS and LBBB pattern

∧ ∿ ∧∧ ∨ ∿

In favor of aberrancy

V₁ ∿ ∿ if in V₆ ∿

VR ∨ ∨ ∿

VF: i) presence of wide QRS and RBBB pattern

∧ ∿ ∿ ∿ ∿ ∧∧ ∿ ∿

ii) presence of wide QRS and LBBB pattern

∿ ∿ ∨

(Figure 5.21). Filtering the T wave is likely to allow us to record the atrial impulse in the case of broad QRS tachycardia. This has already been demonstrated in the case of narrow QRS tachycardia (Goldwasser *et al.* 2008), but has yet to be confirmed in cases of broad QRS tachycardia (see Appendix A-3, Other surface techniques to record electrical cardiac activity, and Figure A-13).

- **Presence of capture and fusion (complexes or beats)** (Figure 5.23)

In the presence of VT recording we can occasionally observe a **narrow premature complex preceded by a**

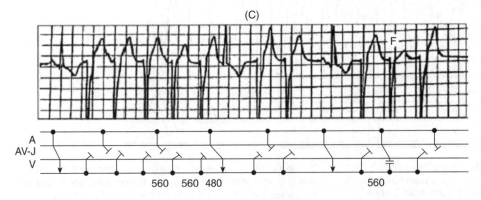

Figure 5.23 After a sinus complex, a ventricular tachycardia (VT) run lasting seven beats occurs. The Lewis diagram represents the complete atrioventricular (AV) dissociation. Between the fifth and sixth complexes of the VT, there is a typical ventricular capture (early QRS with the same morphology as the baseline rhythm). Afterwards, after a normal sinus stimulus (not early), there is a short VT run (three QRS complexes). The complex in the middle is a fusion complex, as it has a different morphology from the other two (narrower QRS and a less sharp T wave), and the RR interval is not modified.

sinus P wave (usually masked within the T wave). This narrow premature complex is the expression of a ventricular capture complex or beat due to a sinus impulse overtaking the baseline VT rhythm. For capture beats to take place, the following should occur: (i) there should not be a complete AV dissociation and (ii) the rate of tachycardia should be relatively slow, so that at a certain point in time a sinus impulse may cross the AV junction and depolarize the ventricles between two ectopic QRS complexes.

Exceptionally, narrow capture QRS complexes may be observed in AV junctional tachycardia with aberrant conduction, in the absence of retrograde atrial activation. However, the presence of capture complexes strongly suggests a tachycardia of ventricular origin.

In most series, **the presence of capture complexes is low (<10%)**. Thus, it is a very specific but not very sensitive sign.

Frequently, the sinus impulse cannot depolarize the whole ventricular myocardium, which is only partially depolarized by the tachycardia impulse. The complex resulting from the ventricular depolarization due to two stimuli – one sinus and the other of ventricular origin – is called **ventricular fusion complex** or beat (Figure 5.23). The ventricular fusion complex is frequently seen in VT and also in many other clinical situations (late ventricular premature complexes, accelerated idiopathic ventricular rhythm (AIVR), ventricular parasystole, etc.) (Figures 5.23 and 5.33). The ventricular fusion complex is nonpremature, or only minimally premature, and its width and morphology are halfway between the sinus and ectopic impulses

(see Figure 3.30). This figure explains that the PR interval of the ventricular fusion complex may be normal (E–H in Figure 3.30) or shorter than the baseline PR interval. However, in the latter case, the PR interval of a fusion complex may not be shorter than 0.06 s with respect to the duration of the PR interval of sinus impulse. This happens because fusion takes place when the ectopic ventricular complex coincides with the sinus complex, simultaneously depolarizing the ventricles, and 0.06 s is the time required by any ventricular impulse to reach the AV junction from any part of the ventricles (Figure 3.30; situations B–D).

In the presence of a bundle branch block, and despite the sinus rhythm and PVC being wide, any fusion ventricular complex originating in the homolateral ventricle to the bundle branch block is narrower than the baseline QRS and the PVC. This is explained because the blocked (homolateral) ventricle is depolarized starting from the extrasystolic focus and, almost simultaneously, the contralateral ventricle is activated by the sinus rhythm (Figure 5.24).

Atrial fibrillation in Wolff–Parkinson–White (WPW) syndrome also shows intermediate-morphology QRS complexes due to different degrees of pre-excitation, or even narrow complexes, such as capture complexes. This happens because the entire ventricle is sometimes depolarized through SCS. The presence of an irregular rhythm, and the fact that narrow QRS complexes are not always premature, as in the capture complexes that occurs during VT, are indicative of atrial fibrillation in the presence of the WPW syndrome (see Figure 4.52) (see Chapter 8).

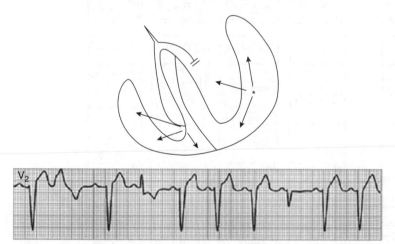

Figure 5.24 A baseline left bundle branch block (LBBB). The second complex in V2 is a premature ventricular complex (PVC) with a wide QRS. The fourth and the eighth are also PVC, although in these beats the QRS is narrow, especially in the eighth once, as they are fusion complexes from a focus starting at the ventricle homolateral to the blocked branch that depolarizes the LV, and a sinus QRS that comes from the contralateral branch (right) and depolarizes the RV (see figure). The fusion PVC is narrow, despite the sinus and ectopic complexes being wide, because the heart activation takes place almost simultaneously from two different foci, sinus and ectopic, which causes the simultaneous ventricular depolarization with shared septal repolarization from both of its sides, and explains why the resulting fusion QRS is narrow.

Differential Diagnosis of Wide Regular QRS Complex Tachycardias: Aberrancy Versus Ectopy

This differential diagnosis is made for fast regular supraventricular tachycardia (SVT) with aberrant conduction. The differential diagnosis between VT and rapid atrial fibrillation in WPW syndrome (irregular tachycardia) is discussed elsewhere (see Chapter 4, Differential Diagnosis, Chapter 8, Arrhythmias and Wolff–Parkinson–White Type Pre-excitation: Wolff–Parkinson–White Syndrome, and Figure 4.52).

Fast regular supraventricular rhythms with aberrant conduction include: (i) Atrial tachycardia, (ii) atrial flutter with 2:1 AV conduction, with advanced bundle branch block pattern, (iii) junctional reentrant tachycardias exclusively (JRFE) (Figure 5.25) or over an according pathway (JRT-AP) (Figure 5.26) (antidromic tachycardia), and (iv), less frequently, atrial flutter or other regular SVT with anterograde conduction over an accessory pathway (Figure 4.66B).

Clinical Criteria

There are some clinical aspects that may help to make a correct differential diagnosis:

○ Wide QRS complex tachycardias occurring in heart disease patients, particularly post-infarction and in cardiomyopathies, are ventricular tachycardias unless proven otherwise.

○ Tachycardia termination through vagal maneuvers or carotid sinus massage (see Table 1.5) is indicative of SVT, although some exceptions to this rule exist.

○ Generally, SVT with aberrant conduction are clinically and hemodynamically better tolerated than VT. However, sometimes fast and prolonged VT episodes are surprisingly well tolerated, even in heart disease patients, whereas episodes of SVT with aberrant conduction may be very badly tolerated.

○ A careful physical examination may be a helpful diagnostic tool for the diagnosis of AV dissociation and, consequently, of VT. Physical examination includes the auscultation of the variable intensity of the first heart sound (S1) (like a cannon shot) (see Figure 1.13), the intermittent presence of cannon A waves in the venous pulse, and the verification of a variable systolic pressure (see Chapter 1, The Physical Examination). However, in the case of a compromised hemodynamic state, an ECG diagnosis should immediately be recorded in order to make the correct diagnosis as soon as possible and to administer

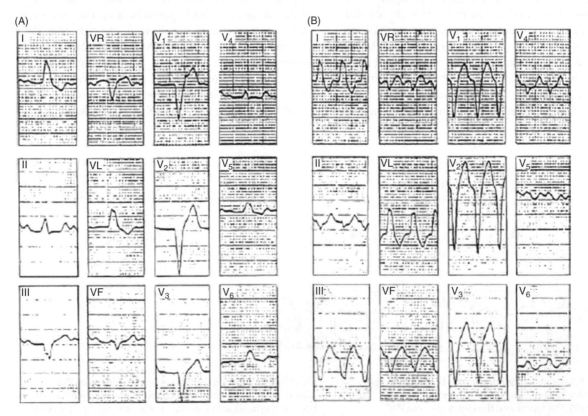

(A)   (B)

Figure 5.25 Taken from a 48-year-old patient with dilated cardiomyopathy and left bundle branch block (LBBB) morphology in the baseline electrocardiogram (ECG) (A). The patient suffered a paroxysmal tachycardia with a wide QRS very similar to the baseline one (B). The supraventricular origin was most likely by the fact that the QRS morphology in all leads (see especially V1) was identical to that present during the sinus rhythm.

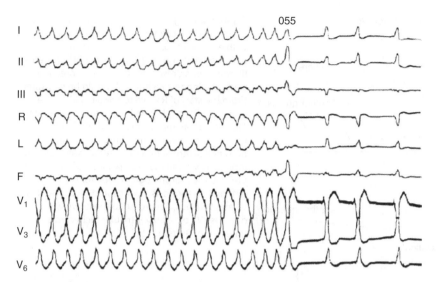

055

Figure 5.26 A broad QRS tachycardia. This is an antidromic supraventricular tachycardia (SVT) over an accessory atrioventricular (AV) pathway (Kent bundle). The morphology is that of a left bundle branch block (LBBB), although the R wave is clearly visible in V3, which is not usual in antidromic tachycardias through an atriofascicular tract (atypical pre-excitation) (Table 8.1 and Figure 4.22). Note the persistence of the Wolff–Parkinson–White (WPW) morphology once the tachycardia disappears. None of the criteria in favor of a VT in the differential diagnosis between VT and antidromic tachycardia are met (see Steurer *et al.*, 1994 and Differential Diagnosis of Wide QRS Complex Tachycardias). All these data suggest that it is a typical antidromic tachycardia (bundle of Kent) with aberrant morphology. Remember that for this differential diagnosis, the algorithm criteria from Figure 5.28 do not apply (see Figure 4.22 and Table 8.1).

the appropriate treatment at the earliest time possible.

Electrocardiographic Diagnostic Criteria

- **Electrocardiographic criteria with a higher positive predictive value (PPV) for the diagnosis of VT are:**
  - The presence of capture and/or fusion complexes (Figure 5.23).
  - The demonstration of AV dissociation (Figure 5.21). This occurs in 50–60% of cases. In other cases, a 1:1 AV conduction is observed. Consequently, in the latter, diagnosis of VT has to be reached using other criteria and complementary techniques, if necessary. Alternatively, carotid sinus massage may be performed to modify the AV relation (Figure 1.15).
  - Evidence of extremely deviated ÂQRS, (between −90° and ±180°).

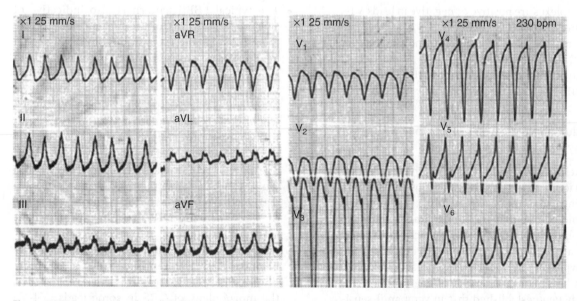

Figure 5.27 An example of a bundle branch ventricular tachycardia (VT) with a typical advanced left bundle branch block (LBBB) morphology (see V1 with a QS pattern). See QRS morphology in V5 with a sharp peak, not usually seen in typical pattern of LBBB.

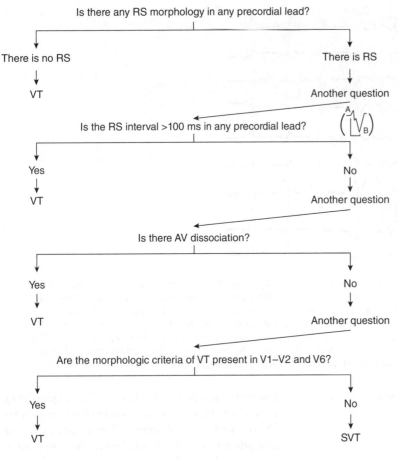

Is there any RS morphology in any precordial lead?

There is no RS → VT

There is RS → Another question

Is the RS interval >100 ms in any precordial lead?

Yes → VT

No → Another question

Is there AV dissociation?

Yes → VT

No → Another question

Are the morphologic criteria of VT present in V1–V2 and V6?

Yes → VT

No → SVT

Figure 5.28 Algorithm for the diagnosis of wide QRS tachycardia. When an RS complex is not visible in any precordial lead, we can make a diagnosis of ventricular tachycardia (VT). When an RS complex is present in one or more precordial leads, the longest RS interval should be measured (from the start of R wave to S wave nadir – see inside the figure). If the RS interval is greater than 100 ms, we can make a diagnosis of VT. If the interval is shorter, the next step is checking the presence of atrioventricular (AV) dissociation. If it is present, we can make a diagnosis of VT. If not present, the morphologic criteria for the differential diagnosis of VT should be checked in V1 and V6 leads. According to these, we will diagnose VT or supraventricular tachycardia (taken from Brugada *et al.*, 1991).

o A markedly wide QRS complex >140 ms in right bundle branch block-like tachycardias, and >160 ms in left bundle branch block-like tachycardias.

o The presence of morphologies that are incompatible with bundle branch block, for example when all QRS complexes are positive or negative in leads V1–V6 (Figure 5.20).

o Determination of QRS complex morphology in leads VF, VR, V1, and V6 (Table 5.5).

o Presence of R wave peak time at lead II ≥50 ms (Pava *et al.*, 2010) (see Electrocardiographic findings).

o Monomorphic aVR configuration (Vereckei, 2014).

- **On the other hand, the best criteria for the diagnosis of tachycardia with aberrancy are:**

o If the tachycardia onset is recorded, the verification of previous atrial activity strongly supports a supraventricular origin (Figure 5.10).

o Morphology resembling a bundle branch block: In this case, the wide QRS complex tachycardia may present a RBBB or LBBB morphology:

- The typical RBBB pattern (rsR′ in lead V1 and qRs in lead V6) is characteristic of aberrancy. It has already been established that in verapamil-sensitive VT, although the morphology is consistent with a RBBB pattern with left ÂQRS deviation, the morphology recorded in lead V1 is not usually an rsR′ wave but a qR or R wave, sometimes with a notch in the descending limb of the R wave (Figure 5.16).

- The typical LBBB pattern is also indicative of aberrancy. However, in the presence of a LBBB, the ÂQRS axis and the morphology of V1 should be checked to ensure that the pattern is due to aberrancy. It should be carefully assessed whether an initial "r" of a relative voltage level (2–3 mm) is observed in V1 (Figure 5.22), which would be very suggestive of VT. The SVT with LBBB aberrant conduction does not usually show an initial r, and on the occasions that it does, it will be minimal r (≥1 mm) (Figure 5.25). On the other hand, the ÂQRS is not usually extremely deviated, as in VT. **Among all types of VT with wide QRS, bundle branch reentrant VT (see before) are the most difficult VT with LBBB morphology to correctly diagnose because they frequently present a QS morphology in V1** (Figure 5.27). In our experience, the morphology of QRS in some leads (V4-V5 with a sharp peak of R-wave especially in lead

V5, see Figure 5.27) is unusual in cases of LBBB aberrancy.

o Morphology of the complexes in VF, VR, V1, and V6 also helps to make a differential diagnosis (see Table 5.5). (Griffith *et al.*, 1991, 1992; Vereckei *et al.*, 2008) (see later).

o Unfortunately, the most specific criteria for VTs are capture complexes, (Figure 5.23), and AV dissociation (Figure 5.21), which, although quite specific (nearly 100%), are not very sensitive criteria.

Practical Approach to Differential Diagnosis Between VT and SVT with Aberrant Conduction

From a practical point of view, and considering the urgency of these cases, the best way to reach a differential diagnosis is to apply an easy sequential algorithm with proven statistical value. Another possibility is to verify whether the morphologies of wide QRS complex tachycardias are consistent with aberrant conduction (morphology similar to that of an RBBB or LBBB). In fact, this last approach constitutes the fourth step of the following sequential algorithm. Also, some other ECG criteria may be useful (see Electrocardiographic Findings).

- **Sequential algorithm**

In 1991, Brugada described an algorithm incorporating the sequential use of many of the aforementioned criteria, which allows for very specific (>95%) and sensitive (>95%) differential diagnosis. Figure 5.28 shows the steps for applying this algorithm and how to measure the RS interval (AB interval, see figure). However, its application is not easy for the emergency physician or the clinical cardiologist, because it is necessary to make an effort to learn how to use this algorithm step by step.

    The algorithm described by Brugada (1991) is not useful in the case of reentrant bundle branch VT (Figure 5.27) **or for differentiating VT from wide QRS complex SVT in WPW syndrome (antidromic tachycardia)** (Figure 5.26). In the latter case, Steurer's sequential approach (Steurer *et al.*, 1994) is sensitive enough and particularly specific. According to the author, the following features are suggestive of VT: (i) negative QRS complex in leads V4–V6, (ii) QR pattern in one of leads V2–V6, (iii) confirmation of AV dissociation (see Chapter 1); (iv) ÂQRS complex < −60° and > +150°. Figure 5.26 shows an example of antidromic SVT with an accessory AV pathway, which does not meet any of these criteria.

    A **new algorithm has been described** (Vereckei *et al.*, 2008), based fundamentally on the **information obtained from the aVR lead**, which features a slightly higher statistical potential. However, it is not valid for tachycardias with aberrant conduction involving an accessory pathway or for reentrant bundle branch VT. According to this algorithm the morphologies of aVR suggestive of aberrancy are usually QS-type complexes with a rapid inscription in the first portion of the QRS complex, which sometimes show an initial "r" ⋎, ⋎, ⋏. The remaining morphologies suggest VT, in particular the morphologies with or without initial R that presents a slow inscription during the first 40 ms of the QRS ⋏, ⋏, ⋎, ⋏, ⋎, ⋎ (Table 5.5).

- **Verify whether the morphologies are consistent with aberrant conduction**

This has already been discussed (Table 5.5). This approach leads to a very high PPV, similar to that obtained through Brugada's algorithm. Because this approach is actually the fourth step of Brugada's algorithm, we think that the most practical method to make this differential diagnosis is to carefully follow this algorithm step by step, incorporating the ECG pattern of VR in the fourth step.

    Figure 5.25 shows a typical example of wide QRS tachycardia due to aberrant conduction. The diagnosis is supported by a comparison between the QRS morphologies of a previous ECG in sinus rhythm, and the QRS morphology of wide QRS tachycardia, which does not meet the abovementioned criteria.

    On the other hand, if we look at Figures **5.21**–5.23 in light of what we have described previously (including Brugada's sequential algorithm), we might quickly discover why these tachycardias are ventricular. If we look at Figure 5.29, we will also understand why it is VT and not SVT with aberrant conduction.

    However, it should be pointed out that the **bundle branch reentrant VT** (Figure 5.27) generally shows a left bundle branch block morphology often with a **QS pattern in V1 that makes the differential diagnosis of SVT with aberrant conduction more difficult.** Sometimes the evidence of **AV dissociation,** if it is present, allows us to reach the correct diagnosis. Surface ECG recordings at high velocity may help in recognizing the "hidden P-waves" (Figure **5.21**).

- **The presence of characteristic ECG pattern in some leads**

There are some ECG criteria that favor VT in cases of broad QRS tachycardia; these have already been discussed (see Electrocardiographic Findings). They include: (i) presence of QR morphology, (ii) presence of R wave peak time at lead II greater than 50 ms, and (iii) concordance of the QRS complex pattern in precordial leads.

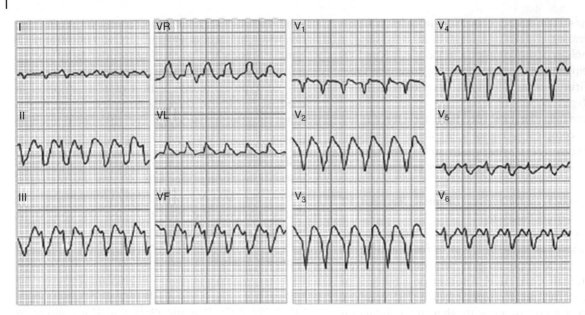

Figure 5.29 Taken from a patient during the subacute phase of a myocardial infarction who showed wide QRS tachycardias at 190 x'. The QRS wideness (0.16 s), the slow inscription of the S wave in V5 (time between the start of R wave to the end of S wave ≥100 ms; second Brugada criterion), and the global QRS morphology (QS or rS from V1 to V6, and slurred R in VR) with an ÂQRS of −90° (fourth Brugada criterion), indicate that this is certainly a ventricular tachycardia (VT), according to the electrocardiographic criteria that have been described beforehand (Figure 5.28 and Table 5.5). In addition, we know that this tachycardia occurs during the subacute phase of a myocardial infarction.

A careful review of surface ECG criteria using the sequential algorithm approach along with the clinical data already discussed may lead to a differential diagnosis between VT and supraventricular tachyarrythmias with aberrant conduction. The diagnosis of bundle branch reentrant VT is certainly challenging.

If a differential diagnosis is not possible, EPS may be performed. However, **when a patient's clinical situation is serious, it is important to rapidly address the problem by performing electrical cardioversion.**

- **In cases of diagnostic uncertainty, which rarely occurs following this approach, invasive electrophysiologic study (EPS) should be carried out** at a reference center in order to make a definitive diagnosis and a better evaluation of the patient.

Prognostic Implications

- **Ventricular tachycardias in heart disease patients**
  In general, classical sustained VT is observed in patients with significant heart diseases, especially post-infarction, in HF and inherited cardiomyopathies. Polymorphic VT more frequently triggers VF in patients with channelopathies. The risk markers for SD (VT/VF) in all these situations are discussed in Chapters 9–11).

  In post-infarction patients, sustained VT is associated with a worse prognosis, especially in the following situations (Wellens, 2001): (i) when it occurs during the first months after MI; (ii) when it is associated with syncope or significant hemodynamic symptoms; and (iii) if there is a history of previous MI. In all these cases, the presence of HF results in a worse prognosis.

  In Chapter 11, we will explain why in large MI patients with the same number of PVC, only those patients who present scars with specific characteristics (fibrosis, more fragmented electrograms, etc.) (Haqqani *et al.*, 2009) present more frequently sustained VT. In this case the anatomic substrate characteristics (scars) are more important than the triggering factor (PVC) in terms of inducing sustained VT.

  It has also been demonstrated (Pascale *et al.*, 2009) that **if MI occurs in the inferior wall, there is an increased risk of VT**. This occurs because the inferior wall is an area with a high density of receptors with vagal activity and after MI there is a lowered protective effect of these vagal responses.

- **Ventricular tachycardia in subjects with no apparent heart disease**
  Sustained VT in subjects with no evidence of heart disease seem to have a better prognosis. They usually present a QRS complex between 0.12 and 0.14 s. Table 5.3 describes the most important characteristics of the three essential types of VT reported in subjects without evidence of heart disease. **Idiopathic VT may be triggered by exercise (adenosine and**

propranolol-sensitive tachycardias) and may also be terminated when during the exercise the sinus heart rate exceeds the VT rate (verapamil-sensitive). The most frequent are those rising from the RVOT (adenosine-sensitive tachycardias) presenting a LBBB morphology. Some occur in repetitive runs (Figure 5.17).

Even though most of these tachycardias have a good prognosis, VT with an LBBB morphology that originate in the RV have occasionally evolved into Torsades de Pointes VT and ARVC VT should always be ruled out (O'Donnell *et al.*, 2003). In ARVC VT, contrary to what is observed in VT with no evidence of heart disease, a left axis deviation of ÂQRS is usually reported (see Figure 9.7B). However, evidence of right ÂQRS axis deviation is also seen in the presence of ARVC (Table 5.4). Furthermore, the use of isotopic techniques has demonstrated an abnormal I-metayodobenzylguanidin (I-MBG) intake, indicative of sympathetic denervation areas, meaning cardiac impairment. The importance of ruling out ARVC VT relies on two factors: (i) this is a progressive disease and may evolve into forms of right or biventricular failure, and (ii) if ablation is consider to control for VT, new techniques of *"dechanneling"* need to be considered (Berruezo *et al.*, 2012).

Treatment

In the presence of broad regular QRS tachycardia, the most important factor for treatment, if the clinical situation of the patient is acceptable, is to perform a good differential diagnosis that includes: (i) VT, (ii) SVT with aberrancy due to BBB (Figure 5.25), (iii) supraventricular antidromic reentrant tachycardia of WPW syndrome (Figures 4.22 and 5.26), (iv) atrial flutter with 2:1, or 1:1 AV conduction with BBB or pre-excitation (see Figures 4.65 and 4.66), and (v) mediated pacemaker tachycardia (see Figure 6.45). The best way to make this differential diagnosis has already been discussed (see Differential Diagnosis of Wide QRS Complex Tachycardias). However, **in cases of hemodynamic compromise it is recommended to proceed immediately to electrical cardioversion (CV).** The correct diagnosis can be made later on. We will now discuss the management of patients with different types of sustained VT.

Ventricular Tachycardia in Heart Disease Patients

- **Drug treatment/electrical CV**
  Lidocaine or procainamide (Gorgels *et al.*, 1996) may be administered to treat VT episodes in stable heart disease patients (Class II a B). Lidocaine is used particularly in the acute phase of IHD (Class II b C) (Table A-11). Beta-blockers and calcium antagonists are contraindicated. However, **electrical CV is the best treatment option in hemodynamically compromised**

patients **(Class IC)**. In cases of VT refractory to electrical CV, intravenous amiodarone (Class II a C) or high-rate pacing (Class II a C) may be considered. To prevent crises of VT, amiodarone may be administered (see Appendix A-5). For more detailed information consult guidelines (Recommended General Bibliography p. xvii).

- **Other treatments**
a) **The implantation of an automatic ICD** as a secondary prevention is necessary in heart disease patients recovering from cardiac arrest due to sustained VT/VF. In the case of previous sustained VT without cardiac arrest, the VT characteristics (duration, hemodynamic tolerance, heart rate) may constitute key parameters when deciding whether an ICD should be implanted (see Table A-5). It is also necessary to consider the great advantages but also the infrequent but possible dangerous side effects of ICD therapy (see Appendix A-4, Automatic Implantable Cardioverter Defibrillator (ICD)) (Connolly *et al.*, 2000).
  - o **After acute MI** with VT/VF in the acute phase, it is recommended to wait several months before deciding if an ICD implant is necessary. This recommendation is discussed in Chapter 11, Ischemic Heart Disease, and Appendix A-4.3, Automatic Implantable Cardioverter Defibrillator (ICD).
  - o **In the presence of HF** with sustained VT and criteria for ICD therapy, the presence of wide QRS complexes with evidence of ventricular dissynchrony, recommend the associated implantation of cardiac resynchronization pacemaker therapy (CRT) coupled with the ICD (ICD-CRT) (see Figure A-15).
  - o Recommendations for ICD therapy in patients with different types of inherited heart diseases and antecedents of VT/VF are discussed in Chapter 9.
b) **Ablation of VT in heart disease patients is currently more feasible (Figure 5.30), especially in cases of endocardial substrate** (i.e., in IHD), if an appropriate protocol is followed and the corresponding algorithms are applied (Miller *et al.*, 1988; Miller and Scherschel, 2009). Ablation of ischemic VT became a more frequent practice after large studies demonstrating feasibility, safety and positive impact on mortality (SMASH VT, VANISH). New techniques that allow for intramyocardial ablation are being developed (Sapp *et al.*, 2013, 2016).
  - o Currently, good results (70% success rate) and few severe complications (<3%), mostly without death, have been obtained following the appropriate protocols in cases of VT of **subepicardial origin, as well as in cases of VT of nonischemic origin** (Cano *et al.*, 2009). Sophisticated techniques are now available to perform ablation of

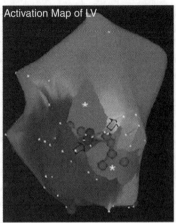

Activation Map of LV

Figure 5.30 Ablation of chronic post-myocardial infarction (MI) ventricular tachycardia (VT). The figure shows the activation map of the left ventricle (LV). The zones marked with asterisks (*) represents scars from old MI. We can see (arrow) that a zone exists with viable myocardium, which explains the start of the reentrant circuit. Ablation in this zone stops the ventricular fibrillation (VF).

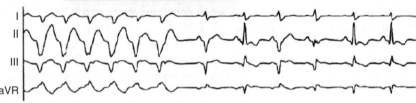

VT rising from the epicardium through a direct epicardium access (Tomassoni *et al.*, 1999). Currently, ablation of epicardial VT through non-surgical procedures is effective; however, it requires a previous coronarography to avoid coronary artery lesions (D'Avila, 2008). Also, an ablation approach performing lines joining different scars has been used successfully (see Appendix A-4, Percutaneous Transcatheter Ablation).

- o **Bundle branch** VT is also easy to treat with ablation of the right bundle branch. This results in circuit interruption and has excellent long-term results (Balasundaram *et al.*, 2008).

c) In each case, the best therapeutic approach depends on the VT characteristics, the patient's clinical situation, and the previous experience of the hospital staff.

Ventricular Tachycardias in Subjects with No Apparent Heart Disease

- • **Drug treatment/electrical CV**
  - o In patients with no apparent heart disease, the well-tolerated sustained VT may be treated with amiodarone and/or β-blockers, especially in cases of RVOT exercise-induced VT. If sustained VT persists, electrical CV is necessary.
  - o To prevent new episodes in these subjects, amiodarone and/or β blockers may be administered.
- • **Ablation**
  - o The introduction of ablation techniques has been a major step forward in the treatment of this type of VT. **Currently, it is the recommended technique in**

most of these cases (Class I C), especially if repetitive episodes are observed or there are significant risk factors for bad prognosis (Klein *et al.*, 1992) (Figure 5.31).

- o Currently, in subjects with no apparent heart disease, ablation techniques may be performed in the majority of cases of sustained VT. However, in order to obtain the best results it is important to determine if the site of origin is endocardial or epicardial. Even the micro-reentry circuit can be ablated by targeting the sites of earliest ventricular activation (Mittal, 2008). The success rate is very high (>80%) and the incidence of severe complications is small, with no procedure-related deaths in many series. Noncontact mapping techniques such as "balloon array" are now available offering the possibility of focal ablations with high success and minor complications rates.
- o However, some authors consider that the incidence of VT recurrence is higher (20% to even 50%) during long-term follow-up. In two-thirds of cases recurrent VT show a different morphology (Ventura *et al.*, 2007). Therefore, a second ablation may be necessary (see Appendix A-4). New available software allows determining the pressure of the tip of the catheter on the endocardial surface, allowing the ablator to determine whether contact will serve the purpose of the ablation. Better interface between the catheter and the endocardial surface results in better long-term results.
- o Surface electrocardiography (Table 5.4 and Figure 5.15) is clearly useful for finding the site of origin of

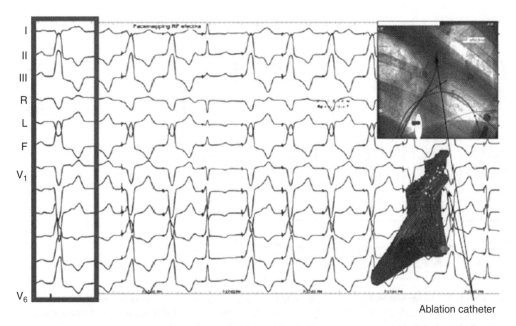

Ablation catheter

Figure 5.31 Ablation of idiopathic right ventricular outflow tract (RVOT) ventricular tachycardia (VT) (Figures 5.15, 5.17, and 5.18). Left: See the surface electrocardiogram (ECG) with left bundle branch block (LBBB) pattern and right ÂQRS. Right above: Position of catheters with the point of effective ablation located below the pulmonary valve. Right below: Reconstruction of the right ventricle (RV) with CARTO may be seen. The ablation catheter is located in the origin of the VT, where the radiofrequency energy stops the VT (see Classical ventricular tachycardia (QRS ≥ 0.12 s): Treatment).

idiopathic VT and for determining the site at which the ablation should be performed. However, it is necessary to perform an electrophysiologic study to confirm the origin of VT. Occasionally, ablation of the right outflow tract for ventricular tachycardia is not successful because the focus of VT is located within the pulmonary artery (Tada *et al.*, 2008). On occasion (i.e., VT originating near the aortic valve leaflets) (see Figure 5.15B), an angiography controlled ablation should be performed to avoid damage of the coronary tree. The same occurs in VT of epicardial origin.

- **ICD therapy**

  o In cases of recurrent VT despite optimal treatment, including VT ablation, ICD therapy may be indicated (Class II a C) (see Appendix A-4.3, Automatic Implantable Cardioverter Defibrillator (ICD))

  For further information regarding the management of patients with sustained VT, please refer to the recommended references and the scientific society guidelines (Recommended General Bibliography p. xvii).

Other Monomorphic Ventricular Tachycardias

Narrow QRS Complex Ventricular Tachycardias (Fascicular Tachycardias) (Hayes et al., 1991; Hanllan and Scheinman, 1996) (Figure 5.32)

Narrow QRS complex VT are infrequent. They represent less than 5% of all VT cases.

Ventricular tachycardias, characterized by a relatively narrow QRS complex (<0.12 s), originate close to the high septum or the fascicular areas (right bundle branch, left bundle branch trunk, or their two divisions). The electrical impulse starting in the site of origin, usually by a reentry mechanism, rapidly spreads through the His–Purkinje system. Narrow QRS complex VT show partial LBBB morphology, if originated in the right bundle branch, and partial RBBB, if originated in the left bundle branch, with evidence of right or left ÂQRS deviation depending on the site of origin (left superior and anterior division or inferior and posterior division, respectively). The cases of VT with partial RBBB patterns plus evidence of left ÂQRS extreme (much more often) deviation are verapamil-sensitive. These VT may have practically the same morphology, but with the QRS complex ≥0.12 s (see Classical VT: Electrocardiographic Findings and Figure 5.16).

In cases of VT with narrow QRS, it is sometimes difficult to make a differential diagnosis with SVT or atrial flutter with aberrancy when only using a surface ECG. The presence of capture and fusion complexes, and the evidence of AV dissociation, are suggestive of a tachycardia of ventricular origin (Figure 5.32). However, sometimes intracavitary electrocardiography is often necessary to reach the correct differential diagnosis.

From a therapeutic point of view, the most reasonable and wise option is to treat narrow QRS VT as a classical wide QRS sustained VT.

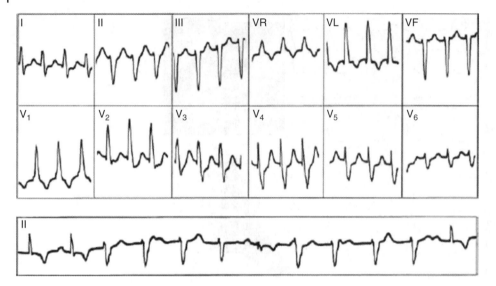

Figure 5.32 The QRS of the tachycardia lasts 110 ms and features a right bundle block and superoanterior hemiblock (RBBB + SAH) morphology. However, the exclusive R wave in V1, and, above all, the presence of captures and fusions (bottom tracing), indicate that this is a narrow fascicular ventricular tachycardia (VT) arising from a zone close to the inferoposterior division.

Idioventricular Accelerated Rhythm (IVAR)
(Figures 5.33 and 5.34)

- **Concept and mechanism**

  This is a ventricular rhythm originating in an automatic ectopic focus with a slightly decreased discharge rate (≈80–100 bpm). Unless heart rate is more than 100 bpm, we should not speak of true VT. Nevertheless, between 80 and 100 bpm is a borderline case. The occurrence of an idioventricular accelerated rhythm during reperfusion is particularly due to increased automatism in the His–Purkinje system. The ectopic focus is visible only when the sinus heart rate has a rate below its discharge rate. This explains the frequent fusion beats that appear, especially at the onset and at the end of the runs. In fact, some cases of suspected slow parasystolic VT correspond to IVAR (see later) (Pèrez-Riera *et al.*, 2010).

- **ECG findings**

  The IVAR appears as an escape but accelerated ventricular rhythm, when the sinus rhythm slows down its rate. Because of this, fusion beats are very frequent (see before) (Figure 5.33).

  - The impulse that initiates the IVAR features a long coupling interval, which is similar to baseline RR interval. Therefore, there are no different coupling intervals of the first PVC of the VT runs, as happens in runs of true parasystolic VT.

  - The IVAR usually shows the same ventricular discharge rate. However occasionally, it may vary in different episodes. Thus, the same focus may, in rare cases, present as a true VT, and in these cases, a treatment similar to that applied to classical sustained monomorphic VT may be necessary.

- **Prognosis and treatment**

  IVAR is a relatively frequent ventricular rhythm occurring in the acute phase of MI, especially during fibrinolytic therapy (Figure 5.34). It may also be seen in other heart diseases, even in young people without evidence of heart disease. In these cases, it is usually sporadic due to some triggering factor (stimulants, surgery, alcohol, etc.). It is usually terminated when the clinical condition of the patient improves or the triggering factor disappears. In the past, it has been considered a "reperfusion rhythm". If it is not well tolerated, amiodarone or β-blockers may be prescribed. If the rate accelerates, it has to be considered as a classical VT.

Repeated Nonsustained Monomorphic Ventricular Tachycardia

Short and infrequent runs of classical monomorphic VT (QRS complex ≥0.12 s) are included in Lown's classification as a type of repetitive PVC (type 4) (Figure 5.3). They have been studied together with isolated PVC (see Premature Ventricular Complexes: Concept and

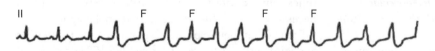

Figure 5.33 Example of a fusion complex. Different fusion degrees (F) in the presence of an accelerated idioventricular rhythm (about 100 bpm).

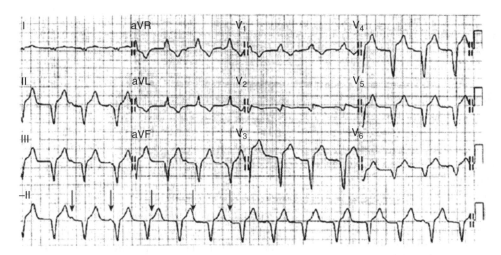

Figure 5.34 Example of an accelerated idioventricular rhythm (90 bpm) in a patient with ST elevation myocardial infarction (STEMI) after fibrinolytic treatment. Arrows show P waves.

Mechanisms). We have already stated that their presence is usually associated with a worse prognosis, both in post-infarction patients and in patients with dilated or hypertrophic hearts. The therapeutic approach in asymptomatic subjects should include the suppression of toxic substances, if these are being administered. Beta-blockers should be given when the number of PVC and runs of VT increase with exercise. Amiodarone and β-blockers constitute the best therapeutic options in post-infarction patients.

In this section, we include frequent VT runs and, in particular, the incessant types (repeated nonsustained VT) (Figure 5.4). These VT tachycardias may cause significant hemodynamic compromise (tachy myocardiopathy),

particularly when the ventricular rate is high. Furthermore, this type of VT may result in sustained VT, which may trigger VF. In order to determine the best treatment option, repeated nonsustained VT should be considered as sustained VT rather than PVC with infrequent VT runs.

Parasystolic Ventricular Tachycardia (Chung et al., 1965; Touboul et al., 1970; Roelandt and Schamroth, 1971) *(Figure 5.35)*

- **Concept and mechanism**

  Parasystolic VT are very infrequent arrhythmias that originate in an automatic focus protected from

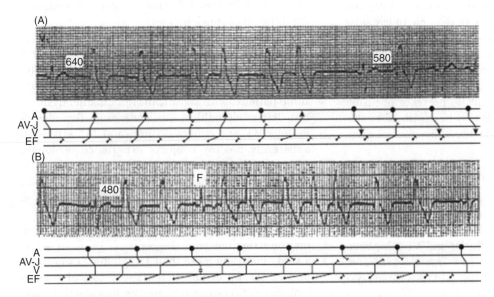

Figure 5.35 (A) and (B) Two strips from a patient with irregular runs of ventricular tachycardia (VT) of parasystolic origin. The electrocardiogram (ECG) characteristics of parasystolic VT may be seen: (i) different coupling intervals of the first premature ventricular complex (PVC) of each run, (ii) the presence of fusion complexes, and (iii) the possible explanation of irregular rhythm due to different grades of exit block of the parasystolic ectopic focus (adapted from Koulizakis *et al.*, 1990).

depolarization by a normal impulse (entrance block). The intrinsic discharge rate is probably high and regular, but also protected with an exit block, due to rate-related refractoriness (Scherf and Bornemann, 1961) or as a consequence of fixed or different degrees of abnormal Phase 4 depolarization of the parasystolic focus (Massumi *et al.*, 1986; Ogawa *et al.*, 1981). Therefore, parasystolic VT usually appears as short runs of VT of ventricular rate <150 bpm and often with an irregular ventricular rate. This is because, in the same ECG recording, the exit block from parasystolic focus transiently appears and disappears suddenly or with progressive degrees of block (Wenckebach-type), resulting in a rate that transiently doubles or splits, or presents some irregularities (sometimes appear as a bigeminal rhythm) with respect to the basal rhythm.

Parasystolic VT usually occur as short runs with special ECG characteristics (see below). As just stated, some reported cases probably correspond to IVAR originating in a ventricular ectopic focus with increased automaticity as a parasystolic focus, but without all other required ECG characteristics of parasystolic VT.

- **ECG findings**
  The following ECG findings are suggestive of typical VT of parasystolic origin: the PVC, which initiate the VT runs, show a variable coupling interval and the runs of VT meet all criteria of parasystole (see PVC: ECG Diagnosis).

  Although the discharge rate of parasystolic VT is relatively fixed, as stated before, different degrees of exit block may explain the presence of irregular RR intervals, as may the presence of fusion and capture complexes. Figure 5.35 shows an example of irregular VT runs due to parasystolic ectopic focus at 140 bpm with different degrees of exit block that explain the irregularity of ventricular rates. This case meets the criteria of parasystolic VT runs: (i) different coupling intervals of the first PVC and (ii) presence of fusion beats. Irregular RR intervals may be explained by different grades of exit block (Figure 5.35).

- **Prognosis and treatment**
  Parasystolic VT prognosis is usually good, due to slow heart rate and the extremely infrequent presence of sustained VT. Parasystolic VT may even disappear over time, because, generally, the exit block becomes more fixed. However, exceptional cases of parasystolic PVC triggering ventricular flutter and VF have been described (Itoh *et al.*, 1996) (see Figure 5.43B) and, theoretically, the same may happen in runs of parasystolic VT.

  The treatment is similar to VT of extrasystolic origin. It depends on the clinical setting, the rate, and

duration of VT. Theoretically, β-blockers may be useful to decrease abnormal automaticity. There is not too much evidence regarding other types of treatment; however, in some cases, verapamil has been given (Massumi *et al.*, 1986). The best approach is to treat as a case of extrasystolic VT.

Polymorphic Ventricular Tachycardia
(Table 5.2)

The QRS of the VT presents polymorphic morphology (see Table 5.2). We will comment on the most characteristics.

- *Torsades de pointes ventricular tachycardia* There are two types: the classical (Dessertene, 1966; Horowitz *et al.*, 1981) and the familiar (Leenhardt *et al.*, 1994) (see p. 332).

Classical Torsades de Pointes Ventricular Tachycardia
This is the most typical and interesting type due to its prognostic and therapeutic implications.

- **Mechanism**
  It was believed to be caused by triggered activity; however, recent publications suggest that Torsades de Pointes VT may be induced by a rotor that produces a spiral wave, which "meanders" in a repetitive fashion (Figure 3.13B).

  The characteristic Torsades de Pointes morphology may be related to a counterclockwise rotation of the wave front along the whole ventricular cavity. Also, it has been demonstrated that global or transmural dispersion of repolarization induces the occurrence of Torsades de Pointes VT. This is especially evident in the different channelopathies.

  Thus, certain degrees of repolarization dispersion may cause Torsades de Pointes VT. However, it is not known what degree of dispersion and ionic channel dysfunction are needed to explain: (i) why some patients with significant ion channel dysfunction (channelopathies) easily develop Torsades de Pointes VT and others do not, and (ii) why some apparently healthy subjects experience prolonged QT intervals that trigger this type of VT after taking specific drugs (see Tables 10.1 and 10.2). Undetermined predisposed genetic factors most likely exist.

  It is well known that Type I antiarrhythmic agents may be arrhythmogenic (Bigger *et al.*. 1984). In fact, in a study including more than 150 Holter ECG recordings of SD, we demonstrated about 15% of cases of ambulatory SD usually triggered by Torsades de Pointes VT. These occurred in patients without severe heart disease, to whom antiarrhythmic agents (generally, type I, such as quinidine, etc.) had been administered to treat the concurrent usually asymptomatic, although frequent, PVC (Bayés de Luna *et al.*, 1989). Because this is a well-known fact, current incidence should be lower. In Chapter 10 (Acquired Long QT), we mention the pharmaceutical agents that most frequently have been associated with Torsades de Pointes VT (see Table 10.2). Furthermore, Table 10.1 shows many predisposing factors that induce a prolonged QT interval and, possibly, trigger Torsades de Pointes VT (for further information see www.qtdrugs.org).

- **Clinical presentation**

Torsades de Pointes VT often precede the development of VF and SD. Patients frequently present dizziness and often syncopal attacks. In its presence we have to urgently take the most appropriate therapeutic measures (see below).

Torsades de Pointes VF episodes may be triggered in patients with bradyarrhythmias (sick sinus syndrome and AV block), that present a very long QT interval, probably due to genetic predisposition (Chevalier *et al.*, 2007).

- **Electrocardiographic findings** (Figures 1.6, 5.36, and 5.37)

Torsades de Pointes VT occur in runs of variable duration (from a few beats to ≥100 beats). The QRS is characteristically not monomorphic, and cyclical changes characterized by a pattern of twisting points (Dessertene, 1966) are observed. However, this characteristic twisting morphology may not be evident in all ECG leads. The baseline ECG presents a long QT interval and the first QRS of the VT has a long coupling interval, but, due to long QT, the PVC usually fall close to the peak of the T (or T+U) wave. Figure 5.37 shows the differences between a classical sustained VT and a Torsades de Pointes VT.

The most important **premonitory ECG signs** of a Torsades de Pointes VF episode are: (i) QTc interval >500 ms, (ii) T-U wave distortion that becomes more apparent in the QRS-T after one pause, (iii) visible macroscopic T wave alternans, and (iv) the presence of evident bradyarrhythmia (sick sinus syndrome or AV block). It is probable that all these ECG signs induce Torsades de Pointes VF due to genetic predisposition, especially in the presence of ionic imbalance and/or the administration of some drugs (Chevalier *et al.*, 2007; Drew *et al.*, 2010).

- **Treatment**

The treatment of classical Torsades de Pointes VT should be considered an emergency treatment, as VF may be triggered at any time.

It is very important to bear in mind that the treatment is **completely different from that administered for runs of monomorphic VT.** First, any drug that has likely induced lengthening of the QT interval should be discontinued, as well as any electrolytic imbalances or other type of anomaly, which may contribute to such lengthening (Class I A).

Cardiac stimulation (pacing) should be performed to speed up the heart rate if it is slow. The most common reason for failing to treat Torsades de Pointes is setting the pacemaker rate below the intrinsic sinus heart rate (Yazdan-Ashoori *et al.*, 2012). Isoproterenol may be administered, especially to patients without the long QT syndrome, but with recurrent pause-dependent Torsades de Pointes episodes (Class II B).

Figure 5.36 A run from a typical Torsades de Pointes ventricular tachycardia (VT). Taken from a patient with long QT syndrome. Note the typical pattern that is particularly evident in some leads (III, VF, and VL).

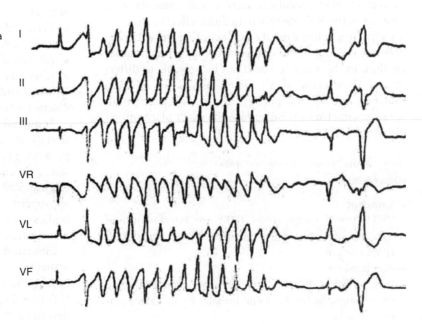

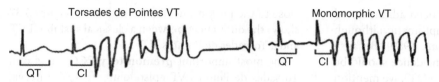

Figure 5.37 Characteristic morphologies of a run of a Torsades de Pointes ventricular tachycardia (VT) and of a classic monomorphic VT. CI: coupling interval.

> Classical Torsades de Pointes polymorphic VT may lead to VF and SD. It is associated with inherited heart diseases such as long QT syndrome, as well as acquired long QT syndrome, which occurs in special circumstances (see Figures 10.17 and Tables 10.1 and 10.2) and/or after administration of certain drugs.

○ Atropine may sometimes be prescribed.
○ Intravenous magnesium sulfate may be administered to patients with long QT syndrome (Class II a B).
○ Finally, it has been demonstrated (Antoons *et al.*, 2010) that ranolazine may be efficient antiarrhythmic agents against drug-induced Torsades de Pointes in experimental models of AV block.

Pleomorphism

Occasionally, sustained VT may alternate morphologies (pleomorphism) such as RBBB and LBBB (Josephson *et al.*, 1979). These changes may be gradual or abrupt and occur over long or short periods of time. They are usually associated with changes in cycle length. Morphologies are considered to be different when they present different patterns, that is, an advanced RBBB or LBBB, or when the ÂQRS deviation changes ≥45°, even if the bundle branch block pattern is unchanged. These changes in the morphology usually occur after the administration of certain pharmaceutical agents, and coincide with changes in the VT rate (proarrhythmic effect).

Often, in a conventional ECG recording we will probably not see more than one morphology with a regular rhythm. In this case, it would not be possible to differentiate from classical VT. Therefore, if we rely too much on one VT morphology at a certain time point, we may sometimes misdiagnose the exact place of origin of the VT.

Bidirectional ventricular tachycardia
(Figure 5.38)

- **Concept**
  Bidirectional tachycardias (BT) are infrequent and may be of supraventricular (BSVT) or ventricular (BVT) origin.
- **Mechanism**
  It is probably delayed after depolarization related to excess digitalis intake, ionic imbalance, or catecholamine levels.

- **ECG findings**
  From an electrocardiographic point of view (Richter and Brugada, 2009), the frontal plane axis (ÂQRS) shows alternative changes of up to approximately 180°, and the RR intervals are usually equal but sometimes present a bigeminal-like pattern (long–short–long).
- **Differential diagnosis**
  The fact that the alternans wide QRS morphology is compatible with an alternating bifascicular block is very suggestive of supraventricular origin (Rosenbaum *et al.*, 1969). In contrast, evidence of AV dissociation supports a diagnosis of ventricular origin (BVT).

  Differential diagnosis of BT also has to be performed with changes of QRS morphology of 2:1 type that may be seen in patients usually with slightly sinus tachycardia (100–130 bpm) (also in cases of AVRT, see Figure 4.18C) and this may lead to a misdiagnosis of slow bidirectional tachycardias. These include all typical cases of **QRS alternans** (see Table 7.1 and Figure 7.5):

  ○ The QRS alternans in AVRT (see Figure 4.18C).
  ○ The cyclical changes in the QRS complex voltage in sinus rhythm as observed in cardiac tamponade (see Figure 7.5).
  ○ Other cases in sinus rhythm that present alternatively (2:1) different QRS morphology (**pseudo alternans**), such as:
    ▪ Ventricular bigeminy with late extrasystoles (in the PR interval).
    ▪ Alternating pre-excitation in WPW syndrome.
    ▪ Alternans bundle branch block QRS complexes (2:1).
- **Clinical and therapeutic implications**
  There are two types of BVT: acquired and inherited.

  Acquired causes. These include digitalis intoxication (Smith *et al.*, 1976), hypokalemia, herbal aconite poisoning (Tai *et al.*, 1992), acute MI, and psychologic stress (Recommended General Bibliography p. xvii) (Figure 5.38). In cases of digitalis intoxication, the appropriate treatment with digoxine-specific antibodies should be administered. However, digitalis intoxication is currently much less frequent.

  Inherited causes. Bidirectional VT is part of an arrhythmia cascade occurring with exercise and preceding the onset of catecholaminergic polymorphic VT (see Figure 9.23). Some cases have also been described in inherited cardiomyopathies (HC, ARVC,

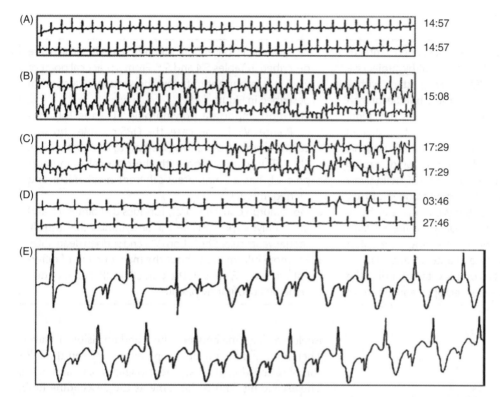

Figure 5.38 (A) Sinus rhythm at rest, with some isolated premature ventricular complexes (PVC). (B) Occurrence of a bi-directional ventricular tachycardia (VT) during psychologic stress testing (bottom, E, at normal speed). (C) Appearance of frequent, polymorphic, and repetitive PVC after the testing. (D) Slower sinus rhythm during sleep, with some isolated PVC. (E) Enlargement of the bi-directional tachycardia.

and Anderson-Tawil syndrome-LQT Type 8) (Bökenkamp *et al.*, 2007) (see Chapter 9).

Catecholaminergic Polymorphic Ventricular Tachycardia
(Leenhardt et al., 1995) (Figure 9.23)

Catecholaminergic polymorphic VT is an infrequent form of polymorphic VT, particularly occurring in young patients with a structurally normal heart. It is usually triggered by exercise; studies have pointed out a genetic origin (Priori *et al.*, 2001).

They may be associated with different active and passive arrhythmias (see Chapter 9, Catecholaminergic Polymorphic Ventricular Tachycardia). As already stated, they are preceded by different exerciseinduced ventricular and supraventricular arrhythmias, usually including bidirectional VT.

In these cases, it might be necessary to implant an ICD because catecholaminergic polymorphic VT may lead to VT/VF (for further details, see Chapter 9, Catecholaminergic Polymorphic Ventricular Tachycardia).

Other Types of Polymorphic Ventricular Tachycardias

Some polymorphic VT may present irregular cadence and different QRS morphologies that usually do not present the typical morphology pattern of Torsades de Pointes. However, in the presence of acute ischemia or in some channelopathies, it may degenerate into VF and SD (Chapters 9 and 11).

In these cases electrical CV should be performed immediately, especially if the patient is unstable (Class I b). In cases of acute ischemia, coronariography should be performed urgently. Beta-blockers (Class I B) or intravenous amiodarone (Class I C) should be given in cases of repetitive episodes and/or to prevent new ones.

Additionally, different morphologies and irregular rhythms are usually observed in patients with sustained VT in the following instances: (i) at the onset of a sustained VT, (ii) when the morphology and heart rate is variable and irregular in the presence of frequent capture and fusion beats, and (iii) when a sustained VT becomes a ventricular flutter. An irregular heart rate after the onset of VT is usually seen in patients taking antiarrhythmic agents.

All cases of polymorphic VT not meeting the criteria for a Torsades de Pointes VT should be treated as classical sustained VT.

Ventricular Tachycardia

- The following are the most frequent sustained ventricular tachycardia (VT) morphologies in healthy subjects: a right bundle branch block (RBBB)-like pattern with a generally left axis deviation and a left bundle branch block (LBBB)-like pattern with variable axis deviation, although usually right (Figures 5.16 and 5.17). Sustained VT usually have a good prognosis, but arrhythmogenic right ventricular cardiomyopathy (ARVC) should be ruled out. An appropriate treatment to prevent definitively further episodes is ablation of the arrhythmogenic focus.

- Classical VT in heart disease patients is a severe arrhythmia. Patients with sustained VT usually require implantable cardioverter defibrillator (ICD) therapy, especially if the ejection fraction is low (see Chapters 9 and 11).

- In the case of wide QRS complex tachycardia, the differential diagnosis between ectopic and aberrant tachycardia is based on different criteria, which are described in Tables 5.4 and 5.5. From a practical point of view, it is important to follow the sequential algorithm described in Figure 5.28.

- The most important polymorphic VT is the Torsades de Pointes VT. In this case, the QRS complex tip successively goes from a low position to a high position. This VT, in comparison with the classical monomorphic VT, has a completely different mechanism and management.

- Monomorphic sustained VT, Torsades de Pointes VT, and other polymorphic VT are the arrhythmias that usually trigger ventricular fibrillation (VF) and sudden death (SD).

- For more information about the management of different types of VF, consult the guidelines (Recommended General Bibliography p. xvii).

Ventricular Flutter

Concept and Mechanism

Ventricular rate is very fast (around 300 bpm) and regular. It is triggered by a PVC that is usually extrasystolic (Figures 5.39 and 5.40) (exceptionally parasystolic, see Figure 5.43) and maintained by a reentry circuit large enough to generate waves, which may trigger very fast yet organized QRS complexes that feature a morphologic pattern. Ventricular flutter is a very fast VT in which the isoelectric space between the QRS complexes is barely observed. Usually, a very quick ventricular flutter triggers VF.

Electrocardiogram

Ventricular flutter is characterized by the presence of QRS complexes of the same morphology and voltage, with no isoelectric baseline between them and no visible T waves. Therefore, there is no clear separation between the QRS complex and the ST-T segment (Figures 5.39 and 5.40). The ascending limb is the same as the descending limb. For this reason, the ECG looks similar when viewed upside down. The ventricular rate is usually 250–300 bpm.

Frequently, it appears that after a few complexes of fast VT, they become ventricular flutter complexes.

Occasionally, some VT show a QRS complex without an evident repolarization wave, at least in some derivations. However, the ventricular rate does not reach 250 bpm.

Nevertheless, there are borderline situations between VT and ventricular flutter, and ventricular flutter and fibrillation, as in the case of atrial fibrillation and atrial flutter.

Ventricular flutter may sometimes be confused with atrial flutter 1×1 with pre-excitation or with bundle branch block aberrancy (Figure 4.65B).

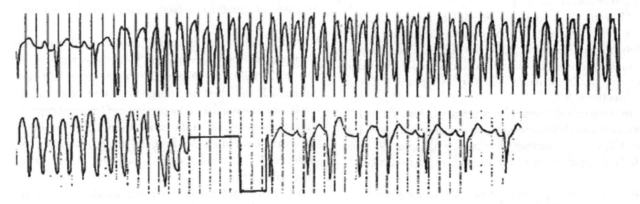

Figure 5.39 Ventricular flutter in a patient with an implantable cardioverter defibrillator (ICD). The discharge from the defibrillator terminates the arrhythmia.

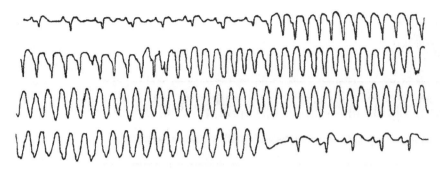

Figure 5.40 A patient with an acute infarction. There are four consecutive strips. A premature ventricular extrasystole triggers a ventricular tachycardia (VT), which, in a short time (third strip), becomes like a ventricular flutter. Fortunately, the arrhythmia was self-limited within a short period.

Prognostic and Therapeutic Implications

Ventricular flutter is a very badly tolerated arrhythmia that usually leads to VF and requires immediate treatment. Except in rare self-limiting cases (Figure 5.40), out of the intensive care unit it results in VF, unless the patient has a defibrillator implanted (Figure 5.39). The therapeutic approach to prevent relapses is the same as for VF (see following section).

Ventricular Fibrillation

Concept

Ventricular fibrillation is a very fast (>300 bpm) and irregular rhythm, with a significant cycle length (RR), morphology, and wave amplitude variability, which does not generate effective mechanical activity and leads to cardiac arrest and death in a short period of time (see

Chapter 6, Cardiac Arrest) unless the patient has an ICD implanted (see Figure A-16) or is resuscitated in a few seconds (Figures 5.42 and 5.44). Exceptional cases of selflimiting VF have been described (Dubner *et al.*, 1983; Castro Arias *et al.*, 2009).

Mechanism

Ventricular fibrillation is triggered by a PVC isolated or repetitive (VT/ventricular flutter) that is usually extrasystolic (Figures 5.42 and 5.44). Exceptional cases of VF triggered by a parasystolic PVC have been published (Figure 5.43). Ventricular fibrillation is maintained as the result of repetitive micro-reentries, a mechanism very similar to the one that causes atrial fibrillation. Although some similarities are observed in terms of how AF and VF are initiated and perpetuated, there are also some differences (Figure 5.45).

It has been suggested (Qu and Garfinkel, 2004) that VF is caused when a spiral wave produced by a rotor becomes

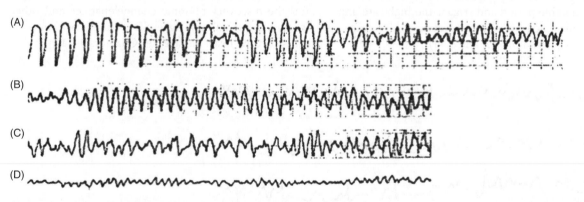

Figure 5.41 (A) Very fast ventricular rhythm of intermediate characteristics between ventricular tachycardia (VT) (it is too fast) and ventricular flutter (typical QRS do not appear in this lead), which quickly turns into ventricular fibrillation (VF). (B), (C) and (D) Different types of VF waves (see text).

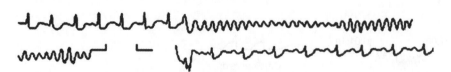

Figure 5.42 Patient with an acute infarction. An isolated premature ventricular complex (PVC) triggers directly a ventricular fibrillation (VF) that ceases after a few seconds (bottom strip) after an electrical cardioversion.

(A)

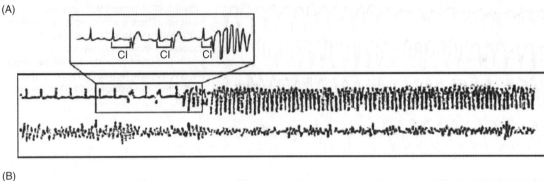

(B)

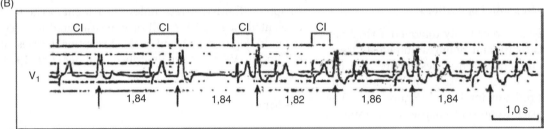

Figure 5.43 (A) Parasystolic premature ventricular complex (PVC) with a premature coupling interval falls on the vulnerable period (T wave) and triggers very quick ventricular flutter/ventricular fibrillation (VF). (B) Frequent PVC of parasystolic characteristics (adapted from Itoh *et al.*, 1996).

unstable, which leads to its singular point displaying a chaotic movement, ultimately breaking up and initiating a VF (see Figure 3.11, and Chapter 3, Reentry).

Ventricular fibrillation may be triggered with or without the presence of acute ischemia when significant heterogeneous dispersion of the repolarization (HDR) of the myocardial fibers exists and one, or more than one, PVC, usually with an R/T phenomenon, fall in the ventricular vulnerable period and trigger the high rate and irregular morphology fibrillatory waves of VF (Adgey *et al.*, 1982) (Figures 1.5, 5.42, and 5.44).

Apart from acute ischemia, VF mainly appears in the presence of HF (see Chapter 11) and inherited heart diseases (see Chapter 9). Ventricular fibrillation may be triggered by isolated PVC, sustained VT or polymorphous VT often of Torsades de Pointes type (Figures 1.4 to 1.6) (Bayés de Luna *et al.*, 1989).

There are still some rare cases of idiopathic VF. However, the number of cases is much lower than some years ago, after the discovery of some channelopathies and other circumstances that may trigger SD in patients without evident structural heart disease (see Chapters 9–11).

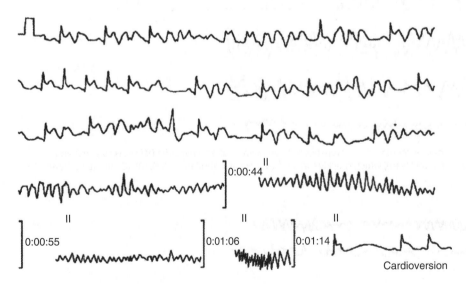

Figure 5.44 A patient with an acute myocardial infarction and frequent, polymorphic, and repetitive PVC, which triggered a ventricular fibrillation (VF) (arrow) that was terminated by cardioversion.

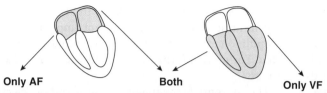

Only AF

1. Mutation of the connexin 40 gene that distorts the conduction.

2. The role of fibrosis in the development of arrhythmias is more relevant.

3. Because the wall is thinner, it is more probably an effective response to sodium channel blockers to terminate the arrhythmia

Both

1. Fibrillation onset by a focal mechanism, spiral (rotors), or micro-reentry

2. Breakage of the excitation wave because of the heterogeneity of refractory periods

3. The possibility of reentries in the ischemic zone is increased.

4. Sometimes gain and sometimes reduction of potassium currents.

Only VF

1. Transmural dispersion of the repolarization heterogeneity.

2. Presence of post-potentials and increase of automaticity ischemic area.

3. Because the wall is thicker, the response to sodium channel blockers is usually inefficacious to prevent ventricular fibrillation

Figure 5.45 Some characteristics are common to atrial and ventricular fibrillation and others only typical of atrial or ventricular fibrillation.

Nevertheless, there is no doubt that the different mechanisms described may interact. Ventricular fibrillation generally occurs in patients with a vulnerable myocardium when some triggering or modulating mechanism acts on it, initiating a sequence of events that lead to VF onset and perpetuation (VF cascade) (Bayés-Genís *et al.*, 1995) (Figure 5.46).

Electrocardiogram

The ECG shows irregular high rate (300–500 bpm) QRS complexes of variable morphology and height, where QRS and ST-T are undistinguishable (Figures 5.41, 5.42, and 5.44). When the waves are relatively broad, recovery prognosis after electric CV is better than when they are slow and not very high (Figure 5.41).

Prognosis and Therapeutic Implications

The greatest significance of VF stems from the fact that it is the final arrhythmia that, in many cases, leads to SD (see Chapter 1, Arrhythmias and Sudden Death (SD)).

The scenario in which VF is most frequently observed is acute ischemia, generally appearing to be triggered by a PVC. Ventricular fibrillation does not usually appear in the first heart attack as a consequence of VT because the appropriate electrophysiologic characteristics (post-infarction scar) promoting the occurrence of reentrant VTs are not present.

Those **patients with MI who are more likely to experience a VT/VF** are those with a greater degree of ischemia associated with the triggering and modulating factors already mentioned (Figures 1.3 and 5.46) and

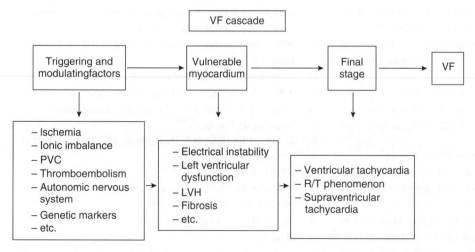

Figure 5.46 Diagram of the precursors of ventricular fibrillation (VF). A triggering factor acts on vulnerable myocardium and provokes the cascade of events leading to VF.

certain genetic and environmental factors. In acute coronary syndrome (ACS), the degree of ischemia with ST elevation may be classified into three groups (Sclarovsky, 1999). According to these authors, Grade 3 ischemia is manifest by an ST elevation that drags the QRS upwards in such a way that the S wave virtually disappears (Bayés de Luna and Fiol, 2008).

In coronary spasm, we have observed (Bayés de Luna *et al.*, 1985) that ventricular arrhythmias appeared, particularly in cases of severe ischemia, manifest by a significant ST elevation and, occasionally, alternans of the ST-QT (see Figure 7.5B). However, due to the brevity of the spasm, sustained VT/VF is not usually triggered (for more information see Chapters 7 and 11, Ischemic heart disease).

In the chronic phase of IHD and in other forms of heart disease, usually in the presence of HF (see Chapter 9.2, WPW-Type Pre-excitation), VF is frequently preceded by a sustained VT (Figure 1.4). Ventricular fibrillation is also responsible for SD in **inherited heart disease**. In these cases VF is also triggered by a VT, most frequently of a polymorphic type. In long QT syndromes it is usually triggered by a Torsades de Pointes VT.

It has been demonstrated that in some patients with **idiopathic VF** triggered by very early PVC, the ablation of the ectopic focus may prevent recurrence in the long-term follow-up (Knecht *et al.*, 2009; Haïssaguerre *et al.*, 2002; Natale and Raviele, 2009). However, ablation alone may not be sufficient to prevent SD and most of the patients will also require implanting an ICD.

As already mentioned, VF leads to SD, except in rare self-limiting cases if an ICD is not implanted or cardiopulmonary resuscitation is not immediately initiated. For more information consult Chapter 6 (Cardiac Arrest).

The appropriate treatment of clinical setting "electrical storm" includes AAA (amiodarone, procainamide, lidocaine, or betablocking agents -propanolol or esmolol-). Probably in the majority of cases the association of amiodarone and betablockers is the best first option. Also the sedation with ansiolitic drugs or even propofol may be useful. In case of bradicardia-dependent "electrical storm", as may happen in LQTS or Brugada syndrome, it may be necessary to increase the heart rate with isoproterenol or pacing. In patients with ICD in the CCU the device may be disconnected, and reprogrammed to avoid the number of discharges. Finally, sometimes a VT ablation may be considered.

With regard to SD prevention and ICD (Moss *et al.*, 2002), we recommend consulting the different aspects related to SD prevention (see Chapters 1, 9, and 11, the Appendix, and the Recommended General Bibliography p. xvii).

Patients who have recovered from VF are candidates for ICD implantation. The ICD implantation has to be delayed some months when VF appears in the acute phase of MI (see Chapter 11, Ischemic Heart Disease, and Appendix A-4, Automatic Implantable Cardioverter Defibrillator (ICD)).

Self Assessment

A. Which is the mechanism that explains the presence of extrasystoles in most cases?

B. How is a differential diagnosis made of extrasystole and parasystole?

C. Describe the premature ventricular complex (PVC) morphology rising from the right ventricle (RV).

D. Describe the morphologic criteria used to differentiate PVC from supraventricular premature complex (SVPC) with aberrant conduction.

E. What are the PVC morphologic characteristics usually observed in patients with advanced heart disease?

F. When do we consider a ventricular tachycardia (VT) a sustained VT?

G. What is a typical monomorphic VT?

H. What are the most frequent electrocardiographic characteristics in the onset and termination of a sustained VT?

I. Describe the most typical morphologies observed in VT in subjects with no evidence of heart disease.

J. Define a bundle branch reentrant VT.

K. Which is the P-QRS relationship in VT?

L. Define capture and fusion concepts.

M. Describe the key diagnostic electrocardiographic signs to perform differential diagnosis when assessing a wide QRS complex tachycardia.

N. What are the markers of a poor prognosis in post-infarction patients?

O. What is accelerated idioventricular rhythm?

P. Define the concept of tachycardiomyopathy.

Q. What are the electrocardiographic characteristics of Torsades de Pointes VT?

R. Discuss the different treatments of classic VT and Torsades de Pointes VT.

S. What is a bidirectional VT?

T. Describe the electrocardiographic and clinical characteristics of ventricular flutter.

U. Define the concept of the ventricular fibrillation (VF) cascade.

References

Adgey AA, Devlin JE, Webb SW. Initiation of ventricular fibrillation outside hospital in patients with acute ischaemic heart disease. Br Heart J 1982;47:55.

Antoons G, Oros A, Beekman JD, *et al.* Late Na(+) current inhibition by ranolazine reduces torsades de pointes in the chronic atrioventricular block dog model. J Am Coll Cardiol 2010 23;55:801.

Balasundaram R, Rao HB, Kalavakolanu S, Narasimhan C. Catheter ablation of bundle branch re-entrant ventricular tachycardia. Heart Rhythm 2008;5 Suppl 6:68.

Baman T, Lange D, Ilg K, *et al.* Relationship between premature ventricular complexes and left ventricular function. Heart Rhythm 2010;7:869.

Bayés de Luna A. Guindo J, Torner P, *et al.* Value of effort testing and acute drug testing in the evaluation of antiarrhythmic treatment. Eur Heart J 1987;8(suppl A):77.

Bayés de Luna A, Coumel P, Leclercq JF. Ambulatory sudden death: mechanisms of production of fatal arrhythmia on the basis of data from 157 cases. Am Heart J 1989;117:151.

Bayés de Luna A, Fiol M. Electrocardiography in ischemic heart disease. Blackwell-Futura, Oxford, 2008.

Bayés de Luna A, Carreras F, Cladellas M, *et al.* Holter ECG study of the electrocardiographic phenomena in Prinzmetal angina attacks with emphasis on the study of ventricular arrhythmias. J Electrocardiol 1985;18:267.

Bayés de Luna A, Goldwasser D, de Porta V, *et al.* Optimizing electrocardiographic interpretation in acute ST-elevation myocardial infarction may be very beneficial. Am Heart J 2011;162(1):e1–2; author reply e5.

Bayés-Genís A, Vinolas X, Guindo J, *et al.* Electrocardiographic and clinical precursors of ventricular fibrillation: chain of events. J Cardiovasc Electrophysiol 1995;6:410.

Bazan V, Gerstenfeld EP, Garcia FC, *et al.* Site-specific twelve lead ECG features to identify an epicardial origin for left ventricular tachycardia in the absence of myocardial infarction. Heart Rhythm 2007;4:1403.

Berruezo A, Mont L, Nava S, *et al.* Electrocardiographic recognition of the epicardial orighin of ventricular tachycardias. Circulation 2004; 109 (15): 1842-1847.

Berruezo A, Fernández-Armenta J, Mont L, *et al.* Combined endocardial an epicardial catheter ablation in arrhythmogenic right ventricular dysplasia incorporating scar dechanneling technique. Circ Arrhythm Electrophysiol 2012; 5 (1): 111-121.

Bigger JT, Fleiss JL, Kleiger R, *et al.* The relationships among ventricular arrhythmias, left ventricular dysfunction, and mortality in the 2 years after myocardial infarction. Circulation 1984;69:250.

Bogun F, Crawford T, Chalfoun N, *et al.* Relationship of frequent postinfarction premature ventricular complexes to the re-entry circuit of scar-related ventricular tachycardia. Heart Rhythm 2008;5:367–74.

Bökenkamp R, Wilde AA, Schalij MJ, *et al.* Flecainide for recurrent malignant ventricular arrhythmias in two siblings with Andersen-Tawil syndrome. Heart Rhythm 2007;4:508.

Brugada J, Berruezo A, Cuesta A, *et al.* Nonsurgical transthoracic epicardial radiofrequency ablation: an alternative in incessant ventricular tachycardia. JACC 2003;41:2036.

Brugada P, Brugada J, Mont L, *et al.* A new approach to the differential diagnosis of a regular tachycardia with a wide QRS complex. Circulation 1991;83:1649.

Cano O, Hutchinson M, Lin D, *et al.* Electroanatomic substrate and ablation outcome for suspected epicardial ventricular tachycardia in left ventricular nonischemic cardiomyopathy. J Am Coll Cardiol 2009;54:799.

Castro Arias JR, López MA, Sánchez LT. Loop recorder documentation of self-terminating cardiac arrest not receiving reanimation manoeuvres. Eur Heart J 2009;30:1702.

Chevalier P, Bellocq C, Millat G, *et al.* Torsades de pointes complicating atrioventricular block: evidence for a genetic predisposition. Heart Rhythm 2007;4:170.

Chung KY, Walsh TJ, Massie E. Ventricular parasystolic tachycardia. Br Heart J 1965;27:392.

Cohen H, Langendorf R, Pick A. Intermittent parasystole. Circulation 1973;48:761.

Cole CR, Marrouche NF, Natale A. Evaluation and management of ventricular outflow tract tachycardias. Card Electrophysiol Rev 2002;6:442.

Connolly SJ, Hallstrom AP, Cappato R, *et al.* Meta-analysis of the implantable cardioverter defibrillator secondary prevention trials. AVID, CASH and CIDS studies. Antiarrhythmics vs implantable defibrillatior study. Cardiac Arrest Study Hamburg. Canadian implantable defibrillator study. Eur Heart J 2000; (24): 2071-2078.

Credner S, Kingerheen T, Mauss O., *et al.* Electrical storm in patients with ICD: incidence, management and prognostic implications. J Am Coll Cardiol 1998;32:1909.

Cygankiewicz I, Zareba W, Vazquez R, *et al.*; MUSIC Investigators. Prognostic value of QT/RR slope in predicting mortality in patients with congestive heart failure. J Cardiovasc Electrophysiol 2008;19:1066.

Cygankiewicz I, Zareba W, Vázquez R, *et al.*; MUSIC Investigators. Risk stratification of mortality in patients with heart failure and left ventricular ejection fraction >35%. Am J Cardiol 2009;103:1003.

D'Avila A. Epicardial catheter ablation of ventricular tachycardia. Heart Rhythm 2008;5 Suppl 6:73.

Dessertene F. La tachycardie ventriculaire à deux foyers opposés variables. Arch Mal Coeur 1966;59:263.

Drew BJ, Ackerman MJ, Funk M *et al.*; on behalf of the American Heart Association Acute Cardiac Care Committee of the Council on Clinical Cardiology, the Council on Cardiovascular Nursing, and the American College of Cardiology Foundation. Prevention of Torsade de Pointes in Hospital Settings: A Scientific Statement. Circulation 2010;121:1047.

Dubner SJ, Gimeno GM, Elencwajg B, *et al.* Ventricular fibrillation with spontaneous reversion on ambulatory ECG in the absence of heart disease. Am Heart J 1983;105:691.

Echt DS, Liebson PR, Mitchell LB, *et al.* Mortality and morbidity in patients receiving encainide, flecainide, or placebo. The Cardiac Arrhythmia Suppression Trial. N Engl J Med 1991 21;324:781.

Goldwasser D, Serra G, Guerra J, *et al.* New computer algorithm to improve P wave detection during supraventricular tachycardias. Eur Heart J 2008; 29(suppl):P472.

Gorgels AP, van den Dool A, Hofs A, *et al.* Comparison of procainamide and lidocaine in terminating sustained monomorphic ventricular tachycardia. Am J Cardiol 1996;78:43.

Griffith MJ, De Belder MA, Linker NJ, *et al.* Difficulties in the use of electrocardiographic criteria for the differential diagnosis of left bundle branch block pattern tachycardia in patients with structurally normal heart. Eur Heart J 1992;13:478.

Griffith MJ, De Belder MA, Linker NJ, *et al.* Multivariate analysis to simplify the differential diagnosis of broad complex tachycardia. Br Heart J 1991;66:166.

Guglin M, Aljayeh M, Saiyad S, *et al.* Introducing a new entity: chemotherapy-induced arrhythmia. Europace 2009 ;11:1579.

Haissaguerre M, Shoda M, Jais P, *et al.* Mapping and ablation of idiopatic ventricular fibrillation. Circulation. 2002;106:962.

Haïssaguerre M, Derval N, Sacher F, *et al.* Sudden cardiac arrest associated with early repolarization. N Eng J Med 2008;358:2016.

Hanllan M, Scheinman M. Uncommon forms of ventricular tachycardia. Cardiol Rev 1996;4:13.

Haqqani HM, Kalman JM, Roberts-Thomson KC, *et al.* Fundamental differences in electrophysiologic and electroanatomic substrate between ischemic cardiomyopathy patients with and without clinical ventricular tachycardia. J Am Coll Cardiol 2009;54:166.

Hayes JJ, Stewart RB, Green HL, Bardy GH. Narrow QRS ventricular tachycardia. Ann Intern Med 1991;114:460.

Hinkle LE Jr, Carver ST, Stevens M. The frequency of asymptomatic disturbances of cardiac rhythm and conduction in middle-aged men. Am J Cardiol 1969;24:629.

Horowitz LN, Greenspan AM, Spielman SR, Josephson ME. Torsades de pointes: electrophysiologic studies in patients without transient pharmacologic or metabolic abnormalities. Circulation 1981;63:1120.

Itoh E, Aizawa Y, Washizuka T, *et al.* Two cases of ventricular parasystole associated with ventricular tachycardia. PACE 1996;19:370.

Janse MJ, Malik M, Camm AJ, *et al.* Identification of post acute myocardial infarction patients with potential benefit from prophylactic treatment with amiodarone. A substudy of EMIAT (THE European Myocardial Infarct Amiodarone Trial). Eur Heart J 1998;19:85.

Josephson ME, Horowitz LN, Farshidi A, *et al.* Recurrent sustained ventricular tachycardia. 4. Pleomorphism. Circulation 1979;59:459.

Jouven X, Zureik M, Desnos M, *et al.* Long-term outcome in asymptomatic men with exercise induced premature ventricular depolarizations. N Engl J Med 2000; 343:826.

Kennedy HL, Whitlock JA, Sprague MK, *et al.* Long-term follow-up of asymptomatic healthy subjects with frequent and complex ventricular ectopy. N Engl J Med 1985 24;312:193.

Kennedy HL. Ventricular ectopy in athletes: don't worry... more good news! J Am Coll Cardiol 2002 7;40:453.

Kinoshita S. Intermittent parasystole originating in the ventricular path of ventricular extrasystoles. Chest 1977;72:201.

Klein LS, Shih HT, Hackett K, *et al.* Radiofrequency catheter ablation of ventricular tachycardia in patients without structural heart disease. Circulation 1992;85:1666.

Knecht S, Sacher F, Wright M, *et al.* Long-term follow-up of idiopathic ventricular fibrillation ablation. J Am Coll Cardiol 2009;52:522.

Koulizakis NG, Kappos KG, Toutouzas PK. Parasystolic ventricular tachycardia with exit block. J Electrocardiol 1990;23:89.

Lamba J, Redfearn DP, Michael KA, *et al.* Radiofrequency ablation for the treatment of idiopathic premature ventricular contractions originating from the right ventricular outflow tract: a systematic review and meta-analysis. PACE 2014; 37 (1): 73-78.

Leenhardt A, Glaser E, Burgera M, *et al.* Short-coupled variant of torsade de pointes. A new electrocardiographic entity in the spectrum of idiopathic ventricular tachyarrhythmias. Circulation 1994;89:206.

Leenhardt A, Lucet V, Denjoy I, *et al.* Catecholaminergic polymorphic ventricular tachycardia in children. Circulation 1995;91:1512.

Lerman BB. Mechanism of outflow tract tachycardia. Heart Rhythm 2007;4:973.

Lerman BB, Stein K, Engelstein ED, *et al*. Mechanism of repetitive monomorphic ventricular tachycardia. Circulation 1995;92:421.

Lown B, Wolf M. Approaches to sudden death from coronary heart disease. Circulation 1971;44:130.

Marrouche NF, Schweikert R, Saliba W, *et al*. Specific surface ECG pattern to predict ventricular tachycardia originating from the aortic cusp. Circulation 2001;104 Suppl II:621.

Massumi RA, Marin J, Udhoji VN. Verapamil in parasystolic ventricular tachycardia and other wide QRS rhythms. Am Heart J 1986;111:400.

McKenna WJ, Behr ER. Hypertrophic cardiomyopathy: management, risk stratification, and prevention of sudden death. Heart 2002;87:169.

Miller JM, Marchlinski FE, Buxton AE, *et al*. Relationship between the 12-lead electrocardiogram during ventricular tachycardia and endocardial site of origin in patients with coronary artery disease. Circulation 1988;77:759.

Miller JM, Scherschel JA. Catheter ablation of ventricular tachycardia: skill versus technology. Heart Rhythm 2009;6:S86.

Mittal S. Focal VT: Insights from catheter ablation. Heart Rhythm 2008;5(Sup): 564.

Mizusawa Y, Saturada H, Nishizaki M, *et al*. Characteristics of bundle branch re-entrant ventricular tachycardia with a right bundle branch block configuration. Europace 2009;11:1208.

Moss AJ. Prognosis after myocardial infarction. Am J Cardiol 1983 1;52:667.

Moss AJ, Zareba W, Hall WJ, *et al*. Prophylactic implantation of a defibrillator in patients with myocardial infarction and reduced ejection fraction. N Engl J Med 2002;346:877.

Moulton KP, Medcalf T, Lazzara R. Premature ventricular complex morphology: a marker for left ventricular function and structure. Circulation 1990;81:1245.

Myerburg RJ, Kessler KM, Luceri RM, *et al*. Classification of ventricular arrhythmias based on parallel hierarchies of frequency and form. Am J Cardiol 1984;54:1355.

Natale A, Raviele A. Ventricular tachycardi/Fibrillation ablation. Oxford: Wiley-Blackwell; 2009.

Niwano S, Wakisaka Y, Niwano H, *et al*. Prognostic significance of frequent premature ventricular contractions originating from the ventricular outflow tract in patients with normal left ventricular function. Heart 2009;95:1230.

Nogami A. Idiopathic left ventricular tachycardia: assessment and treatment. Card Electrophysiol Rev 2002; 6:448.

O'Donnell D, Cox D, Bourke J, *et al*. Clinical and electrophysiological differences between patients with arrhythmogenic right ventricular dysplasia and right ventricular outflow tract tachycardia. Eur Heart J 2003; 24:801.

Ogawa S, Dreifus LS, Watanbe Y. Rapid ventricular parasystole with possible multilevel exit block. J Electrocardiol 1981;14:309.

Opthof T, Coronel R, Wilms-Schopman FJ, *et al*. Dispersion of repolarization in canine ventricle and the ECG T wave: T interval does not reflect transmural dispersion. Heart Rhythm 2007;4:341.

Oreto G, Satullo G, Luzza F, *et al*. "Irregular" ventricular parasystole: the influence of sinus rhythm on a parasystolic focus. Am Heart J 1988;115:121.

Oreto G. Parasystole: Automaticity or reentry?. J Cardiovascular Med 2010;11:336.

Ouyang F, Cappato R, Ernst S, *et al*. Electronatomic substrate of idiopathic left ventricular tachycardia : unidirectional block and macroreentry within the purkinje network. Circulation 2002;105:462.

Pascale P, Schlaepfer J, Oddo M, *et al*. Ventricular arrhythmia in coronary artery disease: limits of a risk stratification strategy based on the ejection fraction alone and impact of infarct localization. Europace 2009; 11:1639.

Pava L, Perafán P, Badiel M, *et al*. R-wave peak time at DII: A new criterion for differentiating between wide complex QRS tachycardias. Heart Rhythm 2010; 7:922.

Pérez-Riera AR, Barbosa Barros R, de Sousa FD, *et al*. Accelerated ideoventricular rhythm: history and chronology of the main discoveries. Indian Pacing Electrophysiol J 2010; 10 (1): 40-48.

Priori S, Napolitano C, Tiso N, *et al*. Mutations in the cardiac ryanodine receptor gene (hRyR2) underlie catecholaminergic polymorphic ventricular tachycardia. Circulation 2001;103:196.

Qu Z, Garfinkel A. Nonlinear dynamics of excitation and propagation in cardiac muscle. In: Zipes DP, Jalife J. (eds). Cardiac electrophysiology. From cell to bedside. Saunders, Philadelphia, 2004, p. 327.

Rabinovich R, Muratore C, Baranchuk A. Initiation mode of ventricular tachyarrhythmias in chronic Chagas' cardiomyopathy. Arch Mex Cardiol 2008; 78 (3): 248-253.

Rasouli M, Ellestad M. Usefulness of ST depression in ventricular premature complexes to predict myocardial ischemia. Am J Cardiol 2001;87:891.

Reddy VY, Reynolds MR, Neuzil P, *et al*. Prophylactic catheter ablation for the prevention of defibrillator therapy. N Engl J Med. 2007; 357 (26): 2657-2665.

Richter S, Brugada P. Bidirectional ventricular tachycardia. Circulation 2009;54:1189.

Roelandt J, Schamroth L. Parasystolic ventricular tachycardia. Observations on differential stimulus threshold as possible mechanism for exit block. Br Heart J 1971; 33(4):505.

Rosenbaum MB, Elizari MV, Lazzari JO, *et al.* Intraventricular trifascicular blocks. The syndrome of right bundle branch block with intermittent left anterior and posterior hemiblock. Am Heart J 1969;78:306.

Sapp JL, Beeckler C, Pike R, *et al.* Initial human feasibility of infusion needle catheter ablation for refractory ventricular tachycardia. Circulation 2013; 128 (21): 2289-2295.

Sapp JL, Wells GA, Parkash R, *et al.* Ventricular Tachycardia Ablation versus Escalation of Antiarrhythmic Drugs. N Engl J Med. 2016 May 5. [Epub ahead of print]

Sarrazin JF, Labounty T, Kuhne M, *et al.* Impact of radiofrequency ablation of frequent post-infarction premature ventricular complexes on left ventricular ejection fraction. Heart Rhythm 2009;6:1543.

Scherf D, Bornemann C. Parasystole with a rapid ventricular center. Am Heart J 1961;62:320.

Sclarovsky S. Electrocardiography of acute myocardial ischaemic syndromes. Martin Dunitz, London, 1999.

Shah RR, Hondeghem LM. Refining detection of druginduced proarrhythmia: QT interval and TRIaD. Heart Rhythm 2005;2:758.

Shimoike E, Ueda N, Maruyama T, Kaji Y. Radiofrequency catheter ablation of upper septal idiopathic left ventricular tachycardia exhibiting left bundle branch block morphology. J Cardiovasc Electrophysiol 2000; 11:203.

Siegal D, Quinlan C, Parfrey B, *et al.* Type II bidirectional ventricular tachycardia as a mechanism of termination of sustained ventricular tachycardia. J Cardiovasc Electrophysiol 2009; 20 (3): 345-346.

Smith TW, Haber E, Yeatman L, *et al.* Reversal of advanced digoxin intoxication with Fab fragments of digoxinspecific antibodies. N Engl J Med 1976 8;294:797.

Steurer G, Gursoy S, Frey B, *et al.* The differential diagnosis on the electrocardiogram between ventricular tachycardia and preexcited tachycardia. Clin Cardiol 1994;17:306.

Tada H, Tadokoro K, Miyaji K, *et al.* Idiopathic ventricular arrhythmias arising from the pulmonary artery: prevalence, characteristics, and topography of the arrhythmia origin. Heart Rhythm 2008;5:419.

Tai YT, Lau CP, But PP, *et al.* Bidirectional tachycardia induced by herbal aconite poisoning. Pacing Clin Electrophysiol 1992 ;15:831.

Tomassoni G, Stanton M, Richey M, *et al.* Epicardial mapping and radiofrequency catheter ablation of ischemic ventricular tachycardia using a three-dimensional nonfluoroscopic mapping system. J Cardiovasc Electrophysiol 1999;10:1643.

Touboul P, Atallah G, Kirkorian G. Bundle branch re-entry: a possible mechanism of ventricular tachycardia. Circulation 1983;67:674.

Touboul P, Delaye J, Clement C, *et al.* Tachycardie ventriculaire parasystolique. Arch Mal du Coeur 1970;63:1414.

Ventura R, Steven D, Klemm HU, *et al.* Decennial follow-up in patients with recurrent tachycardia originating from the right ventricular outflow tract: electrophysiologic characteristics and response to treatment. Eur Heart J 2007;28(19):2338.

Vereckei A, Duray G, Szénási G, *et al.* New algorithm using only lead a VR for differential diagnosis of wide QRS complex tachycardia. Heart Rhythm 2008;5:89.

Vereckei A. Current algorihms for the diagnosis of wide QRS complex tachycardias. Curr Cardil Rev. 2014; 10 (3): 262-276.

Wellens HJ. Electrophysiology: ventricular tachycardia: diagnosis of broad QRS complex tachycardia. Heart 2001;86:579.

Wellens HJ. The value of the electrocardiogram in the differential diagnosis of a tachycardia with a widened QRS complex. Am J Med 1978;64:27.

Yamada T, Litovsky SH, Kay GN. The left ventricular ostium: an anatomic concept relevant to idiopathic ventricular arrhythmias. Circ Arrhyth Electrophysiol 2008;1:396.

Yan GX, Antzelevitch C. Cellular basis for the normal T wave and the electrocardiographic manifestations of the long-QT syndrome. Circulation 1998;98:1928.

Yazdan-Ashorri P, Digby G, Baranchuk A. Failure to treat Torsades de Pointes. Cardiol Res 2012; 1 (1): 34-36.

Zhang F, Chen M, Yang B, *et al.* Electrocardiographic algorithm to identify the optimal target ablation site for idiopathic right ventricular outflow tract ventricular premature contraction. Europace 2009;11:1214.

Zhang L, Mmagu O, Liu LW Li, *et al.* Hypertrophic cardiomyopathy: can the noninvasive diagnostic testing identify high risk patients? World J Cardiol 2014; 6 (8): 764-770.

6

Passive Arrhythmias

This chapter describes the different passive arrhythmias according to the classification in Table 1.1.

Escape Complex and Escape Rhythm

Concept and Mechanism

When heart rate is slow due to depressed sinus automaticity, sinoatrial block, or atrioventricular (AV) block, an AV junction pacemaker at a normal discharge rate (40–50 bpm) may pace the electrical activity of the heart by delivering one or more pacing stimuli (escape beat or complex and escape rhythm) (Figures 6.1–6.5). If the AV junction shows depressed automaticity, an idioventricular rhythm at a slower rate (<30 bpm) would command the heart's activity. Even if the atrial rhythm is atrial fibrillation (AF), the escape rhythm is regular (Figure 6.2). The rhythm is never regular in the presence of AF with normal AV conduction. If the atrial rhythm is atrial flutter, a diagnosis of escape rhythm will be reached based on the slow and regular RR intervals observed, with a variable flutter wave–QRS complex interval (Figure 6.4).

Electrocardiographic Findings

In the electrocardiogram (ECG), the escape complex is recorded as a delayed QRS complex not preceded by a P wave or the preceding P wave has a PR interval <0.12 s (Figure 6.1A). In the ECG the escape rhythm is identified as a sequence of escape QRS complexes (Figures 6.1–6.3), which may be interrupted by sinus captures (Figure 6.1B) and sometimes appear as bigeminal complexes. In this case, a differential diagnosis of bigeminy should be made (Figures 6.1B and 7.6I). The escape rhythm may be fixed, occasionally with retrograde conduction to the atria (Figures 6.1C and 10.1). Sometimes a progressively slower escape rhythm precedes the asystole (Figure 6.5).

The QRS complex is narrow when the escape focus is in the AV junction (Figure 6.1). Conversely, when the escape focus originates from the ventricle or from the AV junction but bundle branch block or Phase 4 aberrancy exists, the resulting QRS complex is wide.

The occurrence of AV junctional escape rhythm or escape complexes at their usual discharge rates should not be considered pathologic, as this is usually observed in athletes or in subjects with increased vagal tone but the escape rhythm disappear with exercise or along the day life. In fact, it warrants protection against a slow rhythm. Frequently, if there is no depression of the AV junction automaticity, the implantation of pacemakers would be neither urgent nor most likely necessary. Obviously, pacemaker implantation is urgent if the slow heart rate is due to a depressed AV junctional or ventricular rhythm.

When the AV junction automaticity is very slow or an infrahisian AV block exists, the heart may be controlled by a slow ventricular pacemaker and in this case implanting a pacemaker is compulsory (Figure 6.3).

Sinus Bradycardia due to Sinus Automaticity Depression
(Figures 6.7 and 6.8)

Concept and Mechanism

The sinus discharge rate is lower than 60 bpm. The following are the mechanisms explaining sinus automaticity depression (see Figure 3.3): 1) decrease of the slope of Phase 4 partly due to the inactivation of the diastolic inward current (If); 2) a threshold potential nearer to zero; and 3) a more negative transmembrane diastolic potential (TPD).

Exercise, emotions, and so on induce a progressive acceleration of the sinus heart rate, which also shows a progressive deceleration when these physiologic stimuli disappear. The sinus node is considered to be pathologically altered when these physiologic changes do not take place.

Frequently, daytime sinus tachycardia alternates with occasional very slow bradycardia during the night, particularly in young athletes. A first-degree and

Clinical Arrhythmology, Second Edition. Antoni Bayés de Luna and Adrian Baranchuk.
© 2017 John Wiley & Sons Ltd. Published 2017 by John Wiley & Sons Ltd.

(A)

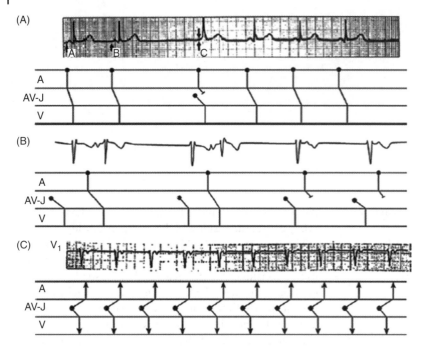

(B)

(C)

Figure 6.1 (A) A 52-year-old patient with bradycardia-tachycardia syndrome. The AB distance is half the BC distance, indicative of a probable 2×1 sinoatrial block. In C, a P wave is initiated, which cannot be conducted because an escape atrioventricular (AV) junctional complex takes place shortly after (third QRS complex). (B) An example of incomplete AV dissociation with slow escape rhythm (first, third, fifth, and sixth complexes) and sinus captures (second and fourth complexes). After the two last QRS complexes, we observe how the P waves are not conducted because they are closer to the QRS complex than the two first P waves, therefore falling in the junctional refractory period. (C) AV junctional rhythm at 64 bpm with retrograde conduction to the atria slower than the anterograde conduction to the ventricles (see the negative P wave following each QRS complex).

(A) 25 mm/s

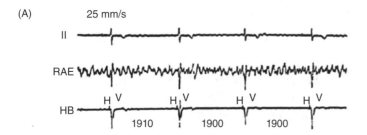

(B) 100 mm/s

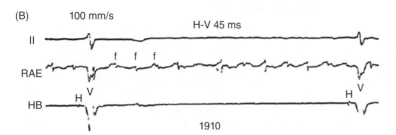

Figure 6.2 (A) Lead II: Regular RR intervals in the presence of underlying atrial fibrillation with narrow QRS complexes. This is indicative of a junctional ectopic rhythm dissociated from the atrial rhythm (atrial fibrillation). See the amplified F waves in the right atrial electrogram (RAE), and how in the His bundle (HB) recording H deflection precedes the narrow ventricular complexes with HV = 45 ms (see B), confirming it is a junctional atrioventricular (AV) block proximal to the bundle of His.

second-degree AV block may even occur at the same time, if right vagal (sinus node) and left vagal (AV node) overdrive exist (Figure 6.6) (see later).

Electrocardiographic Findings

It is manifest by a slow sinus rhythm, which in young athletes or in patients with vagal predominance may even be less than 30 bpm (Bjeregaard, 1983) (Figure 6.7). The sinus discharge rate is not fixed, particularly in children. This is especially evident in the presence of sinus bradycardia. In adults, this variability from one cycle to another is usually less than 10–20%. Sinus arrhythmia may be diagnosed (Figure 6.7B and 6.7C) when RR interval variability from one cycle to another is greater

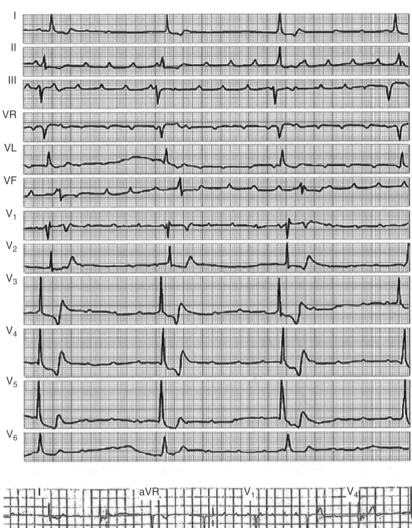

I
II
III
VR
VL
VF
V₁
V₂
V₃
V₄
V₅
V₆

Figure 6.3 Twelve-lead surface electrocardiogram (ECG) in a patient with complete atrioventricular (AV) block (complete dissociated P-QRS relationships), with a somewhat wide (120 ms) QRS complex and a very slow escape rhythm, leading to urgent pacemaker implantation.

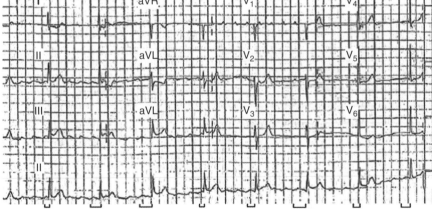

Figure 6.4 Atrial flutter with regular RR at 46 bpm and varying FR distances (see bottom) confirming an atrioventricular (AV) dissociation. This patient suffered from atrial flutter dissociated by AV block of a junctional escape rhythm.

than 20%. The sinus arrhythmia is considered to be mild when the change from one cycle to another is <50%, moderate when the change is between 50% and 100%, and severe if it is over 100%.

Sinus bradycardia is often observed with a normal PR interval (Figure 6.7). Sinus bradycardia and different degrees of AV block are present when a predominant vagal overdrive affects both the right vagus nerve (sinus node) and the left vagus nerve (AV node) (see before) (Figure 6.6).

Finally, it should always be taken into account that a slow sinus rhythm may rarely be explained by the presence of concealed atrial bigeminy (Figures 6.8 and 7.3). It is quite important to consider this possibility and try to identify the

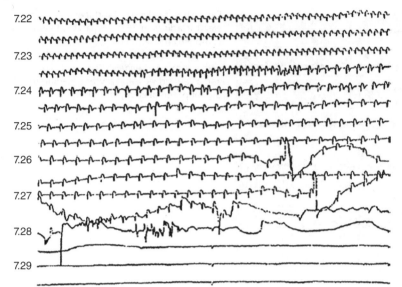

Figure 6.5 A 68-year-old patient who presented sudden death (SD) four days after suffering an acute infarction. In the electrocardiogram (ECG) Holter recording we observe quick progressive automaticity depression with occurrence of a slow escape rhythm leading to cardiac arrest, probably because of an electromechanical dissociation due to cardiac rupture.

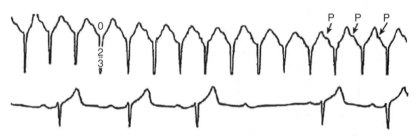

Figure 6.6 A 25-year-old athlete without significant bradycardia with clear electrocardiogram (ECG) signs of sympathetic overdrive during the day (top) and frequent atrioventricular (AV) Wenckebach episodes at night due to the preferential involvement of the left vagus nerve (below).

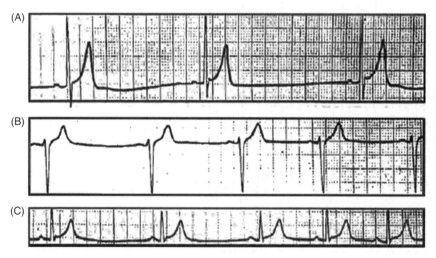

Figure 6.7 (A) Significant sinus automaticity depression. Holter electrocardiogram (ECG) recording (athlete) during sleep showing bradycardia <30 bpm. Note that the PR interval is normal, as the left vagus nerve is not involved. (B) A similar example with a heart rate <40 bpm and somewhat irregular, in a healthy young person. (C) Another example of sinus bradycardia in a healthy young person with significant RR irregularity.

small P′ wave deflection at the T wave (Figure 6.8) or close to the T wave end, which may be confused with the U wave (Figure 7.3) (arrow), as in these cases the therapeutic approach is quite different to that of a slow rhythm due to a sinus bradycardia.

Sinoatrial Block

Concept and Mechanism

In all types of heart block (Chapter 3, Heart Block), we shall discuss first-, second-, and third-degree blocks. In

(A)

(B)

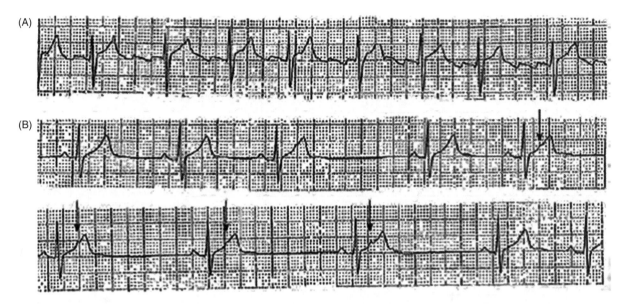

Figure 6.8 (A) Atrial flutter with variable atrioventricular (AV) conduction accounting for the irregular RR and the varying FR. (B) Two continuous strips in sinus rhythm with frequent concealed atrial extrasystoles (notch in T wave ascending limb, see arrow), which give the impression that the basal rhythm, which is already slow, is much more bradycardic.

this case, sinus node stimulus is blocked between the sinus node and the atria. If the sinus stimulus reaches the atria but with delay, a first-degree sinoatrial block is observed, although the AV relation (P wave–QRS complex) is not altered (Figure 6.9). This is not the case in third-degree sinoatrial block, where an AV junctional rhythm is the dominant pacemaker (Figure 6.10). Finally, the second-degree sinoatrial block may be of Mobitz- or Wenckebach-type or Mobitz II, similar to the second-degree blocks of the AV junction (Figures 6.11 and 6.12).

Electrocardiographic Findings

First-degree sinoatrial block
This cannot be detected by conventional ECG (Figures 3.18A and 6.9).

Second-degree sinoatrial block
In the presence of second-degree sinoatrial block, the ventricular rate is half the sinus rate (BC = 2AB in Figures 3.18C

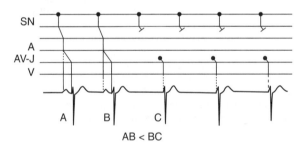

Figure 6.10 Third-degree sinoatrial block. It can be observed how an escape rhythm suddenly appears, with no visible P waves in the ECG. Although it is not shown in the figure, the escape rhythm may retrogradely activate the atria (AB < BC) (see Figure 3.18D).

and 6.11) or much slower (4 times in Figure 6.11 D–E) is of 4:1 type. If the second degree SA block is the type 2:1 fixed, the ECG recording will be similar to that of a sinus bradycardia due to automaticity depression. If the 2:1 block disappears with exercise, an abrupt increase of the heart rate, usually more than double that due to increase of sinus rate, may be observed.

Second-degree sinoatrial block Mobitz I (Wenckebach-type), may also be observed. Usually, this presents a 3:2 (Figure 7.6E) or 4:3 block (Figures 3.18B and 6.12). Figure 6.12 explains why in the second-degree sinoatrial block (Wenckebach-type), the RR intervals progressively shorten. The block increase is gradually less until the complete block initiates a pause. This type of block does not modify the PR interval because the block is at sinoatrial level.

From an electrocardiographic point of view, the 3:2 sinoatrial Wenckebach block shows a sequence and ECG characteristics similar to those of atrial bigeminy due to

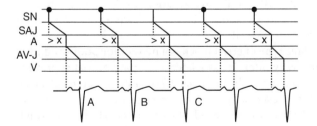

Figure 6.9 First-degree sinoatrial block. Sinoatrial conduction is consistently slowed down (>x). This block is not seen in the surface electrocardiogram (ECG) (x = normal sinoatrial or atrioventricular (AV) conduction time) (AB = BCV) (see Figure 3.18A).

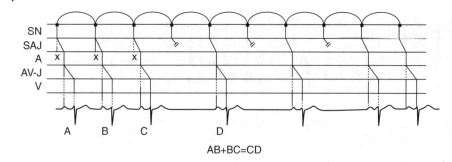

Figure 6.11 Second-degree sinoatrial block type 2:1 or 4:1. Sinoatrial conduction (normal and fixed) (x) before the complete block of the stimuli. The pause generated (CD) in type 2:1 doubles the baseline rhythm (CD = AB + BC) (see Figure 3.18C).

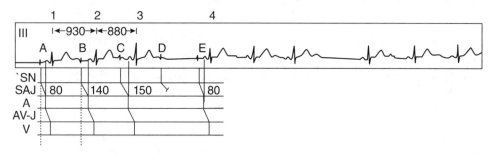

Figure 6.12 Second-degree Wenckebach-type sinoatrial block (4×3). The sinoatrial conduction time progressively increases from normality (80 ms) (from A to onset of first P wave) until a complete block occurs (D not followed by a P wave). The distance between the first two RRs (930 ms) is greater than the distance between the second and third RRs (880 ms). Sinoatrial conduction cannot be determined. Theoretically, A, B, C, D, and E represent the origin of the sinus impulses. A–B, B–C, C–D, and D–E distances are the sinus cadence (870 ms). Additionally, assuming that the first sinoatrial conduction time in the sequence is 80 ms (distance from the arrow, origin of sinus impulse, to A), the successive increases observed in the sinoatrial conduction (80 + 90 = 140 and 140 + 10 = 150) account for the shortening of RR and explain the following pause. Therefore, it is confirmed that the more significant increase in the Wenckebach-type block (a sinoatrial block in this case) occurs in the first cycle of each sequence, following a pause (1–2 > 2–3). PR intervals do not change. The second RR interval (2–3) is 50 ms shorter than the first (930 vs 880 ms), as this is the difference between the sinoatrial conduction increases of the first and second cycles. In fact, the first RR is 870 + 60 = 930 ms, while the second cycle is 930−60 + 10 = 880 ms (see Figure 3.18B).

premature parasinus atrial impulses (P′ wave is identical or almost identical to the sinus P waves). Figure 6.13 explains the key steps for this differential diagnosis (Bayés de Luna *et al.*, 1991).

Third-degree (complete) sinoatrial block

No atrial depolarization due to sinus stimuli is observed. Therefore, the ECG recording shows an AV junctional or ventricular escape rhythm (Figures 3.18D and 6.10).

Atrial Blocks

Concept and Mechanism

We will discuss the block at atrial level, especially between the right and left atrium (interatrial block) (Bayés de Luna *et al.*, 2012a) (see Figure 3.19).

Electrocardiographic Findings

First-degree or partial interatrial block

Diagnostic criteria: (i) the P wave duration is ≥0.12 s, usually with bimodal morphology in the frontal plane and with a variable negative component in lead V1

(Figures 3.19 and 3.20); and (ii) the P wave morphology in the frontal plane is virtually indistinguishable from the P wave of left atrial enlargement, although in the latter, a more negative component of the P wave in V1 is usually seen (Figure 3.20). In fact, interatrial conduction block rather than left atrial dilation is responsible for the ECG signs found in left atrial enlargement especially the increased duration of the P wave.

Third-degree or advanced interatrial block

Diagnostic criteria (Bayés de Luna *et al.*, 1985, 2012a) (Figure 3.19): (i) P wave duration ≥0.12 s; (ii) P ± in leads II, III, and VF; and (iii) in V1–V2 leads a P ± is very often observed as well.

This type of atrial block is a marker for poor prognosis and very often is associated with paroxysmal supraventricular arrhythmia atrial fibrillation or atypical atrial flutter, especially in the presence of: (i) PR duration ≥140ms, (ii) advanced structural heart disease (high CHA_2DS_2-V, and (iii) ambient arrhythmias (Bayés de Luna *et al.*, 1988a, 2012a). Recently, its association with dementia and previous stroke has been confirmed (Martínez-Sellés *et al.*, 2016). The later was already found in all interatrial blocks (Arijarayah *et al.*, 2007). Thus, it

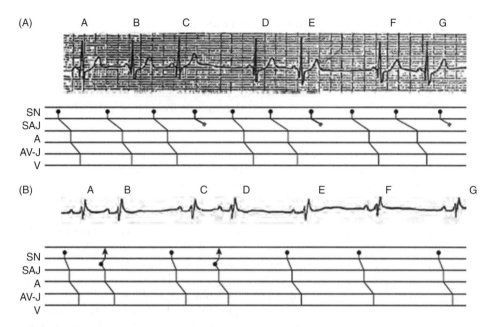

Figure 6.13 Differential diagnosis (Lewis diagrams) between 3×2 sinoatrial block and atrial parasinus bigeminy with very similar or identical P′ waves, and a virtually identical electrocardiogram (ECG) pattern. Above (A): After three sinus impulses conducted to atria, in D a 3×2 sinoatrial block sequence starts. Below (B): Two sequences of atrial bigeminy followed by normal rhythm. In the first case (3×2 sinoatrial block), AB and BC intervals correspond to the baseline rhythm, which is very similar to the shortest RR interval of coupled bigeminal rhythm (DE and FG distances). Conversely, in cases of atrial parasinus bigeminy, the basal rhythm (EF and FG intervals) is very similar to the longest pause observed in the bigeminal rhythm (BC and DE distances) (below). Therefore, in the presence of a bigeminal rhythm with previous basal RR intervals with the same P, PR, and QRS, the diagnosis of a 3×2 sinoatrial block is supported by the fact that the regular RR intervals are very similar to the shortest RR interval corresponding to the bigeminal rhythm (BC similar to DE and FG in A). On the other hand, in B if the regular RR intervals are similar to the longest RR interval of the bigeminal rhythm, it is most likely an atrial parasinus bigeminy (EF o FG similar to BC in B).

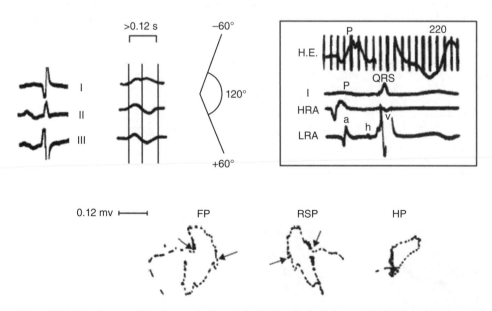

Figure 6.14 Top: P wave with +/− morphology in II, III, VF typical of advanced (third degree) interatrial block with retrograde conduction to the left atrium. See how the ÂP of the first and second part of the P wave have to be measured. To the right we see how the impulse travels from the high right atrium (HRA) to the low right atrium (LRA), and finally to the high esophageal leads (HE). The estimulus goes first from HRF to LRA and later to HE. Below: The P loop in the three planes with the second part of the loop upwards is shown (see Figures 5.6, 10.4 and 10.5) (Bayés de Luna *et al.*, 1985).

is an arrhythmologic syndrome (Daubert, 1996; Bayés de Luna *et al.*, 1988a, 1989) that has recently been named Bayes' Syndrome (Conde and Baranchuk, 2014a, 2014b; Bacharova and Wagner, 2015) (see Chapter 10, Advanced interatrial Block with Left Atrial Retrograde Conduction, and Figures 3.19, 6.14, 10.4–10.7).

Second-degree interatrial block

This corresponds to the cases of partial or advanced IAB that are transient. These cases form part of the atrial aberrancy concept (Chung, 1972). This concept includes not only cases of transient IAB (Figure 6.15) but also of transient P wave change without morphology of IAB, probably due to RA intermittent block (see Chapter 3) that may not be ectopically induced, and may appear in the same tracing (Figures 3.23, 6.16) or in two different tracings (see Figure 3.24) and at interatrial level or in one atrium (Figure 3.24) (Enríquez *et al.*, 2015; Marano *et al.*, 2015).

Atrioventricular Block

Concept and Mechanism

Conduction block is observed in the AV junction. As in other types of heart block, we shall refer to first-, second-, and third-degree blocks (see Chapter 3, Heart Block). The exact location of the block (suprahisian, hisian, or infrahisian block) is accurately determined only by intracavitary studies (see Figure 6.21). However, the presence of a narrow QRS complex escape rhythm and a second-degree Wenckebach-type AV block suggests that the block is located in the AV junction, whereas the presence of a wide QRS complex favors evidence of a block below the His bundle.

Electrocardiographic Findings

Discuss here are the key diagnostic criteria of the different AV blocks that may be found in a surface ECG.

First-degree AV Block

A first-degree AV block occurs when the PR interval is greater than 0.18 s in children, 0.20 s in adults, and 0.22 s in elderly patients (Figures 3.21A and 6.17).

Second-degree AV block

One or more P waves are not conducted to the ventricles despite being beyond the physiologic AV junctional refractory period (Figure 3.21B and C). Second-degree AV block may be of a Wenckebach-type, (also known as Mobitz I), or of a Mobitz-type block (Mobitz II). **In the Wenckebach-type AV block** (Figure 6.18), the progressive shortening of the RR intervals is due to a progressive reduction of the AV block increase (180–260–300 ms) until a complete AV block is reached. The latter initiates a pause that is longer than any other RR interval.

Therefore, a Wenckebach-type AV block is characterized by: (i) a progressive lengthening of the PR interval, starting from the first PR interval after the pause; (ii) the most significant increase being observed in the second PR interval after the pause (Figures 3.21B and 6.18); and (iii) the pause being a longest RR interval. However, for different reasons, these rules are not always followed. Figure 3.21E shows two forms of atypical Wenckebach-type AV block.

In the second-degree AV block of Mobitz II type, the AV block and consequent pause occur abruptly without

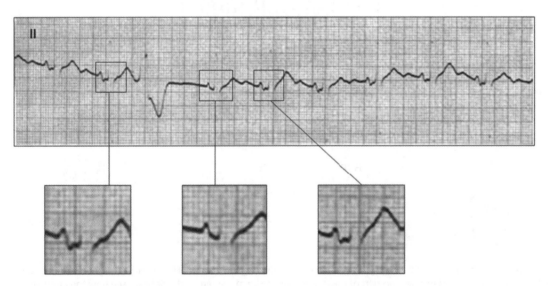

Figure 6.15 Patient with A-IAB (P ± in lead II). After a premature ventricular pause followed by a normal P wave appears. Then the image reappears IAB-A.

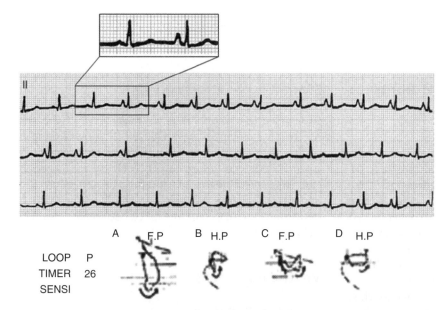

Figure 6.16 Top: Continuous recording of lead II. Note the repetitive changes in the P wave morphology and polarity in a heart disease patient with chronic bronchitis. Observe the abrupt change in P morphology that lasts several seconds and is not related to respiration. Two types of P wave are clearly defined: a peaked P wave and a flat and somewhat bimodal P wave. Below:

Vectocardiogram showing the two P wave morphologies observed in this patient. One P wave (A–B) downwards in the frontal plane (FP) and, therefore, very positive in II, III, and VF, with figure-eight shaped rotation in the horizontal plane (HP); the other P wave is shown in (C) and (D) with a different axis in FP (C) and a lack of figure-eight form in the loop in HP (D).

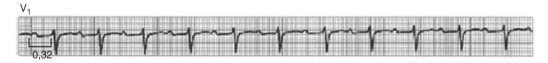

Figure 6.17 First-degree AV block (PR 0.32 s).

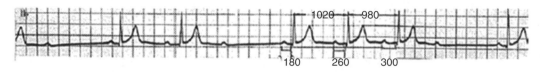

Figure 6.18 Second-degree AV block (Wenckebach-type Mobitz I). PR interval increases are progressively smaller (80 ms (260–180) and 40 ms (300–260)) and, consequently, RR intervals are successively shorter (1020 and 980).

progressive lengthening of the PR interval. As a result, one or several P waves may be blocked (paroxysmal AV block) (Figures 3.21C and 6.19). The second-degree 2×1 AV block (one out of two P waves is blocked) may be explained by both Mobitz I and Mobitz II-type blocks (Figure 6.20).

On rare occasions, in the presence of a 2×1 block in the AV junction (high part), the Wenckebach phenomenon may arise from the conducted P waves themselves occurring in the lower part of AV junction (**alternating Wenckebach phenomenon**) (Halpern *et al.*, 1973; Amat y Leon *et al.*, 1975; Garcia-Niebla and Sclarovski, 2013).

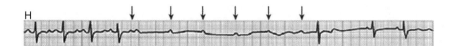

Figure 6.19 Paroxysmal second-degree AV block (Mobitz II type). Note the six blocked P waves without a prior increase of the PR interval. The first QRS complex following the pause is an escape QRS complex as it features a very long PR interval. The last two P waves are conducted.

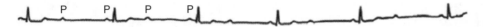

Figure 6.20 Second-degree 2×1 AV block.

Figure 3.21F shows an example of this odd electrophysiologic phenomenon.

Third-degree AV block

In this type of block a complete dissociation between the P waves and the QRS complexes exists, thus it is frequently named complete AV block (Figures 3.21D, 6.3, and 6.22). The escape rhythm is slow (usually less than 45 bpm), except in some patients with congenital AV block (Figure 6.23), and it is almost always lower than the sinus rate. When the escape ventricular rhythm is greater than the sinus rhythm, we cannot be sure that the AV block is complete, as some P waves may not be conducted as a result of an interference phenomenon (the P waves falls in the AV node physiologic refractory period).

The wideness of QRS may be narrow if the AV block is high (suprahisian), or wide if it is infrahisian, or aberrant conduction exists.

The exact location of the block place

This can only be determined by means of a His bundle ECG (see Appendix A-3, Intracavitary ECGs and Electrophysiologic Studies). Figure 6.21 shows examples of first-degree AV block after His level (prolonged HV interval) (A), second-degree 2×1 block before His deflection (B), second-degree block (after His deflection) (C), and second-degree AV block at His level (see two H deflections – H–H′– and the block between the two His deflections H–H′) (D).

Ventricular Blocks

Concept and Mechanism

The intraventricular conduction system is formed by the right bundle branch, left bundle branch, and the

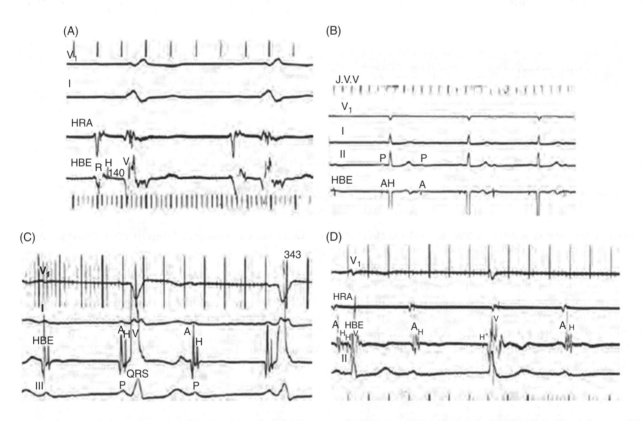

Figure 6.21 (A) Infrahisian first-degree block. In the His lead (EHH) a very long HV is observed (140 m). The high right atrium (HRA) deflection coincides with the onset of the P wave. (B) Pre-hisian second-degree 2×1 atrioventricular (AV) block. The stimulus is blocked after the A deflection and before the H deflection as this is not recorded in the bundle of His lead (EHH). (C) Infrahisian second-degree 2×1 AV block. The P wave is blocked after the deflection of the His bundle. (D) Intrahisian second-degree AV block. Note the split H deflection in the first complex (but with AV conduction), followed by a block after the H deflection. Later, an escape complex is observed, preceded by the second deflection of the His bundle (H′). Finally, there is a block after the first His deflection.

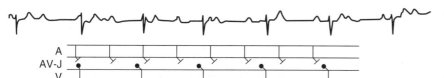

Figure 6.22 Third-degree or advanced atrioventricular (AV) block. A complete AV dissociation is observed.

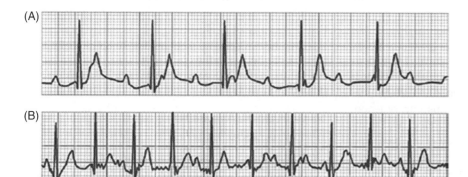

Figure 6.23 (A) Congenital atrioventricular (AV) block with clear AV dissociation in a 20-year-old patient. P waves are independent from QRS complexes, with an escape rate >60 bpm. Note the high and sharp T waves. (B) During exercise there is still AV dissociation, although the sinus heart rate is >130 bpm (see P–P) and the accelerated escape rhythm is over 100 bpm. This is a clear example of congenital AV block not yet requiring pacemaker implantation.

superoanterior, inferoposterior and septal divisions of the left bundle (Figure 2.7).

A. Ventricular blocks may occur on the right side of the heart (Table 6.1) or on the left side of the heart (Table 6.2) at different levels (proximal-proximal part of right or left bundle, or distal – at Purkinje level) depending on where the delay of conduction occurs. It may affect the whole ventricle (global block) or only part of it (regional or divisional block).

Table 6.1 Right ventricular block.

Global (right bundle branch block): this is usually a block located in the proximal part of the right bundle branch and, less frequently, on the right side of the His bundle or at distal level (parietal or peripheral block)

- Advanced (third-degree): this corresponds to the Mexican school type III (QRS ≥0.12 s)
- Partial (first-degree): this corresponds to the Mexican school types I and II (QRS <0.12 s)
- Second-degree block: this corresponds to some type of aberrant ventricular conduction (see Chapter 3, Aberrant Conduction)

Regional

- No evident r′ in V1. The delay of conduction may be located in the anterosuperior zone – SI, SII, SIII morphology or less often in the posteroinferior zone – S1, R2, R3 morphology always with QRS <0.12 s. These morphologies may be due to other causes (Bayés de Luna *et al.*, 1987; Bayés de Luna, 2011).

Table 6.2 Left ventricular block.

Global (left bundle branch block): this is usually a proximal block located in the main trunk or, rarely, on the left side of the His bundle or at distal level (parietal or peripheral block)

- Advanced (third-degree): this corresponds to the Mexican school type III (QRS ≥0.12 s)
- Partial (first-degree): this corresponds to the Mexican school types I and II (QRS <0.12 s)
- Second-degree block: this corresponds to some type of aberrant ventricular conduction (see Chapter 3, Aberrant Conduction)

In the divisions of the left bundle branch:

- Block of superoanterior o inferoposterior fascicle (hemiblocks according to the Rosembaum's School, 1968)
- Block of middle fibers (see the text)

B. The blocked area shows a delayed depolarization and, in patients with advanced global ventricular block, the blocked ventricle, either right or left is the last area of the heart to be depolarized.

C. In the global ventricular block (Sodi-Pallares *et al.*, 1964), the stimulus delay usually occurs in the proximal portion of the right or left bundle branch (RBB and LBB respectively). For this reason, in the presence of a global ventricular block, the denomination is "bundle branch blocks".

D. Advanced (third-degree) right and left bundle branch blocks are characterized by:
  o The diagnosis is made essentially through the horizontal plane (V1 and V6 leads).
  o The QRS complex duration measuring at least 0.12 s.
  o Slurring of the QRS complex usually being in the opposite direction of the T wave.
  o Depolarization of the homolateral ventricle to the blocked branch taking place through the septum, starting from the contralateral ventricle. The widening of the QRS complex and the particular ECG morphologies, in the case of both right and left bundle branch blocks, are explained by this phenomenon. The results of LV activation with endocardial mapping in the case of LBBB (Aurichio *et al.*, 2004) and with computer simulation (Strauss *et al.*, 2011) show that the presence of mid-QRS notches with slurring are the result of abnormal activation of the LV. The first notch corresponds to the transeptal activation arriving to the endocardium and the second to the epicardium. This process lasts about 130 ms.
  o The septum repolarization dominates the left ventricular free wall repolarization, being responsible for the ST-T changes observed in bundle branch blocks.
  o Generally, the anatomic abnormalities are more diffuse than the ones suggested by the electrocardiographic changes.
E. Partial (first-degree) bundle branch blocks originate morphologies usually indistinguishable from the corresponding ventricular enlargements.
F. Left divisional blocks (previously called "hemiblocks" now called "fascicular blocks") (Rosenbaum and Elizari, 1968) have been studied in more detail, both from anatomic and electrophysiologic points of view, than the right regional blocks (Cosín *et al.*, 1983; Bayés de Luna *et al.*, 1987) (Table 6.1). We will also briefly discuss the block of middle (or septal) fibers of the left bundle branch (see Chapter 3, Third-degree Block).

We will now look at the different intraventricular blocks and especially the right bundle branch block, left bundle branch block, and anterosuperior and posteroinferior divisions of the left bundle (hemiblocks). In addition to isolated blocks, bifascicular and trifascicular blocks will be discussed (Bayés de Luna, 2011).

Different Types of Ventricular Block: Ventricular Activation and Diagnostic Criteria
(Sodi-Pallares and Calder, 1956; Sodi-Pallares et al., 1964; Bayés de Luna, 2011)

Third-degree (advanced) RBBB
Ventricular activation
This is a block of the activation process of the whole right ventricle (RV) (global block) (Table 6.1 and Figures 3.26 and 6.24A).

Figure 3.26 shows the four characteristic activation vectors in this type of block at the proximal level resulting from the depolarization of the whole RV through the septum. The typical electrocardiographic morphologies, a result of the loop–hemifield correlation in the frontal and horizontal planes, are also shown.

Global blocks at a distal level also feature an advanced RBBB morphology, However, they often present more slurring in the "plateau" as in arrhythmogenic right ventricular cardiomyopathy (see Figure 9.6), or more inflexion points in the QRS morphology, as in Ebstein's disease (Bayés de Luna, 2011).

Diagnostic criteria (Figure 6.24A)
These are as following:

  o QRS complex ≥0.12 s and mid-final QRS slurrings. After the paper of Strauss, probably 130 ms for women and 140 ms for men (Strauss *et al.*, 2011).
  o Lead V1: rsR' pattern with a slurred R' wave and negative T wave.
  o Lead V6: qRs with evident slurring of S wave and positive T wave.
  o VR: QR with evident slurring of R wave and negative T wave.
  o T wave polarity opposite to the slurring of the QRS complex.

First-degree (partial) right bundle branch block
Ventricular activation
In this case, the delay of all RV activation (block) exists but is less significant.

Diagnostic criteria (Figure 6.24B)
The QRS complex duration is less than 0.12 s, although morphology in lead V1 still remains rsR' or rsr', but with fewer notches and less slurring. This is due to a decreased transeptal depolarization, as part of the RV depolarization is made through the right bundle branch (Figure 6.24B).

A tall R wave or an rsR' pattern in lead V1 not due to a typical bundle branch block may be observed in different situations, such as: (i) right ventricular hypertrophy, (ii) pre-excitation, (iii) lateral wall infarction, and (iv) different normal variant patterns (Bayés de Luna, 2011). Baranchuk published an algorithm that allows the differential diagnosis of all ECG pattern with r' in V1 to be performed (Baranchuk *et al.*, 2015).

Second-degree right bundle branch block
This is a type of aberrant ventricular conduction (see Chapter 3, Aberrant Conduction, and Figures 3.32 and 3.33).

Regional right ventricular block
The regional right ventricular block may occur in the anterosuperior or posteroinferior zone of the RBB,

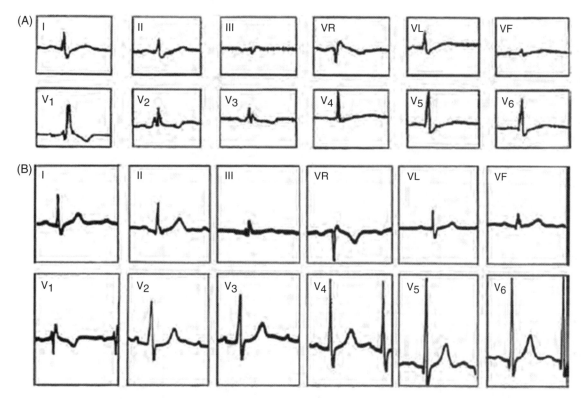

Figure 6.24 (A) Electrocardiogram (ECG) of a patient with advanced right bundle branch block (RBBB). (B) ECG of a patient with partial RBBB (see text and Figures 3.22 and 3.26). Note how all the criteria are met.

originating type S1, S2, S3, and sometimes S1, R2, R3 morphologies respectively, with narrow QRS complexes (Cosín *et al.*, 1983; Bayes de Luna *et al.*, 1987). However, the diagnosis of this type of block is practically impossible as these morphologies may be seen in different processes and also as normal variant patterns (Bayes de Luna *et al.*, 1987; Bayés de Luna, 2011).

Third-degree (advanced) left bundle branch block
Ventricular activation
This is a block of the whole left ventricle activation process (global block) (Table 6.2, and Figures 3.27 and 6.25A).

Figure 3.27 shows the typical four activation vectors for this type of block and the corresponding electrocardiographic morphologies resulting from the loop–hemifield correlation in the frontal and horizontal planes.

Distal LBB blocks occur less frequently than proximal blocks. The morphology in cases of distal block is usually similar to a proximal advanced LBBB, although more mid-final slurring is present, and sometimes are accompanied by very wide QRS (Bayés de Luna, 2011). Meanwhile, when the LBBB block pattern is due to involvement of both divisions, the ECG pattern is very similar to the proximal advanced LBBB pattern. However, experimentally a narrow "q" wave sometimes may be seen in I, VL, and V6, after the block of SA+IP divisions, which may be explained by the initial activation of the LV through the middle

fibers, although the overall ventricle activation is made from the RV through the septum.

To summarize, all types of global advanced LBBB, proximal or distal, share a pattern characterized by R in lead V6, and QS (rS) in lead V1, with QRS complex duration ≥0.12 s.

Diagnostic criteria (Figure 6.25A)
These are:

- o QRS complex duration ≥0.12 s, and sometimes >0.16 s, with mid-final slurring. More recently (Strauss *et al.*, 2011) may be considered ≥130 ms for women and ≥140 ms for men.
- o Lead V1: QS or rS complexes with an embryonic r wave and positive T wave.
- o Lead I and V6: single R wave, with R wave peak occurring after 0.08 s.
- o Lead VR: QS complex with positive T wave.
- o T wave with polarity opposite to the slurring of the QRS complex.

First-degree (partial) left bundle branch block
(Table 6.2 and Figure 6.25B)
Ventricular activation
In this situation, the delay in the overall left ventricular activation is less important as part of the LV depolarization is made through the left branch and therefore the transeptal depolarization is less important.

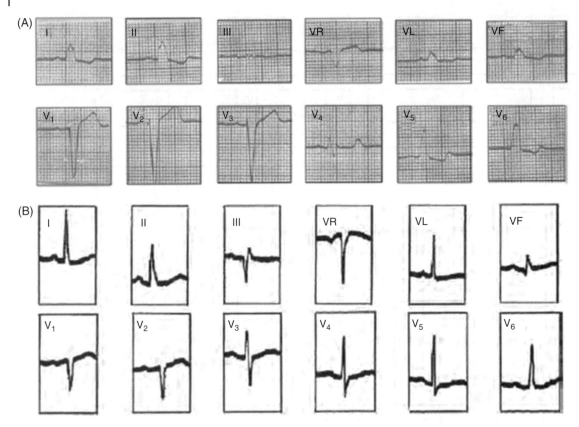

Figure 6.25 (A) Electrocardiogram (ECG) of a patient with advanced left bundle branch block (LBBB). (B) ECG of a patient with partial LBBB (see text and Figures 3.22 and 3.27). Note how all the criteria are met.

Diagnostic criteria (Figure 6.25B)

QRS complex duration <0.12 s, with a QS morphology in V1 or an embryonic "r" wave, and an isolated R wave in leads I and V6. This is probably due, at least in part, to the presence of septal fibrosis (absence of the first vector) (Bayés de Luna *et al.*, 1988b).

Second-degree left bundle branch block

It corresponds to a type of aberrant ventricular conduction (see Chapter 3, Aberrant Conduction). This type of LBBB may appear suddenly (Figure 3.25B) or progressively (Wenckebach-type) (Figure 3.25A). The latter occurs very rarely. Frequently, when the transient LBBB disappear, a negative T wave can be seen (cardiac memory or electrotonic modulation) (Rosenbaum *et al.*, 1982; Chiale *et al.*, 2010). Cardiac memory, frequently seen after resolution of bundle branch blocks, is represented by inverted T waves in the same leads where the maximum deflection vectors were seen.

Regional left ventricular block

Concept The stimulus is blocked in one of the two divisions (anterosuperior and posteroinferior) of the LBB (hemiblocks) (commonly called fascicular blocks)

(Rosenbaum and Elizari, 1968). Only the electrocardiographic criteria of advanced hemiblocks are discussed here. The electrocardiographic criteria of the block of middle fibers of LBB have been published by the Brazilian School (Pérez Riera, 2009; Pérez Riera *et al.*, 2016); they are briefly discussed later.

In both hemiblocks, the left intraventricular activation is modified due to the delayed depolarization of the blocked area; this accounts for the typical electrocardiographic changes observed.

Anterosuperior hemiblock (ASH) or left anterior fascicular block (LAFB)

Figure 3.28 shows the activation in the case of an ASH and the typical ECG patterns, a result of the loop–hemifield correlation in the three keys leads of the frontal plane. The diagnosis of ASH may be done only with the ECG in the presence of specific ECG criteria (Figure 6.26) as follows.

o QRS complex duration <0.12 s.
o Extreme left deviation of ÂQRS (between −45° and −75°). Inferior necrosis, Wolff–Parkinson–White (WPW) syndrome type II, as well as the SI, SII, SIII pattern should be ruled out (Figure 6.26, below).

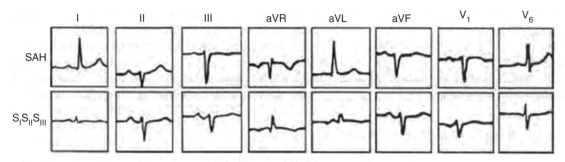

Figure 6.26 Electrocardiogram (ECG) of a patient with superoanterior hemiblock and a differential diagnosis with SI, SII, SIII morphology (see text and Figure 3.28).

- Leads I and VL: qR morphology.
- Leads II, III and VF: rS morphology with S3 > S2 and R2 > R3.
- S wave present up to lead V6 with intrinsicoid deflection in lead V6 < in VL.

Posteroinferior hemiblock (PIH) or left posterior fascicular block (LPFB) Figure 3.26 shows the activation in cases of posteroinferior hemiblock, as well as the typical electrocardiographic morphology resulting from the loop–hemifield correlation in the frontal and horizontal planes.

In this case, to establish this diagnosis, in addition to the typical electrocardiographic pattern, some clinical information is necessary, such as the absence of right ventricular hypertrophy and lean body built, that may also present rightward ÂQRS. Evidence of LV involvement is also probably necessary.

Diagnostic criteria (Figure 6.27) are:

- QRS complex <0.12 s.

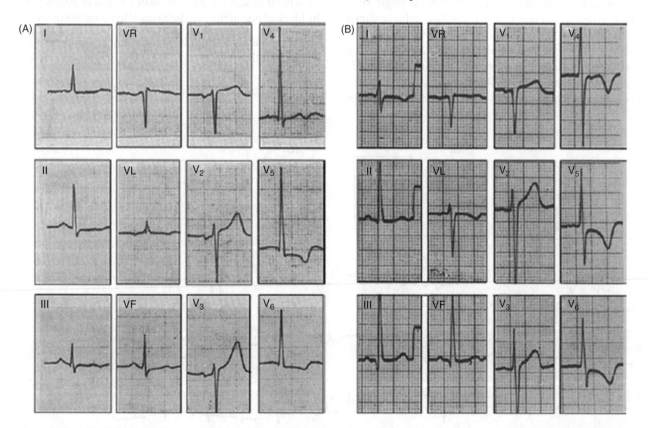

Figure 6.27 Left: (A) Electrocardiogram (ECG) of a 55-year-old patient with hypertension + ischemic heart disease. Despite no clinical evidence of myocardial ischemia, a significant electrocardiographic change was observed after a few days. (B) (ÂQRS leftwards direction turned rightwards; Rs in VF turned into qR, with intrinsecoid deflection time = 0.06 s, whereas qR in V6 turned into Rs) probably due to the establishment of posteroinferior hemiblock (PIH) (see text and Figure 3.29).

o Right deviation of ÂQRS (between +90° and +140°; ≥110° for some authors).

o Lead I, VL: RS or rS.

o Leads II, III, and VF: qR.

o Precordial leads: S wave present up to lead V6 with intrinsicoid deflection in leads V6 and VF > in VL.

Block of middle fibers or left septal fascicular block (LSFB) As already mentioned in Chapter 2, for some authors the intraventricular conduction system could be considered a quadrifascicular system (RBB, anterosuperior and posteroinferior divisions of the LBB and middle fibers). Applying programmed electrical stimulation to healthy subjects, Kulbertus *et al.* (1976) demonstrated that ventricular loops of different types of aberrant conduction, including a morphology with a significant forward location in the horizontal plane, are recorded. The latter loop correlates with an increase of R wave amplitude in V1 and particularly in V2. These loop–ECG changes may be explained by a block of the middle fibers located at the LV anterior and septal areas (Hoffman *et al.*, 1976; Pérez Riera, 2009).

Diagnosis that these pattern only corresponds to a block is rather difficult, and can only be strongly supported when a transient electrocardiographic pattern switch from rS to Rs morphology in leads V1–V2 is observed (Bayés de Luna and Fiol-Sala, 2008), with no other apparent cause that may explain it (i.e., severe transient lateral ischemia) (Pérez-Riera *et al.*, 2015). An example of an ECG featuring these characteristics is shown in Figure 6.28 (see legend). If the block of middle fibers alone or associated to RBBB or bifascicular block occurs, a tall R or qR pattern in V1–V2 is most likely recorded. A consensus paper devoted to this controversial topic has been published. In this it said that, in fact, the presence of intermittent R in V1 is due to conduction delay but we cannot assure at which level. It probably involves fibers of right bundle and some of the middle septal zone (Bayés de Luna *et al.*, 2012b). A recent book was completely devoted to this topic, and interested readers should be directed to this reference (Pérez-Riera *et al.*, 2016).

Block in more than one bundle

The following possibilities may exist: (i) a delay of conduction in the RBB and in one of the two divisions of LBB (bifascicular blocks); (ii) the conduction of impulses is intermittently blocked in one or the other bundle branches (bilateral bundle branch block); and (iii) finally, a trifascicular block may also exist.

Now, we will discuss the electrocardiographic criteria of these different types of intraventricular blocks in more than one bundle (see Chapter 10).

Bifascicular blocks

We will comment on the diagnostic criteria of RBBB with the block of one of the two divisions of left bundle branches.

A. Advanced right bundle branch block + anterosuperior hemiblock (Figure 6.29A). The diagnostic criteria are:

o QRS complex duration ≥0.12 s.

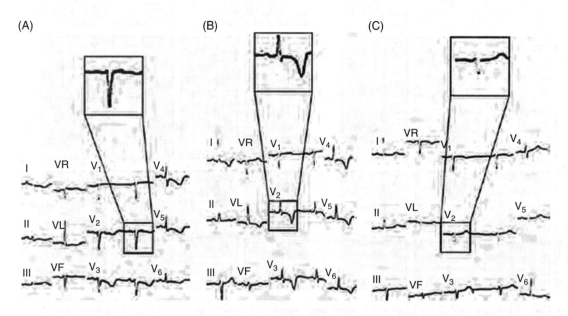

(A) (B) (C)

Figure 6.28 (A) Electrocardiogram (ECG) from an ischemic heart disease patient who, during an acute coronary syndrome (B), showed a significant morphology change in V2 (high transitory R), with very negative T wave in right precordial leads (left anterior descending (LAD) coronary artery involvement), which disappeared after some hours (C). As there is not any evidence of transient lateral ischemia, the transient pattern of V2 (tall R wave) (B) may be explained by a block of the middle fibers of left bundle branch, and/or right bundle (see text).

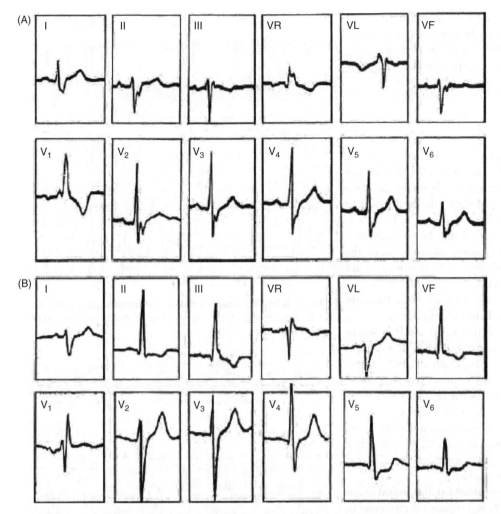

Figure 6.29 (A) A 70-year-old patient with no apparent heart disease showing the typical morphology right bundle branch block and superoanterior hemiblock (RBBB + SAH). (B) A 76-year-old patient suffering from ischemic heart disease (IHD) and hypertension without right ventricle pathology or asthenic habitus that shows a typical morphology right bundle branch block and inferoposterior hemiblock (RBBB + IPH) (see text). The ST segment is decreased in the left precordial leads due to the underlying disease.

- ○ QRS complex morphology: the first part, upward and leftward shift, is similar to that of the anterosuperior hemiblock. The second part similar to a global advanced RBBB morphology presents a forward and rightward shift (Figure 6.29A).
- ○ When a significant left ventricular delay exists, it may compensate the rightwards forces. The final result is forward-deviated left forces. As a consequence, the ECG pattern will show a high R wave in lead V1 with no S wave in lead I and VL, but occasionally an S wave in lead V6. Thus, the frontal plane looks as if an advanced left bundle branch block exists, whereas the horizontal plane shows an advanced RBBB pattern **(masked block)** (Bayés de Luna *et al.*, 1988c) (see Figure 10.10).

B. Advanced right bundle branch block + posteroinferior hemiblock (Figure 6.29B). The diagnostic criteria are as follows:
- ○ QRS complex duration >0.12 s.

- ○ QRS complex morphology: the first part of the QRS complex shifts downwards, as in posteroinferior hemi-block, whereas the second part shows a forward and rightwards shift, as in advanced RBBB (Figure 6.29B).
- ○ If the block occurs at the same time in both proximal branches, it is equivalent to advanced AV block.

Bilateral block In this case the patient sometimes shows advanced RBBB and LBBB patterns alternatively (see Chapter 10, High Risk Ventricular Block, and Figure 10.14).

Trifascicular blocks A trifascicular block is a delay of conduction in three fascicles. The most frequent combinations are:

- ○ Advanced RBBB alternating with SA and IP hemiblock (Rosenbaum-Elizari syndrome) (see Figure 10.13, and Chapter 10, High Risk Ventricular Block).

o Bifascicular blocks with a long PR interval. It should be considered that long PR may be due to AV junctional delay. However, intracavitary electrophysiologic studies are necessary to locate exactly the place of block that explains the long PR interval.

Cardiac Arrest

A diagnosis of cardiac arrest is reached when the patient carotid pulse is not palpable and no cardiac sounds are heard by auscultation. The presence of brain anoxia leads to pupil dilation and, a few minutes after the cardiac arrest, respiratory arrest also occurs. In a continuous ECG recording it is observed how cardiac arrest may be preceded by a progressive bradyarrhythmia (Figure 6.5) or tachyarrhythmia, usually ventricular fibrillation (VF) (see Figures 1.4 and 1.5). Sometimes, ventricular tachycardia (VT) may directly trigger the cardiac arrest (Figure 5.14C). **Patients in coronary Intensive Care Units** usually are recovered with electrical cardioversion if the cardiac arrest is due to primary VF (see Figures 5.42 and 5.44, and Table 11.1).

Hospitalized patients suffering from a cardiac arrest should be treated as emergency patients (cardiac arrest protocol, thoracic compression + electrical CV<5'). This measure could lead to an acceptable number of recoveries (consult advanced cardiac life support pulseless arrest algorithms, Circulation 2005, Europace 2006, and other guidelines produced by scientific societies, see General Recommended Bibliography p. xvii).

The fight against out-of-hospital cardiac arrest often also due to VF (see Chapter 1) is a significant challenge in modern cardiology. Its efficacy has been proven but its efficiency is limited (PAD Trial, 2004). Automated external defibrillators (AED) available at selected locations (airports, sport stadiums, enterprises) must be our aim. However, at present logistic and economic problems make universal implementation impossible. Another objective is that the time elapsed before resuscitation by AED not be too long because still many cardiac arrest survivors suffer from neurologic sequel. Finally, it would be desirable if there was an AED in every home and that it could be used with efficacy, but this is difficult to achieve (Bardy *et al.*, 2008).

The Pacemaker Electrocardiography
(Garson, 1990; Kasumoto and Goldschlager, 1996; Hesselson, 2003; Baranchuk, 2013) (Figures 6.30–6.38)

Components of the Pacemaker ECG

A pacemaker ECG comprises three components: the stimulation spike, the subsequent ventricular depolarization, and, finally, the repolarization wave.

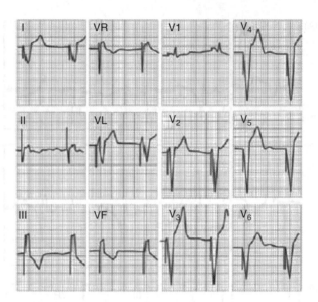

Figure 6.30 Pacemaker rhythm with electrode implanted in the left ventricle (right bundle branch block (RBBB) morphology) and qs in lead I.

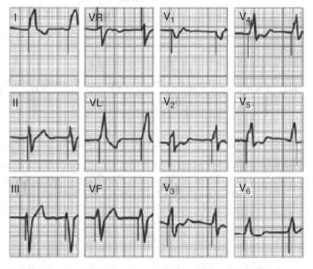

Figure 6.31 Pacemaker rhythm with electrode implanted in the apex of the right ventricle (left bundle branch block (LBBB) morphology).

Spikes may be either monopolar or bipolar. Monopolar spikes show a higher voltage. Bipolar spike voltage may increase due to pacemaker dysfunction. Nonstimulating monopolar spikes may shift the isoelectric line due to their high voltage, mimicking a QRS complex and thus appearing to be normal (Figure 6.38). Patients with pacemakers may show different types of fusion complexes (Figure 6.39A).

The QRS complex morphology and the ÂQRS vector direction depend on the pacing site (Figures 6.30–6.33). Currently, stimulation is almost always made from the RV (transvenous-endocardic pacing), and the ECG recording morphology is similar to that of an advanced

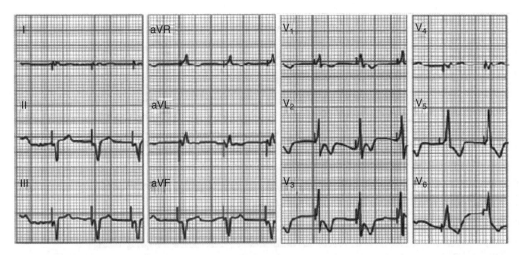

Figure 6.32 Patient with biventricular stimulation (resynchronization pacemaker). The QRS is definitively shorter than the previous QRS in sinus rhythm. The left ventricular stimulation explains the ÂQRS and the QRS complex morphologies (R in V1 and QR in VL) in the different leads.

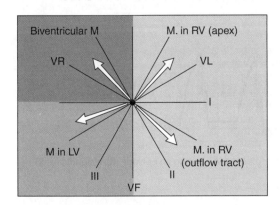

Figure 6.33 ÂQRS in the different types of ventricular stimulation (see Figures 6.30, 6.31, and 6.32).

LBBB (Figure 6.31). Resynchronization pacemakers (see Appendix A-4.2.2.) ideally must show a morphology characterized by a narrower QRS complex than that observed at baseline (Figure 6.32). However, different QRS morphologies may be found (Barold *et al.*, 2006a; Steinberg *et al.*, 2004) (Figure 6.33 shows the QRS axis in the different types of ventricular stimulation).

Bicameral (dual chamber) DDD pacemakers feature two consecutive spikes, corresponding to atrial and ventricular activation respectively (Figure 6.39C).

Esp-qR morphology observed in I, VL, and V6 usually with "q" ≥0.03 s is suggestive of old anterior infarction (Figure 6.34). A review of ECG diagnosis of myocardial infarction (MI) and ischemia during cardiac pacing has been previously published (Barold *et al.*, 2006b).

On the other hand, in patients with intermittent pacing it is observed, as in intermittent LBBB and right-sided accessory pathway (WPW pattern), that the nonpacing complexes present negative T waves that are not due to myocardial ischemia (electrical memory phenomenon) (Figure 6.35). Repolarization disorders are

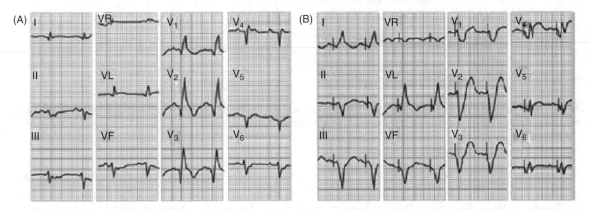

Figure 6.34 (A) Patient with anteroseptal and lateral infarction and advanced right bundle branch block (RBBB) in whom a pacemaker was implanted. (B) Note that Esp-qR morphology is not only recorded in I and VL, but also in V5–V6, suggestive of necrosis in patients with pacemaker.

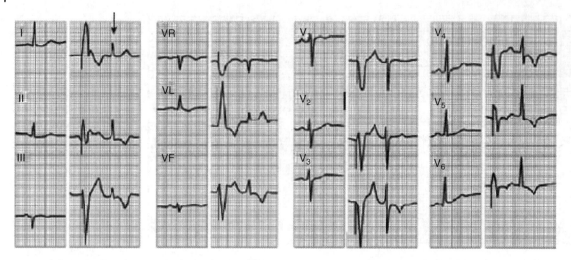

Figure 6.35 Patient with sick sinus in whom a pacemaker was implanted. The left panel of each trace pair shows the basic electrocardiogram (ECG), whereas the right panel shows the pacemaker ECG, followed in each lead by spontaneous complexes. An alteration in the repolarization of the spontaneous complexes (negative T waves) is observed, which is not due to the presence of ischemia but to the phenomenon of "electrical memory".

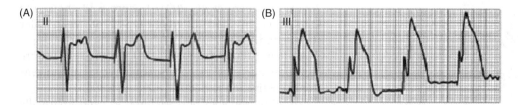

Figure 6.36 Patient with episode of Prinzmetal angina in whom a pacemaker was implanted (A). During an episode (B), a significant ST elevation is observed.

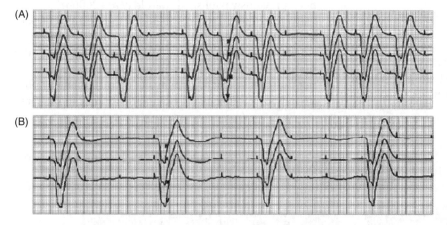

Figure 6.37 (A) A 57-year-old patient with a pacemaker in a cardiogenic shock with spike-myocardium block and some nonstimulating spikes. (B) After a few minutes, agonic rhythm is present (most of the spikes do not stimulate).

not easily discerned in patients with pacemakers and, thus, in the presence of precordial pain, pacemakers usually hinder the diagnosis. However, when ST changes are significant, they may be clearly observed in the ECG (Figure 6.36).

When patients with pacemakers develop cardiogenic shock, spikes not followed a paced QRS may occur in the final Phase (Figure 6.37). A lack of conduction between the pacemaker spike and the myocardium may also be observed due to pacemaker malfunction (Figure 6.38) (see later).

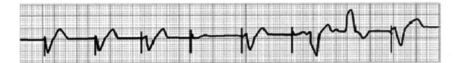

Figure 6.38 Fourth and sixth spikes are not followed by QRS complexes. Note the spike morphology with isoelectric baseline distortion, which may be mistakenly interpreted as a genuine QRS complex. The sixth spike is not conducted and after a ventricular escape and then a sinus capture occurs.

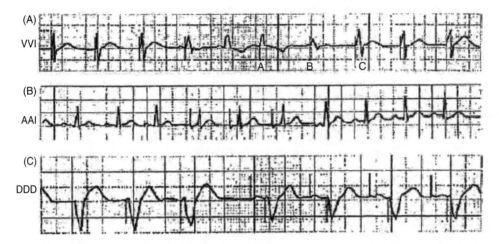

Figure 6.39 (A) VVI pacemaker. Ventricular on-demand pacemaker. The pacemaker is activated when the spontaneous rhythm is slower than its discharge rate. There are fusion impulses (4 and 7). After two sinus impulses (5 and 6), the pacemaker rhythm starts again. The first pacemaker impulse is delayed with regard to the programmed stimulation rate (hysteresis) (AB>BC). (B) AAI pacemaker. The three first complexes and the three final complexes are sinus complexes, inhibiting the discharge of the atrial pulse generator. Complexes 4–7, due to the normal heart rate being slowed down, start with an atrial spike, followed by an atrial depolarization wave (P wave). From the eighth complex, the sinus activity is again predominant and the pacemaker is inhibited. (C) DDD pacemaker. Example of physiologic (sequential) pacemaker. First, we observe three complexes caused by the pacemaker ventricular stimulation ("atrial sensing"). Next, the sinus rate decreases and starts the pacing by complexes initiated by the physiologic atrioventricular sequential stimulation (two spikes).

Evolution of Pacemaker Technology

The first pacemakers were fixed-pace devices and could not detect the electrical activity of the heart in the patient (sensing capacity), nor could they be inhibited in the presence of spontaneous electrical activity. Thus, the spontaneous electrical activity of the heart interfered with pacemaker activity. According to the three- and five-letter codes (Parsonnet *et al.*, 1981; Bredikis and Stirbys, 1985) (Table 6.3), these pacemakers delivered ventricular (V) pacing but did not have a sensing function (O) and, therefore, no automatic response (O) to the sensing capacity. This type of pacemaker (VOO) is no longer used.

To overcome this, pacemakers with the sensing capacity to detect spontaneous electrical activity of the heart were designed. The most commonly used pacemaker displays an automatic response to this sensing capacity by inhibiting its discharge. Later, a new response cycle is initiated, which starts a pacemaker impulse, provided that a spontaneous QRS complex does not occur before. This type of pacemaker is called a **VVI pacemaker** (Figure 6.39A) (V = ventricular pacing; V = ventricular sensing; I = demanded response (inhibition)). In cases of sinus node disease without AV block, single-chamber pacemakers (**AAI**) (Figure 6.39B) have been used. However, the progression to AV block in patients with sinus node dysfunction is about 2%/year (Andersen *et al.*, 1998), thus, in patients with sick sinus syndrome, rather than implanting AAI pacemakers, DDD pacemakers are currently recommended to provide ventricular pacing back up if necessary. This has triggered the need to implement different algorithms to prevent unnecessary RV pacing (Baranchuk, 2013). Each company has its own algorithm and physicians involved in device follow-up should be aware of the functioning of each algorithm (Baranchuk, 2013). When the sinus node function is normal but an AV block exists, VDD and now more frequently, **DDD** pacemakers may be implanted (Figure 6.39C) (see Choosing the Best Pacemaker in Different Clinical Settings).

Currently, the most commonly used pacemakers are sequential (dual-chamber) pacemakers, which pace and sense both atria and ventricles, and may display inhibition or other types of response. These are DDD pacemakers (Table 6.4 and Figure 6.39C) with two spikes (see

Table 6.3 Pacemakers: three- and five-letter identification codes.

Types	Category	Letters
I	Chamber(s) paced	V: ventricle A: atrium D: dual (A+V)
II	Chamber(s) sensed	V: ventricle A: atrium D: dual (A + V) O: none
III	Modes of response	T: triggered I: inhibited (on demand) D: dual (triggered/inhibited) O: none (asynchronous) R: reverted
IV	Programmable antiarrhythmic functions	P: single programmable M: multiprogrammable C: communicating R: rate modulation O: none
V	Special functions	P: pacing S: shock D: dual (P + S)

Table 6.4 Characteristics of the main types of pacemakers currently used.

Letter position (I II III)	Mode description	Use
VVI	Ventricular on demand pacemaker (inhibited by R wave) (Figure 6.39A) On-demand rate-response or rate-modutalion (type VVI-R biosensors) (Figure 6.41)	Currently, the most used pacemaker. The spontaneous QRS complex is sensed by the device and the following pacemaker impulse is inhibited. The generator output circuit is recycled and a pacemaker stimulus is generated at a given rate, unless a spontaneous QRS is generated before. It is especially indicated for patients with atrial arrhythmias, particularly atrial fibrillation (AF), slow ventricular rate, advanced age, sedentary lifestyle, infrequent bradycardia episodes and recurrent tachycardia mediated by the pacemaker
AAI	Atrial on-demand pacemaker (inhibited P wave) (Figure 6.39B). Rate response or rate-modulation AAI-R	Especially indicated for sinus node disease with intact atrioventricular (AV) conduction, and presumably with no AF in the short-term follow-up
DDD	Universal. Atria and ventricles sensed and paced (Figure 6.39C). Different types of programmable parameters may be included. Rate response or rate-modulation (DDD-R type) (Figure 6.40)	Sinus node disease and all types of AV block. It does not provide additional benefits over the VVI in case of persistent AF. Pacemaker-mediated tachycardias may occur in the presence of retrograde conduction, which could be prevented by programming the pacemaker without atrial detection

before), which initiate atrial and ventricular depolarization in a sequential mode.

Today, many pacemakers adapt to normal everyday life because they may increase the heart rate on demand. They include biosensors, the most commonly used being the "accelerometer", a small sensor able to detect movement. It allows the pacemaker to regulate the heart rate according to demand by exercise. Tracking the P wave and pacing the ventricle in cases of AV block with intact sinus node is a common way of pacing. Both VVI and DDD pacemakers may present this type of response (**DDDR and VVIR**) (Figures 6.40 and 6.41). External programmers may modify all the pacemaker parameters when necessary. Moreover, advances in the field of multiprogramming systems and telemetric interrogation may facilitate the correction of the different pacemaker dysfunctions and allow better pacemaker monitoring. Arrhythmias may also be memorized and diagnosed

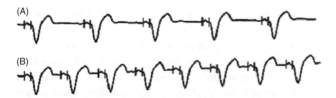

Figure 6.40 (A) DDDR pacemaker in a patient with sick sinus and atrioventricular (AV) block. Note how the pacemaker pacing increases with exercise (B).

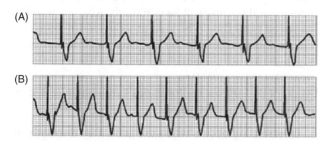

Figure 6.41 (A) VVIR-type pacemaker in a patient with atrial fibrillation (AF) and atrioventricular (AV) block. Note how the pacemaker pacing increases with exercise (B).

(Holter function). Likewise, implantable defibrillators may be monitored and controlled. Currently, home monitoring allows "distance" interrogation of both pacemakers and defibrillators without moving the patients from their homes of nursing care facilities. It is currently under development the possibility of "programming" the devices at distance (already available in some countries).

As a result of all these advances, indications for pacemakers have also been changed. Today, they are not only used to prevent SD secondary to bradyarrhythmias but also to better treat some tachyarrhythmias or improve ventricular function. Some examples of available "hybrid" techniques to treat arrhythmias using cardiac devices are:

- **AV node ablation + VVIR pacemaker implantation** in patients with rapid persistent AF in whom the AV node conduction cannot be well controlled with drugs. This approach allows for improvement of the ventricular function and quality of life in AF patients with a very fast ventricular rate. Currently, the AV node ablation is combined with biventricular pacing (cardiac resynchronization therapy (CRT)), with success in cases of very advanced heart failure (HF) + AF + QRS >120 ms (Gasparini *et al.*, 2006) (see Chapter 4, Ablation Techniques).
- **Ventricular resynchronization pacemakers** (Figure 6.32) are indicated for refractory HF patients who have received optimized pharmacological treatment despite of which they persist in functional class II to IV (Zareba *et al.*, 2011; Healey *et al.*, 2012). These pacemakers deliver electrical stimulating pulses to both ventricles to coordinate contraction of the

chambers. Therefore, these pacemakers correct the dyssynchrony generated by pacemakers located in the right ventricle and/or by the underlying LBBB, improving ventricular contractility and HF (CRT). Resynchronization pacemakers are implanted in the left ventricle using a catheter, which is introduced in a coronary vein (ideally the postero-lateral branch) through the coronary sinus to stimulate the ventricular free wall. Excellent reviews (Steinberg *et al.*, 2004; Barold *et al.*, 2006a) have been published commenting on assessment of biventricular pacing and the diagnostic value of 12-lead ECG during biventricular pacing for cardiac resynchronization. The indications for CRT are discussed in Appendix A-4, Cardiac Resynchronization Therapy (CRT). New techniques implanting the right ventricular lead in the outflow tract of the RV are being associate with better response to resynchronization (Stavrakis *et al.*, 2012).

Stepwise Approach to Interpret an Unknown ECG Pacemaker: a Pacemaker Clinic

To interpret the ECG tracing of a patient with a pacemaker we can use the following stepwise approach: (i) determine the mode of operation of the pacemaker (VVI, DDD, etc.); (ii) measure pacemaker parameters (rate, AV intervals, etc.); and (iii) evaluate the pacemaker function output (spike characteristics), sensing capacity, and ventricular capture (triggering).

Today's advanced pacemaker technology and increased cost of sophisticated devices require methodical long-term follow-up in order for the patient to receive the optimum pacing benefit and for the treatment to be as cost effective as possible. For these reasons, a well-organized Pacemaker Clinic is needed.

For a more detailed description of pacemaker ECG, as well as all related main components, goals, logistical needs, and functional aspects of a Pacemaker Clinic, including the assessment of pacemaker malfunctioning, it is advised to consult other specialized publications (Garson, 1990; Hesselson, 2003; Crossley *et al.*, 2011) as well as those of scientific societies (Recommended General Bibliography p. xvii). We will now comment only briefly on some different aspects of pacemaker complications.

Pacemaker complications

The complications include those related to implantation, those related to dysfunction of some components of the pacing system, the pacemaker-induced arrhythmias, the pacemaker syndrome and the pacemaker system infection.

Implant-related complications
These are very infrequent in experimented implanters. Only qualified physicians should undertake pacemaker

(or ICD, CRT) implantation. The pacemakers are now nearly always implanted transvenously. The insertion of a transvenous pacing catheter and the creation of the pocket for the pulse generator do not usually require difficult surgical procedures. Although multiple venous routes have been used for lead placement, the subclavian vein is most commonly used. Potential, but rare, complications include pneumothorax, subcutaneous emphysema, vein thrombosis, and the most dangerous, cardiac tamponade due to lead perforation, among others. (For more information consult the Recommended General Bibliography p. xvii.) More recently, the "leadless" pacemaker has been released. This is a small device that is inserted via the femoral vein using a long introducer. It is deployed in the apex of the right ventricle, and then the system is retrieved via the femoral vein. It allows sensing and pacing in the RV and it is indicated when accessing the subclavian is not possible or when having leads in the venous system is contraindicated. Both, St Jude and Medtronic have released their products and two large trials are ongoing (Reddy *et al.*, 2015).

Pacemaker dysfunction

In pacemaker-dependent patients, a dysfunction due to a failure of a component of the pacemaker may induce syncope, hemodynamic disorders, and even SD. Therefore, early detection is very important. There are many different reasons for pacemaker dysfunction. We shall briefly look at some electrocardiographic clues that may reveal different pacemaker dysfunctions due to stimulation and sensing problems, which usually are due to badly positioned or fractured leads. Further information on the subject can be found elsewhere (Hesselson, 2003; Barold *et al.*, 2006a, 2008; Hayes *et al.*, 2008; Recommended General Bibliography p. xvii. A full book on these issues was written by Oswaldo Gutierrez and can be found in the SIAC website (www.siacardio.com)).

Pacemaker stimulation problems

These are generally due to failure of spike generation or transmission. Spikes are generally assessed through a signal-averaging analysis, which allows for identification of the most important abnormalities. It is particularly important to check the changes of voltage, as well as the spike duration and transmission. Impedance measurement also helps to diagnose these problems. The most important stimulation problems occur in the following situations:

o The spike falls outside the myocardial refractory period and, therefore, has the potential to stimulate. Despite this, it is not followed by a QRS complex, due to an exit block (Figure 6.38).
o The spike is not permanently or intermittently detected (Figure 6.44).

o Sometimes a spike presenting a different morphology initiates a subthreshold stimulation (Figure 6.43).
o In many leads, spike polarity changes are observed (it may be normal if occurring in only one lead), initiating an exit block and occasionally a sensing problem (Figure 6.45). In the Holter ECG recording, spike polarity changes frequently occur, although generally they are not clinically significant.
o This function of the device can be easily tested with the magnet function (place a magnet on top of the device and sensing will be inhibited). After each spike, a paced QRS should be seen at a rate of 100 bpm × 3 beats and then back to the magnetic rate ~85 bpm).

Pacemaker sensing problems

Different pacemaker malfunctions can be manifested as oversensing or undersensing.

A. Oversensing occurs when the generator responds to signs different from the QRS complex (or the P wave in the case of atrial pacemakers), which leads the pacemaker discharge rate to be prolonged because other signs are inappropriately perceived. Some of the reasons are:
   o The T wave is sensed (t-wave oversensing (Baranchuk *et al.*, 2007; Almehairi *et al.*, 2015).
   o The pacemaker wire is partially broken and sensing any type of muscle fasciculation.
   o Interference of myopotentials produced by pectoral muscle contractions (the most common form of oversensing). The pacemaker senses the muscle contraction as an intrinsic cardiac activity and becomes inhibited (Figure 6.46).
   o External interference, such as electromagnetic or radio frequency interference (particular interest should be paid to electric blades during thoracic surgery in patients dependent on pacing).
   o Oversensing accounts for most of the cases of abnormal pauses observed in patients with permanent pacemakers.
B. Undersensing occurs when a pacemaker is unable to sense the underlying signal (either atrial or ventricular). This may be due to:
   o A failure in the pacemaker system (generator or electrode).
   o A cardiac problem generally related to a transitory or permanent QRS voltage decrease. The spike appears regularly, even though there are sinus QRS complexes. These QRS have not been sensed by the VVI system because of their low voltage (Figure 6.47).
   o Changes of the intrinsic signal such as in new myocardial infarct, hyperkalemia, hypothermia, and so on.
   o Programming defects (always test for the sensing of intrinsic signal when undersensing is detected).

o An electrode displacement that may occur early after implantation.

Pacemaker-induced arrhythmias (Figure 6.42)

The development of DDD-type dual chamber pacemakers involves the generation of an artificial reentry circuit. An anterograde loop comprises the dual chamber generator with the atrial sensor, whereas the retrograde arm is either the specific conduction system (SCS) or an accessory pathway allowing only retrograde conduction (Figure 6.42).

These circuits may account for the occurrence of pacemaker-mediated supraventricular tachycardias. Figure 6.42 explains how the tachycardia is initiated and perpetuated. During tachycardia, every pacemaker QRS complex is paced and there is ertroconduction to the atrium that is sense, triggering a new paced ventricular circuit. This problem may occur in DDD pacemakers if the pacemaker atrial refractory period (RP) is shorter than the duration of ventricle–atrial conduction. It has also been called endless-loop tachycardia (Baranchuk, 2013).

Several methods have been designed to prevent pacemaker-mediated tachycardias. Some models automatically prolong the atrial RP after sensing the ventricular premature extrasystole, a function which may be programmable. Generators have been designed to interrupt the tachycardia and restore the normal heart rate through a periodic ventricular impulse that transiently interrupts the AV conduction, leading to the reversion of the tachycardia. These tachycardias may be easily terminated by the application of a magnet over the pacemaker, thus inhibiting atrial sensing and producing an asynchronous stimulation. Next, it is necessary to reprogram the pacemaker and increase the atrial refractory period (PVARP).

On some occasions other supraventricular tachyarrhythmias may be triggered (fibrillation, flutter, etc.). Sometimes, an extracardiac cause is involved in the development of these arrhythmias (it may be triggered by myopotentials, magnets, electrocauterization, etc.).

With current lower output pacemakers, the risk of VF is practically zero, even though the electrical stimulus of the pacemaker may coincide with the patient's T wave (vulnerable ventricular period).

Frequently, ventricular extrasystoles are observed in patients with implantable pacemakers. Although they may disappear when heart rate increases, they often require antiarrhythmic treatment. Patients with a doubtful indication for pacemaker implantation are frequently taking antiarrhythmic agents that depress conduction and/or automaticity. This is an important factor when considering pacemaker implantation (see When a Pacemaker has to be Implanted).

Pacemaker syndrome

This is due to retrograde AV conduction that occurs particularly in type VVI pacemakers, causing a "negative atrial kick" that produces a more important hemodynamic impairment than simple loss of AV synchrony and include hypotension, fatigue, dizziness, and so on (see Choosing the Best Pacemaker in Different Clinical Settings) (Rodriguez *et al.*, 2014).

Pacemaker system infection

The overall incidence of infection is less than 1%. The most common clinical presentation is localized pocket infection. It may also present as erosion of part of the pacemaker system with secondary infection, or even a sepsis with or without positive blood culture, but often with vegetations found by echocardiography. Late infections are usually caused by staphylococcus epidermitis. In case of sepsis the treatment requires the removal of the entire infected pacing system by simple traction, other techniques (lasser-sheath, etc.) and even open surgical techniques (for more information see the Recommended General Bibliography p. xvii). Pacemaker replacement carry on a risk of serious infection up to 3%. The more complex the procedure, for example, upgrading a pre-existent dual chamber ICD to a CRT-D device, the risk of infection increases, (depending on the series to approximately 8-10%). New, ongoing trials are testing different ways to prevent infection (Connolly *et al.*, 2013) by using pre, post or pre-post IV antibiotics and/or local antibiotics in the pocket before closing.

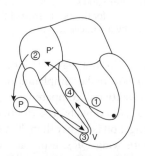
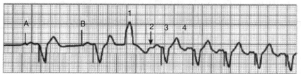

Figure 6.42 Diagram explaining how pacemaker-mediated (DDD) tachycardias are triggered. Note how after two impulses from a sequential pacemaker (A and B), a PVC (1) is conducted retrogradely to the atrium. The retrograde P (2) is sensed by the pacemaker, generating, after a delay in the AV conduction, a new paced QRS complex (3) that may be retrogradely conducted again (4), perpetuating the repetitive phenomenon of the tachycardia. In the case of a VVI pacemaker no tachycardia would occur, because this type of pacemaker does not sense the atria (Table 6.4), preventing the occurrence of subsequent QRS stimulation.

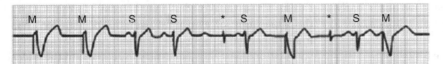

Figure 6.43 Pacemaker complexes (M) alternating with sinus complexes (S). Two different spikes (*) are observed, with a subthreshold stimulation not followed by QRS.

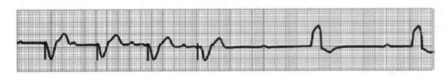

Figure 6.44 After four pacemaker complexes, the spike is not observed and a very slow escape rhythm appears, probably due to cable rupture.

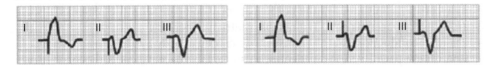

Figure 6.45 Significant changes of spike polarity in many leads. This is an abnormal pattern.

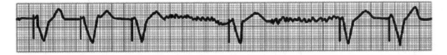

Figure 6.46 Example of oversensing: typical interference by myopotentials. The pacemaker perceives the muscular contraction to be intrinsic activity and becomes inhibited.

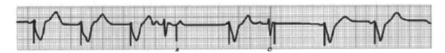

Figure 6.47 Example of undersensing. Sensing failure in a patient with a VVI pacemaker. The fourth and sixth spikes fall on the ST of prior complexes and are not followed by new QRS as the myocardium is in refractory period. The reason for the occurrence of these spikes is the failure in the detection of prior QRS because they have a low voltage that is not perceived by the pacemaker.

Clinical, Prognostic, and Therapeutic Implications of Passive Arrhythmias

Clinical and Prognostic Implications

1) In patients with physiologic sinus bradycardia, the heart rate progressively accelerates with exercise and emotions, and decelerates during rest and sleep. It also presents certain RR interval variability due to the vagal modulation of the heart rate, which increases with breathing. Occasionally, the heart rate variability is greatly increased, evolving into an arrhythmia that is usually not severe because it does not involve significant pauses (Figure 6.7). In contrast, it is known that a decreased heart rate variability (HRV) (<50 ms) is associated with a worse prognosis in different types of patients (post-infarction or HF patients, etc.).

2) The prospective Framingham study (Cheng *et al.*, 2009), which included a follow-up period of more than 20 years, has demonstrated that patients with first-degree

AV block have a twofold higher risk of AF, a threefold higher risk of pacemaker implantation, and a slight increase in mortality risk compared with patients in the control group. Additionally, risk increases if the PR interval prolongation is higher than 20 ms/year.

3) In patients with wide QRS, especially with advanced LBBB or bifascicular block, the mortality rate is higher than in the general population due to a higher incidence of advanced heart disease, HF or renal failure. Masked bifascicular block is particularly associated with a worse prognosis (see Chapter 10, High Risk Ventricular Block). One study (Marti-Almor *et al.*, 2009) demonstrated that the overall mortality rate in patients with chronic bifascicular block is lower than expected (a 2-year mortality rate of 6%) and that the most important mortality predictive factors are advanced heart disease and renal failure. An ongoing trial (Krahn *et al.*, 2012) is testing whether patients with bifascicular block and syncope would benefit from pacemaker implantation and no further testing or an implantable loop recorder (ILR) would

be necessary to determine whether and advanced form of AV block is responsible for the symptoms.

4) The differential diagnosis of very slow sinus bradycardia with third-degree AV block is essentially made by electrocardiography. However, it may be presumed from palpation of a very slow pulse rate that does not increase with exercise and by cardiac auscultation of the first heart sound of variable intensity (the cannon first heart sound). It may also be detected by inspection of the venous pulse, as a cannon wave that has a different electrophysiologic explanation from the cannon first heart sound (see Chapter 1, The Physical Examination). These physical explorations may still be useful for clinicians and do not have to be left behind in cardiology history (Garrat *et al.*, 1994).

5) he incidence of partial interatrial block increases with age. In a general population sample of individuals aged >65 years old, it was found that more than 50% of patients had a partial interatrial block (Spodick and Ariyarajah, 2008, 2009). It has been demonstrated that these patients present a greater incidence of AF in a long follow-up (Holmqvist *et al.*, 2009) (see Chapter 4, New Concepts).

6) The prevalence of patients with advanced IAB increases with age, being 8% in the 70s to 25% in centenarians. Furthermore, patients with A-IAB present higher incidence of dementia and stroke (Martínez-Sellés *et al.*, 2016). Also, patients with advanced interatrial block with left atrial retrograde conduction (P ± in leads II, III, VF) usually have supraventricular paroxysmal arrhythmias, atrial fibrillation/flutter, which constitutes an arrhythmologic syndrome named Bayes Syndrome (Conde and Baranchuk, 2014a, 2014b; Conde *et al.*, 2015; Bacharova and Wagner, 2015; Bayés de Luna *et al.*, 1988a; Sadiq *et al.*, 2015) (Chapter 10, Advanced Interatrial Block with Left Atrial Retrograde Conduction). Thus, its presence may be considered a risk marker for future tachyarrhythmia and, consequently, the administration of a preventive antithrombotic treatment to avoid stroke and arrhythmias may be recommended if its efficacy is demonstrated in a trial. It is not clear that a treatment to avoid atrial fibrillation may be useful.

7) Sudden death secondary to bradyarrhythmias may be due to: (i) a progressive depression of sinus and AV junctional automaticity, often related to an electro-mechanic dissociation in patients with MI or cardiogenic shock with a progressively slower escape rhythm (Figure 6.5); and (ii) an advanced AV block.

8) The diagnosis of AV block as the cause of symptoms such as dizziness or even syncope is suspected when the ECG shows an advanced LBBB or a bifascicular block, especially with long PR interval. In this case, the demonstration by electrophysiologic studies (EPS) that the long PR interval is due to an infrahisian block may lead us to think that symptoms may be attributed to an advanced paroxysmal AV block. Confirmation of level of block by EPS is currently not recommended as patient are candidates to pacemaker regardless the level of block.

9) The passive arrhythmias may be due to different etiologies.

A. Acute ischemic heart disease. The impairment of perfusion in some part of the SCS and/or the vagal overdrive that may be present in acute MI may explain the appearance of some passive arrhythmias, including:

o Sinus bradycardia, which occurs very frequently, particularly in patients with MI involving the inferior wall of the heart (Chapter 11, Ischemic Heart Disease).

o In the acute phase of MI, partial AV block progressing to a complete AV block may occur, especially in acute MI of the inferior wall of the heart, due to the occlusion of the right coronary artery (generally one of its branches perfuses the AV node). It is usually a transient suprahisian block, frequently due to a great vagal overdrive, therefore not usually requiring pacemaker implantation. However, when AV block occurs during acute anterior MI, the area involved is usually greater, and an advanced infrahisian AV block may occur abruptly. In the latter, bradyarrhythmic escape rhythm is slower and pacemaker implantation is often urgent. Prognosis is poorer due to a greater extension of infarction.

o An advanced RBBB may be observed in patients with occlusion of the left anterior descending coronary artery above the first septal branch, the artery perfusing the RBB.

o Even in the case of acute ischemia in the absence of infarction (i.e., spasm of the right coronary artery proximal to the artery that perfuses the AV node), a transient AV block may be seen (Figure 6.48).

o The appearance of AV block during exercise has been considered suggestive of ischemic origin. This is not always the case, however (Wissocq *et al.*, 2009).

B. Chronic ischemic heart disease, valvular heart disease, cardiomyopathies, and congenital heart disease may induce not only frequent paroxysmal active arrhythmias but also different types of passive arrhythmias. Occasionally these passive arrhythmias are worsened by the depressive effect of some drugs on the SCS.

C. Progressive blocks of the SCS may also occur in relatively young subjects without evidence of heart

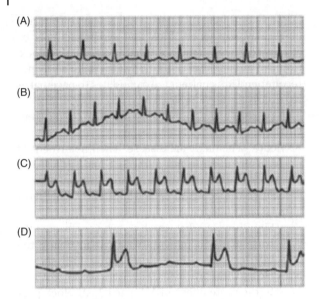

Figure 6.48 Exercise stress test in a patient with precordial anginal pain. Before the test (A) and at the end (B), the ST segment is normal. A few minutes later a coronary spasm is observed with significant ST elevation associated with precordial pain (C), followed by a transient AV block (D).

disease due to familial SCS structural disorders (Lenegre syndrome) (see Chapter 9, Specific Conduction System Involvement: Lenegre Syndrome).

D. Atrioventricular or ventricular blocks without evidence of heart disease may occur in elderly people due to SCS degenerative intrinsic disease (Lev disease) (see Chapter 9, Specific Conduction System Involvement: Lenegre Syndrome).

E. Cases of AV block and/or intraventricular block may be found after surgery for aortic valve disease or different congenital heart diseases. Peripheral RBBB is the rule after surgery of Fallot's tetralogy (see Chapter 11, Congenital Heart Disease).

F. Some degenerative and inflammatory diseases may provoke different types of AV block. One case of SD due to acute AV block in a child with influenza A virus associated to fulminant myocarditis has been reported (Bratincsák *et al.*, 2010).

G. Rheumatic fever, unfortunately still frequent in many developing countries, may result in different degrees of AV block, especially transient first-degree AV block (long PR interval).

H. The occurrence of AV junctional escape impulses at their normal discharge rate should not be considered pathologic. They are frequent in athletes or in subjects with a significant vagal overdrive. In fact, they warrant protection against a slow rhythm. If depression of the AV junction automaticity does not occur, the implantation of a pacemaker is not urgent and probably not necessary. Some athletes and subjects with pronounced vagal overdrive may show significant sinus bradycardia and/or even second-degree AV block (Wenckebach-type) during rest and sleep (see Chapter 11, Athletes). Atrioventricular block in the absence of marked bradycardia is indicative of a left vagus overdrive predominance (Figure 6.6).

I. A new alternative to treat aortic stenosis via transfemoral approach (TAVI) carries on the risk of complete AV block, particularly those with pre-existent LBBB (Schwerg *et al.*, 2013).

When a Pacemaker has to be Implanted

Which passive arrhythmias (sinus bradycardia, sinoatrial and AV block, and high-risk ventricular blocks) require pacemaker implantation will now be discussed. The use of resynchronization pacemaker is discussed in Chapter 11 and the Appendix.

1) The requirement for pacemaker implantation is obviously urgent when the heart rate is very slow as a result of a sinus dysfunction (sick sinus syndrome and brady-tachy syndrome) (see Chapter 10, Severe Sinus Bradycardia) or AV block, and a slow junctional or ventricular escape rhythm occurs. In the case of slow ventricular rhythm the patient usually has severe symptoms (decreased cardiac output, dizziness, and even syncope, sometimes with Stokes–Adams episodes: transient abrupt loss of consciousness followed by the resumption of heart beats and flushing of the face). In many other circumstances the decision to implant a pacemaker is doubtful or not urgent (see below).

2) Physiologic sinus bradycardia should not be treated, and it even constitutes a good prognostic marker during the acute and chronic phases of ischemic heart disease (Bjeregaard, 1983). However, the implantation of a pacemaker may be considered in the presence of sinus bradycardia: (i) when sinus bradycardia is associated with pauses >3 s, (ii) when sinus rate does not appropriately accelerate with exercise, and (iii) when an abrupt twofold increase in heart rate occurs. This constitutes the evidence of a sinoatrial 2×1 block which disappears with exercise. The need for a pacemaker is especially evident when the bradycardia is due to a sinoatrial block and/or there are clinical signs of low cardiac output. The administration of drugs, or the presence of other factors such as concealed atrial extrasystoles, that may induce the development of important sinus bradycardia should be ruled out before taking the decision (Figures 6.8 and 7.3). In case of syncope, sometimes implanting a subcutaneous loop recorder to demonstrate the final cause of the symptom may be necessary.

3) Pacemaker implantation is not required in the presence of asymptomatic bifascicular block or advanced LBBB, especially if the PR interval is normal. However, it is recommended to carry out periodic monitoring according to the patient's clinical condition. In this group of patients the annual incidence of progression to advanced AV block is <1%. However, in the presence of syncopal episodes it is much higher (≈10%) (McAnulty *et al.*, 1982). Thus, an EPS is recommended in patients with advanced LBBB or bifascicular block, in the presence of alerting symptoms such as dizziness and syncope, especially if PR interval is long, to confirm if an infrahisian block exists. Other tests (tilt test, see Appendix A3, Tilt table test, etc.) may be carried out to determine the origin of symptoms and to help to take the appropriate decision.

4) Evidence of trifascicular block (Rosenbaum syndrome) or bilateral block (see Chapter 10, High-risk Ventricular Block) requires, without any other test, prompt pacemaker implantation, considered urgent in the presence of symptoms.

5) Pacemaker implantation is clearly not indicated in the case of asymptomatic isolated first-degree AV block, but the patient should be routinely followed-up (see Clinical and Prognostic Implications) However, if during exercise testing the PR interval shortens, it is indicative of a vagal origin. It is also important to determine whether paroxysmal blocks in the Holter ECG recording exist.

6) On occasion, a second-degree Mobitz II-type AV block is associated with block of more than one or two P waves (paroxysmal AV block) (Figure 6.19). In these situations, syncope may occur, and pacemaker implantation is required. It is impossible to know when new episodes will occur or what the rate of the escape rhythm will be (Rosenbaum *et al.*, 1973; Lee *et al.*, 2009).

7) In other cases of second-degree AV block where no severe symptoms are present and no more than one P wave is blocked, pacemaker implantation is usually not urgent. However, further studies (Holter ECG, EPS, etc.), may recommend it. In some young asymptomatic subjects with significant vagal overdrive, episodes of second-degree AV block (Wenckebach-type) occur only during rest or sleep. This is not a serious condition, thus pacemaker implantation is not required. However, a periodic follow-up is recommended (Figure 6.6).

8) We have already established that in advanced AV block pacemaker implantation is mandatory, although there are some exceptions. Such is the case of the AV block that appears in acute inferior MI and is usually transient, and also in transient AV block that occurs in acute ischemia due to right coronary spasm (Figure 6.48). In congenital AV block, pacemaker implantation largely depends on the rate of the escape rhythm (Figures 6.23 and 10.15). Pacemaker implantation, even in the absence of symptoms, is recommended, due to the potential risk of SD (Friedman, 1995), if there is a mean heart rate during exercise <100 bpm, and in Holter ECG recording evidence of slow escape rhythm (<35 bpm at night), and mean heart rate <45–50 bpm or evidence of abnormalities of QT interval, or an important ventricular arrhythmias (see Chapter 10, Advanced AV block).

9) Slow escape rhythm or bradyarrhythmias, including cases of slow AF and bradycardia-tachycardia syndrome (Chapter 10, Advanced Atrioventricular Block), frequently present alarming symptoms, such as dizziness or even syncope. There is usually time for pacemaker implantation, a measure that will not only prevent SD but also improve patient quality of life.

10) In contrast, pacemaker implantation is sometimes indicated even in AF that sometimes presents a fast ventricular rate where drug therapy to block the AV conduction is needed. However, this treatment is not possible because at times during the day or night the ventricular rate is spontaneously very slow. Pacemaker implantation allows for the administration of appropriate drugs because the patient is then protected from inadequate slow rhythm. If the ventricular rate is not controlled with drugs, AV node ablation may also be necessary.

11) The treatment of passive arrhythmias, including pacing indications, in the acute phase of MI, is shown in Table 11.1.

Choosing the Best Pacemaker in Different Clinical Settings *(Figures 6.49 and 6.50)*

We must consider: (i) the appropriate pacemaker function for each case and (ii) implantation protocols.

Appropriate pacemaker function for each case

The appropriate pacemaker function depends on many factors:

- **Preservation of normal atrial contraction and an appropriate AV conduction synchrony**.
  An appropriate atrial contraction does not occur in the presence of advanced interatrial block with retrograde left atrial activation (P± leads II, III, VF). In this situation, the atrial electrode should be preferentially located in the upper septal region, so that both atria may depolarize at the same time.
  An appropriate AV synchrony is very important, as without it atria contracts against closed AV valves and venous

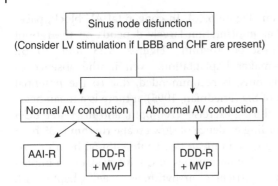

Figure 6.49 Decision tree. Selection of stimulation mode in sinus node dysfunction. AAIR: AAI with rate response; DDD: dual chamber; DDDR: dual chamber with rate response; LVF: left ventricular function; HF: heart failure; MVP: algorithms minimizing ventricular pacing, allowing for maximum stimulation from the specific conduction system (see Implantation protocols and Nielsen DANPACE TRIAL 2010).

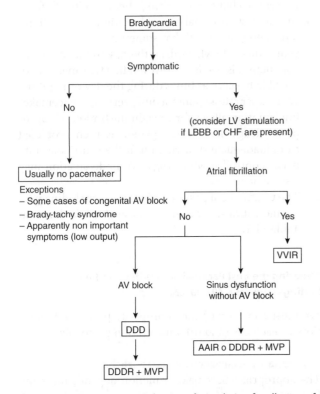

Figure 6.50 Decision tree. Selection of stimulation for all cases of bradycardia, regardless of their origin (see Figure 6.49, and Implantation protocols).

congestion occurs. The inadequate timing of atrial and ventricular contractions may set off a constellation of signs and symptoms known as pacemaker syndrome (see Pacemaker Complications). This includes a decreased cardiac output, hypotension, fatigue, exercise intolerance, dizziness, lightheadedness, and even near-syncope. **Pacemaker syndrome** usually occurs when stimulation is VVI with 1×1 retrograde AV conduction.

Retrograde AV conduction causes a "negative atrial kick" with a more profound hemodynamic disadvantage than simple loss of AV synchrony. Pacemaker syndrome may also occur in the presence of VDD stimulation with retrograde conduction, and also in the case of DDD pacemakers with inappropriate AV synchrony due to incorrect programming. Pacemaker syndrome due to VVI pacing with AV 1×1 conduction can be eliminated by restoring AV synchrony with atrial pacing, if AV conduction is normal, or dual-chamber pacing with an appropriate AV delay.

- **Preservation of the normal ventricular activation sequence**

Changes in this sequence originated by pacemaker stimulation in the right ventricular apex or in the case of advanced LBBB may induce hemodynamic alterations and even trigger heart failure (Stockburger *et al.*, 2009; Tops *et al.*, 2009). In consequence, when the AV conduction is normal, maintenance of a normal ventricular activation sequence is recommended. In the case of sick sinus syndrome this may be achieved by monocameral atrial pacing usually with rate-responsive capability (AAI-R) because there is cronotropic incompetence, and by dual chamber rate-responsive (DDDR) pacing (Table 6.3 and Figure 6.49). The rate of progressive AV block in patients with sinus node dysfunction has already been explained, and this is why AAIR pacemakers are rarely used. Dual chamber rate-responsive pacing maintains the AV synchrony but it is not a physiologic pacing modality. When dual chamber pacemakers pace the RV unnecessarily, the incidences of AF and HF increase. New pacing algorithms were designed to avoid unnecessary RV pacing. Hence, in patients with sick sinus syndrome requiring DDDR pacing (i.e., AV block), implanting a pacemaker with algorithms allowing a maximum pacing through the normal SCS, so that the pacing ventricular stimulation is kept to a minimum, is recommended (algorithms minimizing ventricular pacing (MVP)) (Figure 6.49). However, in patients with normal AV conduction and no left bundle branch block or other severe complication, it has been demonstrated in a long follow-up trial (Nielsen, 2010) that although there is no difference in mortality in either group (AAI-R and DDD-R) the number of crises of paroxysmal AF and of reintervention was lower in the group of DDD-R. Furthermore, the DDD pacemaker protects from the small possibility (≈2% of annual risk) of future AV block development (see Implantation Protocols). It is important to note that in current dual chamber pacemakers, the mode of pacing is automatically adjusted in response to the stability of intrinsic conduction. For example, a patient with sick sinus syndrome will be pacing predominantly in AAI-r mode, however; if paroxysmal AV block occurs, it will automatically switch to DDD-R mode in order to provide ventricular support.

There is considerable evidence (Zhang *et al.*, 2008; Sanna *et al.*, 2009) that apical right ventricular pacing (ARVP) originates abnormal heart contractions, and favors left ventricular dysfunction and HF. In patients with normal EF, in a 12-month follow-up, ARVP induces adverse LV remodeling and a decrease in EF when compared with biventricular pacing (Yu *et al.*, 2009). Some authors believe that from a hemodynamic point of view, stimulation from the right ventricular outflow tract may be better than that from the right ventricular apex (Cock *et al.*, 2003). It has been shown that even survival may improve (Vanerio *et al.*, 2008). The parahisian technique is appropriate to preserve a physiologic AV synchrony and prevent inter- and intraventricular asynchrony (Occhetta *et al.*, 2006). Further improvement in the use of appropriate electrodes to stimulate the His region will minimize the current technical limitations.

Therefore, in patients with LBBB and/or depressed ventricular function requiring pacemaker implantation, biventricular pacing should be recommended. Pacing should reach the LV through the coronary sinus via a cardiac vein contacting the left ventricular lateral wall (Cazeau *et al.*, 2001). This leads to resynchronization of the cardiac activation (CRT) and prevents abnormal activation (LBBB-type), occurring with right ventricular activation (Moss *et al.*, 2009) (see Chapter 11 and Appendix A-4.2 Pacemakers).

- **Maintenance of a normal physiologic chronotropic function**

  This currently may be achieved with modern technologies (progressive rate-responsive pacemakers) (AAI-R, VVI-R and DDD-R) (Vardas *et al.*, 2007).

Implantation protocols

Different protocols, including guidelines for implantation and selection of the appropiate cardiac pacemakers, are now available (see guidelines scientific societies, Recommended General Bibliography p. xvii; Vardas *et al.*, 2007; Epstein *et al.*, 2008; Martínez Ferrer *et al.*, 2009).

Figures 6.49 and 6.50 show the respective algorithms used to determine the best pacemaker for sick sinus syndrome and bradycardia due to any cause.

o In patients with sick sinus syndrome without AV block, the first choice of pacing currently after the DANPACE trial (Nielsen, 2010) is probably the DDD-R (Figure 6.49). Furthermore, the AAI-R has the inconvenience that eventually AV block may occur. However, if AV block is not present at the time of implantation (a progressive atrial stimulation warranting a 1×1 AV conduction up to a rate of 140 bpm should be made), the annual risk of AV block is 2%.

o When symptomatic bradycardia occurs in the presence of slow AF, VVIR mode pacemakers are the most widely used option (Figure 6.50). In patients with AV block and normal sinus function, DDD pacemakers are the first choice. In the presence of sinus node dysfunction, a DDDR pacemaker with MVP function should be implanted (Figure 6.50).

Passive arrhythmias

- Passive arrhythmias include both decreased sinus automaticity and all block types: sinoatrial blocks, atrial blocks, AV blocks, and ventricular blocks.

- A hisiogram is necessary to establish the precise location of the AV blocks (see Appendix A-3, Intracavitary ECGs and Electrophysiologic Studies).

- Athletes and vagotonic subjects may alternate tachycardia during daytime activities and bradycardia (sometimes very significant), or even second-degree Wenckebach-type AV block, at night.

- Surface ECG allows for the correct diagnosis of the different types of SA blocks, atrial blocks, AV blocks, first-, second-, and third-degree ventricular blocks (except first-degree SA blocks) (Figure 6.9), as well as passive arrhythmias due to depressed sinus automaticity.

- In some cases of bradycardia, the ECG is especially useful to reach the differential diagnosis between active and passive arrhythmias. Figure 6.12 shows an ECG recording of bigeminal rhythm, where a 3×2 sinoatrial block may be distinguished from parasinus bigeminy. Figure 6.8 shows how a slow rhythm may be explained by a concealed atrial bigeminy (active arrhythmia).

- In patients with terminal heart failure from any cause, the most frequent cause of SD is a progressive depression of automaticity leading to a cardiac arrest.

- The ECG allows the type of implanted pacemaker to be identified, and pacemaker dysfunctions, and stimulation and sensing problems, to be detected.

- The correct function of pacemakers depends on: (i) the maintenance of a normal atrial activation sequence and AV synchrony, (ii) the preservation of a normal ventricular activation sequence, and (iii) the preservation of a chronotropic physiologic function.

- In the case of slow heart rate (regardless of its origin) leading to low cardiac output or symptoms that may progress to a syncope, or those representing a high risk of SD, pacemaker implantation is mandatory and often should be carried out immediately.

Self Assessment

A. Define the escape complex and describe its electrocardiographic characteristics.

B. How can decreased heart rate (bradycardia) be accounted for when the AV junctional conduction speed is not reduced (normal PR interval)?

C. What are the diagnostic key points used to identify second-degree sinoatrial blocks (Wenckebach-type), and why is the differential diagnosis of the sinoatrial junction block much more complicated than that of the atrioventricular junction block?

D. What is the difference between a bigeminal sequence due to a 3×2 SA block and a bigeminal sequence resulting from parasinus atrial bigeminy?

E. Describe the diagnostic criteria used to identify advanced interatrial block.

F. How is AV junctional Wenckebach phenomenon diagnosed?

G. What characteristics of intracavitary ECG permit a differential diagnosis in suprahisian, infrahisian, and intrahisian AV blocks?

H. Describe the diagnostic criteria used to identify advanced or third-degree LBB.

I. Which are the components of the pacemaker ECG?

J. What are the three- and five-letter codes?

K. What are the main types of sequential pacemakers?

L. Define resynchronization pacemakers and explain their specific indications.

M. Discuss the most important forms of dysfunction in pacemakers.

N. What are pacemaker-induced arrhythmias?

O. When should a pacemaker be implanted?

P. What is the best pacemaker for different clinical settings?

Q. May apical right ventricular pacing favour left ventricular dysfunction?

References

Almehairi M, Somani R, Ellenbogen K, *et al*. Inappropriate detection of ventricular fibrillation in the presence of T-wave oversensing algorithm. PACE 2015;38(3):407.

Amat y Leon F, Chuquimia R, Wu D, *et al*. Alternating Wenckebach periodicity: a common electrophysiologic response. Am J Cardiol 1975;36:757.

Andersen HR, Nielsen JC, Thomsen PE, *et al*. Atrioventricular conduction during long-term follow-up of patients with sick sinus syndrome. Circulation 1998;98(13):1351.

Ariyarajah V, Puri P, Apiyasawat S, *et al*. Interatrial block: a novel risk factor for embolic stroke? Ann Noninvasive Electrophysiol 2007;12:15.

Auricchio A, Fantoni C, Regoli F, *et al*. Characterization of left ventricular activation in patients with heart failure and left bundle-branch block. Circulation 2004;109:1133.

Bacharova L, Wagner GS. The time for naming the interatrial block Syndrome: Bayes Syndrome. J Electrocardiol 2015;48:133.

Baranchuk A. Atlas of advanced ECG interpretation. REMEDICA, London, UK, 2013.

Baranchuk A, Ribas S, Divakaramenon S, Morillo CA. An unusual mechanism causing inappropriate implantable cardioverter defibrillator shocks: transient reduction in R-wave amplitude. Europace 2007;9(8):694.

Baranchuk A, Enriquez A, García-Niebla J, *et al*. Differential diagnosis of rSr′ pattern in leads V1-V2. Comprehensive review and proposed algorithm. Ann Noninvasive Electrocardiol 2015;20(1):7.

Bardy G, Lee K, Mark D, *et al*. Home use of automated external defibrillators for cardiac arrest. N Eng J Med. 2008;358:1793.

Barold SS, Giudici MC, Herweg B, *et al*. Diagnostic value of the 12-lead electrocardiogram during conventional and biventricular pacing for cardiac resynchronization. Cardiol Clin 2006a;24:471.

Barold SS, Herweg B, Curtis AB. Electrocardiographic diagnosis of myocardial infarction and ischemia during cardiac pacing. Cardiol Clin 2006b;24:387.

Barold SS. Cardiac pacemakers and resynchronizaiton therapy: Step by step. An illustrated guide, 2nd edn. John Wiley & Sons Ltd, Chichester, 2008.

Bayés de Luna A. Clinical Electrocardiography. John Wiley & Sons Ltd, Chichester, 2011.

Bayés de Luna A, Fiol-Sala M. Electrocardiography in ischemic heart disease. Clinical and imaging correlations and prognostic implications. Blackwell Futura, Oxford, 2008.

Bayés de Luna A, Fort de Ribot R, Trilla E, *et al*. Electrocariographic and vextorcardiographic study of interatrial conduction disturbances with left atrial retrograde activation. J Electrocardiol 1985;18:1.

Bayés de Luna A, Carrio I, Subirana MT, *et al*. Electrophysiological mechanisms of the SI SII SIII electrocardiographic morphology. J Electrocardiol 1987;20:38.

Bayés de Luna A, Cladellas M, Oter R, *et al*. Interatrial conduction block and retrograde activation of the left atrium and paroxysmal supraventricular tachyarrhythmia. Eur Heart J 1988a;9:1112.

Bayés de Luna A, Serra-Genis C, Gix M, *et al.* Septal fibrosis as determinant of Q wave in patients with aortic valve disease. Eur Heart J 1988b;4(Suppl E):86.

Bayés de Luna A, Torner P, Oter R, *et al.* Study of the evolution of masked bifascicular block. PACE 1988c;11:1517.

Bayés de Luna A, Cladellas M, Oter R, *et al.* Interatrial block with retrograde activation of the left atrium: Influence of preventive antiarrhythmic treatment. Int J Card 1989a;22:147.

Bayés de Luna A, Guindo J, Homs E, *et al.* Active vs. passive rhythms as an explanation of bigeminal rhythm with similar P waves. Chest 1991;99:735.

Bayés de Luna A, Platonov P, G. Cosio F, *et al.* Interatrial blocks. A separate entity from left atrial enlargement: a consensus report. J Electrocardiol 2012a;45:445.

Bayés de Luna A, Pérez-Riera A, Baranchuk A, *et al.* Electrocardiographic manifestation of the middle fibers/septal fascicle block. A consensus report. J Electrocardiol 2012b; 45: 454.

Bjeregaard P. Incidencia y significacion clinica de las bradiarritmias en individuos sanos. Rev Latina Card 1983;4:47.

Bratincsák A, El-Said HG, Bradley JS, *et al.* Fulminant myocarditis associated with pandemic H1N1 influenza A virus in children. J Am Coll Cardiol 2010;55:928.

Bredikis JJ, Stirbys P. A suggested code for permanent cardiac pacing leads. Pacing Clin Electrophysiol 1985 8:320.

Cazeau S, Leclercq C, Lavergne T, *et al.* Effects of multisite biventricular pacing in patients with heart failure and intraventricular conduction delay. N Engl J Med 2001;344:873.

Cheng S, Keyes M, Larson M, *et al.* Long-term outcomes in individuals with prolonged PR interval. JAMA 2009;301;2571.

Chiale PA, Pastori JD, Garro HA, *et al.* Reversal of primary and pseudo-primary T wave abnormalities by ventricular pacing. A novel manifestation of cardiac memory. J Interv Card Electrophysiol 2010;28(1):23.

Chung EK. Aberrant atrial conduction. Unrecognized electrodardiographic entity. Br Heart J 1972;34:341.

Cock CC, Giudici MC, Twisk JW. Comparison of the haemodynamic effects of right ventricular outflow-tract pacing with right ventricular apex pacing: a quantitative review. Europace 2003;5:275.

Conde D, Baranchuk A. Bloqueo interauricular como sustrato anatómico-eléctrico de arritmias supreventriculares: Sindrome de Bayés. Arch Cardiol Mex 2014a;84(1):32.

Conde D, Baranchuk A. What a cardiologist must know about Bayes's Syndrome. Rev Argent Cardiol 2014b;82:220.

Conde D, Baranchuk A, Bayés de Luna A. Advanced interatrial block as a substrate of supraventricular tachyarrhythmias: a well recognized syndrome. J Electrocardiol 2015;48:135.

Connolly SJ, Philippon F, Longtin Y, *et al.* Randomized cluster crossover trials for reliable, efficient, comparative effectiveness testing: design of the Prevention of Arrhythmia Device Infection Trial (PADIT). Can J Cardiol 2013;29(6):652.

Cosín J, Gimeno JV, Ramirez A, *et al.* Estudio experimental de los bloqueos parcelares de la rama derecha. Rev Esp Cardiol 1983;36:125.

Crossley GH, Poole JE, Rozner MA, *et al.* The Heart Rhythm Society (HSR)/American Society of Anesthesiologists (ASA) Expert Consensus Statement on the perioperative management of patients with implantable defibrillators, pacemakers and arrhythmia monitors; facilities and patient management this document was developed as a joint project with the American Society of Anesthesiologists (ASA), and in collaboration with the American Heart Association (AHA), and the Society of Thoracic Surgeons (STS). Heart Rhythm 2011;8(7):1114.

Daubert J-C. Atrial flutter and interatrial conduction block. In: Waldo A, Touboul P (eds) Atrial flutter: advances in mechanisms and management. Futura Publishing Company, New York, 1996, p. 331.

Enriquez A, Marano M, D'Amato A, *et al.* Second-degree interatrial block in hemodialysis patients. Case Rep Cardiol 2015; Article ID 468439. Epub 2015 Feb 10.

Epstein AE, DiMarco JP, Elenboge KA, *et al.* Guidelines for device-based therapy of cardiac rhythm abnormalities: a report of the American College of Cardiology/American Heart Association task force on practice guidelines (writing committee to revise the ACC/AHA/NASPE 2002 Guideline update for implantation of cardiac pacemakers and antiarrhythmia devices): developed in collaboration with the American Association for Thoracic Surgery and Society of Thoracic Surgeons. Circulation 2008;117:350.

Friedman RA. Congenital AV block. Pace me now or pace me later? Circulation 1995;92:283.

García-Niebla J, Sclarovski S. Wenckebach periods of alternate beats. In: Baranchuk A (ed) Atlas of advanced ECG interpretation. REMEDICA, London, UK, 2013, Chapter 4, case 25.

Garrat CJ, Griffith MJ, Young G, *et al.* Value of physical signs in the diagnosis of ventricular tachycardia. Circulation 1994;90:3103.

Garson A. Stepwise approach to the unknown pacemaker ECG. Am Heart J 1990;118:924.

Gasparini M, Auricchio A, Regoli F, *et al.* Four-year efficacy of cardiac resynchronization therapy on exercise tolerance and disease progression: the importance of performing atrioventricular junction ablation in patients with atrial fibrillation. J Am Coll Cardiol 2006;48:734.

Halpern MS, Nau GJ, Levi RJ, *et al.* Wenckebach periods of alternate beats. Clinical and experimental observations. Circulation 1973;48:41.

Hayes DL, Friedman PA. Cardiac pacing, defibrillation and resynchronization: A clinical approach, 2nd edn. John Wiley & Sons Ltd, Chichester, 2008.

Healey JS, Hohnloser SH, Exner DV, *et al.* Cardiac resynchronization therapy in patients with permanent atrial fibrillation: results from the Resynchronization for Ambulatory Heart Failure Trial (RAFT). Circ Heart Fail 2012;5(5):566.

Hesselson AB. Simplified interpretation of pacemaker ECGs. Futura/Blackwell Publishing, New York, 2003.

Hoffman I, Mehta J, Hilsenrath J, *et al.* Anterior conduction delay: a possible cause for prominent anterior QRS forces. J Electrocardiol 1976;9:15.

Holmqvist F, Platonov PG, Carlson J, *et al.* Altered interatrial conduction detected in MADIT II patients bound to develop atrial fibrillation. Ann Noninvasive Electrocardiol 2009;14:268.

Kasumoto FM, Goldschlager N. Cardiac pacing. N Engl J Med 1996;334:89.

Krahn AD, Morillo CA, Kus T, *et al.* Empiric pacemaker compared with a monitoring strategy in patients with syncope and bifascicular conduction block – rationale and design of the Syncope: Pacing or Recording in The Later Years (SPRINTELY) study. Europace 2012;14(7):1044.

Kulbertus HE, de Laval-Rutten F, Casters P. Vectorcardiographic study of aberrant conduction anterior displacement of QRS: another form of intraventricular block. Br Heart J 1976;38:549.

Lee S, Wellens HJJ, Josephson ME. Paroxysmal atrioventricular block. Heart Rhythm 2009;6:1229.

Marano M, D'Amato A, Bayés de Luna A, *et al.* Hemodialysis affects interatrial conduction. Ann Noninv Electrocardiol 2015;20(3):299.

Marti-Almor J, Cladellas M, Bazan V, *et al.* Long-term mortality predictors in patients with chronic bifascicular block. Europace 2009;11:1201.

Martínez Ferrer J, Fidalgo Andres ML, Barba Pichardo R, *et al.* Novedades en estimulacion cardiaca. Rev Esp Cardiol 2009;62:117.

Martínez-Sellés M, Massó-van Roessel A, Alvarez-García J, *et al.* Interatrial block and atrial arrhythmias in centenarians: prevalence, associations, and clinical implications. Heart Rhythm 2016;13:645.

McAnulty JH, Rahimtoola SH, Murphy E, *et al.* Natural history of "high-risk" bundle-branch block: final report of a prospective study. N Engl J Med 1982;307:137.

Moss AJ, Hall WJ, Cannom DS, *et al.* Cardiac-resynchronization therapy for the prevention of heart-failure events. N Engl J Med 2009;361:1329.

Nielsen JC. The Danish multicenter randomized trial on single atrial (AAAIR) versus dual chamber pacing in sick sinus syndrome. 2010. http://spo.escardio.org/eslides/view.aspx?eevtid=40&fp=3764 (last accessed 24 April 2017).

Occhetta E, Bortnik M, Magnani A, *et al.* Prevention of ventricular desynchronization by permanent para-hisian pacing after atrioventricular node ablation in chronic atrial fibrillation. J Am Coll Cardiol 2006;47:1938.

Parsonnet V, Furman S, Smyth NP. A revised code for pacemaker identification. Pacing Clin Electrophysiol 1981;4:400.

Pérez Riera A. Learning easily Frank vectorcardiogram. Editora e Graficas Mosteiro Ltda, Sao Paulo, 2009.

Pérez Riera AR, Baranchuk A, Chiale PA. About left septal fascicular block, Ann Noninv Electrocardiol 2015;20(2):202.

Pérez Riera AR, Barbosa-Barros R, Baranchuk A. Left septal fascicular block. Springer, 2016.

PAD Trial (Public Access Defibrillation Trial Investigators). Public access defibrillators and survival after out-of-hospital cardiac arrest. N Eng J Med 2004;351:637.

Reddy VY, Exner DV, Cantillon DJ, *et al.* Percutaneous implantation of an entirely intracardiac leadless pacemaker. N Engl J Med 2015;373:1125.

Rodriguez LD, Conde D, Baranchuk A. Pacemaker syndrome: an underdiagnosed cause of cardiac heart failure. Rev Insuf Card 2014;9(1):31.

Rosenbaum MB, Elizari MV. Los hemibloqueos. Editorial Paidos, Buenos Aires, 1968.

Rosenbaum MB, Elizari MV, Levi RJ, *et al.* Paroxysmal atrioventricular block related to hypopolarization and spontaneous diastolid depolarization. Chest 1973;63:678.

Rosenbaum MB, Blanco HH, Elizari MV, *et al.* Electrotonic modulation of the T wave and cardiac memory. Am J Cardiol 1982;50:213.

Sadiq Ali F, Enriquez A, Conde D, *et al.* Advanced interatrial block is a predictor of new onset atrial fibrillation in patients with severe heart failure and cardiac resynchroniztion therapy. Ann Noninv Electrophysiol 2015;20(6):586.

Sanna I, Franceschi F, Pevot S, *et al.* Right ventricular apex pacing: it is obsolete? Arch CV Dis 2009;102:135.

Schwerg M, Baldenhofer G, Dreger H, *et al.* Complete atrioventricular block after TAVI: when is pacemaker implantation safe? Pacing Clin Electrophysiol 2013;30(7):898.

Sodi-Pallares D, Calder R. New bases of electrocardiography. Mosby, St Louis, 1956.

Sodi-Pallares D, Bisteni A, Medrano G. Electrocardiografia y vectocardiografia deductivas. La Prensa Medica Mexicana, Mexico, 1964.

Spodick DH, Ariyarajah V. Interatrial block: a prevalent, widely neglected, and portentous abnormality. J Electrocardiol 2008;41:61.

Spodick DH, Ariyarajah V. Interatrial block: the pandemic remains poorly perceived. Pacing Clin Electrophysiol 2009;32:667.

Stavrakis S, Garabelli P, Reynolds DW. Cardiac resynchronization therapy after atrioventricular junction ablation for symptomatic atrial fibrillation: a meta-analysis. Europace 2012;14(10):1490.

Steinberg JS, Maniar PB, Higgins SL, *et al*. Noninvasive assessment of the biventricular pacing system. Ann Noninvasive Electrocardiol 2004;9:58.

Stockburger M, Celebi O, Krebs A, *et al*. Right ventricular pacing is associated with impaired overall survival, but not with an increased incidence of ventricular tachyarrhythmias in routine cardioverter/defibrillator recipients with reservedly programmed pacing. Europace 2009;11:924.

Strauss DG, Selvester RH, Wagner GS. Defining left bundle branch block in the era of cardiac resynchronization therapy. Am J Cardiol 2011;107:927.

Tops LF, Schalij MJ, Bax JJ. The effects of right ventricular apical pacing on ventricular function and dyssynchrony. J Am Coll Cardiol 2009;54:764.

Vanerio G, Vidal JL, Fernandez P, *et al*. Medium- and long-term survival after pacemaker implant: Improved survival with right ventricular outflow trac pacing. J Interv Card Electrophysiol 2008;21:195.

Vardas PE, Auricchio A, Blanc JJ, *et al*. Guidelines for cardiac pacing and cardiac resynchronization therapy: The Task Force for cardiac pacing and cardiac resynchronization therapy of the European Society of Cardiology. Developed in collaboration with the European Heart Rhythm Association. Eur Heart J 2007;28:2256.

Wissocq L, Ennezat PV, Mouquet F. Exercise-induced high-degree atrioventricular block. Arch Cardiovasc Dis 2009;102:733.

Yu CM, Chan JY, Zhang Q, *et al*. Biventricular pacing in patients with bradycardia and normal ejection fraction. N Engl J Med 2009;361:2123.

Zareba W, Klein H, Cygankiewicz I, *et al*. Effectiveness of cardiac resynchronization therapy by QRS morphology in the Multicenter Automatic Defibrillatior Implantation Trial-Cardiac Resynchronization Therapy (MADIT-CRT). Circulation 2011; 123(10):1061.

Zhang XH, Chen H, Sin CW, *et al*. New-onset heart failure after permanent right ventricular apical pacing in patients with acquired high-grade atrioventricular block and normal left ventricular function. J Cardio Electrophysiol 2008;18:136.

7

Analytical Study of an Arrhythmia

In this chapter, the different steps to be taken to properly diagnose an arrhythmia are discussed.

Determining the Presence of a Dominant Rhythm

It is generally easy to identify whether the dominant rhythm is of sinus or ectopic origin and, in this particular case, to know what kind of arrhythmia it is. Occasionally, however, it may be difficult to determine which rhythm is dominant, for instance:

o In the case of chaotic atrial tachycardia (see Figure 4.31). In this arrhythmia, by definition, there is no dominant rhythm (see Chapter 4, Chaotic Atrial Tachycardia).

o At times it may also be difficult to distinguish between sinus rhythm and 2:1 flutter (see Figure 4.20).

o In particular, when atrial rate is around 200 bpm. It is impossible to distinguish between atypical flutter and tachycardia due to an atrial macro-reentry (MAT-MR). In fact, these two arrhythmias may be considered the same (see Chapter 4, Atrial Flutter: ECG Findings).

o When atrial activity is not observed it may also be quite difficult to determine with certainty which is the dominant rhythm. In this case we can perform carotid sinus massage and other maneuvers (see Figure 4.10), or use T wave filtering techniques, if available (see Figure A-13).

Atrial Wave Analysis

Be Sure that the Atrial Activity is Visible in the Electrocardiogram (ECG)

In an ECG tracing with narrow or broad QRS tachycardia, relatively frequently atrial activity is not observed in the surface ECG because the atrial wave is hidden in the QRS complexes (see Figure 4.19A). On some occasions it may be useful to take an ECG during deep breathing (see Figure 4.10) or during carotid sinus compression (see Table 1.5). If, despite all these measures, the atrial wave is not seen, it is useful to use voltage amplification techniques (see Figure 4.38) and, if possible, to apply the T wave filter (Goldwasser *et al.*, 2008) (Figure A-13). However, the fact that no atrial activity is detected in the surface ECG even in the presence of slow heart rate is not conclusive evidence for atrial paralysis (see Figure 4.62), because the atrial rhythm may be concealed. Atrial paralysis is only confirmed when no atrial activity is observed in intracavitary ECGs.

Once Atrial Activity has been Determined

Several aspects of the atrial wave should be focused on when atrial activity has been determined.

Morphology and Polarity

The atrial wave morphology suggests sinus or ectopic origin. During sinus rhythm, it is positive in leads V2–V6 and I, and negative in lead VR; it is frequently ± in lead V1, whereas in rare cases it is ± in leads II, III, and VF (Bayés de Luna *et al.*, 1985); finally, it is negative or ± in VL.

In the case of monomorphic atrial tachycardia of ectopic focus (MAT-EF), the algorithm shown in Figure 4.15 allows us to localize the atrial origin of the ectopic P′ wave (Kistler *et al.*, 2006). On the other hand, a very narrow P wave (<0.06 s) is indicative of ectopic origin (see Figure 4.13), although it should be pointed out that many ectopic P′ waves are wide (see Figure 4.11).

F waves of atrial fibrillation (AF) show variable voltage from practically concealed to more than 2mm, and being more evident in V1 (see Figures 4.36 and 4.37). The frequency of F waves also is variable being the outcome of HF worse (Platonov *et al.*, 2012) in cases of low heart rate of "f" waves.

The typical common flutter waves display a sawtooth morphology with a predominant negative component in leads II, III, and VF (see Figure 4.57).

Figure 4.69 shows the morphology of atrial activation waves in the different supraventricular tachycardias with regular and monomorphic waves. In contrast, in Chapter 4

Clinical Arrhythmology, Second Edition. Antoni Bayés de Luna and Adrian Baranchuk.
© 2017 John Wiley & Sons Ltd. Published 2017 by John Wiley & Sons Ltd.

(Monomorphic Atrial Morphology), we describe the different atrial monomorphic and polymorphic activation waves typical of the different active supraventricular rhythms. In this regard, it should be remembered that P′ waves located after but close to the previous QRS complex are usually due to paroxysmal atrioventricular (AV) junctional re-entrant tachycardias (JRT) with accessory pathway involvement (see later). Finally, Figures 4.70 and 4.71 show the different algorithms that, depending on whether atrial activity is present or not, allow us to determine the type of active supraventricular arrhythmia with narrow QRS and regular or irregular RR. For the sake of convenience, those figures are also included in this chapter (Figures 7.1 and 7.2).

Cadence

The cadence of ectopic atrial activity may be regular or irregular. In sinus rhythm, the cadence is regular, although it usually presents a little variability, especially during respiration (see Chapter 4, Sinus Tachycardia). Ectopic atrial waves may show a regular or irregular cadence. The cadence of atrial activity is regular in all ectopic forms or reentrant tachycardias (of atrial or junctional origin) and in atrial flutter, whereas cadence is irregular in chaotic atrial tachycardia and AF (Figures 7.1 and 7.2). Relatively often, ectopic atrial tachycardias present some changes in the heart rate at the onset or end of the crisis (see below), in relation to some stimuli (exercise, etc.) or after some drugs (digitalis) (see Figure 11.13).

Rate

Sinus rate during rest is not usually faster than 80–90 bpm, although this rate may be higher in sympathetic overdrive or in different pathologic situations (fever, acute myocardial infarction, hyperthyroidism, heart failure, etc.). Exercise and emotions (see Figures 4.7 and 4.8) lead to a progressive increase of up to 180–200 bpm in young people, whereas a progressive slowing down is observed when the stimuli disappear. The rate is also increased in inappropriate sinus tachycardia and in sinus reentrant tachycardia (see Chapter 4, Sinus Tachycardia). The sinus rate during sleep or rest may be slower than 50 or even 40 bpm (see Chapter 6, Sinus Bradycardia Due to Sinus Automaticity Depression).

In MAT-EF, the P′ wave ranges between 100 and 200 bpm. In some cases its rate increases during exercise and at the onset of tachycardia (warming up) (see Table 4.6, and Figure 4.11).

In MAT-MR the atrial rate that usually is fast does not change with exercise. If it reaches ≈200 bpm, it may resemble an atypical flutter. In fact, both names probably correspond to the same arrhythmia (see Chapter 4, Atrial Flutter).

On the other hand, the rate of AF waves has prognostic implications. Platonov showed that in heart failure the presence of slow heart rate of AF waves is sign of good prognosis (Platonov *et al.*, 2012).

The rate of two types of AV junctional tachycardias due to reentrant mechanism (JRT), exclusively junctional and with accessory pathway is usually high (≈150–170 bpm).

The regular ventricular rate of an irregular atrial rhythm during atrial fibrillation is explained by AV dissociation and may be the consequence of the effect of some drugs (i.e., digoxin).

A not very fast but fixed rate (100–130 bpm) both during the day and night, supports diagnosis of ectopic rhythm (atrial tachycardia or 2:1 flutter instead of sinus rhythm) (see Figure 4.20).

A slow regular atrial rate (<60 bpm) is indicative of sinus bradycardia or, in rare cases, of a sinoatrial 2:1 block. In the latter case, the heart rate may double with exercise, whereas in sinus bradycardia the heart rate increases progressively.

Location of the Atrial Wave in the Cardiac Cycle (RR)

The sinus P wave and most MAT P′ waves precede the QRS complex, with a PR<RP relationship (Figure 4.19D).

In paroxysmal junctional tachycardias, where the reentrant circuit exclusively involves the AV junction (AVNRT or JRT-E), the P′ wave is located within the QRS complex (and is therefore not visible) or it is attached to its end, resulting in morphology distortion (Figure 4.19A and 4.19B). If the reentry involves an accessory pathway (AVRT or JRT-AP), the P′ follows the QRS complex closely so that, in the slow-fast tachycardia RP′ < P′R (Figure 4.19C), or the p′ may be located before the QRS (RP′>P′R) in the fast–slow type (Coumel type) (Figure 4.21).

In junctional ectopic tachycardia when there is VA conduction, the P′ may be located before or after, or be hidden within the QRS complex (see Chapter 4, AV junctional tachycardia due to ectopic focus).

QRS Complex Analysis

Width and Morphology

The QRS complexes may be narrow or wide.

Narrow QRS complexes are the result of normal ventricular activation due to sinus rhythm if they are preceded by a sinus P wave, or due to different types of supraventricular tachyarrhythmias (see Table 4.2). Narrow qRS complexes in the case of slow rates not preceded by sinus P waves correspond to junctional escape complexes or rhythm.

Wide QRS complexes may be the result of intraventricular aberrant conduction, over an accessory pathway, or due to ectopy (see later).

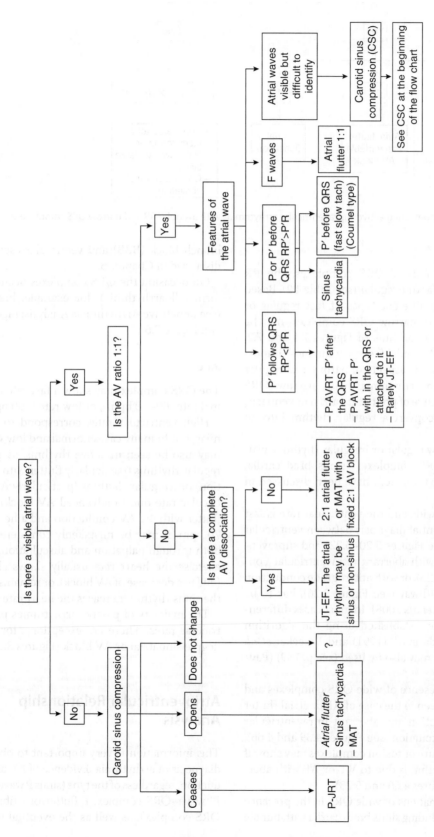

Figure 7.1 Algorithm for detecting active supraventricular arrhythmias with regular RR intervals and narrow QRS complexes.

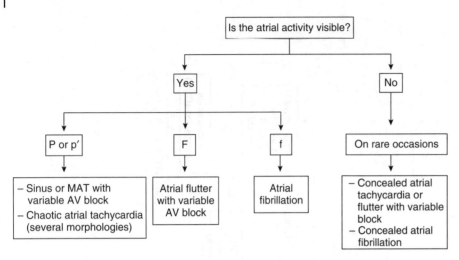

Figure 7.2 Algorithm for detecting active supraventricular arrhythmias with irregular RR and narrow QRS complexes.

Cadence

In the presence of narrow QRS complexes, the RR cadence may be regular or irregular (see Table 4.2). Based on this premise, the different types of fast regular or irregular rhythms with narrow QRS complexes may be diagnosed using the algorithms of Figures 7.1 and 7.2. Additionally, Tables 4.4 and 4.5 display the most important electrocardiographic aspects of paroxysmal regular supraventricular tachyarrhythmias with narrow QRS complexes. The presence of premature atrial or ventricular complexes may convert a regular rhythm into an irregular one.

All the types of slow regular or irregular rhythms, usually with narrow QRS complexes (sinus bradycardia, escape functional rhythm, etc.), have been discussed in Chapter 6.

When the QRS is wide and the ventricular rate is fast and regular, a differential diagnosis between ventricular tachycardia (VT) (see Figures 5.20–5.22) and supraventricular tachycardia with aberrant intraventricular conduction (see Figure 5.25), or with anterograde conduction over an accessory pathway (see Figure 5.26), has to be performed (Vereckei *et al.*, 2008). In most cases differential diagnosis may be established using the algorithm developed by Brugada *et al.* (1991) and Vereckei *et al.* (2014); other criteria may also be used (see p. 189) (Pava *et al.*, 2010).

Meanwhile, the presence of wide QRS complexes and irregular rhythm is seen in the case of AF or atrial flutter with variable conduction and aberrant intraventricular conduction or pre-excitation (see Figures 4.39 and 4.66). The presence of capture or fusion complexes may show if the fast irregular rhythm is due to VT or AF with aberrant conduction (Figures 4.66 and 5.23).

The possible explanations of wide QRS in the presence of slow heart rate, including sinus bradycardia with bundle branch block (BBB) and ventricular escape rhythm, are discussed in Chapter 6.

On occasion the QRS complexes occur in a repetitive form (alloarrhythmia), for example, bigeminal rhythm (see Repetitive Arrhythmias Analysis: Bigeminal Rhythm, and Figure 7.6).

Rate

The QRS complex may show a fast rate (>90 bpm), normal rate (60–90 bpm), or low rate (<60 bpm).

High ventricular rates correspond to active arrhythmias, but in many cases normal and low ventricular rates may also be seen in active rhythms, as is the case with regular rhythms (particularly flutter with 4:1 AV conduction) or irregular rhythms (particularly AF with low ventricular rate due to advanced AV block). In the case of flutter with 4:1 AV conduction and a heart rate of about 70 bpm, it may be mistakenly considered sinus rhythm both through palpation and auscultation. However, with exercise the heart rate usually shows abrupt increases (due to a decrease of AV block), or remains stable, whereas the sinus rhythm increases the heart rate progressively.

The majority of passive arrhythmias present low ventricular rates. There are exceptions, for example, first-degree sinoatrial or AV block (Figures 3.18A and 3.21A).

Atrioventricular Relationship Analysis

This information is very important to obtain the correct diagnosis of arrhythmia. Evidence of AV anterograde conduction, regardless of the type (sinus P wave–QRS complex, P′ wave–QRS complex, F flutter or f fibrillation waves–QRS complex), as well as the eventual ventriculo-atrial

(VA) retrograde activation, is often a key parameter to correctly diagnose properly the arrhythmias (Figure 7.1).

If no AV or VA relationship is observed, we may state that AV dissociation is present, which may be due to a block or interference (see Chapter 3, Decreased Conduction: Blocks). In the first case, the ventricular rate is slow, due to an advanced block or a complete block (see Figures 3.21D, 6.3, and 6.22), whereas in the second case the ventricular rate is fast. If the QRS is wide it is very suggestive of VT (see Figure 5.21). Less often, it may be due to junctional ectopic tachycardia with aberrant conduction.

Premature Complex Analysis

These may show normal or wide QRS morphology (aberrant or ventricular ectopy).

The most frequent causes of premature complexes are extrasystoles of supraventricular or ventricular origin (see Figures 4.1 and 5.1).

Other possible causes of premature QRS complex should be considered:

o Parasystolic complexes (see Figures 4.2 and 5.2).
o Reciprocating complexes (if they are repetitive, they are indicative of a reentrant tachycardia) (see Figures 1.17, 3.8–3.10, and 4.16–4.18).
o Sinus captures in the presence of VT (see Figure 5.23) or escape rhythm (see Figure 6.1).
o Premature complexes in the case of atrial flutter with variable conduction, or in cases of AF.
o Premature complexes due to sinus arrhythmia (see Figure 6.7).

Pause Analysis

The presence of a pause is generally due to a passive rhythm, (second-degree or transient advanced sinoatrial or AV block, or sudden depression of the sinus node automatism). In children and athletes, pauses are occasionally due to a marked physiologic sinus arrhythmia (see Figure 6.7).

Rarely, they are due to an active rhythm, such as a blocked supraventricular extrasystole (Figures 6.8 and 7.3), or even due to a concealed junctional extrasystole that is not conducted to the atria or the ventricles (Figure 1.17 B-4).

Delayed Complex Analysis

Late QRS complexes are usually escape complexes (see Figure 6.1B), which may be narrow or wide (aberrant Phase 4 junctional escape complexes or ventricular escape complexes).

They may also be sinus complexes, as a result of a sudden decrease in sinus automatism with delayed normal P wave. Sometimes delayed sinus complexes occur after a sinoatrial or second- or third-degree AV block (Figures 6.12, 6.13, and 6.18), or after a tachyarrhythmia episode that may be followed by a long pause (brady-tachy syndrome), after which a sinus P wave or an escape complex occurs (Figure 4.42). To be sure that the delayed complex is of sinus origin, the preceding P wave should be conducted to the ventricles (PR interval ≥120 ms). Often, the sinus P wave occurs simultaneously with the escape complex. This diagnosis is made because the PR interval is ≤120 ms, or the QRS complex overlaps the P wave (coincident complex) (Figure 6.1A).

Analysis of the P Wave and QRS-T Complexes of Variable Morphology
(Figures 7.4 and 7.5, Table 7.1)

Morphology changes in the same tracing frequently affect QRS complexes, although occasionally the P wave and ST/T segment may also present changes.

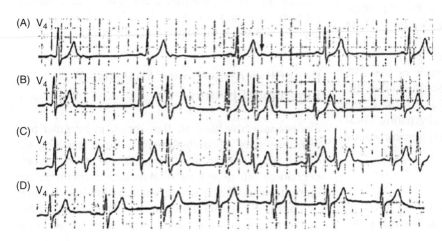

Figure 7.3 (A) Significant sinus bradycardia featuring small sharp and short waves after the T wave (arrow), corresponding to concealed atrial extrasystoles, very different from the smooth and longer U wave. In (B) and (C) the same extrasystoles are observed after being conducted. After administration of propafenone (D), the extrasystoles disappeared and the heart rate decreased.

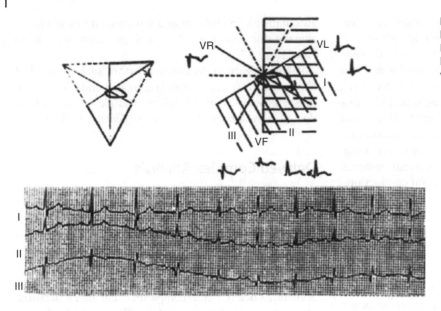

Figure 7.4 Above: See the position of the loop in II, III, and VF, before deep inspiration. Below: QRS-T changes during deep breathing in III (Qr turns into qR). The loop verticalizes, and the Q in III became, qR or R.

QRS Complexes of Variable Morphology

The most frequent types are due to:

o The presence of a QRS complex with different degrees of ventricular fusion, particularly observed in relatively slow VT (see Figure 5.23), accelerated idioventricular rhythm (see Figure 5.33), or in ventricular extrasystoles in the PR interval (see Figure 5.6). Different degrees of fusion may also be found in parasystolic rhythms (see Figure 5.2).

o Capture complexes may also be considered to have a variable morphology. They have already been discussed when referring to premature complex analysis (see Premature Complex Analysis).

o The rare cases of Wenckebach-type BBB QRS complexes of variable morphology may also appear (see Figure 3.25).

o Sometimes, QRS complexes with variable morphology are observed, especially in the precordial leads V2 to V5, due to respiratory changes. A clear example of this is when a QS complex in lead

o III turns into qR with a deep breath (positional change) (Figure 7.4), which rules out that the Q wave is due to necrosis.

o QRS complexes with variable morphology also include the different types of electric alternans of the QRS complex that may be seen in sinus rhythm and in different arrhythmias (Figure 7.5). Table 7.1 shows the most frequent situations in which alternating QRS/ST-T are seen (Bayés de Luna, 2011; Recommended General Bibliography p. xvii).

ST-T Morphology Changes

These may be irrelevant when associated with QRS complex morphology changes during deep breathing (for instance, in lead III (Figure 7.4)). In this case, changes do not show alternans but a cyclical pattern related to respiration.

When evident ST-T electrical alternans are observed, as in the case of important acute ischemia (Figure 7.5B), in the presence of electrolyte and/or serious metabolic disorders (Figure 7.5D), as well as in the long QT syndrome (Figure 7.5C), they constitute a marker for malignant arrhythmias and sudden death (see Chapter 9, Long QT Syndrome).

P Waves with Variable Morphology

In some instances they may be due to different degrees of atrial fusion, as in the case of atrial parasystole (Figure 4.2), or when late junctional extrasystoles are present (Figure 4.30). If these are bigeminal, they may originate an evident alternans of the P wave.

Different changes in the P wave morphology due to other causes may also be found in the same ECG tracing (wandering sinus pacemaker, respiratory movements, artifacts, aberrant atrial conduction, and so on (see Figures 3.23 and 6.15) (Bayés de Luna, 2011).

Repetitive Arrhythmias Analysis: Bigeminal Rhythm

Occasionally, the heart rhythm shows an irregular pattern over time (alloarrhythmia). If short and long RR alternate, we refer to this as bigeminal rhythm. On rare occasions, the sequences of repetitive arrhythmia are due to trigeminal or quadrigeminal rhythm (for instance, two or three normal QRS complexes followed by a third or fourth premature complex). The latter are generally

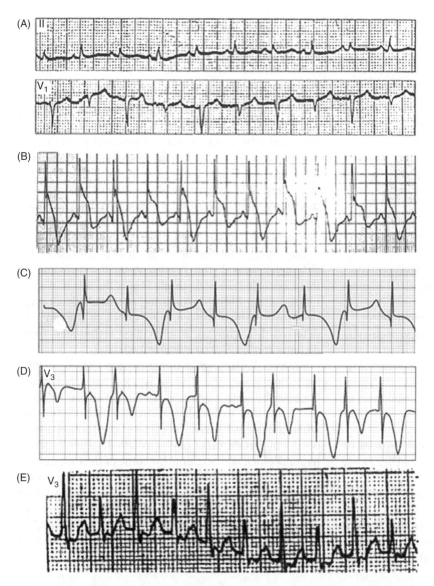

Figure 7.5 Typical examples of electrical alternans (Table 7.1). (A) QRS alternans in a patient with pericardial tamponade. (B) ST/T alternans in Prinzmetal angina. (C) Repolarization alternans in a congenital long QT syndrome. (D) Repolarization alternans in significant electrolytic imbalance in a patient with atrial fibrillation. (E) QRS alternans during a reentrant AV junctional tachycardia involving an accessory pathway (see Table 4.5).

explained by the same mechanisms accounting for bigeminal rhythm, which will be described in the following paragraphs.

Figure 7.6 shows different examples of bigeminal QRS complex, with repetitive short and long RR intervals. This figure illustrates the more common mechanisms, according to our experience, explaining the different causes of bigeminal rhythm that may be determined by the surface ECG. We also encourage the reader to make the correct diagnosis in the last tracing (k) marked with a question mark (see the figure legend) and to practice by placing the corresponding Lewis diagram (Chapter 1, Preliminary Considerations) for each example. We will

now briefly comment on the key signs used for obtaining the correct diagnosis in the different examples:

C. Atrial bigeminy: the atrial bigeminal wave (P′) is different from the sinus P wave, as is the case when atrial premature systoles are observed.

D. Ventricular bigeminy: the bigeminal QRS complexes are wide and show a fixed coupling interval.

E. Concealed atrial trigeminy: the T wave of the bigeminal complexes is slightly different from the T wave of the sinus wave due to the presence of a concealed P′ wave.

F. Escape-ventricular extrasystole sequence: the first QRS complex of the bigeminal rhythm is not preceded by a P wave.

Table 7.1 Most frequent causes of QRS-T alternans.

QRS alternans	ST-T alternans
– Cardiac tamponade	– Serious hyperacute ischemia
– Presence of AVRT	– Long QT syndrome
– False alternans:	– Electrolyte imbalance
• Related to breathing (in precordial leads)	
• Bundle branch block or WPW 2×1	
• Late bigeminal PVC. QRS complexes in the PR interval	

JRT-AP, junctional reentrant tachycardia with accessory pathway; PVC, premature ventricular complex; WPW, Wolff–Parkinson–White syndrome.

G. 3×2 sinoatrial block: this should be differentiated (differential diagnosis) from parasinus atrial bigeminy (see Figure 6.13).

H. 2×1 atrial flutter alternating with 4×1 atrial flutter.

I. Sinus rhythm with second-degree Wenckebach-type AV block with 3×2 AV conduction.

J. AV junctional ectopic rhythm with a 3×2 Wenckebach-type AV block. There is no evident atrial activation. The patient also showed an ECG with regular junctional tachycardia with a relatively slow rate (110 bpm) (not included in the figure).

K. Escape–capture sequence with different degrees of aberrant sinus complex (captures) (Lopez-Diez *et al.*, 2010).

L. Atrial fibrillation may occasionally and randomly show apparently bigeminal complexes.

M. We expect the reader to detect the subtle T wave morphology changes in the bigeminal rhythm, a key factor in determining that it is caused by concealed atrial trigeminy (see C).

The most frequent cause of bigeminal rhythm is supraventricular or ventricular extrasystoles. However, as already discussed, there are many other active and passive arrhythmias that may initiate bigeminal rhythm (Figure 7.6). Obviously, sometimes the diagnosis is uncertain. In this case it is advisable to review the previous chapters and to use Lewis diagrams to determine the type of arrhythmia. If needed, other complementary techniques should be used (atrial wave amplification, T wave filtering, intracavitary ECG, etc.).

Differential Diagnosis Between Several Arrhythmias in Special Situations

If the ECG knowledge set out throughout this book is applied, it should not be difficult to determine the type of a given arrhythmia. However, we would like to review the ECG clues for some situations where reaching a correct diagnosis is somewhat difficult.

Sinus Rhythm Misdiagnosed as Ectopic Rhythm

The patient may show moderate tachycardia (100–130 bpm) with no visible atrial activity. In this situation, it is useful to perform maneuvers that lead to rhythm changes (for instance, deep breathing) to assess whether the P wave appears, in which case it is probably sinus rhythm (see Figure 4.10). Occasionally, atrial rhythms may feature subtle changes with such maneuvers, but the P wave polarity and characteristics will usually allow for distinction between sinus and ectopic atrial tachycardia.

Very rarely, misdiagnosis is due to the fact that although a sinus rhythm is present, the P wave is not visible (concealed sinus rhythm). This is the result of a significant atrial fibrosis generating potentials that cannot be measured by a surface ECG, although they may be detected through wave amplification techniques (Bayés de Luna *et al.*, 1978) (see Figure 4.62).

Sinoventricular conduction is a rare type of cardiac activation where the P wave is sometimes not visible because the sinus rhythm is conducted to the AV node and ventricles with delayed atrial activation, or even without evident P wave. This type of conduction usually occurs in certain cases of electrolyte disorders, such as hyperkalemia, and accounts for some of the rare cases of sinus rhythm with short PR interval or nonvisible P wave. This is due (Figure 7.7) to delayed atrial activation, which may explain a short PR interval, and may be confused with a pre-excitation with short RR intervals (Figure 7.7B), or even with AV junctional rhythm when the P wave is hidden by the QRS (Figure 7.7C).

Differential Diagnosis Between 2:1 Flutter and Sinus Rhythm

This confusion may occur when the flutter rate is slow (around 200 bpm) and, therefore, the QRS complex is around 100 bpm. In this situation, one "f" wave may be hidden within the QRS complex or it may not be appropriately observed, whereas the other "f" wave may be mistaken for a sinus P wave (see Figure 4.20). For a correct diagnosis to be reached it is important: (i) to be aware of this possibility (i.e., that flutter waves may be concealed in the QRS complex) and (ii) to assess whether the patient has a fixed heart rate over time, which is usually not the case in sinus rhythm, and this therefore supports a diagnosis of 2:1 flutter. Again, vagal maneuvers (such as carotid sinus compression, Valsalva, ocular compression) or drugs that depress AV conduction (i.e., Adenosine) may help slowing the conduction over the AV node, allowing the flutter waves to be detected.

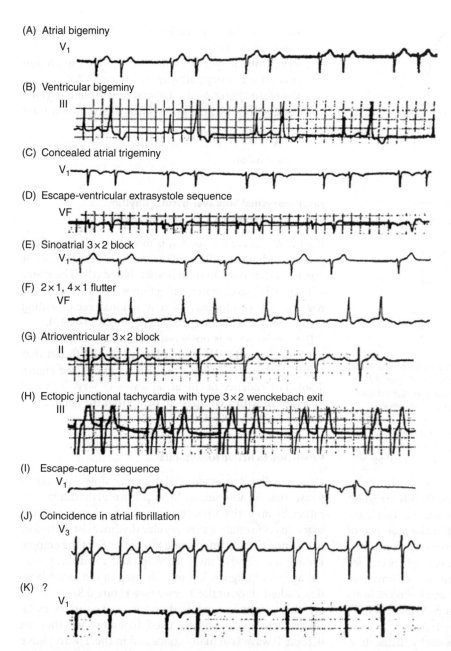

(A) Atrial bigeminy
V₁

(B) Ventricular bigeminy
III

(C) Concealed atrial trigeminy
V₁

(D) Escape-ventricular extrasystole sequence
VF

(E) Sinoatrial 3×2 block
V₁

(F) 2×1, 4×1 flutter
VF

(G) Atrioventricular 3×2 block
II

(H) Ectopic junctional tachycardia with type 3×2 wenckebach exit
III

(I) Escape-capture sequence
V₁

(J) Coincidence in atrial fibrillation
V₃

(K) ?
V₁

Figure 7.6 Different types of bigeminal QRS complexes. The different mechanisms are shown within the figure, except for the case K, which corresponds to a concealed atrial trigeminy (similar to case C). Note that in K the second T wave of each QRS bigeminy is less deep, as it is hidden a positive P wave. Other parts of the ECGs tracing show atrial trigeminy. This subtle T wave alteration led us to reach the correct diagnosis.

Meanwhile, as previously discussed, it is often very difficult to distinguish between a slow atypical flutter and a fast monomorphic atrial tachycardia (see Chapter 4, Atrial Flutter). From a clinical point of view, the latter is not a relevant problem, because both may be considered the same arrhythmia, in contrast to the case where 2×1 flutter is misdiagnosed as sinus rhythm, because this mistake may lead to incorrect diagnosis and management. However, in the EP lab, the distinction is of utmost importance as different ablative options should be considered for each arrhythmia.

Aberrant Supraventricular Tachycardia Misdiagnosed as Ventricular Tachycardia

In this situation, regardless of the diagnostic criteria already discussed (see Chapter 5, Classical Monomorphic Ventricular Tachycardias, Table 5.5, and Figure 5.28), when assessing a wide QRS complex tachycardia it is useful to remember:

- In the presence of heart disease, and above all in ischemic heart disease, the arrhythmia is most likely of ventricular origin.

(A)

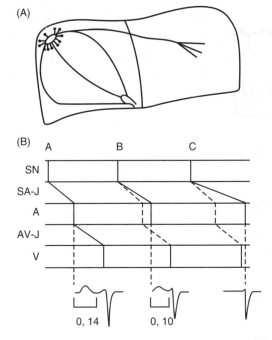

(B)

Figure 7.7 Sinoventricular conduction. Above: Scheme of activation. Below: Lewis diagram: (A) Sinoatrial (SA) and atrioventricular (AV) normal conduction. (B) Normal internodal conduction (dotted line), originating a QRS complex as expected. Sinoatrial conduction is slow, thus delaying the onset of the P wave, and therefore the PR is short, not because of an accelerated conduction, but because of a delayed conduction between the sinus node and the atria (short PR). (C) If the SA conduction is still longer, the P wave may be hidden in the QRS, mimicking AV junctional rhythm.

- Ventricular tachycardias may present slightly irregular patterns, especially at onset. However, when a significant rhythm irregularity is observed, and in the presence of dominant wide QRS complexes, narrow QRS complexes are present at random and do not meet the criteria for captures (in VT the narrow sinus captures are always premature) because they appear early or late; it is most likely AF in a patient with Wolff–Parkinson–White (WPW) syndrome, rather than VT (see Figure 4.52).
- In the case of wide QRS complex tachycardia, it is sometimes difficult to perform the correct differential diagnosis. The following supraventricular tachycardias may present wide QRS complexes:

  - ○ Atrial 2:1 flutter in patients with WPW syndrome (see Figure 4.66B).
  - ○ Reentrant tachycardia with anterograde conduction over an accessory pathway (see Figure 5.26).
  - ○ Reentrant junctional tachycardia with anterograde conduction through an atypical preexcitation tract (see Figure 4.22).
  - ○ Typical supraventricular tachycardia with BBB (see Figure 5.25).

Fast Paroxysmal Supraventricular Rhythm with QRS Complex <0.12 s and r′ in Lead V1

If atrial waves are not seen, it is most likely that the ECG pattern with terminal r′ in V1 sometimes very tiny is not due to partial right bundle branch block (r′). The cause of terminal QRS complex deflection is a P′ wave with retrograde VA conduction of a junctional reciprocating tachycardia of AVNRT type (see Figures 4.17–4.19).

If an atrial wave is observed preceding the QRS complex, the r′ may be the second F wave of a 2:1 flutter that is attached to the end of the QRS complex. (see Figure 4.56). The cadence of the atrial waves (F waves) should be assessed with a compass to prove that the apparent r′ wave in lead V1 is, in fact, an F wave.

Pause Due to Active Arrhythmia

Occasionally, concealed atrial extrasystoles initiate a pause that is not caused by a passive arrhythmia, but rather by an active one. In some cases, when concealed bigeminy is present, a slow regular rhythm exists. The key in diagnosis is to demonstrate the presence of the ectopic P wave at the end of the T wave as a short and sharp low-voltage wave (Figure 7.3) or a slurring in the ascendant-descendent slope of the T wave (see Figure 6.8).

If this cannot be suggested by means of a surface ECG, other techniques may be used to assess whether an ectopic P wave is actually concealed in the T wave: wave amplification, faster registration speed (see Figure 4.62), T wave filtering (Figure A-13) and special lead tracing (Lewis lead) (Bakker *et al.*, 2009) (see Appendix A-3).

Self Assessment

A. How is a dominant rhythm assessed?

B. Describe the different morphologies of monomorphic atrial activity.

C. What are the different possible diagnoses when wide QRS complexes are present?

D. How may atrioventricular (AV) dissociation due to a block be differentiated from AV dissociation due to interference?

E. When may a pause be explained by an active rhythm?

F. What is a coincident complex?

G. What are the most frequent QRS complexes featuring a variable morphology?

H. Describe the different types of bigeminal QRS complexes.

I. Define the sinoventricular conduction.

References

Bakker AL, Nijkerk G, Groenemeijer BE, *et al*. The Lewis lead. Making recognition of P waves easy during wide QRS complex tachycardia. Circulation 2009;119:92.

Bayés de Luna A. Electrocardiography: John Wiley & Sons Ltd, Chichester, 2011.

Bayés de Luna A, Boada FX, Casellas A, *et al*. Concealed atrial electrical activity. J Electrocardiol 1978;11:301.

Bayés de Luna A, Fort de Ribot R, Trilla E, *et al*. Electrocardiographic and vectorcardiographic study of interatrial conduction disturbances with left atrial retrograde activation. J Electrocardiol 1985;18:1.

Brugada P, Brugada J, Mont L, *et al*. A new approach to the differential diagnosis of a regular tachycardia with a wide QRS complex. Circulation 1991;83:1649.

Goldwasser D, Serra G, Guerra J, *et al*. New computer algorithm to improve P wave detection during supraventricular tachycardias. Eur Heart J 2008;29(suppl): P472.

Kistler PM, Roberts-Thomson KC, Haqqani HM, *et al*. P-wave morphology in focal atrial tachycardia: development of an algorithm to predict the anatomic site of origin. J Am Coll Cardiol 2006;48:1010.

Lopez-Diez JC, Femenia F, Baranchuk A. Diagnóstico diferencial de latidos agrupados; bigeminia escape-captura como manifestación de enfermedad del nódulo sinusal. Rev Arg Fed Cardiol 2010;39(4):324.

Pava LF, Perafan P, Badiel M, *et al*. R-wave peak time at DII: a new criterion for differentiating between wide complex QRS tachycardias. Heart Rhythm 2010;7(7):922.

Platonov P, Cygankiewicz I, Stridh M, *et al*. Low atrial fibrillatory rate is associated with poor outcome in patients with mild to moderate heart failure. Circ Arrhythm Electrophysiol 2012;5:77.

Vereckei A, Duray G, Szénási G, *et al*. New algorithm using only lead a VR for differential diagnosis of wide QRS complex tachycardia. Heart Rhythm 2008;5:89.

Vereckei A. Current algorithms for the diagnosis of wide QRS complex tachycardias. Curr Cardiol Rev 2014;10(3):262.

Part III

The ECG and Risk of Arrhythmias and Sudden Death in Different Heart Diseases and Situations

8

Ventricular Pre-Excitation

Concept and Types of Pre-Excitation

The term ventricular pre-excitation implies that the myocardium depolarizes earlier than expected if the stimulus follows the normal pathway through the specific conduction system (Wolff *et al.*, 1930). In actual fact, this is not really what happens before excitation (pre-excitation). Instead, it refers to ventricular excitation occurring earlier than expected.

Three types of pre-excitation have been defined (Table 8.1, and Figures 8.1 and 8.2):

1) **Wolff–Parkinson–White pre-excitation (WPW)**, in which the pre-excitation is due to muscular connections composed of working myocardial fibers that connect the atrium and ventricle, bypassing the atrioventricular (AV) nodal conduction delay. They comprise the accessory AV pathways (AP) that are known as Kent bundles.
2) **Atypical pre-excitation**, encompassing different long anomalous pathways or tracts showing decremental conduction, localized on the right side of the heart. This type of pre-excitation includes the classical Mahaim fibers (Sternick and Wellens, 2006) (see Atypical Pre-Excitation).
3) **Short PR pre-excitation** (Lown *et al.*, 1957), where the early excitation is due to an accelerated conduction through the AV node and, in some cases, is due to the presence of an atriohisian tract (Figure 8.2) (see Short PR Interval Pre-Excitation).

A recently identified genetic mutation in the ionic channels is responsible for some complex forms of WPW syndrome that are accompanied by heart blocks and atrial fibrilloflutter episodes (Gollob *et al.*, 2001). For the time being, these findings should not be extrapolated to the classical WPW-type pre-excitation. We have, therefore, not included ventricular pre-excitation in the section dealing with inherited diseases, but we imagine that in the future it may be possible.

WPW-type Pre-Excitation (Type 1)

Concept and Mechanism

WPW-type pre-excitation occurs by means of the presence of accessory AV pathways, which, in the classical form, correspond to the so-called Kent bundle. These bundles directly connect the atria to different parietal or septal areas of the ventricular myocardium (Figure 8.1A and 8.1B).

Generally, only one accessory pathway (AP) exists (>90% of cases) and conduction is usually fast and in both directions (anterogradely and retrogradely) (≈2/3 of cases). On certain occasions (20%), the conduction of the AP occurs only retrogradely (concealed WPW). Other WPW-type pre-excitations are much infrequent (Table 8.1).

These APs of conduction form a circuit (specific conduction system (SCS)–ventricle –AP–atrium–SCS) with anterograde or retrograde conduction, which constitutes the anatomic substrate of reentrant arrhythmias that are frequently observed in the presence of WPW-type pre-excitation (WPW syndrome) (see Arrhythmias and Wolff–Parkinson–White Type Pre-Excitation: Wolff–Parkinson–White Syndrome). Table 8.1 shows the most characteristic electrocardiographic morphologies in sinus rhythm and during a tachycardia episode, according to the anatomic and functional properties of the different types of pre-excitation (anterograde and/or retrograde conduction, and fast or slow conduction). Figures 8.3–8.7 show the four different electrocardiogram (ECG) patterns observed in WPW-type pre-excitation, depending on the location of the AV AP (Kent bundle).

Electrocardiographic Characteristics

The ECG alterations are only observed when anterograde conduction exists. They consist mainly of a short PR interval and an abnormal QRS complex presenting initial slurrings (δ wave).

Clinical Arrhythmology, Second Edition. Antoni Bayés de Luna and Adrian Baranchuk.
© 2017 John Wiley & Sons Ltd. Published 2017 by John Wiley & Sons Ltd.

Table 8.1 Pre-excitation types. 1: Wolff–Parkinson–White (WPW)-type pre-excitation; 2: atypical pre-excitation; 3: short PR-type pre-excitation. Surface ECG rate and characteristics in sinus rhythm and during paroxysmal tachycardia episodes, according to the functional characteristics of the different types of pre-excitation.

Accessory pathway		Frequency	ECG in sinus rhythm	ECG during tachycardia
Type 1	a) Fast conduction in both ways: atrioventricular (AV) accessory pathway (classical Kent bundle) (Figures 9.1–9.7)	60–65%	Short PR. δ wave	No δ wave. RP' < P'R
	b) Fast conduction in the AV accessory pathway (only in retrograde direction) (concealed pre-excitation)	20–30%	Normal PR. No δ wave	No δ wave. RP' < P'R
	c) Fast conduction in the AV accessory pathway (only in anterograde direction) (frequently two or more bundles involved)	5–10%	Short PR. δ wave	Wide QRS due to an anterograde conduction of the stimuli through the accessory pathway (antidromic tachycardia)
	d) Only retrograde and slow conduction through AV accessory pathway	≈5%	Normal PR. No δ wave	Frequently incessant tachycardia with RP' > P'R.
	e) Presence of >1 accessory pathway	5–10%	May switch from one to another QRS morphology qrs or qRs in V1 This diagnosis is generally difficult based only on a surface ECG	Antidromic tachycardia or alternating antidromic/orthodromic tachycardia Alternation of short and long PR Morphology changes in ectopic P wave Electrophysiologic studies confirm this diagnosis
Type 2	Slow anterograde conduction, generally through a long atriofascicular tract (distal right branch), or AV without retrograde conduction (including classical Mahaim* fibers – node ventricular or fasciculoventricular) (atypical pre-excitation)	Rare	Nonexistent or slight pre-excitation (i.e., no Q in V5–V6, with borderline PR and uncertain δ wave, and rS in III. This is due to the slow conduction through the abnormal tract Globally, the ECG is normal or presents different grades of bundle branch pattern	Antidromic tachycardia with anterograde conduction through the right atriofascicular tract and retrograde conduction through the right bundle branch. Therefore, it features a left bundle branch block morphology. Compared with the antidromic tachycardias (generated due to anterograde conduction through a right AV accessory pathway – Type 1 c) in this table), features a narrower QRS complex and a thinner r wave in V1–V4, with a delayed transition to RS in precordial leads (compare Figures 4.22 and 5.26)
Type 3	AV node accelerated conduction, sometimes due to an atriohisian tract (short PR pre-excitation)	Rare	Short PR interval No δ wave	Normal QRS complex No δ wave

* Today it is believed that the classical Mahaim fibers (nodoventricular and fasciculoventricular fibers) initiate paroxysmal tachycardias less frequently than the right atriofascicular tracts. Currently considered that they are not involved in the circuit that triggers the tachycardia, which is usually due to a right atriofascicular tract, as previously mentioned.

The short PR interval occurs because the sinus stimulus reaches the ventricles through the AP sooner than through the specialized conduction system (SCS). The presence of an abnormal QRS complex is the result of the ventricular activation taking place through two pathways, the normal AV conduction and the AP (a Kent bundle). This results in a slightly early activation of the ventricles in subepicardial zones where there are very few Purkinje fibers. This explains not only the early QRS complex (short PR interval) but also the δ wave as the result of the slow activation of the myocardial tissue. The rest of the myocardial mass is activated through the normal pathway (SCS). **The QRS complex is thus a genuine fusion complex.**

Depending on what myocardial areas are activated through one pathway or the other, the QRS complex will show a greater or lesser degree of abnormality and, therefore, a greater or lesser degree of pre-excitation.

In the rare cases of Type 2 pre-excitation (Table 8.1), the baseline ECG may present morphologies varying

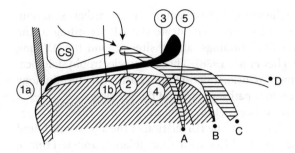

*A, B, C, D, Points of onset of ventricular activation

▨▨▨ Cardiac muscle

██ Central fibrous body

1. Bundle of Kent is ventricular wall 'a' and 'b'
2. AV node
3. Atriohisian (Short PR interval preexcitation)
4. His/fascicle
5. Atrium fascicle (Atypical preexcitation)

Coronary sinus (CS)

Figure 8.1 Right lateral view of the accessory pathways.

from normal to subtle evidence of minimal pre-excitation to cases with left bundle branch block (LBBB) pattern (see Atypical Pre-Excitation). In Type 3 pre-excitation,

the only anomaly of the ECG is the short PR interval (see Short PR Pre-Excitation).

A. PR interval (Figure 8.1)

This generally ranges from 0.08 to 0.11 s. Cases with a normal PR interval are rare and are explained by the presence of a long left AV AP Kent bundle type with delayed atrial conduction. In this scenario, even though the ventricular activation is performed through a classical Kent bundle, the PR interval is usually at the lower limit of normality (0.12–0.13 s), and therefore is not considered short. It is, however, shorter than when no pre-excitation occurs, as conduction through the normal pathway would present a longer PR interval.

A normal PR interval may also exist in the following cases: atypical long atriofascicular/atrioventricular anomalous tracts with slow conduction or other atypical tracts, including the classical Mahaim fibers (atypical pre-excitation) (very rare). These tracts may partially or completely prevent the slow intranodal conduction (Sternick and Wellens, 2006) (see Atypical Pre-Excitation).

B. Ventriculogram alterations (Figures 8.3–8.7)

The QRS complexes show an abnormal morphology wider than the baseline QRS complex (frequently ≥0.11 s) with characteristic initial slurrings (δ wave) due to (see before)

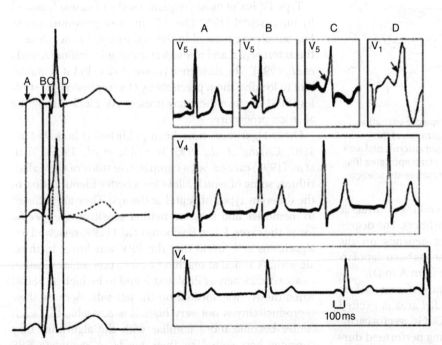

Figure 8.2 Top left: Diagram of the P-QRS relationship in normal cases. AB: P wave; BC; PR segment; CD: QRS. Middle panel: Wolff–Parkinson–White (WPW)-type pre-excitation (the broken line represents the QRS complex if no pre-excitation occurred). AD distance is the same as under normal conditions, with a wide QRS complex in detriment to the PR segment (BC distance), which partially or totally coincides with the δ wave. Below: In cases of short PR segment, the QRS complex is shifted forward because

the PR segment is shortened or may even disappear. Top right: Four examples of δ wave (arrow) by increasing order of relevance. D pattern. Atrial fibrillation patient in whom the first QRS is conducted over the normal pathway, whereas the second QRS is conducted over the accessory pathway with maximum pre-excitation. Middle panel: Example of four complexes with pre-excitation, with an average-sized δ wave. Below: Four complexes in a case of short PR pre-excitation.

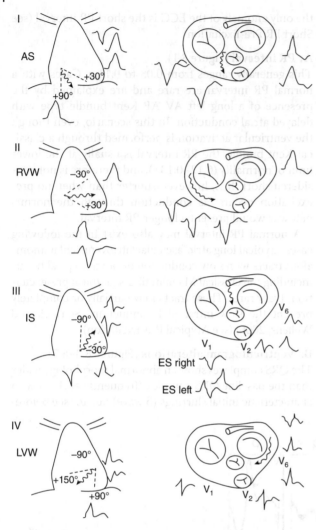

Figure 8.3 Wolff–Parkinson–White (WPW)-type pre-excitation morphologies according to the different localization of the atrioventricular (AV) accessory pathway. I: Right anteroseptal area (RAS); II: right ventricular free wall (RFW); III: inferoseptal area (PS); and IV: left ventricular free wall (LFW). PS: Premature stimulation.

the activation being initiated at the working contractile myocardium in an area poor in Purkinje fibers. The degree of abnormality of the QRS complex depends on the amount of ventricular myocardium that has been depolarized through the AP (Figure 8.2, arrow from A to D).

The QRS complex morphology in the different surface ECG leads depends on which epicardial area is excited earliest. Studies correlating surface ECGs, vectorcardiography (VCG), and epicardial mapping performed during surgical ablation of APs by the Gallagher group (Tonkin *et al.*, 1975) have shown the value of studying δ wave polarity to identify the site of earliest ventricular epicardial excitation. The first 20-ms vector in the ECG (first δ wave vector that can be measured on the ECG) is situated in different places on the frontal plane (in the horizontal plane it is always directed forward), depend-

ing on the site of earliest ventricular epicardial excitation. These studies precisely locate the AP according to the surface ECG findings, at ten sites around the AV ring (Gallagher *et al.*, 1978). There is an electrophysiological statement (Cosio, 1999) to standardize the terminology of accessory pathways around the AV rings.

Later, Milstein (1987) (Figure 8.8) described an algorithm that allows the correlation of the alterations found in the surface ECG with four ablation zones. From a practical point of view, the WPW-type pre-excitation may be classified into four types based on these findings: anteroseptal, right ventricle (RV) free wall, inferoseptal, and left ventricle (LV) free wall (Bayés de Luna, 2011) (Figure 8.3). In Figures 8.4–8.7, we can see examples of QRS morphologies in these four electrocardiographic modalities of WPW-type pre-excitation. Types I and II mimic a LBBB, with a more deviated left axis (ÂQRS beyond +30°) in Type II, whereas in Type I the ÂQRS is usually between +30° and +90°. In Type III the QRS is predominantly negative in inferior leads, especially in III and VF, with R or RS morphology in V1 or V2, and the ÂQRS is between –30° and –90°. Type IV has a predominant negative morphology in lateral leads (I, VL) and a generally high R wave in leads V1 or V2, with a right axis deviation (ÂQRS beyond +90° up to +150°).

Type IV is the most frequent (≈50% of cases) followed by inferoseptal (25%).The APs in close proximity to the His bundle are located in the anteroseptal zone, close to the anteroseptal and midseptal tricuspid annulus (Arruda *et al.*, 1998). The incidence is rare (1–2%) but it is important to localize them precisely by electrophysiologic studies (EPS) because they may present AV block during the ablation procedure.

Other algorithms have been published (Lindsay *et al.*, 1987; Chiang *et al.*, 1995; Iturralde *et al.*, 1996). Yuan *et al.* (1992) carried out a comparative study of eight algorithms, some of which allow for a better identification of the different types of septal pathways. They are difficult to memorize and they are neither sensitive nor specific for all the cases. Later, Basiouny *et al.* (1999) reviewed ten algorithms and found that the PPV was lower in those algorithms aimed at reaching a more precise localization (> six sites), whereas PPV was found to be higher (>80%) when the AP was located on the left side. Because their reproducibility is not very high, it is advisable that each center become more familiar with the algorithm they consider best suited to their needs. A complete EPS should, therefore, be carried out to precisely identify the exact location of the AP before performing an ablation.

C. Repolarization alterations

Repolarization is altered except in those cases with minor pre-excitation. These changes are secondary to depolarization alterations and become more pathologic

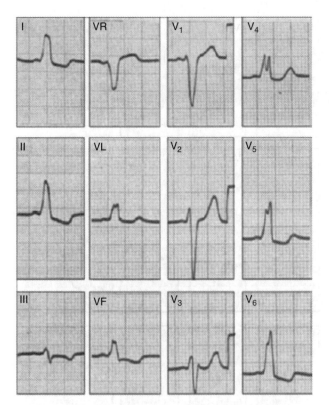

Figure 8.4 A 65-year-old patient with Wolff–Parkinson–White (WPW) syndrome involving an atrioventricular (AV) accessory pathway in the right anteroseptal area according to the Milstein classification (Type I WPW). It shows considerable pre-excitation. These cases are similar to Type II (Figure 8.5), but when compared to those with advanced left bundle branch block (LBBB) with a left deviation the ÂQRS does appear ≈ +40° (Figure 8.3(I)).

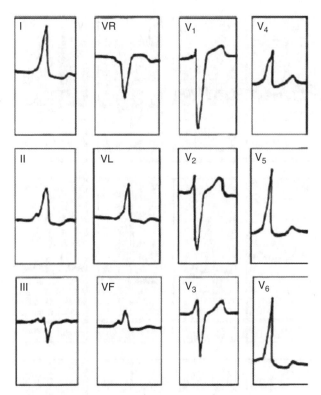

Figure 8.5 A Wolff–Parkinson–White (WPW) patient with the accessory pathway located in the right ventricular free wall (Type II WPW). It shows a pattern of advanced left bundle branch block (LBBB) similar to Type I, but has a more significant left ÂQRS deviation (rS in III) (Figure 8.3(II)).

(more significant opposing polarity when compared with that of the R wave) as the degree of pre- excitation increases (Figure 8.2).

When pre-excitation is intermittent, the complexes conducted without pre-excitation may show repolarization alterations (negative T wave), which are explained by an "electrical memory phenomenon" (Chatterjee *et al.*, 1969; Nicolai *et al.*, 1981; Rosenbaum *et al.*, 1982). The concept of cardiac memory or electronic modulation was recently reviewed by Chiale and Elizari, representatives of the Buenos Aires' School of electrocardiology (Chiale *et al.*, 2014).

D. ECG diagnosis of more than one AP (Wellens *et al.*, 1990)

Approximately 5–10% of cases involve more than one AP. This may be clinically suspected when the patient suffers from syncope or malignant ventricular arrhythmia, or wide QRS complex paroxysmal tachycardia (antidromic tachycardia).

Some ECG data are indicative of this association, both in sinus rhythm and during tachycardia. These are:

- **In sinus rhythm**: (i) QrS or qRs morphology in lead V1; and (ii) morphology changes from one to the other type of pre-excitation (Figure 8.11).
- **During tachycardia**: (i) wide QRS complex or alternating wide and narrow QRS complexes; (ii) alternating long and short RR; and (iii) changes in the P' wave morphology. Generally, this diagnosis suspicion should be confirmed with intracavitary EPS.

E. *Differential diagnosis of WPW-type pre-excitation*

Wolff–Parkinson–White Type I and II pre-excitation may be mistaken for LBBB (Figures 8.4 and 8.5). We have already seen that in Type II pre-excitation, a left axis deviation of ÂQRS beyond +30° is observed.

Type III pre-excitation with an inferior MI, a right bundle branch block (RBBB) or a right ventricular hypertrophy (Figure 8.6).

Type IV pre-excitation with a lateral MI or right ventricular hypertrophy (Figures 8.7 and 8.12).

It is very important to know the different signs that allow us to suspect the presence of acute or chronic ischemia when pre-excitation is present. In the acute phase, the repolarization changes, especially the ST segment elevation, may lead us to suspect acute coronary syndrome (ACS) with ST elevation. It is more difficult to

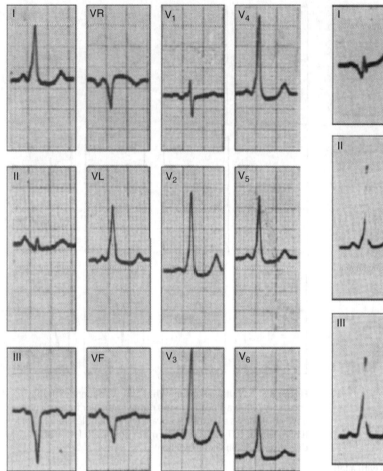

Figure 8.6 A Wolff–Parkinson–White (WPW) patient with the accessory pathway located in the inferoseptal heart wall (Type III WPW). This case (and also Type IV cases) may be mistaken for an inferior or inferolateral infarction, right ventricular hypertrophy, or right bundle branch block (RBBB) (Figure 8.3(III)).

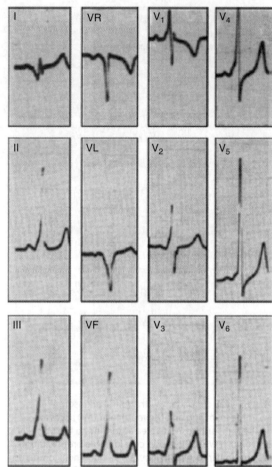

Figure 8.7 A Wolff–Parkinson–White (WPW) patient with the accessory pathway located in the left ventricular left wall (Type IV WPW). This case may be mistaken for a lateral infarction, right ventricular hypertrophy, or right bundle branch block (RBBB) (Figure 8.3(IV)).

make the correct diagnosis in ACS without ST elevation. In the chronic phase of Q wave myocardial infarction, the association may sometimes be suspected when repolarization shows more symmetrical T waves (Bayés de Luna and Fiol, 2008; Bayés de Luna, 2011) (Figure 8.13).

In any case, the presence of a short PR interval and/or a δ wave, always keeping in mind the possibility of WPW-type pre-excitation, is key ECG data for the correct diagnosis of this condition.

F. Spontaneous or induced changes of the abnormal morphology

The pre-excitation may be intermittent (Figures 8.9–8.11). Sometimes the degree of pre-excitation progressively changes (concertina effect) (Figure 8.9).

The pre-excitation may increase if stimulus conduction through the AV node is depressed (vagal maneuvers, some drugs such as digitalis, β-blockers, calcium antagonists, adenosine, etc.), and vice versa. It may decrease when the AV node conduction is facilitated (i.e., through exercise, etc.).

We have already commented on how the presence of sudden changes in the QRS complex morphology with the δ wave remaining present, or changes from the typical WPW pattern to short PR interval alone, demonstrate that two pathways of pre-excitation exist (Figure 8.11).

G. How to confirm or exclude the presence of pre-excitation

Some patients are referred with suspected WPW pre-excitation when none exists and others have a genuine pre-excitation and are considered normal. Using a selective AV node blocking agent, such as adenosine, may confirm or exclude the presence of pre-excitation (Belhassen *et al.*, 2000).

On the other hand, the presence of the septal Q wave in V6 is considered to be evidence that excludes minimal pre-excitation in doubtful cases (Bogun *et al.*, 1999).

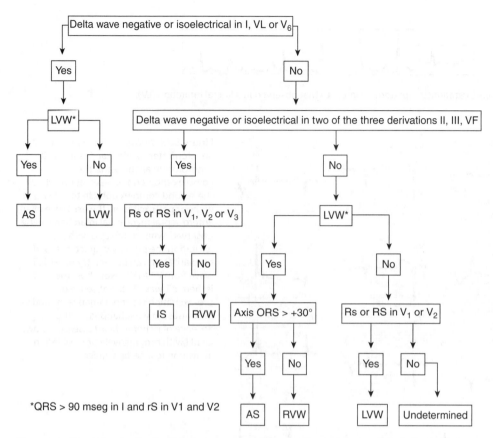

Figure 8.8 Algorithm used to localize the accessory pathway in one of the four surgical areas: right anteroseptal (RAS); right ventricular free wall (RVW); inferoseptal area (IS); and left ventricular free wall (LVW).

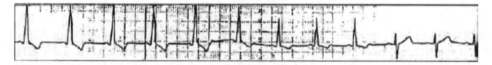

Figure 8.9 Concertina effect. The five first complexes are identical and show short PR and pre-excitation. In the next four complexes, pre-excitation decreases with a shorter PR (0.12 s). The three last complexes do not show any pre-excitation and the PR = 0.16 s.

Holt.

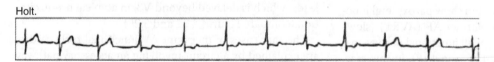

Figure 8.10 Conduction occurs via both the normal and the accessory pathway. When the stimulus is conducted over the accessory pathway, the PR interval is shorter than when the stimulus is conducted over the normal pathway (0.15 s).

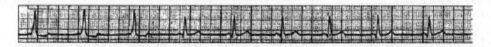

Figure 8.11 Intermittent pre-excitation. In the first three complexes the PR interval is short (80 ms) and the δ wave is observed. In the rest of the tracing the δ wave disappears, but a short PR interval is still observed (100 ms). Thus, this surface ECG suggests the presence of two accessory pathways, one of which short-circuits the AV node (short PR, QRS with no δ wave), whereas the other pathway is located in the ventricular myocardium (Kent bundle), as the PR interval is very short and a clear δ wave is seen.

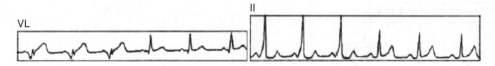

Figure 8.12 Intermittent Type IV pre-excitation: the pattern is similar to that observed in a lateral infarction (LV).

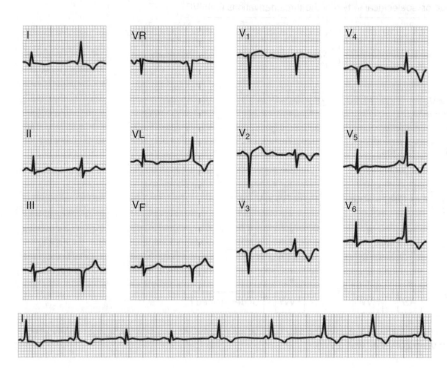

Figure 8.13 Above: ECG of a patient with an intermittent Wolff–Parkinson–White syndrome. In all the leads, the first complex shows no pre-excitation, while the second complex does. In the ECG without pre-excitation, the existence of an antero septal myocardial infarction can be observed, while in the ECG with pre-excitation the primary characteristics of repolarization can be seen (symmetric T wave from V2 to V4). Note how the ischemic T wave in the absence of pre-excitation is flat or negative in I and VL, in contrast to what happens in the absence of ischemic heart disease. Below: Lead I with progressively pre-excitation activation (concertina effect).

Finally, Eisenberger *et al.* (2010) have shown a stepwise approach that is very sensitive and specific for excluding or confirming WPW pre-excitation.

Arrhythmias and Wolff–Parkinson–White-Type Pre-Excitation: Wolff–Parkinson–White Syndrome

Patients with WPW pre-excitation show paroxysmal junctional re-entrant tachycardia with an AP (AVRT) (slow-fast type), accounting for 50% of all junctional paroxysmal tachycardias (see Figures 3.9, 4.16, and 4.18). In this case, during tachycardia, ventricular depolarization usually occurs through the normal pathway, and the AP is the retrograde path of the macro-reentrant circuit (see Figure 3.9). For this reason, the QRS complex does not show pre-excitation at this time (orthodromic tachycardia).

In less than 10% of cases of paroxysmal tachycardia, antegrade ventricular depolarization takes place over the AP, initiating a very wide QRS complex (antidromic tachycardia) (see Figure 5.26). Antidromic tachycardia involves the presence of two pathways, one with anterograde conduction over the accessory pathway and the other with retrograde conduction over the AV node-His. When antidromic tachycardia is the result of an atypical pre-excitation (long atriofascicular pathway with decremental conduction) (Type 2 pre-excitation in Table 8.1), the QRS complex morphology of the tachycardia presents some differences with respect to the QRS morphology in cases of typical AV AP (Kent bundle). The differences particularly concern the R/S transition in precordial leads, which is delayed beyond V3, in atypical pre-excitation (compare Figures 4.22 and 5.26).

The rare cases of incessant AV junctional tachycardias are explained by a circuit involving an accessory pathway with slow retrograde conduction (fast-slow type) (Farré *et al.*, 1979; Critelli *et al.*, 1984) (see Figures 3.10 and 4.21).

Patients with WPW-type pre-excitation present atrial fibrillation and flutter episodes more frequently than the general population (Figures 4.52, 4.66, and 8.13). This happens because patients with WPW often present a shorter atrial refractory period and higher atrial vulnerability (Hamada *et al.*, 2002). All these properties favor the triggering of atrial fibrillation (AF) when a fast retrograde conduction of a premature ventricular complex over the AP falls in the atrial vulnerable period (AVP), or because a patient with paroxysmal reentrant tachycardia triggers AF (Peinado *et al.*, 2005).

In the presence of rapid AF or flutter, more stimuli are conducted to the ventricles through the AP than through the normal pathway. If one of them falls in the vulnerable ventricular period, it may trigger ventricular fibrillation (VF) and SD (Figure 8.13C) (Castellanos *et al.*, 1983). This phenomenon accounts for some cases of SD, especially in young people, although this is fortunately rare. Figure 4.66 shows a patient with WPW syndrome and AF (top) and atrial flutter (bottom) episodes. In both cases, the differential diagnosis with ventricular tachycardia (VT) is difficult, even more in cases of atrial flutter because the heart rate is regular (Figure 4.66B) (see Chapter 4, Atrial Fibrillation: ECG Findings). In cases of AF, the diagnosis is based on the irregularity of the rhythm and the presence of narrow QRS complexes, sometimes premature and sometimes late, whereas in VT the rhythm is regular and, if narrow QRS complexes are present, they are always premature (captures) (see Figure 4.52). However, in a 2:1 atrial flutter with pre-excitation these key points for differential diagnosis do not exist. We have to take into consideration other clinical and ECG data (history taking, AV dissociation, etc.). Figure 8.13A and 8.13B shows a patient with both a paroxysmal tachycardia and an AF episode:

o The WPW-type pre-excitation is characterized by specific ECG changes.
o The WPW syndrome is a combination of the WPW ECG pattern (the result of the WPW-type pre-excitation) and different arrhythmias.

Clinical, Prognostic, and Therapeutic Implications

The significance of WPW-type pre-excitation may be seen in two ways:

i) If it is not correctly diagnosed it may be mistaken for different and serious problems (myocardial infarction, BBB, and/or ventricular hypertrophy) (see before).
ii) Its relationship with supraventricular arrhythmias and SD. Approximately 30–35% of paroxysmal junctional re-entrant tachycardias are due to a circuit including an AP (AVRT) (see Junctional Reentrant Tachycardia) (see Figures 3.8–3.10, 4.16, and 4.18). Paroxysmal tachycardia episodes in patients with WPW syndrome may lead to important hemodynamic alterations, although generally they have a good prognosis. They are, however, potentially dangerous because they may trigger a fast AF, which may lead exceptionally to SD (Figure 8.13C). Thus, it is not recommended to treat paroxysmal episodes of AVRT with drugs (i.e., digitalis, calcium antagonists, β-blockers, adenosine, etc.) that slow conduction over the AV node more than over the APs (see Chapter 4, Junctional Reentrant Tachycardia: Prognostic and Therapeutic Implications).

Electrocardiographic criteria have been described to allow for the identification of patients at higher risk for SD during an AF episode or other supraventricular tachyarrhythmia episodes. They include the following (Klein *et al.*, 1979; Torner-Montoya *et al.*, 1991):

o A very short RR interval (≤220 ms) during spontaneous or induced AF (Figure 8.13C).
o The presence of two or more types of supraventricular tachyarrhythmias.
o The presence of underlying heart disease.
o The presence of permanent pre-excitation during a Holter recording, exercise test, and after the administration of certain drugs.
o The presence of more than one AP. This is frequent in the presence of antidromic AVRT.

In addition, there are electrophysiologic criteria during sinus rhythm allowing for the identification of patients at higher risk, including the presence of a short refractory period over the AP and the presence of multiple APs (Klein *et al.*, 1979; Torner-Montoya *et al.*, 1991).

Today, performing ablation of the AP with radio-frequency techniques (see Figure 4.25) is very successful (≈95%) and recommended, not only in cases of patients meeting high-risk criteria for developing malignant arrhythmias (see before) but also in any patient who experiences paroxysmal arrhythmia episodes. However, it has to be explained to the patient that the ablation technique, although very safe, presents in a small number of cases (<2%) severe complications, such as AV block in rare cases of septal APs and the incidence of death is extremely low (<1‰). The rate of recurrence is also low (<5%) (see Appendix A-4, and consult specific references (Recommended General Bibliography p. xvii)).

It is debatable whether ablation in patients with a WPW ECG pattern without symptoms (paroxysmal tachycardia) is recommendable due to the potential likelihood of the first episode being a fast AF. Ablation was recommended in certain situations, such as in the case of athletes, high-risk activities (divers), or professions that entail a potential danger to the public (airplane pilots), especially in the presence of permanent pre-excitation in Holter and exercise testing.

Santinelli *et al.* (2009) studied the natural history of 100 young patients with asymptomatic pre-excitation over 10 years. This study demonstrated that 30% presented some type of arrhythmia and that in ≈10% of cases the arrhythmia was potentially very dangerous. An EPS gave the best information to stratify risk. The short refractory period over AP (<240 ms) and the presence of multiple APs were the most important risk factors for future events. Therefore, an EPS has to be performed, especially in young patients with an asymptomatic WPW pattern. If the patient presents a short refractory period and/or multiple APs, ablation of the APs is highly recommended.

In fact, ventricular pre-excitation is now a nonfrequent problem, because over the last 20 years ablation has solved the majority of these cases, and now the problem may be solved even in the new born.

In cases where the AP is located in the right anteroseptal position, near the His bundle, in order to reduce the risk of inadvertent AV block, cryoablation is available. A stepwise approach to these pathways may prevent delivering full cryo (−80°) if transient AV block is observed at intermediate temperatures (−30°).

Atypical Pre-Excitation

Concept and Mechanism

This group includes those cases of pre-excitation not included in the classical Kent bundle group (AV APs) or the short type PR pre-excitation group.

It has been observed that long anomalous tracts, with slow anterograde decremental conduction only, exist from the atrium to the RV, known as atriofascicular and atrioventricular tracts, which constitute 80% of atypical tracts. Short bundles with slow decremental conduction (nodeventricular or fasciculoventricular Mahaim-type) formed by Mahaim fibers have also been described (Table 8.1, Type 2) (Sternick and Wellens, 2006; Recommended General Bibliography p. xvii).

Electrocardiographic Characteristics

In sinus rhythm, most atypical pre-excitation cases present a normal ECG or an ECG with subtle evidence of minimal pre-excitation (absence of "q" wave in V6 and I and presence of rS morphology in III lead).

During tachycardia, in general, slow decremental right atriofascicular or rarely atrioventricular tracts participate in re-entrant antidromic tachycardias. Anterograde conduction is usually over the abnormal tract, whereas retrograde conduction is through the right bundle, depolarizing the whole left ventricle through the septum. This accounts for the morphology of wide QRS complexes with LBBB and left axis deviation of ÂQRS. Characteristically, a late R/S precordial transition is observed (V4–V6) (see Figure 4.22). Meanwhile, in cases of antidromic WPW-type tachycardia (AV AP) (Kent bundle), the precordial R/S transition occurs earlier (V3) (see Figure 5.26).

If the long tract is atriofascicular, the QRS of the tachycardia is relatively narrow (<140 ms). In the rare cases when the long tract is atrioventricular, the QRS is wider because the pathway inserts directly into the ventricular muscle and the LBBB pattern is less characteristic.

Clinical, Prognostic, and Therapeutic Implications

Today, it is thought that even in the absence of definite anatomic correlations, the long right atriofascicular tracts with only anterograde conduction probably account for most antidromic tachycardias with LBBB morphology, which until recently were considered to be related to classical Mahaim fibers (Table 8.1, Type 2).

It is currently believed that classical nodoventricular or fasciculoventricular fibers described by Mahaim, although they exist, are not involved in the tachycardia circuit, which, in most cases, comprises a right atrioventricular pathway (Table 8.1, Type 2).

The best treatment in these patients with paroxysmal tachycardia is ablation of the anomalous tract (Cappato *et al.*, 1994; Haïssaguerre *et al.*, 1995).

Short PR Interval Pre-Excitation
(Lown et al., 1957) (Figures 8.14 and 8.15)

Concept and Mechanism

The short PR interval is generally due to the presence of a hyperconductive AV node, usually related to an anomaly in the AV node that allows rapid conduction to occur.

Occasionally, it may be due to the presence of an anomalous atriohisian bundle that short-circuits the slow conduction zone of the AV node. Unlike the WPW syndrome, characterized by an AP (Kent bundle) that is implanted in the ventricular working myocardium, in this case the anomalous bundle is implanted in the bundle of His (Figures 8.1 and 8.2).

The likelihood that re-entrant paroxysmal arrhythmias are generated is lower than in WPW-type pre-excitation.

Electrocardiographic Characteristics

In this case, the only ECG manifestation is a short PR interval (Figure 8.14, and Table 8.1, Type 3). Based on the surface ECG, it is impossible to confirm that the short PR is due to a genuine pre-excitation from an atriohisian tract or an accelerated conduction through the AV node, as is the case with some subjects (with or without heart disease) (sympathetic overdrive).

An intracavitary ECG shows a short atrio-His (AH) interval (see Figure 9.15A) in the presence of accelerated AV conduction, whereas in the case of an atriohisian tract, it shows a short hisian-ventricular (HV) deflection, or no inscription of the H deflection. On the other hand, the hisiogram will allow us to identify those cases with short concealed PR interval (Figure 8.15) (Ruiz-Granell *et al.*, 2000).

When confronted with a short PR interval, we should rule out other causes that may initiate such a pattern. In exceptional cases, generally with important electrolytic disorders, it may be due to a disturbance in the atrial muscle activation (sinoatrial block), in the absence of a sinus-AV node block. This is known as sinoventricular conduction, in which the QRS complex is normal, although the P wave onset is delayed, resulting in a shorter PR interval that is not due to

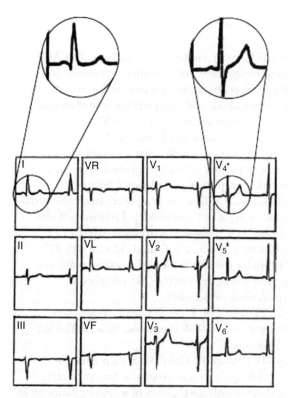

Figure 8.14 Example of typical short PR interval pre-excitation syndrome (0.10 s).

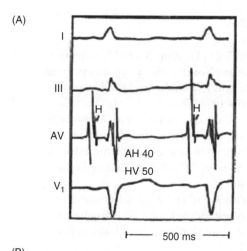

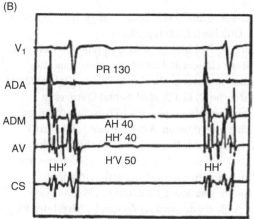

Figure 8.15 (A) A hisiogram showing a typical case of short PR syndrome. The PR shortening is due to the AH interval shortening (40 ms). (B) Concealed short PR syndrome. Although AH is short (50 ms), it is counterbalanced by an intrahisian block (HH′ = 40 ms) and a His–Purkinje (H′V) conduction rate of 50 ms, resulting in a normal PR (Ruiz-Granell *et al.*, 2000).

an accelerated AV conduction but rather to the late inscription of the P wave (see Chapter 7, and Figure 7.7). The differential diagnosis of the different types of short PR intervals may only be done through intracavitary EPS (Figure 8.15).

Clinical, Prognostic, and Therapeutic Implications

Short PR-type pre-excitation is also sometimes associated with arrhythmias, mainly reentrant supraventricular arrhythmias, and occasionally with AF that, given AV conduction characteristics, may be very rapid.

In comparison with WPW-type pre-excitation, fewer cases of re-entrant paroxysmal tachyarrhythmias are observed and the risk of sudden death is probably lower, although the occurrence of AF with rapid ventricular response is a potential risk.

The hyperconductive AV node may sometimes be controlled with β blockers. Patients with an anomalous atriohisian bundle and atrial flutter or fibrillation with rapid ventricular response, require urgent treatment with drugs, such as amiodarone, that can suppress this rapid AV conduction and/or prevent the arrhythmia. In cases of atrial flutter, catheter ablation is possible and highly successful. Ablation of AF may also be feasible. If these efforts are not successful, ablation of the AV node with RV pacing may be considered.

Self Assessment

A. List the different types of pre-excitation.

B. What are the electrocardiogram (ECG) characteristics of Wolff–Parkinson–White (WPW) type pre-excitation?

C. Define the four types of WPW syndrome according to the morphology of QRS.

D. Describe the most important differential diagnosis of WPW syndrome.

E. Which are the most frequent arrhythmias in WPW pre-excitation?

F. What are the criteria for risk of sudden death based on the ECG?

G. What is the definition of atypical pre-excitation?

H. What is the definition of short PR interval pre-excitation?

References

Arruda M, McClelland J, Wang X, *et al.* Development and validation of an algorithm identifying accessory pathway ablation site in WPW syndrome. J Cardiovasc Electrophysiol 1998;9:2.

Basiouny T, De Chillou C, Fareh S, *et al.* Accuracy and limitations of published algorithms using the twelve-lead electrocardiogram to localize overt atrioventricular accessory pathways. J Cardiovasc Electrophysiol 1999;10:1340.

Belhassen B, Fish R, Viskin S, *et al.* Adenosine-5'-triphosphate test for the noninvasive diagnosis of concealed accessory pathway. J Am Coll Cardiol 2000;36:803.

Bayés de Luna A. Clinical electrocardiology. John Wiley & Sons Ltd, Chichester, 2011, p.203.

Bayés de Luna A, Fiol M. Electrocardiography in ischemic heart disease: clinical and imaging correlations and prognostic implications. Blackwell-Futura, Oxford, 2008.

Bogun F, Kalusche D, Li YG, *et al.* Septal Q waves in surface electrocardiographic lead V6 exclude minimal ventricular pre-excitation. Am J Cardiol 1999;84:101.

Cappato R, Schlüter M, Weiss C, *et al.* Catheter-induced mechanical conduction block of right-sided accessory fibers with Mahaim-type pre-excitation to guide radio-frequency ablation. Circulation 1994;90:282.

Castellanos A, Bayés de Luna A, Zaman L., Myerburg RJ. Risk factors for ventricular fibrillation in pre-excitation syndromes. Practical Card 1983;9:167.

Chatterjee K, Harris AM, Davies JG, *et al.* T-wave changes after artificial pacing. Lancet 1969;1:759

Chiale PA, Etcheverry D, Pastori JD, *et al.* The multiple electrocardiographic manifestations of ventricular repolarization memory. Curr Cardiol Rev 2014;10(3):190.

Chiang C, Chen S, Teo W, *et al.* An accurate stepwise ECG algorithm for localization of accessory pathway during sinus rhythm. Am J Card 1995;76:40.

Critelli G, Gallagher JJ, Monda V, *et al.* Anatomic and electrophysiologic substrate of the permanent form of junctional reciprocating tachycardia. J Am Coll Cardiol 1984;4:601.

Eisenberger M, Davidson NC, Todd DM, *et al.* A new approach to confirming or excluding ventricular pre-excitation on a 12-lead ECG. Europace 2010;12:119.

Farré J, Ross D, Wiener I, *et al.* Reciprocal tachycardias using accessory pathways with long conduction times. Am J Cardiol 1979;44:1099.

Gallagher JJ, Pritchett EL, Sealy WC, *et al.* The pre-excitation syndromes. Prog Cardiovasc Dis 1978;20:285.

Gollob MH, Seger JJ, Gollob TN, *et al.* Novel PRKAG2 mutation responsible for the genetic syndrome of ventricular pre-excitation and conduction system disease with childhood onset and absence of cardiac hypertrophy. Circulation 2001;104:3030.

Haïssaguerre M, Cauchemez B, Marcus F, *et al.* Characteristics of the ventricular insertion sites of accessory pathways with anterograde decremental conduction properties. Circulation 1995;91:1077.

Hamada T, Hiraki T, Ikeda H, *et al.* Mechanisms for atrial fibrillation in patients with Wolff–Parkinson–White syndrome. J Cardiovasc Electrophysiol 2002;13:223.

Iturralde P, Araya-Gomez V, Colin L, *et al.* A new ECG algorithm for the localization of accessory pathways using only the polarity of the QRS complex. J Electrocardiol 1996;29:289.

Klein GJ, Bashore TM, Sellers TD, *et al.* Ventricular fibrillation in the WPW syndrome. New Engl J Med 1979;301:1080.

Lindsay BD, Crossen KJ, Cain ME. Concordance of distinguishing electrocardiographic features during sinus rhythm with the location of accessory pathways in the Wolff–Parkinson–White syndrome. Am J Cardiol 1987;59:1093.

Lown B, Ganong W, Levine S. The syndrome of short PR interval, normal QRS and paroxysmal rapid heart rate. Circulation 1957;5:693.

Milstein S, Sharma AD, Guiraudon GM, Klein GJ. An algorithm for the electrocardiographic localization of accessory pathways in the Wolff–Parkinson–White syndrome. Pacing Clin Electrophysiol 1987;10:555.

Nicolai P, Medvedowsky JL, Delaage M, *et al.* Wolff–Parkinson–White syndrome: T wave abnormalities during normal pathway conduction. J Electrocardiol 1981;14:295.

Peinado R, Merino JL, Gnoatto M, *et al.* Atrial fibrillation triggered by postinfarction ventricular premature beats in a patient with Wolff–Parkinson–White syndrome. Europace 2005;7:221.

Rosenbaum MB, Blanco HH, Elizari MV, *et al.* Electrotonic modulation of the T wave and cardiac memory. Am J Cardiol 1982;50:213.

Ruiz-Granell R, Garcia Civera R, Morel S, *et al.* Electrofisiologia cardíaca clínica. Editorial McGraw Hill – Interamericana, 2000.

Santinelli V, Radinovic A, Manguso F, *et al.* The natural history of asymptomatic ventricular pre-excitation a long-term prospective follow-up study of 184 asymptomatic children. J Am Coll Cardiol 2009;53:275.

Sternick E, Wellens H. Variants of ventricular pre-excitation. Blackwell-Futura, Oxford, 2006.

Tonkin A, Wagner G, Gallagher J, *et al.* Initial forces of ventricular pre-excitation in WPW syndrome. Circulation 1975;52:1030.

Torner-Montoya P, Brugada P, Bayés de Luna A, *et al.* Ventricular fibrillation in the WPW syndrome. Eur Heart J 1991;12:144.

Wellens HJ, Atié J, Smeets JL, *et al.* The ECG in patients with multiple accessory pathways. J Am Coll Cardiol 1990;16:745.

Wolff L, Parkinson J, White PD. Bundle branch block with short PR interval in healthy young people prone to paroxysmal tachycardia. Am Heart J 1930;5:685.

Yuan S, Iwa T, Tsubota M, Bando H. Comparative study of eight sets of ECG criteria for localization of the accessory pathway in Wolff–Parkinson–White syndrome. J Electrocardiol 1992;25:203.

9

Inherited Heart Diseases

Introduction

In each of these processes (Table 9.1), the importance of the electrocardiogram (ECG) to reach a diagnosis and to determine prognosis will be emphasizeed. We will also briefly discuss the molecular and genetic basis, as well as the most important clinical, diagnostic, and therapeutic implications, and the different aspects related to sudden death (SD) or serious arrhythmia (Antzelevitch, 2003). It is important to emphasize that genetic studies are still in the preliminary stage and that they should not be performed systematically in all cases of recovered cardiac arrest, as already discussed in Chapter 1, Arrhythmias and Sudden Death. Genetic tests have to be performed on survivors and some of their relatives when a genetic disease appears to be responsible for the cardiac arrest, according to the clinical test results, and especially when genetic testing may help to correctly identify the cause and to take a better decision for patient management. When an inherited heart disease is suspected, the genetic study has to be focused on that. This means studying three to five genes in cases of hypertrophic cardiomyopathy (HC), five to six genes in cases of arrhythmogenic right ventricular dysplasia/cardiomyopathy (RVD/C), five to eight genes in long QT syndrome, or at least one gene in Brugada's syndrome, for example. However, when we suspect an inherited disease but we do not know which, we have to study more than ten genes. When genetic studies may be performed very quickly and economically, they will be much more widely used (Wordsworth et al., 2010).

Cardiomyopathies

Hypertrophic Cardiomyopathy
(Table 9.2 and Figures 9.1–9.5)

Concept: Genetic Alterations
Hypertrophic cardiomyopathy (HC) is usually a familial disease of genetic origin, characterized by alterations in proteins of the myocardial cell leading to myocardial fiber disarray, hypertrophy of the heart, and an increased SD incidence. This hypertrophy may often cause a dynamic obstruction of the left ventricle (LV) outflow tract and on some occasions it leads to delayed cardiomyopathy (DC) and heart failure (HF). When the apex is preferentially involved in the hypertrophic CM, the ECG pattern shows typical features (see later).

More than 500 genetic mutations and nine genes have been described. Currently, genetic tests help to reach a diagnosis and to choose the appropriate treatment in around 50% of cases (Bos et al., 2009; Wordsworth et al., 2010). The more frequent mutations include troponin T (TNNT2) and β-myosin heavy chain (MYH7). It has been proven that **patients with troponin T mutations show more electrical instability** and SD, with less hypertrophy in young patients (Varnava et al., 1999). In contrast, alterations of the β-myosin heavy chain result in more hypertrophy and fibrosis and a lower risk of SD, although they may occasionally cause HF in adults (Geisterfer-Lowrance et al., 1990; Epstein et al., 1992). Some carriers of β-myosin heavy chain mutations with apical hypertrophy may have a poor prognosis (see later).

Electrocardiographic findings
(Figures 9.1–9.4)
Pathologic ECGs are observed in approximately 95% of cases (Table 9.2), although there is no characteristic ECG alteration indicative of a specific mutation.

As opposed to what is observed in the inherited long QT syndrome, **in HC it is not possible to predict the phenotype based on the different mutations,** except perhaps for some types of predominantly apical HC (Arad et al., 2005).

However, on certain occasions some electrocardiographic patterns are clearly indicative of HC, in particular, a large negative and sharp T wave that is typical of apical HC (Figure 9.2), as well as a narrow and deep Q wave associated with a positive T wave, suggestive of septal hypertrophy. In HC patients, especially in apical HC patients, RS morphology is often observed in V1. This may be mistakenly diagnosed as right ventricular hypertrophy, but is in fact caused by septal hypertrophy.

Table 9.1 Inherited induced heart diseases with risk of sudden death.

Cardiomyopathies (alterations in myocardial protein)

- Hypertrophic cardiomyopathy (HC)
- Arrhythmogenic right ventricular dysplasia/CM
- Spongiform cardiomyopathy (noncompacted)
- Dilated cardiomyopathy (sometimes)

Specific conduction system involvement: Lenegre syndrome

No apparent structural involvement: channelopathies (isolated alterations in ionic channels)

- Long QT syndrome
- Short QT syndrome
- Brugada's syndrome
- Catecholaminergic ventricular tachycardia
- Familial atrial fibrillation
- Torsades de Pointes ventricular tachycardia with short coupling interval (probably)
- Idiopathic ventricular fibrillation (probably)
- Others

Table 9.2 Electrocardiographic (ECG) alterations in hypertrophic cardiomyopathy (HC) (Figures 9.1–9.4).

Abnormal ECG

- Abnormal in 95% of the cases
- Sometimes with normal or slightly changed echocardiogram especially in the first years of the disease.

Signs of left ventricular enlargement

- Frequent. Sometimes characteristic repolarization alterations are observed (Figure 9.2) (large negative T wave, frequently very symmetrical and sharp). However, often the ECG is not distinguished from other processes that involve left ventricular enlargement (aortic stenosis, hypertension) (Figure 9.3)
- QRS voltage is usually increased. If it is relatively low (SV1 + RV6 <35 mm), the patient is likely to suffer from heart failure in the future (Figure 9.4)

Pathological Q wave

- Not very frequent but if exist: **a)** It is observed in leads where it is usually not seen. **b)** Narrow and sometimes very deep. Generally, the T wave is positive (Figure 9.1)

Repolarization alterations

- Very frequent (see before), sometimes with large negative but sharp T waves (Figure 9.2)

Thanks to the relationships between ECG and magnetic resonance imaging (MRI), it has been possible to localize with the ECG the more hypertrophic areas (Dumont *et al.*, 2006). More recently, a comprehensive review on the value of non-invasive methodologies for diagnosis and prognosis of HC has been published (Zhang *et al.*, 2014).

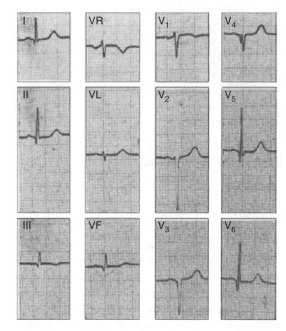

Figure 9.1 Hypertrophic cardiomyopathy (HC). Deep "q" waves in anterolateral leads, which may be mistaken for those observed in ischemic heart disease.

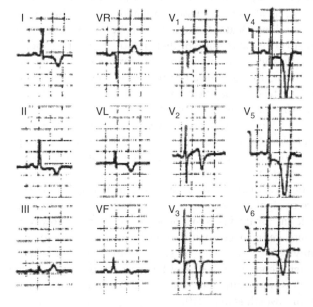

Figure 9.2 Apical hypertrophic cardiomyopathy (HC). The large negative T waves lead us to make a differential diagnosis with ischemic heart disease (IHD).

- **At times the ECG alterations are observed before the echocardiogram shows any changes**. Therefore, an abnormal ECG may be the only evidence suggesting the presence of HC in a patient's relatives, or may oblige us to rule it out when it is a casual finding.

Patients frequently show ECG signs of left ventricular enlargement, which are impossible to distinguish

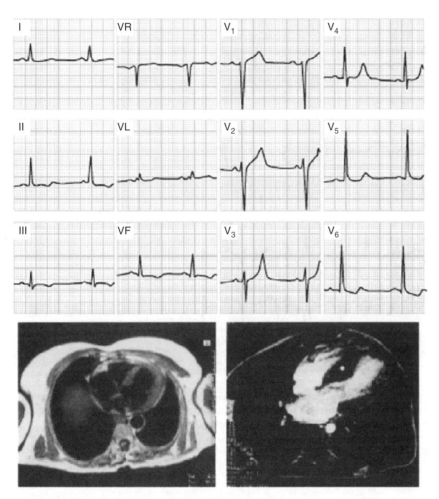

Figure 9.3 Top: Electrocardiogram (ECG) with left ventricular enlargement pattern not specific of any heart disease. Below: Cardiovascular magnetic resonance (CMR) (right) showing an asymmetric septal hypertrophy (asterisk), which confirms the diagnosis (HC). Left: CMR with normal left ventricle (LV) image (for comparative purposes). It should be pointed out that echocardiography allows us to reach the same diagnosis.

from those found in other heart diseases. In these cases, imaging techniques play a major role in establishing the correct diagnosis (Figure 9.3).

Fragmentation of the QRS (fQRS) in patients with HC has been found to be a predictor of ventricular arrhythmias ion patients already implanted with an ICD (Femenia *et al.*, 2103).

The QRS voltage is usually increased, whereas low voltage is associated with a higher incidence of dilated cardiomyopathy (DC) during follow-up (Ikeda *et al.*, 1999) (Figure 9.4).

- **Arrhythmias**. Often patients with HC present arrhythmias in the ECG. The most frequent supraventricular arrhythmia is atrial fibrillation (AF) (≈10% of patients). The resulting loss of the atrial contribution to the filling of a hypertrophied and stiff left ventricle results in clinical deterioration.

The presence of PVCs is also common; they are found in more than three-quarters of patients wearing a Holter device. Runs of nonsustained VT are found in one-quarter of patients and its presence has prognostic implications (see later). The presence of sustained VT is infrequent.

Very often, different types of blocks, especially interauricular and intraventricular blocks (left bundle branch block, LBBB) are present in advanced cases.

Clinical Presentation and Prognosis

Most HC patients will likely develop LV outflow obstruction (Maron *et al.*, 2009a), although a clear **dynamic pressure gradient in the LV outflow tract is only seen in** ≈**30%**. Some patients with HC present predominant apical involvement, which is more frequently observed in Japan (Suzuki *et al.*, 1993).

Often, HC patients present progressive dyspnea, especially after 40–50 years, due to diastolic dysfunction. Sometimes it is related to the appearance of AF. However, only about **10–15% of HC patients will develop dilated cardiomyopathy** (DC). The underlying physiopathologic mechanism that explains this evolution is not known with certainty. However, it has been shown that at 10-year follow-up the incidence of heart failure is higher in patients with low voltage QRS complexes (SV1 + RV6 <35 mm) (Figure 9.4). This is probably because the low voltage is a marker of increased fibrosis (Ikeda *et al.*, 1999).

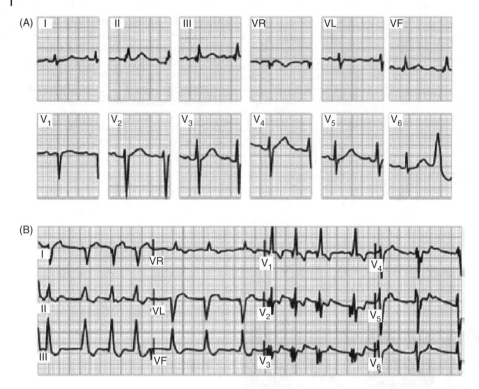

Figure 9.4 A 50-year-old patient with familial hypertrophic cardiomyopathy. (A) Note the low voltage QRS and the diffuse repolarization alterations, as well as the presence of premature ventricular complexes (PVC). Patients with hypertrophic cardiomyopathy usually exhibit a high voltage. It has been shown that the presence of relatively low voltages is associated with congestive heart failure (CHF) in the long-term follow-up. (B) In this case, after 15 years the patient suffered from advanced CHF with atrial fibrillation (AF), resulting in a very abnormal electrocardiogram (ECG): advanced right bundle branch block (RBBB) with pseudonecrosis q waves and a significant right QRS deviation due to right heart failure.

Angina-like precordial pain, especially with exercise, is frequently present. This is often related to an imbalance between oxygen supply and demand as a consequence of great myocardial hypertrophy. Other symptoms include fatigue, palpitations, and dizziness, and can be exacerbated by exercise.

However, **patients are very often asymptomatic,** especially before the age of 40–50 years, and the first symptom may be syncope, or the disease may be discovered in a routine screening or stemming from family history.

The few cases with normal ECG have a better prognosis (McLeod *et al.*, 2009), even though some exceptions have been found in patients with troponin T alterations, family history and evidence of fibrosis by MRI (see later).

The cases with predominant apical hypertrophy have a good prognosis, except those with β myosin heavy chain mutations (see before). The 15-year survival rate was found to be 95%. Younger age, HF NYHA ≥ Class II, and enlarged left atrium are predictors of cardiovascular complications (Eriksson *et al.*, 2002).

- **The differential diagnosis of an athlete's heart constitutes an interesting challenge**. There are clinical,

ECG, and echocardiographic data on which we could base our differential diagnosis (Maron *et al.*, 1981). If necessary, other techniques may be used to diminish the doubtful cases (gray zone in Figure 9.5) (Bayés de Luna *et al.*, 2000).

It is also important to perform the differential diagnosis with aortic valve stenosis. Usually this is relatively easy by auscultation and, if necessary, echocardiography.

- **Sudden death is the most important risk in this patient population.** The yearly mortality rate is around 1%. Sudden death usually occurs during exercise due to a sustained VT leading to ventricular fibrillation (VF). This is *the most common cause of SD in athletes*. However, based on the experience of Maron *et al.* (2009b), more than 30 years may elapse before another cardiac arrest occurs.
  - The most useful main risk factors of SD (McKenna and Behr, 2002; Maron, 2003, 2010) are:
    - Familial history of SD.
    - Personal antecedents of unexplained syncope.
    - Multiple-repetitive non-sustained ventricular tachycardia (NSVT) in Holter recordings.

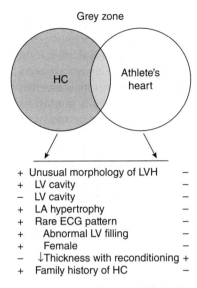

Grey zone

HC   Athlete's heart

+ Unusual morphology of LVH	–
+ LV cavity	–
– LV cavity	–
+ LA hypertrophy	–
+ Rare ECG pattern	–
+ Abnormal LV filling	–
+ Female	–
– ↓Thickness with reconditioning	+
+ Family history of HC	–

Figure 9.5 Criteria used to distinguish hypertrophic cardiomyopathy (HC) from an athlete's heart when the left ventricular wall thickness is within the gray zone, consistent with both diagnoses (adapted from Bayés de Luna, 1999).

- Abnormal blood pressure response during exercise testing.
- Massive right ventricle hypertrophy. The incidence of SD increases with septum thickness ≥20 mm, and especially ≥30 mm.

 The presence of two of the abovementioned factors, or even one for some authors (Maron, 2010), especially when accompanied with genetic alterations (troponin T mutations), **is associated with an increased risk of SD and requires implantable cardioverter defibrillator (ICD) implantation** (see later). Meanwhile, absence of the abovementioned risk factors, especially family history of SD in patients older than 50–60 years, is indicative of a better prognosis (see later).

- o **Other described markers of poor prognosis are:**
  - ST segment depression in I and VL leads.
  - A QRS duration >110 ms (Hombach *et al.*, 2009).
  - The presence of T wave alternans.
  - Evidence of serious arrhythmias in an implantable loop recorder (see Appendix A-3).
  - Serious ventricular arrhythmias during exercise testing (Gimeno *et al.*, 2009).
  - Fibrosis shown by contrast enhanced CV magnetic resonance (CE-CMR) (Leonardi *et al.*, 2009; Maron *et al.*, 2009a). Even asymptomatic patients with no left ventricular hypertrophy (LVI) but with troponin T mutations (TNNT2), significant family history, and electrophysiologic study (EPS)-induced VT/VF, show extensive fibrosis in the CE-CMR as the only pathologic abnormality (Ariyarajah *et al.*, 2009).

- o It is necessary to acknowledge that risk stratification in children is more difficult. Elderly people without previous syncope or malignant ventricular arrhythmias (VA) in the last 10–15 years have a better prognosis.
- o Unfortunately, electrophysiologic testing (Spirito *et al.*, 1997) and the tilt test are not very useful in identifying high-risk patients (Class II Bc).

Treatment

From a therapeutic point of view, it is important to improve symptoms, especially dyspnea, and to relieve a dynamic obstruction of the LV outflow tract. This is achieved with the administration of β-blockers (first-choice treatment) and, sometimes, calcium channel blockers, aimed at improving diastolic function. The latter are especially indicated if β-blocker intolerance is observed.

- o **In very symptomatic patients, septal myectomy (SM)** should be performed. This is still the first-choice treatment for patients with a very significant LV outflow tract obstruction despite receiving the optimal pharmacologic treatment.
- o **In very symptomatic cases** unresponsive to medication, **the implantation of a dual-chamber pacemaker** (DDD) with a very short AV distance to prevent LV outflow tract obstruction was considered an option. However, this is almost never used today (McKenna and Kaski, 2009).
- o **Septal ablation** (SA) with alcohol is currently standardized and presents a mortality rate similar to SM. Because of the increased risk of conduction disorders and the persistence of a post-intervention LV gradient, **SA should be considered an alternative to SM only when SM cannot be performed, or when SA is performed in very experienced centers** (Agarwal *et al.*, 2010).

It is also important to **avoid AF episodes**. Ablation of AF may be considered, even if AF is permanent, especially in cases where left ventricular systolic function worsens and sinus rhythm is not restored with drugs and/or electrical cardioversion, and/or it is difficult to control the average ventricular rate. Ablation is not usually successful in the presence of atrial fibrosis detected by CE-CMR (see Chapter 4, Ablation Techniques).

Implantable cardioverter defibrillator (ICD) implantation as a secondary prevention measure is mandatory in cases of recovered cardiac arrest or previously sustained VT (Class IB recommendation). In this setting, the yearly incidence of appropriate ICD discharge is around 4%. In primary prevention, ICD implantation in the presence of evident markers of risk for SD is considered necessary (Maron *et al.*, 2000; Maron, 2003) (Class II aC). In this setting, the yearly incidence of appropriate discharge is around 2%. However, **there is no clear consensus about the number of risk factors (RF) that have to be present in order to take this approach.** It was thought that ICD implantation may be performed in the presence of only one of the main risk factors previously described (Maron *et al.*, 2007; Maron, 2010). We consider that this depends on the risk factor, but certainly the decision may be taken in the presence of two (see before). In fact, no definitive "risk score" has been established, probably due to the difficulty of organizing trials with high statistical power, taking into account the relatively infrequent incidence of this disease (Maron, 2010). However, when deciding whether to proceed with ICD implantation it must be taken into account that the morbidity of ICD therapy is substantial, especially in young people, who will need several changes of generator, and so on. It is necessary to have a strategic programming for detection and reduction of inappropriate shocks that are troublesome and even dangerous (Wikoff *et al.*, 2008) (see Appendix A-4).

Amiodarone may be given if ICD implantation is not feasible, or in doubtful cases (Class II bc) or to prevent new shocks or crises of AF (see Appendix A-5).

Hypertrophic cardiomyopathy

Hypertrophic cardiomyopathy (HC) is usually a familial disease of genetic origin, which frequently shows evident electrocardiogram (ECG) alterations but no well defined genotype–phenotype relationship in the ECG.

There are different types of septal involvement. The apical form presents with the most characteristic ECG pattern (negative and profound T wave and often RS in V1) generally associated with a good prognosis (see text).

Hypertrophic cardiomyopathy patients show different risk markers of SD. The trigger usually is ventricular tachycardia (VT) generally related to exercise and/or an intraventricular gradient increase.

Sudden death (SD) may be prevented in at risk patients with the implantation of an implantable cardioverter defibrillator (ICD). It is mandatory to implant an ICD in patients who survived a first episode of cardiac arrest, whereas it is recommended if there are clear risk markers, including a family history of SD, to prevent new syncope or SD.

Arrhythmogenic Right Ventricular Dysplasia Cardiomyopathy (ARVC)
(Tables 9.3 and 9.4, Figures 9.6–9.8)

Concept: Genetic Abnormalities
This is a familial disease of genetic origin, comprising both a recessive form and a dominant form. There are at least five genes involved, and in half of the cases it is due to a mutation involving the protein plakophilin (Grosman *et al.*, 2004). It has been demonstrated that patients with this mutation suffer from arrhythmia at an early age (Dalal *et al.*, 2006). The genetic diagnosis may be performed in around 50% of cases. Due to the great number of loci involved in the disease, there are at least 11 different types of phenotype. Type 2 is due to a

Table 9.3 ARVC: summary of revised Task Force Criteria (Marcus *et al.*, 2010).

I.	Global or regional dysfunction And structural alterations	• By 2D echo, MRI or RV angiography: A Regional RV akinesia, dyskinesia or aneurysm • By MRI: ↓RV ejection fraction (<40% major, 40–45% minor dysfunction)
II.	Repolarization abnormalities	• Major: Inverted T wave (V1–V3) or beyond in individuals >14 y. No RBBB (Figure 9.7A) • Minor: Inverted T wave only in V1–V2 in individuals >14 y. No RBBB Inverted T waves in V1–V4 individuals >14 y, in presence of RBBB (Figure 9.6)
III.	Depolarization abnormalities	• Epsilon wave in V1–V3 (Figure 9.8) • Localized prolongation of QRS in V1–V3 (>110 ms) • Late potentials. In the absence QRS ≥110 ms
IV.	Arrhythmias	• Non-sustained or sustained VT (LBBB morphology superior axis) Major criteria (Figure 9.7) • Non-sustained or sustained VT (LBBB morphology inferior axis). Minor criteria • >500 PVC per 24 h. (Holter) Minor criteria
V.	Family history	• History of ARVC/D in a first-degree relative • Premature sudden death (<35 years of age) due to suspected ARVC/D in a first-degree relative • ARVC/D confirmed pathologically or by current Task Force Criteria in second-degree relative

ARVC, arrhythmogenic right ventricular dysplasia cardiomyopathy; MRI, magnetic resonance imaging; PVC, premature ventricular complex; RBBB, right bundle branch block; RV, right ventricle; VT, ventricular tachycardia.

Table 9.4 Diagnosis of familial ARVC (Hamid *et al.*, 2002).

Diagnostic criteria for ARVC in first-degree relatives
(Hamid et al., 2002)

The degree of familial relationship should be associated with one of the following criteria:

Repolarization alterations: negative T wave (V1–V3).

In 20% of the cases the ECG is normal Arrhythmias:

- VT with a LBBB pattern in the surface ECG, Holter ECG or during the exercise stress test
- PVC >200 in 24 h. Holter ECG
- Positive late potentials
- Structural or functional alterations of the RV

ARVC, arrhythmogenic right ventricular dysplasia cardiomyopathy; ECG, electrocardiogram; LBBB, left bundle branch block; PVC, premature ventricular complex; RV, right ventricle; VT, ventricular tachycardia.

mutation in a calcium channel, the ryanodine receptor (Tiso *et al.*, 2001).

The disease is characterized by fatty infiltration and fibrosis localized especially in the right ventricle (RV), leading to electrical instability and risk of SD.

In 50% of cases, RV dyssynchrony associated with RV dysfunction exists. This is related to late activation of the distal part of right bundle branch that explain the ECG changes (Tops *et al.*, 2009).

Frequently (>80% of cases), left ventricle (LV) involvement exists as well, often developing before the RV is involved. Evidently, from a prognostic and therapeutic point of view, it is very important to define the degree of LV involvement accurately (Sen-Chowdhry *et al.*, 2007) (see later). Rarely, in cases of genetically proven ARVC (mutation of the desmoplakin gene), isolated LV involvement is detected by the presence of a negative T wave in left lateral leads, PVC of left ventricle origin and imaging signs (CMR) of LV dysfunction, without the evidence of RV abnormalities (ECG, CMR) (Coats *et al.*, 2009).

Electrocardiographic Findings

The following are the electrocardiographic signs most frequently observed in ARVC (Jain *et al.*, 2009):

- **QRS complex width in lead V1>V6** (Fontaine *et al.*, 2004). This is due to late RV depolarization and explains that late potentials are in fact frequently positive (see Appendix) (Figure 9.6). This is reported in 80% of the cases.
  - **Atypical pattern of RBBB**. This is generally manifest as a wide R wave of relatively low voltage in lead V1 (Figure 9.6). It is due to late RV depolarization. This is found in 35% of cases.
  - **Negative T wave in precordial** V1 to V3–5 leads (Figures 9.6 and 9.7), sometimes with mild ST segment elevation. This is observed in 50% of cases.
  - **Epsilon wave** occasionally (≈10% of cases), the late depolarization of the upper RV wall is recorded as separate from the end of the QRS complex, showing subtle notches/undulations epsilon (**ε**), especially in right precordial leads and in frontal plane leads (Figure 9.8). Recently, has been published (García-Niebla *et al.*, 2016) that the incidence of epsilon wave may be conditioned by the type of filter used.
  - **Anomalous P wave** in more than 10% of cases.
  - It is important to remember that the **ECG may be normal in 20% of cases even in presence of sudden death**.
  - Frequently, **ventricular arrhythmias** are present. They originate in the RV as isolated or repetitive (VT runs) PVC with LBBB morphology (Figure 9.6), generally with left axis deviation of ÂQRS, although a right axis deviation is also possible (see Table 5.4). Sustained VT, sometimes at very high rate, are observed (Figure 9.7B), which may lead to VF.

Clinical Presentation and Prognosis

Arrhythmogenic right ventricular dysplasia cardiomyopathy (ARVD) is a serious condition that may lead to a sustained and generally monomorphic VT with LBBB morphology, eventually leading to VF and SD.

The diagnosis must be made according to the criteria of the Task Force for Cardiomyopathy (McKenna *et al.*, 1994). Recently, revised **Task Force Criteria** (Marcus *et al.*, 2010) have been published (Table 9.3).

Arrhythmogenic right ventricular dysplasia cardiomyopathy may initially mimic myocarditis (Pieroni *et al.*, 2009). This should be taken into account, as myocarditis is not mentioned in the guidelines for differential diagnosis.

Different anatomoclinical types of presentation exist and some are confined to specific geographic areas (Venice and Naxos Island) (Naxos is a beautiful small island in Greece where Protonotarios and Tsatspoulous first described the disease (Protonotarios *et al.*, 1986). Naxos syndrome is an autosomal recessive variant associated with cutaneous abnormalities (palmoplantar keratosis and woolly hair), in which penetrance is higher than that of classical ARVC. The clinical presentation and ECG abnormalities are similar, but the prognosis is usually worse (Protonotarios *et al.*, 1986). Naxos syndrome is also associated with deletion of the plakoglobulin protein. Other cases have been reported in different parts of the world, especially in Mediterranean countries

A new histochemical test (myocardial biopsy) has been developed that identifies immunohistochemical abnormalities before histologic abnormalities occur. If proven reliable, it would be very useful in reaching an early diagnosis, which is a key strategy in preventing SD (Asimaki *et al.*, 2009).

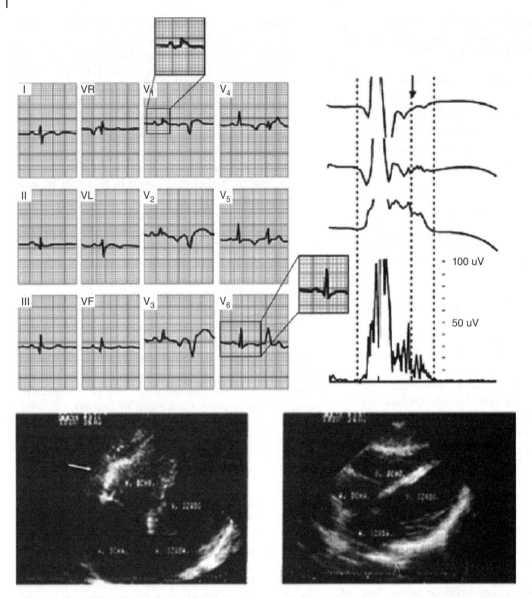

Figure 9.6 Typical electrocardiogram (ECG) pattern of a patient with arrhythmogenic right ventricular cardiomyopathy (ARVC). Note the atypical right bundle branch block (RBBB), premature ventricular complexes (PVC) from the right ventricle and negative T wave in V1–V4. We also see how QRS duration is clearly longer in V1–V2 than in V6. The patient showed very positive late potentials (right). Below: typical echocardiographic pattern showing the distortion of the right ventricular contraction (arrow).

It is important to remember that small repolarization changes (Figure 9.7A) are enough to suspect the condition and that the ECG may be normal in about 20% of cases.

Left ventricle involvement (as proven by imaging studies) in patients with ventricular arrhythmias of RV origin supports a diagnosis of ARVC (actually with biventricular involvement) and is a marker of bad prognosis (Sen-Chowdhry *et al.*, 2007) (see before).

When active arrhythmias of RV origin are present (PVC occurring frequently, above all during exercise, and runs of VT), and symptoms, such as syncope during exercise, are observed, a CMR should be performed to

confirm the ARVC. This technique is very useful with athletes suffering from this condition, and also to rule out HC or an anomalous origin of the coronary arteries.

Diagnosis of ARVC in relatives of patients with this heart disease may be reached according to the criteria described by Hamid *et al.* (2002) (Table 9.4).

A differential diagnosis with Brugada's syndrome has to be performed. Generally, this may be done based on ECG data (see Brugada's syndrome: Electrocardiographic Findings). More recently, Baranchuk *et al.* (2015) has published an algorithm that facilitate the differential diagnosis of all cases with r′ in V1.

(A)
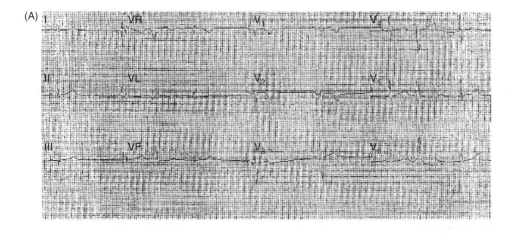

(B)
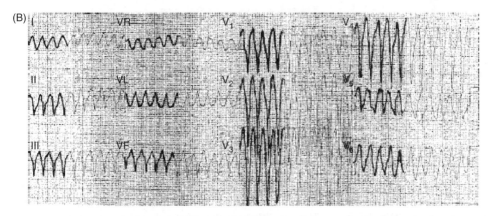

Figure 9.7 (A) Arrhythmogenic right ventricular cardiomyopathy (ARVC). Note that apart from the premature ventricular complexes (PVC), the only electrocardiogram (ECG) abnormality is the symmetric and negative T wave in V1–V2, with flat T wave in V3–V4. It is important to assess these subtle changes when suspecting the diagnosis. (B) Very fast and not well-tolerated ventricular tachycardia (VT) in the same patient. It is initiated in the apex (left VT ÂQRS), a different site from where PVC are generated (see the different morphology in VF). Implantable cardioverter defibrillator implantation was performed. The differential diagnosis of VT associated to ARVD needs to be done with right ventricular outflow ventricular tachycardia (RVOT VT). Sometimes, the analysis of the ECG in sinus rhythm provides the clue to the diagnosis of ARVD (Gottschalk *et al.*, 2014).

Treatment

In the presence of sustained VT or frequent PVC, ablation of the arrhythmogenic focus is usually indicated, even though frequent recurrences have been observed (Dalal *et al.*, 2007). A technique called "de-channeling" has been created by the Catalan group and consist in finding critical isthmuses in between the fatty tissue, responsible for reentry VT (Berruezo *et al.*, 2012). The technique has been proved to be safe and effective, however may not always prevent the implant of an ICD.

Implantable cardioverter defibrillator therapy is considered the best treatment option particularly in patients with a history of sustained VT/VF (Class I B), patients with extensive LV involvement, affected siblings, and those with a history of syncope (Class II a C). Ablation may be recommended if frequent ICD discharge is observed (Class II a C).

Arrhythmogenic right ventricular cardiomyopathy

- Arrhythmogenic right ventricular cardiomyopathy is an inherited disease comprising different anatomic and clinical presentations.
- There are ECG signs that support this diagnosis, although the ECG may be normal in 20% of cases.
- The diagnostic criteria for ARVC (McKenna *et al.*, 1994; Marcus *et al.*, 2010) and for suspecting its presence in first-degree relatives has been established (Table 9.3 and 9.4).
- Arrhythmogenic right ventricular cardiomyopathy is a serious condition that may lead to sustained VT, eventually leading to VF and SD. In the presence of sustained VT or frequent PVC, ablation of the arrhythmogenic focus is usually indicated, even though frequent recurrences have been observed (Dalal *et al.*, 2007). Therefore, often ICD implantation may be the best treatment option.

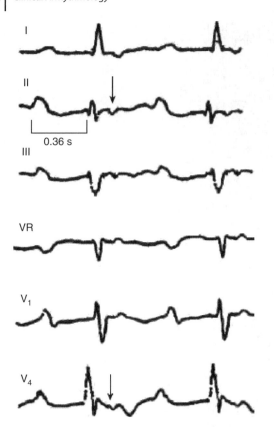

Figure 9.8 Example of delayed depolarization wave (ε) following the QRS complex with a small separation and, generally, low voltage (arrow). It is mainly observed in right precordial leads and in I, II, III, and VR in some cases of arrhythmogenic right ventricular cardiomyopathy (ARVC). It is sometimes mistakenly taken for a very premature concealed atrial extrasystole. Note that in this case a high-voltage P wave is observed and that a first-degree atrioventricular (AV) block exists.

Spongiform or Noncompacted Cardiomyopathy
(Figure 9.9)

Concept and Mechanism

This is a rare familial cardiomyopathy of uncertain etiology, for which a genetic origin has been proposed (Murphy *et al.*, 2005). In some cases that present catecholaminergic VT, genetic mutations in the ryanodine gene have been found.

From an anatomopathologic point of view, it is characterized by an increase in the trabecular mass of the LV (noncompacted), contrasting with a thin and compacted epicardial layer that may be visualized with imaging techniques (echocardiography and, above all, CMR).

Electrocardiographic Findings

Initial diagnosis is based on the following surface ECG features (Steffel *et al.*, 2009):

o Intraventricular conduction disturbances (50%).
o Repolarization disorders, manifest especially as negative and symmetric T waves in precordial leads (70%) (Figure 9.9).
o Prolonged QT interval (50%).
o Left ventricular hypertrophy (30%).
o Normal ECG in 5% of cases.

Occasionally, the ECG is similar to that of some cases of ARVC (Figure 9.7A). As many of the patients are adolescents, the repolarization disorder (negative T wave) present in the precordial leads may also be mistaken for normal ECG variations. This is a very serious mistake as a consequence of misdiagnosing the disease. The ECG we describe (Figures 9.7A and 9.9) shows a deeper and more symmetrical T wave when compared to normal variations and this is often, but not always, present up to lead V5 (Figure 9.9).

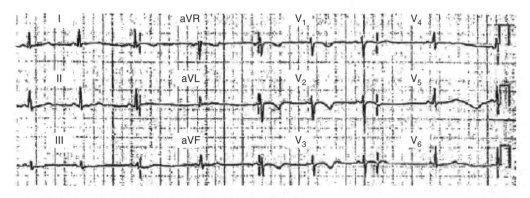

Figure 9.9 Electrocardiogram (ECG) of an 18-year-old patient with repetitive sustained ventricular tachycardia (VT). In sinus rhythm a clear QT prolongation is observed (>500 ms), as well as a negative T wave up to lead V3 with a flat T wave in V4–V6. This ECG may be mistaken for a normal ECG variant in a healthy subject. However, the long QT interval, the negative T wave up to V3 and the flat T wave in V4–V6 raise the suspicion of abnormal pattern. The echocardiogram allows for the diagnosis of spongiform cardiomyopathy.

The morphology of PVC and sustained VT usually suggests a RV origin, although PVC frequently do not display the same morphology as the VT (Paparella *et al.*, 2009).

Clinical, Prognostic, and Therapeutic Implications

The patient may remain asymptomatic for many years, but usually this cardiomyopathy eventually evolves into DC and HF. Sometimes embolism and/or ventricular arrhythmias appear in the follow-up. Ventricular arrhythmias may trigger sustained VT/VF and SD.

Therefore, the clinical presentation is very variable, from asymptomatic cases to cases with severe HF or sustained VT. In cases with sustained VT, ICD implantation has to be performed. In some cases, the ablation of the arrhythmic focus may be attempted (Hong *et al.*, 2006; Paparella *et al.*, 2009). Finally, some cases with HF may be candidates for heart transplantation.

Dilated Cardiomyopathy

(Figures 9.10 and 9.11)

Concept and Mechanisms

Dilated cardiomyopathy is characterized by ventricular dilatation, especially of the LV, featuring a generally progressive impairment of ventricular function that frequently leads to HF.

Dilated cardiomyopathy may be idiopathic (30–40% of cases), or due to many etiologies, such as infections, toxic agents, drugs, autoimmune processes, and neuromuscular, metabolic, or mitochondrial diseases, although the condition most frequently associated with DC is chronic ischemic heart disease (IHD) and/or arterial hypertension. In our opinion, the new classification of cardiomyopathies (Maron *et al.*, 2006), without a convincing rationale, has excluded the cases of myocardial

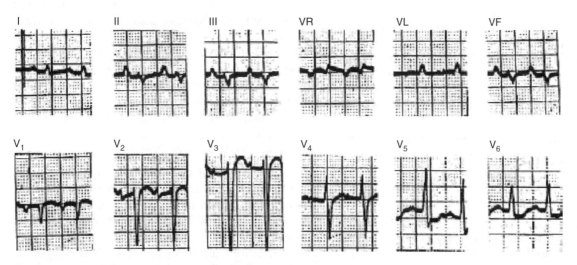

Figure 9.10 Typical electrocardiogram (ECG) pattern corresponding to idiopathic dilated cardiomyopathy in heart failure (HF). Note the low voltage in the frontal plane, the significant alterations in the P wave and the QRS complex (atypical left bundle branch block, LBBB, with QRS ≈0.12 s), as well as the abnormal repolarization. The high voltage in V3 (with no notching) supports the idiopathic nature of the condition (see Figure 9.11).

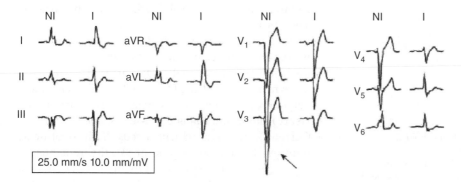

Figure 9.11 Electrocardiogram (ECG) of two patients with dilated cardiomyopathy one with ischemic (I) and the other with nonischemic (NI) heart disease. Note the different QRS complexes in V3: in one patient a notched low-voltage QRS complex is present consistent with ischemic dilated cardiomyopathy (I), whereas the other patient shows a high-voltage QRS complex, which is consistent with nonischemic dilated cardiomyopathy (NI).

involvement that are a direct consequence of other cardiovascular diseases, such as hypertension, IHD, and congenital or valvular heart disease.

There is evidence that up to 35% of patients with idiopathic DC have a family history or share environmental surroundings (Towbin and Bowles, 2002). Some genetic predisposition has already been established.

More than 20 mutations in different genes have been identified, including the AIC lamine gene, which is present in 30% of cases and is related to high incidence of SD. Additionally, the genetic relationship between DC and muscular dystrophies (such as Duchenne, Emery-Dreifuss, and Becker dystrophies) has also been reported. Each dystrophy may lead to cardiac alterations, evolving into DC and HF (Burkett and Hersberger, 2005).

Electrocardiographic Findings

Table 9.5 shows the ECG abnormalities most suggestive of DC (Figure 9.10).

Heart failure patients with DC and advanced LBBB + AF (about 5% of all the cases) have a higher mortality rate, both in terms of death from any cause or from SD (Baldasseroni *et al.*, 2002; Vázquez *et al.*, 2009) (see Chapter 11, Heart Failure).

In contrast, we have described (Bayés-Genís *et al.*, 2003) how in DC patients with LBBB, the QRS complex voltage in lead V3 is useful to differentiate idiopathic and ischemic etiology of DC (Figure 9.11, see legend).

Table 9.5 Suspected dilated cardiomyopathy, based on the electrocardiogram (Figure 9.10).

Sinus tachycardia: often atrial fibrillation (10–20%)

Anomalous P wave with often advanced intertatrial block pattern (17% of cases) (Alvarez-Garcia *et al.*, 2016)

Anomalous QRS complex with:
Very frequently, ≥0.12 s. Patients with very wide QRS complexes (≥140 ms) have worse ventricular function
Frequently low voltage in the frontal plane, with high voltages in V1–V4, mainly in the cases of idiopathic dilated cardiomyopathy (Figures 9.10 and 9.11)
Significant left or right ÂQRS deviation
Sometimes a pathologic Q wave

Anomalous repolarization

Premature ventricular complexes of special morphologic characteristics (wide QRS complex with slurred and low-voltage R), sometimes with Q wave and frequently with symmetrical T wave (Figure 5.9). These complexes are observed in any type of advanced heart disease with ventricular dysfunction

In patients with dilated cardiomyopathy and heart failure, a left bundle branch block plus atrial fibrillation pattern is a marker for poor prognosis (Baldasseroni *et al.*, 2002; Vázquez *et al.*, 2009).

Clinical, Prognostic, and Therapeutic Implications

Both idiopathic and secondary DC (ischemia, alcohol, etc.), present a high incidence of SD because DC frequently presents HF and is related to ventricular arrhythmias and SD (see Chapter 11, Heart failure). The likelihood of developing SD depends on the presence of different risk factors (chain of events) (Figure 11.5). Fibrosis, autonomic nervous system alterations, ionic/metabolic abnormalities, lengthening of repolarization as a result of the prolongation of the K current function, and many other triggering/modulating factors are involved.

We have published (Vázquez *et al.*, 2009) (see Chapter 11, Heart Failure) a "risk score" for the identification of cases with DC and HF that present a higher risk of SD. This score is based on clinical (age, heart rate, gender), electrocardiographic (QRS complex width, presence/absence of sinus rhythm, PVC on Holter recording), echocardiographic (LA size, ejection fraction), and blood test (proBNP, renal function) data. These data are available for any clinical cardiologist, and allow cases at high and low risk for SD to be identified (Figure 11.6).

Very recently, we have demonstrated that the patients with HF and A-IAB pattern present a progressive worse prognosis (Alvarez-Garcia *et al.*, 2016).

Heart failure should be prevented and treated according to guidelines produced by scientific societies (Recommended General Bibliography p. xvii).

○ In cases of ventricular asynchrony (wide QRS complex (≥130 ms) due to LBBB or apical RV pacing), cardiac **resynchronization therapy (CRT)** is very useful in improving LV function in patients with depressed ejection fraction (EF) <35%. Its usefulness has been already proved in patients with mild HF (Healey *et al.*, 2012, RAFT Study) and there are promising results in cases with relatively preserved EF. However, it should be remembered that the number of nonresponsive remains at about 25–30% (see Chapter 11, Heart Failure, and Appendix A-4, Cardiac Resynchronization Therapy (CRT).

○ Implantable cardioverter defibrillator implantation to prevent SD is based on the ejection fraction, as well as the history of a recovered cardiac arrest, sustained VT or syncope (see Chapter 5, Classical Ventricular Tachycardia, Chapter 11, Ischemic Heart Disease and Heart Failure, and Appendix A-4, Implantable CD).

○ Currently, when a patient needs both treatments (improve LV function + prevent SD) the implantation of a unique device with both functions (ICD-CRT), if the requirements for this treatment exist, may be the best option.

For more information see Chapters 5 and 11, the Appendix, and the guidelines given in the Recommended General Bibliography p. xvii.

Specific Conduction System Involvement: Lenegre Syndrome

Lenegre syndrome is a rare disease that consists of a progressive intraventricular conduction block without apparent heart disease. It appears in members of the same family at a relatively young age (Lenegre, 1964). On certain occasions a relationship with SCN5A mutations has been shown (Schott *et al.*, 1999). It is known that different electrocardiographic phenotypes (long QT syndrome, Brugada's syndrome and Lenegre syndrome) may be related to mutations in the same gene (SCN5A) (Bezzina *et al.*, 1999).

Thus, from a genetic point of view, the Lenegre syndrome is caused by a sodium channel dysfunction (decreased Na inflow into the cell) due to gene SCN5A mutations, accounting for the progressive decrease in the conduction of the stimulus (Probst *et al.*, 2003).

Histological studies show that a **diffuse fibrotic degeneration of the whole intraventricular SCS exists**, which may lead to an AV block without involvement of the sinus node and the fibrous skeleton of the heart. The presence of this evident pathologic involvement differentiates the Lenegre syndrome from channelopathies (see later).

Lenegre syndrome should be distinguished from Lev disease (Lev, 1964). The latter is additionally characterized by the progressive occurrence of intraventricular conduction defects, frequently with a concurrent advanced AV block. Lev disease, which is found in older patients, is, however, due to a noninherited senile degeneration of the SCS and the fibrous skeleton of the heart.

Usually, pacemaker implantation becomes necessary during the course of both Lenegre syndrome and Lev disease.

Ionic Channel Disorders in the Absence of Apparent Structural Heart Disease: Channelopathies

In this section we will include heart diseases with no apparent structural involvement and related to gene mutations leading to defects of ionic transport. In particular, these include defects in sodium, potassium, and calcium transport through the corresponding ionic channels (Marbán, 2002; Brugada *et al.*, 2007). Demonstration of gene alteration is not found in all cases. It is believed that channelopathies are not characteristically accompanied by structural heart abnormalities (see later) and that their first clinical manifestation may be a syncope or SD. Due to the presence of definitive ultrastructural abnormalities in the intraventricular conduction system, the Lenegre syndrome, even if related to the Na$^+$ channel defect, is not considered a channelopathy (see before and later).

Exclusive alterations of the ionic channels are observed in long and short QT syndrome, Brugada's syndrome and catecholamine-sensitive VT. They are also probably present in familial AF and other cases of SD due to other malignant ventricular arrhythmias (MVA), such as familial Torsades de Pointes VT, and cases of VT that until now were considered idiopathic VF. Additionally, ionic channel alterations are involved in some cases of sinus bradycardia of genetic origin and in WPW syndrome (see Chapter 8, Concept and Types of Pre-Excitation, and Chapter 10, Severe Sinus Bradycardia).

Some of the most well-known channelopathies show a typical phenotypic ECG pattern, which frequently allows for a correct diagnosis and even identification of the gene involved. Recently, some evidence has been published showing that initially isolated ionic alterations (true channelopathies) may present some ultrastructural changes in the follow-up. Some histological alterations (Frustaci *et al.*, 2009), as well as subtle abnormalities of RV morphology, detected by CMR, have been described (Catalano *et al.*, 2009) in asymptomatic relatives of patients with Brugada's syndrome who carried SCN5A mutations. This confirms that the phenotypic manifestation of Brugada's syndrome and its physiopathology might be more complex than first thought, and that the **initially isolated ionic alterations may induce evident ultrastructural changes in the future.**

All channelopathies may increase the risk of developing different types of VT/VF, eventually leading to SD. In catecholaminergic-sensitive VT this is related to defects in excitation–contraction coupling and to exercise-induced catecholamine discharge (Liu *et al.*, 2008). In long QT, short QT, and Brugada's syndromes, occurrence of VT/VF could be due to heterogeneous dispersion of repolarization (HDR), occurring in transregional (Opthof *et al.*, 2007) or transmural areas (Antzelevitch *et al.*, 2007). This HDR favors a premature ventricular complex to induce VT/VF, probably due to a Phase 2 reentrant phenomenon (see Table 3.1).

In Chapter 3 (Figure 3.11E), we described how ventricular HDR is responsible for the increased T wave peak/T wave end interval, and that this parameter is a marker of poor prognosis and the development of ventricular arrhythmias. We also mentioned that some evidences suggest that HDR occurs not at the transmural level as proposed by Antzelevitch *et al.* (2007) in several studies carried out in wedge preparations, but rather at a transregional level, as suggested by different experiments done in dogs (Opthof *et al.*, 2007).

Now we will look at the most important aspects of the different channelopathies, explaining the underlying genetic alterations and the ionic mechanisms, as well as their electrocardiographic characteristics and their clinical prognostic and therapeutic implications.

Long QT Syndrome

(Figures 9.12–9.14)

Concept: Genetic and Molecular Basis

(Moss et al., 1985; Moss and Kan, 2005; Zareba et al., 2003; n)

This is a genetically induced syndrome characterized by a long QT interval due to dispersion of the repolarization that may also present other repolarization alterations (Table 9.7). This syndrome presents syncope attacks that eventually lead to SD. It may encompass two congenital long QT syndromes: Jervell and Lange-Nielsen syndrome, a very rare autosomal recessive disorder that causes congenital deafness (Jervell and Lange-Nielsen,1957), and the autosomal-dominant Romano-Ward syndrome (Vincent, 1986), somewhat more common.

It has been demonstrated that this syndrome is caused by a defect in the ionic channels. Until now at least 500 mutations in at least six genes have been described in an ever-increasing list (Kapplinger *et al.*, 2009), resulting in 10 different phenotypes (long QT 1–10) (Morita *et al.*, 2008a). This represents a genetic identification in 50% of cases.

The ultimate ionic mechanism underlying the repolarization dispersion is the result of a genetic mutation that leads to a slow and late activation of K channels (IKr, IKs), along with an incomplete inactivation of Na$^+$ and Ca^{++} channels with a late Ca^{++} and Na$^+$ inward current (Moss and Kan, 2005). Most of the mutations result in K channel alterations, which eventually lead to long QT syndrome. In some cases (i.e., LQT3), long QT syndrome is fundamentally the result of incomplete inactivation of the Na channels. It has even been described that LQT8 (Timothy syndrome) (Splawsky and Timothy, 2004) is due to an L-type Ca channel alteration (gene CACCNAIC).

We are only going to discuss the three best-known variants of long QT syndrome in which there is a **good genotype/phenotype correlation (ECG expression). These are LQT1, LQT2, and LQT3** (Table 9.7, Figures 9.12 and

9.13) (Zareba *et al.*, 1998) (see later). In all these LQT syndrome variants, a more significant myocardial transmembrane action potential (TAP) lengthening is appreciated in the area, which was already more prolonged (in wedge preparations the M cell tissue). This entails a prolongation of the QT interval, as well as an increase of the T wave peak (end of the area with shorter TAP) to T wave end (end of the area with longer TAP) (T peak/T end interval) (see Figure 3.11E). This HDR is accompanied by a long QT (with different phenotypic expressions) (Figure 9.12). The presence of HDR is associated with a greater likelihood of developing VT (Torsades de Pointes) caused by reentry Phase 2, due to the voltage gradient originating between both TAP. Rotors with unstable spiral waves have also been involved in the mechanism of VT/VF (see Figures 3.11–3.13).

Electrocardiographic Findings

(Figures 9.12 and 9.13, Tables 9.6–9.8)

Table 9.6 shows QTc values that are considered pathologic according to age and gender. QT interval measurement should be done in leads II and V5 or V6, taking the mean value of the QT interval measurements in five RR cycles, from the earliest QRS onset until the end of the T wave. It is very important to recognize a long QT when examining an ECG recording (Viskin *et al.*, 2005, Postema, 2008). We can only speak about **long QT syndrome** when a patient presents a nonacquired long QT interval with syncopal attacks or recovered cardiac arrest due to Torsades de Pointes VT often leading to SD, or a family history of this syndrome.

In cases with borderline QTc interval, epinephrine QT stress testing may be useful in the evaluation of a possible congenital long QT syndrome, especially in LQT1 and LQT2 (Vyas and Ackerman, 2006). Changes of QTc with exercise or standing, evaluating the changes occurring with tachycardia, may also help in cases of borderline QTc duration, (Zareba, 2010). Currently, the observation of QT prolongation after standing up, is known as the "Viskin maneuver" (Viskin *et al.*, 2010).

Table 9.7 and Figure 9.12 show the characteristic electrocardiographic alterations of LQT1, LQT2 and LQT3 syndromes (Zareba *et al.*, 1998; Moss, 2002). All these alterations (QT prolongation, QT dispersion, T peak/T end interval, and other repolarization anomalies) are

Long QT1 Chromosome 11	Long QT2 Chromosome 7	Long QT3 Chromosome 3
V$_5$	V$_5$	V$_5$

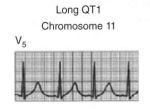 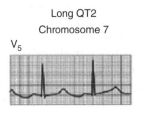 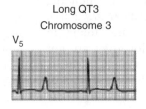

Figure 9.12 Three examples of electrocardiogram (ECG) patterns in long QT syndrome clearly associated with different chromosomal alterations: LQT1 (1), LQT2 (B), and LQT3 (C).

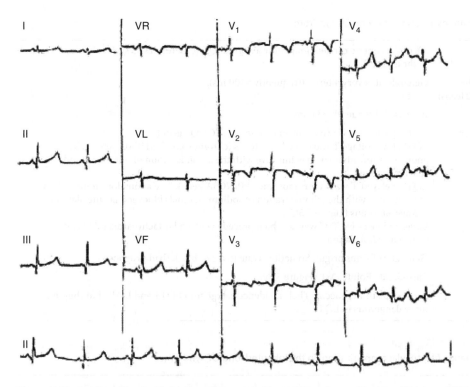

Figure 9.13 A child with a family history of congenital long QT syndrome. The long QT interval (QT = 520) allows us to reach a diagnosis of congenital long QT syndrome. However, at first glance as the T wave morphology is not very typical of long QT syndrome this may not have been diagnosed. Therefore, that highlights the need to perform systematic measurements of the QT interval in all ECG tracings.

more striking than those observed in other pathologic conditions with a long QT.

Table 9.8 shows the genotype/phenotype correlation (repolarization) in the long QT syndromes mentioned (long QT1, LQT2 and LQT3). Each shows a definitely long QTc (the longest QTc is observed in the LQT3 variant) and in many cases the repolarization alterations allow for the recognition and identification of the genotype. LQT1 has wide high-voltage T waves, while LQT2 features low voltage and frequently notched T waves and LQT3 late T waves (Figure 9.12). Although the genotype/phenotype correlation is generally good in these three long QT syndromes (Figure 9.12), on certain occasions there are some poorly defined forms (Figure 9.13). Table 9.8 also shows the percentage of carriers of the genetic mutation displaying such ECG morphology, the percentage of carriers with a normal

ECG and the drugs that improved morphology (Zareba *et al.*, 1998; Moss, 2002).

In wedge preparations it has been demonstrated that Torsades de Pointes VT is triggered when HDR is >90 ms (Antzelevitch *et al.*, 2007). Clinical studies confirmed (Takenaka *et al.*, 2003) that an increased T peak/T end interval during exercise is a marker of bad prognosis in LQTS1 patients.

Fatal arrhythmia (Torsades de Pointes VT) leading to ventricular fibrillation and SD (especially in LQT2) frequently begins in the presence of large negative (but not sharp) T-U waves after a premature ventricular complex, followed by a long pause before the onset of the Torsades de Pointes VT (Kirchhof *et al.*, 2009) (see Chapter 5, Ventricular Tachycardia).

Patients with long QT syndrome usually do not reach the heart rate adjusted by age during exercise testing.

Table 9.6 QTc prolongation in different age groups, based on the Bazett formula: values within the normal interval, borderline values, and altered values.

Value	1–15 years old	Adult (men)	Adult (women)
Normal, ms	<440	<430	<450
Borderline, ms	440–460	430–450	450–470
Altered (prolonged), ms	>60	>450	>470

Table 9.7 Electrocardiogram (ECG) alterations in congenital long QT syndrome.

• QT prolongation	3% of the genetic carriers may show a normal QT (different ECG series should be done in these cases)
• QT dispersion (difference between the longest and the shortest QT in the 12 leads)	Generally it is very altered (frequently >100 ms).
• T peak/T end interval	Increased. Frequently >90 ms
• Morphologic repolarization alterations (Zareba *et al.*, 1998) (Figure 9.12)	LQT1: prolonged T wave (chromosome 11) (KCNQ1 gene) LQT2: low-voltage T wave and/or notches (chromosome 7) (HERG gene). The anomalous morphology may improve with the administration of potassium and spironolactone LQT3: delayed T wave (chromosome 3) (SNC5A gene). The anomalous morphology may improve with the administration of sodium channels blockers (i.e. mexiletine) T wave alternans (Figure 7.5C) Large and negative T/U waves, which precede ventricular tachycardia (VT) and ventricular fibrillation
Bradycardia	Generally of sinus origin. Sometimes due to a 2×1 block (bad prognosis)
Arrhythmias	Torsades de Pointes VT (Figure 5.36)
	Sudden death may occur. Their incidence is higher in LQT1 and LQT2 but they are more dangerous in LQT3

Table 9.8 Genotypic–phenotypic correlation (ventricular repolarization) in the inherited long QT syndrome.

	Genetic mutation	More typical T wave morphology[*]	Mutation carriers with typical abnormal ECG (long QT and ST/T alteration)	Mutation carriers with normal ECG (QTc <440 ms and normal ST/T)	Improved pattern after drug administration
LQT1	Chromosome 11, KCNQ1 gene	Wide base	<80%	≈3%	—
LQT2	Chromosome 7, HERG gene	Low voltage and bimodal	>80%	≈3%	K and spironolactone
LQT3	Chromosome 3, SCN5A gene	Delayed onset and sharp	≈65%	0%	Sodium channels antagonists (mexiletine, flecainide)

[*] Occasionally other abnormal morphologies may be observed (Moss, 2002).

Furthermore, cases of LQT1 prolong the QT interval with exercise (Medeiros-Domingo *et al.*, 2007; Zareba, 2010). Exercise testing may produce T wave alternans that are indicative of electrical instability.

Holter monitoring is very useful to monitor the QT interval and also to record different arrhythmias, especially ventricular arrhythmias and some bradyarrhythmias, including 2×1 AV block.

Diagnosis and Prognosis
A "point score" diagnostic criteria for long QT syndrome (LQTS) has been proposed (Table 9.9) (Schwartz *et al.*, 1993). The diagnostic criteria are listed in this table with points assigned to various electrocardiographic, clinical, and familial findings. The score ranges from a minimum value of 0 to a maximum value of 9 points. The point score is divided into three probability categories: ≤1 point = low probability of LQTS;

>1–3.0 points = intermediate probability of LQTS; and ≥3.5 points = high probability of LQTS. As QTc overcorrects at fast heart rates, additional diagnostic caution is necessary when dealing with tachycardic patients or infants with fast heart rates.

The overall population with LQTS who receive β-blockers have a good prognosis (SD = 0.1% yearly). The presence of syncope during β-blocker therapy represents a subgroup of a risk of life-threatening events (≥2% yearly).

Figure 9.14 shows the global risk stratification in LQTS patients, including the three types of risk (low, high and very high-risk of VT/VF). It is based on the studies carried out by the Moss group (Goldberger and Moss, 2008). Silvia Priori has established a similar risk pyramid that is currently accepted in the medical community (Priori *et al.*, 2003). Nevertheless, it should be pointed out that in some forms of long QT syndromes (such as LQT1 and LQT2), the prognosis may vary substantially depending

---

Long QT syndrome

Diminishing and slowing of the outward currents of the repolarization together with an increase in the inward $[Ca^{2+}]$ and late $[Na^+]$ currents.
All of this is mediated by mutations in various genes (Table 9.8)

Heterogeneous dispersion of the Repolarization (DHR)

The TAP of the longer zone* extends further than that of the shorter zone which initiates a heterogeneous dispersion of the repolarization (HDR), manifesting itself as an increase in the length from T peak to T end

Lengthening of the QT
- Genotype/phenotype correlation (typical ECG morphologies in LQT1, LQT2 and LQT3.
- At times there may be electrical alternans.

The voltage gradient originated by the HDR can trigger a re-entry in phase 2 than gives rise to VT/VF

Long QT syndrome

Scheme 9.1 Long QT Syndrome. *According to the Gussak group (Gussak *et al.*, 2008), heterogeneous dispersion occurs on a transmural level and the zone with the longest TAP is the zone with M cells. Other authors support the existence of heterogeneous dispersion of the repolarization but question whether it is at a transmural level (Ophof, 2007).

Table 9.9 Long QT syndrome (LQTS) diagnostic criteria (1993).

	Points
1. Electrocardiographic findings*	
– QTc[†]	
>480 ms	3
460–470 ms	2
450 (male) ms	1
– Torsades de pointes[‡]	2
– T wave alternans	1
– Notched T wave in three leads	1
– Low heart rate for age[§]	0.5
2. Clinical history	
– Syncope[‡]	
With stress	2
Without stress	1
– Congenital deafness	0.5
– Family history[¶]	
A. Family members with definite LQTS	1
B. Unexplained sudden cardiac death below age 30 among immediate family members	0.5

* In the absence of medications or disorders known to affect these electrocardiographic features.
† QTc calculated by Bazett's formula where $QTC=QT/\sqrt{RR}$.
‡ Mutually exclusive.
§ Resting heart rate below the 2nd percentile for age.
¶ The same family member cannot be counted in A and B.
Score: <1 point = low probability of LQTS; 2–3 points = intermediate probability of LQTS; ≥3.5 points = high probability of LQTS.

and stress (tachycardia-dependent arrhythmias), whereas in LQT2 and LQT3 types they are more related to rest, sleep or acoustic stimuli (pause-dependent arrhythmias) (Schwartz *et al.*, 2006). Competitive sports are contraindicated for patients with congenital LQTS.

It has been demonstrated that an increased T peak/T end interval is a marker of poor prognosis (Yamaguchi *et al.*, 2003) (see before).

The exercise test and Holter monitoring may be useful in detecting risk markers (see before).

Electrophysiologic testing does not generally induce arrhythmias.

It has been recently shown that risk also depends on the type of mutation in certain genes (*KCNQ1*) and their biophysical function (see before) (Moss *et al.*, 2007; Vincent *et al.*, 2009, Yang *et al.*, 2009).

Treatment
Treatment includes β-blockers, left-sided stellate ganglion denervation, and, with increasing frequency, implantation

on the K⁺ channel dysfunction derived from the genetic mutation (Moss *et al.*, 2007; Vincent *et al.*, 2009).

The incidence of arrhythmias, especially Torsades de Pointes VT, (see Chapter 5, Torsades de Pointes Polymorphic Ventricular Tachycardia) that often induce syncopal attacks and, unfortunately, may trigger SD is higher in LQT1 and LQT2 types. However, arrhythmias observed in the LQT3 type are potentially more dangerous. Meanwhile, in LQT1, arrhythmias occur mainly as a result of physical exercise

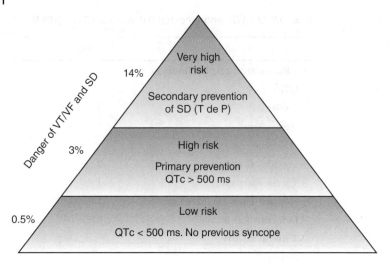

Danger of VT/VF and SD

14% Very high risk
Secondary prevention of SD (T de P)

3% High risk
Primary prevention QTc > 500 ms

0.5% Low risk
QTc < 500 ms. No previous syncope

Figure 9.14 Risk stratification in long QT syndrome (Goldberger and Moss, 2008) (See text).

of automatic ICD (Goldberger and Moss, 2008; Viskin and Halkin, 2009). Other therapeutic approaches will be also mentioned.

At the present time, and based on the global risk stratification, we may assert that in the cases at **very high risk** shown in Figure 9.14, an ICD should be implanted and β-blockers should be administered (Class IA).

In **high-risk cases** (Figure 9.14), β-blocker treatment should be given and an ICD implanted if symptoms (syncope) persist despite treatment (Class I B). Patients with QTc ≥450 ms and with syncope during β-blocker therapy are at high risk for VT/VF (SD ≥2% yearly), and ICD therapy is recommended (Class II a B). Women and children in particular should be recommended for this treatment (Jons *et al.*, 2010). Dual chamber ICDs are preferred as they could be used to pace the atrium preserving the intrinsic AV conduction and reducing the QTc length.

For the time being, **low-risk patients** (Figure 9.14) should receive β-blockers (Class I B), unless they are contraindicated. These are especially effective in LQT1 (mean dose 2.2 ± 1.2 mg/kg). In LQT1 syndrome, β-blockers are very effective if they are taken regularly and drugs that lengthen the QT interval are avoided. If no symptoms are present (syncope), ICD implantation is not necessary (Vincent *et al.*, 2009). Some evidence supports that β-blockers, if administered correctly, are also effective in LQT2 and LQT3, although to a lesser degree than in LQT1 (Viskin and Halkin, 2009). Recently (Horner *et al.*, 2010) questioned the need of ICD implant in many patients with LQTS. This study showed that the greatest save rate occurs among LQT2 women, who were assessed to be at high risk. It is necessary to balance the advantages of ICD implant with the complications (inappropriate shocks) that may occur even in 20–30% of cases in some series. Subcutaneous implants may offer protection with less number of complications.

The implantation of a pacemaker, along with the administration of β-blockers, has been a helpful measure in patients with bradycardia, AV block, and, above all, pause-dependent VT Torsades de Pointes. At present, they are rarely implanted alone and are instead incorporated into the ICD.

The left-sided stellate ganglion denervation should be applied to patients experiencing an electrical "storm" despite taking β blockers and having an ICD implanted (Class II b B). It is currently carried out through video surgery, a technique that has drawn more attention to this indication (Collura *et al.*, 2009).

Ablation of the extrasystolic focus triggering the VT/VF has also been described as another promising technique to prevent ventricular arrhythmias (Haïssaguerre *et al.*, 2003).

Today, a new therapeutic option is being discussed: ranolazine or other similar drugs has been reported that significantly shortens the QTc interval in LQT3 patients.

Finally, the dawning of genetic therapy (K$^+$ channel activators, Na$^+$ channel knockers, etc.), although still in the experimental phase (Khan and Gowda, 2004), should be acknowledged.

Short QT Syndrome
(Figure 9.15)

Concept: Genetic and Molecular Basis

Two families showing a QT interval of ≤300 ms regardless of the heart rate with no apparent cause (i.e., electrolyte imbalance) have been described (Gaita *et al.*, 2003). This is a very infrequent new inherited disease in which mutations in various genes have been described, including: HERG (IKr gain-of-function mutation) (short QT syndrome 1), KCNJ2 (Iki gain-of-function mutation) (short QT syndrome 3), and KCNQ1 (IKs gain-of-function mutation) (short QT syndrome 2).

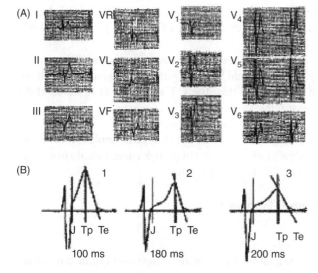

Figure 9.15 (A) Short QT syndrome. A typical electrocardiogram (ECG) pattern with QT <300 ms and high, sharp T waves. (B) Symptomatic short QT pattern (1), asymptomatic (II), and normal QT (control) (III) (see text) (adapted from Anttonen *et al.*, 2009).

These K$^+$ channel mutations lead to a HDR with a greater TAP shortening in an area that already had a shorter TAP compared to the area with the baseline longest TAP. According to some authors, this HDR occurs at a transmural level (Extramiana and Antzelevitch, 2004; Anttonen *et al.*, 2008).

As a result of the different degrees of shortening between the two TAP lengths, a voltage gradient is generated. This may trigger the occurrence of VT/VF through a reentrant mechanism in TAP Phase 2 (see Figure 3.11E and scheme).

Short QT syndrome may be associated with AF and Brugada's syndrome (alteration of L-type Ca channels) (Antzelevich *et al.*, 2007) and also with early repolarization pattern (Watanabe *et al.*, 2010).

A clinical score to determine the risk associated with short QT syndrome has been published (Gollob *et al.*, 2011) See Table 9.10.

Electrocardiographic Findings

o **Short QT interval**. The short QT syndrome should be considered when the QT interval is between 320 and 350 ms without an apparent cause. The diagnosis is certain when a QT interval below 300 ms is confirmed.
o A very tall and sharp T wave is recorded in virtually all cases of symptomatic short QT. The tall T wave presents especially in right precordial leads, almost equally in ascending and descending limbs (almost-symmetrical T wave), with a J point–T peak distance <150 ms. This allows it to be differentiated from other asymptomatic short QT cases that present J point–T

peak interval >150 ms (Figure 9.15B). The normal J-Tp is >200 ms (Anttonen *et al.*, 2009).
o Virtual absence of ST segment.
o An increase in the T peak/T end ratio (Anttonen *et al.*, 2008).
o An early repolarization pattern may be found in patients with short QT syndrome (Watanabe *et al.*, 2010).
o The ECG occasionally resembles a hyperkalemia tracing. However, potassium concentrations are not measured in the cases reported.
o Electrophysiologic studies show that the atrial and ventricle refractory periods are short and that in most cases there is an increased susceptibility to develop atrial or ventricular fibrillation.

Table 9.10 Short QT syndrome: diagnostic criteria.

ECG findings[a]	Points
QTc	
<370 ms	1
<350 ms	2
<330 ms	3
J point-T peak interval[b] < 120 ms	1
Clinical history[c]	
History of sudden cardiac arrest	2
Documented polymorphic VT or VF	2
Unexplained syncope	1
Atrial fibrillation	1
Family history[d,e]	
First-or second-degree relative with high-probability STQS	1
First- or second-degree relative with autopsy-negative sudden cardiac death	
Sudden infant death syndrome	1
Genotype[e]	
Genotype positive	
Mutation of undetermined significance in a culprit gene	2
High-probability SQTS:≥4 points, intermediate-probability	1
SQTS: 3 points, low-probability SQTS: ≤ 2 points	

a) Must be recorded in the absence of modifiers known to shorten the QT.
b) Must be measured in the precordial lead with the greatest amplitude T wave.
c) Events must occur in the absence of an identifiable etiology, including structural heart disease. Points can only be received for cardiac arrest, documented polymorphic VT, or unexplained syncope.
d) Points can only be received once in this section.
e) A minimum of 1 point must be obtained in the ECG section in order to obtain additional points.

VF: ventricular fibrillation; VT: ventricular tachycardia.

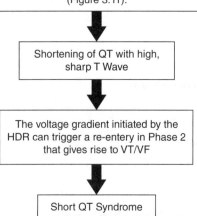

Scheme 9.2 Short QT Syndrome.

Clinical, Prognostic, and Therapeutic Implications

First, it is necessary to exclude all possible causes that may shorten the QT interval, especially electrolyte alterations, such as hypomagnesemia, acidosis, digitalis intoxication, androgenic anabolics, and so forth (Biggi *et al.*, 2009). Because of the significant T wave height, a differential diagnosis should be performed to rule out all other possible causes of tall T wave (Bayés de Luna, 2011). In all the other cases of tall T wave, the QT interval is not short and there is no familial history of SD.

Sudden death triggered by VT/VF due to a reentry Phase 2 mechanism, is the most severe complication of short QT syndrome.

It has been known for several years that the presence of a short QT interval may be related to SD. In a study with Holter monitoring (Algra *et al.*, 1993), the short QT interval was considered a marker of poor prognosis.

Diagnosis of inherited short QT syndrome is based on: (i) symptoms, especially syncopal attacks; (ii) familial history of short QT/SD; and (iii) QT with special electrocardiographic characteristics (point J–peak T <150 ms) (Figure 9.15).

Because it is sometimes associated with AF, short QT syndrome should be ruled out in young patients with AF. In order to do this, the QT interval has to be carefully measured.

Despite a lack of experience due to the scarce number of cases, there is no doubt that ICD implantation is the treatment of choice for high-risk cases (family history of SD and/or serious syncope).

Brugada Syndrome
(Figures 9.16–9.21)

Concept

This is a familial genetically determined syndrome, characterized by an autosomal dominant inheritance and variable penetrance. The incidence rate is higher in young men (because the Ito current is more predominant in men) without apparent structural heart disease (see later). Syncope or SD is usually triggered during rest or sleep, sometimes without any isolated, previous PVC. Most often polymorphous VT trigger VF (Brugada and Brugada, 1992) (see Diagnosis and Differential Diagnosis).

Genetic and Molecular Basis

More than 70 mutations generally related to Na$^+$ channels have been described. It has been demonstrated that in at least 20% of cases there are SCN5A gene mutations. GPDIL and SNCIB gene mutations are less common. These mutations explain loss-of-function of the sodium channel (accelerated inactivation of these channels). Patients who are carriers for SCN5A mutations present a longer PR interval and QRS duration and a higher incidence of AF (Smits *et al.*, 2002). Additionally, loss-of-function mutations in genes encoding L-type calcium channels have been described in Brugada's syndrome, as well as in short QT syndrome (Antzelevitch *et al.*, 2007).

As we have already discussed, mutations in the same gene (SCN5A) may cause different diseases, such as long QT syndrome, Brugada's syndrome and Lenegre syndrome (Bezzina *et al.*, 1999). Brugada's syndrome has also been also associated with sudden infant death syndrome (SIDS) (Priori *et al.*, 2000).

In contrast with LQTS, in which the phenotype is much clearer and genetic testing is able to provide a positive genotype in more than 70% of patients, in Brugada's syndrome no more than 25–30% of patients are currently genotyped.

Pathophysiologic Basis

Based on the evidence that ECG abnormalities are found in right precordial leads and VT/VF mostly originates from the RV, the Brugada pattern was considered to be the phenotypic ECG expression of ionic channel alterations of the RV in the beginning of repolarization, without structural associated changes. However, subtle ultrastructural and cardiovascular magnetic resonance alterations have been discovered (Papavassiliu *et al.*, 2004; Coronel *et al.*, 2005; Frustaci *et al.*, 2009). Therefore, it would appear that some types of structural alterations may be present in Brugada's syndrome.

However, **there are currently three pathophysiologic hypotheses used to explain the ECG changes in Brugada's syndrome** (Meregalli *et al.*, 2009): (i) the repolarization hypothesis already mentioned, involving the presence of transmural or transregional dispersion of RV action potential morphology in the beginning of repolarization; (ii) the depolarization hypothesis, involving a RV conduction delay at the end of depolarization combined with subtle structural RV anomalies; and (iii) the theory of abnormal neural crest development.

(i) **The repolarization hypothesis**. This best-known hypothesis is supported by basic scientific experiments. According to this theory, ECG findings, especially coved–ST elevation (Type I Brugada pattern), and the increased likelihood of SD are due to the accelerated inactivation of the inward Ina current in the RV. Because of this, the early transient outward K^+ repolarization current (Ito), which predominantly acts on the RV epicardium, remains dominant (Antzelevitch, 2001) (see Figure 2.13). This explains how the TAP of the RV epicardium (not the TAP of the endocardium) loses its dome (Phase 1 shortening) and presents low voltage during Phase 2. This occurs because the early transient ionic outward current (Ito) of the RV epicardium initiates a certain degree of premature and transient repolarization, which manifests itself as a notch in the TAP, expressed as changes in the early ST segment. In typical cases of Brugada's syndrome, the subepicardial TAP duration is greater than the subendocardial TAP duration (Figure 3.11E–4). This HDR between RV endocardium and epicardium (transmural dispersion) generates a voltage gradient that triggers VT/VF through a reentrant Phase 2 mechanism (Yan and Antzelevitch, 1999; Antzelevitch, 2007) (see Chapter 3, Reentry, and Figure 3.11E).

It has been suggested (Lambiase *et al.*, 2009) that HDR may be generated at transregional rather than at transmural level, contrary to what was traditionally believed (Yan and Antzelevitch, 1999). Mapping studies with Brugada's syndrome patients, which also involved control subjects (Lambiase *et al.*, 2009), documented significant differences in the repolarization

of different zones of the RV endocardium, and this may play a key role in triggering VT/VF.

(ii) **The depolarization hypothesis**. This hypothesis is based on clinical-electrophysiologic studies. During ajmaline provocation testing in simultaneously recorded 12-lead ECGs, VCGs, and body surface maps, it was demonstrated that the high take-off of QRS-ST junction in V1, occurs earlier than the end of QRS in V6 (Figure 9.20). Therefore, it may be presumed that some degree of RV conduction slowing is essential in the development of a Type I Brugada pattern (Postema *et al.*, 2010). This depolarization abnormality, rather than abnormal repolarization, is according these authors the primary pathophysiologic basis of the coved–type ST segment elevation.

Borggrefe and Schimpf (2010) comment on different arguments in favor of and against these two hypotheses. Both mechanisms may play a role in the genesis of the ECG pattern; however, the mechanism responsible for triggering VT/VF is most likely a voltage gradient due to HDR (transmural or transregional). Recently, it has been shown in models with structural RV disease that excitation failure, by current-to-load mismatch, especially when cardiac sodium current is reduced, may trigger VT/VF in patients with Brugada pattern (Hoogendijk *et al.*, 2010). This author attempts to find a unifying mechanism for Brugada pattern based on this study and previous depolarization hypothesis studies (Hoogendijk *et al.*, 2010). It would seem, however, that although scientifically attractive, it may be too premature due to the limited knowledge we have about this syndrome today (Brugada, 2010).

(iii) **The theory of abnormal neural crest development.** According this theory postulated by Elizari (2007) a few years ago, the two mechanism discussed before may be explained by RVOT anomalies due to abnormal neural crest development.

At present (April 2017) the current debate between these different hypotheses clearly illustrates the need for further studies to better understand the mechanisms underlying Brugada's syndrome.

Electrocardiographic Findings
(Table 9.11)

According to the repolarization hypothesis, the ionic channel alterations and the HDR explain the typical ECG findings of Brugada's syndrome: ST segment elevation followed by a final negative T wave in the right precordial leads (Kurita *et al.*, 2002; Scheme 9.3). However, in a Type I pattern the RV epicardial TAP is usually longer than the endocardial TAP (Figure 3.11E and Scheme 9.3), although no QT interval changes

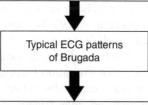

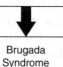

Scheme 9.3 Brugada Syndrome.

should be observed (except sometimes in right precordial leads), because the left ventricular TAP is not altered, and thus there is no universal prolongation of repolarization. The differences observed in the RV TAPs (HDR) and the evidence of zones of RV with a different delay of conduction support the increased likelihood of developing VT/VF. The depolarization hypothesis (Postema *et al.*, 2010) proposes that all patterns are explained by RV conduction delay, with the ST-T being secondary to changes due to RV delay. However, according to these authors the possibility that the ECG and the origin of VT/VF may be explained by the repolarization hypothesis may be feasible.

ECG patterns
(Table 9.12 and 9.13)
It is currently accepted after the consensus paper published in 2012 (Bayés de Luna *et al.*, 2012) that there are

Table 9.11 Electrocardiogram alterations in Brugada's syndrome.

A. ECG criteria

1. Changes in precordial leads

- **Morphology of QRS-T in V1–V3: ST elevation** (sometimes only in V1 and exceptionally also in V3 (Brugada electrocardiographic pattern – BP)
- **Type 1 Coved pattern:** initial ST elevation ≥2 mm, slowly descending and concave (sometimes rectilinear) respect to the isoelectric baseline, with negative symmetric T wave.
- **Type 2 saddleback pattern:** ST elevation, convex respect to the isoelectric baseline, with positive T wave in V2. The elevation, that usually is ≥1 mm, is preceded by an r′ wave, generally wide compared with the r′ wave in athletes or *pectus excavatum*.

2. Duration of QRS:

- Mismatch between the end of QRS pattern in V1–V2 (longer) and V6.

3. New ECG criteria

- **The ST is downsloping:** The index: height of ST in V1–V2 at high take-off/at 80 ms.later >1 (in other cases is upsloping and the index is <1). The end of QRS (J point) usually is later (Bayés de Luna, 2011) than the high take-off of QRS-ST (according to corrado coincides with J point – Corrado *et al.*, 2010) but the index is still valid.
- **The ß angle formed by ascending S and descending r′ is > 58° in type 2 BP** (in athletes is much lower) (Chevalier *et al.*, 2011) (SE 79%, SP 83%).
- **The duration of base of triangle of r′** at 5 mm from the high take-off is much longer in BP type 2 than in athletes (usually >3.5 mm – SE: 79.3%, SP: 84%) (Serra *et al.*, 2014).

B. Other ECG findings:

3. **QT generally normal.** May be prolonged in right precordial leads (Pitzalis *et al.*, 2003)
4. **Conduction disorders:** Sometimes prolonged PR interval (long HV interval) or delayed RV conduction (VCG) (Pérez-Riera, 2009)
5. **Supraventricular arrhythmias.** Especially atrial fibrillation (Schimpf *et al.*, 2008, Pappone *et al.*, 2009)
6. **Some other ECG findings** may be seen: Early repolarization pattern in inferior leads (Sarkozy and Brugada, 2005), fractioned QRS (Morita *et al.*, 2007), alternans of T wave after ajmaline injection (Tada *et al.*, 2008), etc.

only two well-defined ECG patterns with characteristic morphology in V1–V3.

(i) **Type I pattern (coved)** (Figure 9.16A): a rounded ascent appears at the end of QRS with a height that is generally ≥2 mm (dubious cases between 1 and 2 mm) followed by a concave or rectilinear descending curve. May mimic an ACS-STE like pattern in asymptomatic patients. This pattern is the most dangerous which presents as VT/VF.

(ii) **Type II pattern (saddle-back pattern)** (Figure 9.16B): this presents r′ (sometimes called the J wave) that is rounded and ≥2mm, followed by a downsloping descending branch that gives way to ST elevation

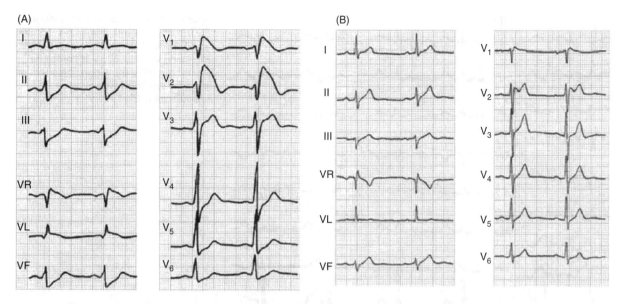

Figure 9.16 Typical ECG patterns of Brugada type I (coved) and type II (saddle-back) (see text, Table 9.10 and 9.11).

measuring at least 0.5mm. ST is followed by a T wave that is positive in V2 and varies in morphology in V1.

In both types QRS is longer in V1 than in V6, as occurs in ARVD. This is not observed in cases with r′ in V1, due to variants of normality, such as pectus excavatum, athletes, or patients with partial RBB.

Characteristically, **the QRS morphology can vary from one intercostal space to another.** It is always necessary to record V1–V2 in the second and fourth intercostal spaces (Figure 9.17).

The ECG pattern is dynamic and may be intermittent (Figure 9.18). There are various factors behind it (e.g., fever, some drugs) (Antzelevitch and Brugada, 2002; Samani *et al.*, 2009) (see www.brugadadrugs.org). Drugs that act on the sodium channels (ajmaline or some equivalent) are useful in determining whether a change from type I to type II pattern occurs (Postema *et al.*, 2009; Yap *et al.*, 2009).

(iii) **Brugada phenocopies** (Figure 9.19): this term, proposed by Perez-Riera, represents ECG patterns identical to Brugada patterns (Baranchuk *et al.*, 2012; Gottschalk *et al.*, 2016a) that correspond to underlying causes, and resolution of the abnormal ECG occurs upon resolution of the underlying cause (i.e., electrolyte disorder, ischemia, etc. See the Educational Portal and International Registry at www.brugadaphenocopy.com). These patterns appear transiently, usually in relation with environmental factors that preferentially affect the RV outflow tract, such as ischemia, tumors, pulmonary embolism, drugs, and so on (Gottschalk *et al.*, 2016b). The prognosis of this pattern is not well established; it is most probably that it depends of the underlying associated process (at the present time, there were no arrhythmic deaths in the International Registry (Anselm *et al.*, 2014).

Figure 9.17 A patient with syncope episodes and an atypical ECG that present a clearly more typical pattern of Brugada type 2 in the second ICS (B) than in the 4th ICS (A)

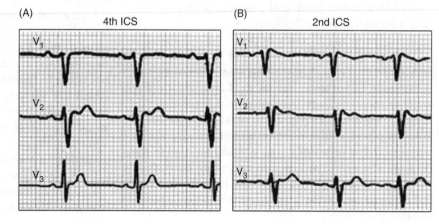

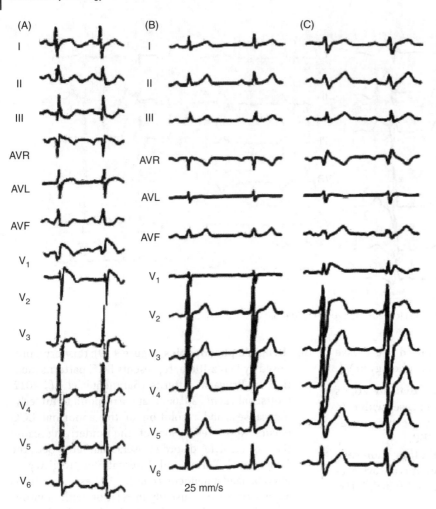

(A)

(B)

(C)

25 mm/s

Figure 9.18 (A) 12-lead electrocardiogram (ECG) in a patient with Brugada's syndrome who lost consciousness some days before. A few days later, the ECG was normal (B), but it showed the characteristic features of Brugada's syndrome after ajmaline administration (C).

Differential diagnosis for the Brugada pattern in the ECG

Figure 9.20 shows different morphologies of rSr′ in lead V1 (García-Niebla and Serra-Autonell, 2009). The bottom four patterns are pathologic (Brugada type I and II), arrhythmogenic RV dysplasia (aRVD), and hyperkalemia, and the last four are variants of normality (lead V1 located in a higher precordial position, pectus excavatum, athletes and partial RBBB).

The differential diagnosis between type II Brugada pattern and other patterns with r′ in V1 is sometimes very difficult. Evaluating the characteristics of r′ is of paramount importance (Bayés de Luna, 2012). The angle of the ascendant and descendent branch of r′ is wider in the Brugada pattern (Chevalier *et al.*, 2011). We have proposed the measurement of the base of r′ at 5 mm from the vertex of r′ that is usually ≥4 mm in the Brugada II pattern and <4 mm in pectus excavatum, partial RBBB and athletes (Bayés de Luna *et al.*, 2010, 2012; Serra *et al.*, 2014). This criterion is easier to measure that the ß angle.

ARVD may present a positive wave in V1 (ε wave) that is somewhat separate from the QRS and generally without ST elevation. Positioning the leads in the "Fointaine" position may help to exacerbate the visualization of the Epsilon-wave (Gottschalk *et al.*, 2014).

In pectus excavatum, the P wave is usually negative in V1 and r′ is narrow. This is also seen in athletes and partial RBB.

Figure 9.20 also shows, in the first vertical line, the differences in duration of QRS between V1 and middle/left leads in the ECG of the two types of Brugada pattern, hyperkalemia and ARVD (Ozeke *et al.*, 2009). This does not occur in the four remaining examples of rSr′ in V1, which are variants on normality. The second vertical line, located 80 ms from the first, shows how in the two Brugada patterns the curve of S-T in V1–V2 descends, while in athletes, pectus excavatum, and partial RBB it is ascending, at least in V2 (Corrado index) (Corrado *et al.*, 2010; Bayés de Luna *et al.*, 2012).

Figure 9.21 shows the algorithm that we consider most useful for this differential diagnosis (Baranchuk *et al.*, 2015).

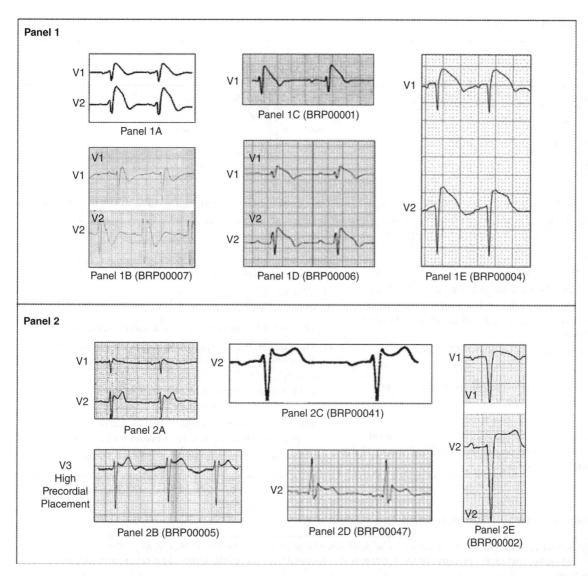

Figure 9.19 *Panel 1*: Comparison of various type 1 Brugada phenocopies. (A) True congenital type 1 Brugada syndrome electrocardiogram shown in comparison to (superior left); (B) congenital hypokalemic periodic paralysis (type 1B BrP) (inferior left); (C) acute inferior ST-elevation myocardial infarction with right ventricular involvement (type 1A BrP) (superior middle); (D) concurrent hyperkalemia, hyponatremia, and acidosis (type 1A BrP) (inferior middle); and (E) acute pulmonary embolism (type 1B BrP) (right). *Panel 2*: Comparison of various type 2 Brugada phenocopies. (A) True congenital type 2 Brugada syndrome shown in comparison (superior left) to (B) congenital pectus excavatum causing mechanical mediastinal compression (type 2A BrP) (inferior left); (C) acute pericarditis (type 2A BrP) (middle superior); (D) after accidental electrocution injury (type 2A BrP) (middle inferior); and (E) as a result of using inappropriate high-pass electrocardiographic filters (type 2C BrP) (right). Numbers under figures are International Registry of Brugada Phenocopies identification numbers. BrP, Brugada phenocopy.

Brugada pattern versus Brugada syndrome: Table 9.13 shows the different genetic and clinical criteria that associated to the ECG pattern allow the diagnosis of Brugada syndrome to be performed.

Prognosis

The following considerations have to be taken into account for risk stratification (Figure 9.22 and Treatment):

- It is important to have in mind the family history (SD or syncope) and that the prognosis is worst in men and in the age window between 20–60 years.

- On the bases of ECG type (I or II) and the presence or not of symptoms, we may have the following groups (Garrat and Elliot, 2010) (Figure 9.22):

  - On the benign side of the spectrum there are **asymptomatic individuals presenting a fixed Type II Brugada pattern.** Usually, they have a good prognosis, especially in the absence of family history of SD or syncope (Oto, 2004). The annual incidence of SD is close to 0% per annum. However, as the typical Brugada morphology (Type I) is sometimes intermittent, it cannot be ruled out based

Table 9.12 ECG patterns of Brugada syndrome in V1-V2.

Type 1 Coved pattern	Type 2 Saddle back pattern
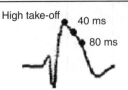	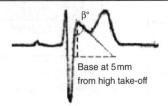

This typical coved pattern present in V1–V2 the following:

a) At the end of QRS an ascending and quick slope with a high take-off ≥ 0.2 mv followed by concave or rectilinear downsloping ST

b) There is no clear r' wave

c) The high take-off often does not correspond with the J point

d) At 40 ms of high take-off the decrease in amplitude of ST is ≤ 0.4mv (Nishizaki 2010). In RBBB and athletes the decrease is much higher

e) ST at high take-off $>$ ST at 40ms $>$ ST at 80ms

f) ST is followed by negative and symmetric T wave

g) the duration of QRS is longer than in RBBB and there is usually a mismatch between V1 and V6

h) The index of Corrado >1. In athletes is <1

i) There are few cases of coved pattern with a high take off <2 mm >1mm that needs, for clear identification of type 1 BP of complementary exams

This typical saddle-back pattern present in V1–V2 the following:

a) High take-off of r' (that not necessary coincides with J point) ≥ 2mm

b) Descending arm of r' coincides with beginning of ST (sometimes is not well seen)

c) Minimum ST ascent ≥ 0.05 mv

d) ST is followed by positive T wave in V2

(T peak $>$ ST minimum >0) and of variable morphology in V1

e) The characteristics of triangle formed by r' allow to define different criteria useful for diagnosis
- β angle $>58°$ (Chevallier 2011)
- duration of the base of triangle of r' at 5 mm from the high take-off >3.5 mm (Serra 2012)

f) The duration of ORS is longer in BP2 than in other cases with r' in V1 and there is a mismatch between V1 and V6

g) The index of Corrado in V1–V2 >1. In non BP patients is <1

Table 9.13 Diagnostic criteria of Brugada's syndrome.

1. **Concave Type I ST elevation in V1–V3** (Figure 9.16) with no other cause accounting for the ST morphology. The **electrocardiographic pattern is indicative of the syndrome if associated with one of the following electrocardiographic/clinical factors**:

   Survivors of cardiac arrest
   Polymorphic ventricular fibrillation (VF)
   Familial history of sudden death (SD) in patients <45 years old
   Type I ST pattern in relatives
   Inducible malignant ventricular arrhythmias
   History of syncope

2. **Non-concave Type II ST elevation in V1–V2–V3** (Figure 9.17), turning into Type I after administering sodium channel blockers. The scenario is identical to the previous case

3. **If there is an ST elevation ≥2 mm after drug administration** but it is nonconcave, the diagnosis is probable if any or more of the clinical criteria mentioned are present

4. **If the morphology is unclear** (either the baseline morphology or the morphology observed after drug administration), the diagnosis may be confirmed, apart from the electrocardiographic/clinical criteria put forward in the first paragraph, by the presence of the following parameters among others (see text):

   a) ST anomaly not observed beyond V3
   b) Wide r' in V1 (see text)
   c) Late positive potentials
   d) Occurrence of a more typical pattern in high precordial leads
   e) Other ECG methods (Bayés de Luna, 2012) exercise test, Holter monitoring, VCG, EPS, genetic test

Figure 9.20 This figure shows clearly (first vertical line) the difference in the duration of QRS in V1 compared to V3 in Brugada patterns 1 and 2 ARVD and hyperkalemia (lower row). However, in four variants of normality (upper row) the duration of QRS in V1–V3 is the same. The second vertical line, measured 80 ms later, clearly shows that in the two Brugada patterns the ST segment is downsloping (ratio ST↑ at J point / ST↑ 80 ms later >1) (Corrado index), but it is upsloping in at least V2 in normal variants (upper row) (ratio <1).

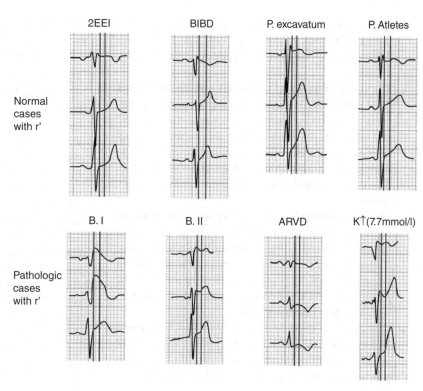

Figure 9.21 (Baranchuk algorithm) Flow chart for performing differential diagnosis of patients with r' in V1–V2 based on the measurement of the base of triangle of r'. If the base of triangle (above) is ≥ 4 mm, this is very suggestive of Brugada type 2 (Serra *et al.*, 2014).

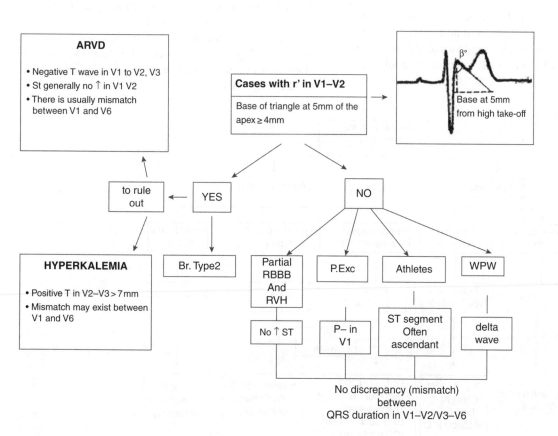

only on one ECG. Therefore, to determine whether the ECG pattern is in fact a fixed type II Brugada ECG pattern, the ajmaline injection test may be necessary.

- The cases of **asymptomatic drug-induced Type I ECG pattern** usually present a relatively good prognosis with a SD incidence of <1% per annum (Garrat and Elliot, 2010). However, in this group, as in all asymptomatic cases, the prognosis depends on the associated markers (result of EPS, genetic test, etc.). Therefore, to establish a "risk score" would be very useful.

- **The asymptomatic cases of Type I spontaneous pattern** present, in some series, <1% risk of SD, and in others the risk is 7%. It depends on the presence of risk markers, (age, gender, etc.) the evaluation of symptoms, and the presence of fixed or intermittent pattern. Clearly, it is necessary to stratify these cases with a better "risk score" (see Figure 9.22).

- **The cases of drug-induced Type I ECG pattern and symptoms** (syncope or VT) present a real risk of SD (around 2% yearly). If the type I ECG pattern is spontaneous, the risk is higher (around 4% yearly).

- **The patients with the highest risk are symptomatic** (syncope/previous cardiac arrest) and with a fixed Type I pattern. The incidence of SD per annum is between 10% and 14%, according to different series.

The following ECG parameters have been recently described as **risk markers of VT/VF**, and may be used for better stratification:

- The presence of prolonged QRS. Symptomatic patients with Brugada syndrome present QRS longer compared with asymptomatic ones (115 ± 6 ms vs 104 ± 19 ms) (p <0.01) (Juntilla *et al.*, 2008).
- The presence of a final R wave >3 mm in the VR lead is a marker of future arrhythmias (Babai Bigi *et al.*, 2007). Howeve,r the value of this sign as risk marker was not confirmed in other study (Juntilla *et al.*, 2008).
- The presence of a fragmented QRS, which is a marker of delayed conduction (as previously mentioned), is also a marker of ventricular arrhythmias and syncope (Morita *et al.*, 2008b). The presence of long QT in right precordial leads (Pitzalis *et al.*, 2003). In fact, this is related to longer duration of epicardium TAP of RV in the Type I Brugada pattern (see before, Electrocardiographic Findings).
- The presence of conduction disturbances in different parts of RV (Benito *et al.*, 2009).
- The presence of the T wave alternans (Tada *et al.*, 2008).
- The presence of an early repolarization pattern in inferior leads (Sarkozy *et al.*, 2009).
- T peak–T end interval dispersion (Castro *et al.*, 2006), increased T peak–T end interval in leads V2 and V6 (Letsas *et al.*, 2010), and the T peak–T end/QT ratio (Lambiase, 2010).

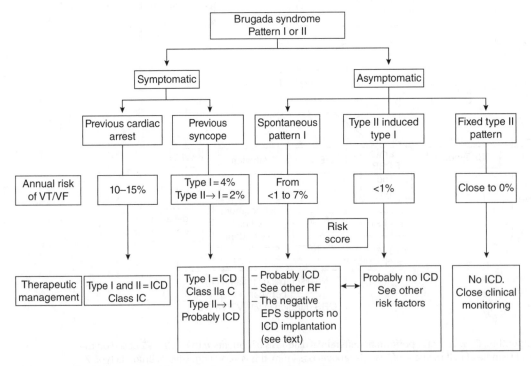

Figure 9.22 Decision tree algorithms in patients with Brugada's syndrome.

Other useful techniques for risk stratification are:

o It has been shown that the presence of **late potentials** detected by a signal-averaged ECG may be a marker of future arrhythmic events (Huang *et al.*, 2009).

o ST-segment elevation during the recovery phase of **exercise** occurs in 30% of cases and is a strong predictor of spontaneous VF (Makimoto *et al.*, 2010).

o Impaired QT dynamicity with respect to heart rate variations in **Holter recordings** has also been associated with arrhythmic events.

o **The role of EPS** study for risk stratification is debatable (Priori *et al.*, 2002b; Brugada *et al.*, 2003; Gehi *et al.*, 2006; Paul *et al.*, 2007; Benito *et al.*, 2008; Probst *et al.*, 2010). According to Brugada, the EPS has a pivotal role in risk stratification (Casado-Arroyo *et al.*, 2016). In this large study EPS had a low PPV (23%) but over three years of follow-up it had a very high NPV (93%). In contrast, Priori (Priori and Napolitano, 2005) considers EPS to have a low accuracy in predicting VT/VF, and Probst *et al.* (2010) affirm in the FINGER trial that symptoms and spontaneous Type I ECG were predictors of arrhythmic events, whereas gender, family history of SD, inducibility by EPS, and the presence of SCN5A mutations were not predictive of arrhythmic events. Also, Kamakura *et al.*, (2009), in Japan, reach similar conclusions. It is clear that there is not a consensus about the need to perform an EPS in these patients. However, if we perform an EPS a negative result is probably in favor of do not implant an ICD (Sacher *et al.*, 2006). Therefore, we consider that we need a risk score that help to decide the best management of difficult cases of Brugada syndrome. New results published recently increases the value of EPS but for some authors (Havakuk and Viskin, 2016) still are some aspects that have to be clarified.

o It has been demonstrated with **tissue Doppler echocardiography** that a delay between RV and LV contraction ($\geq$40 ms) is a risk marker of cardiac events (Biggi *et al.*, 2008).

> A risk score that includes the epidemiological (age, gender) clinical (symptoms) genetic and ECG parameters would be very useful.

Treatment

The most challenging task is to decide whether an ICD should be implanted or not. An implantable cardioverter defibrillator is recommended after risk has been appropriately stratified (see Prognosis), taking especially the following parameters into account: (i) family history; (ii) personal history of syncope or resuscitated cardiac arrest (in fact, it is very important to recognize the clinical characteristics of syncope, because it is crucial to determine if it is of cardiac origin); and (iii) the presence of typical electrocardiographic morphology (or that induced by ajmaline injection). Other risk factors used for stratification include inducible VT/VF during EPS, result of exercise testing, Holter, LP, and echocardiography and other risk markers of bad prognosis (see before).

The ESC/AHA/ACC guidelines of 2006 recommend ICD implantation in the following cases:

(i) Class IC, Brugada's syndrome with previous cardiac arrest (CA).

(ii) Class II a C, cases with spontaneous type I ECG pattern and previous syncope (be sure that is not vasovagal), or documented sustained VT.

The guidelines consider it reasonable to closely monitor clinical patients with a Type I pattern induced by drugs only, to demonstrate if this Type I pattern appears spontaneously.

Before taking the final decision in asymptomatic cases with or without spontaneous typical ECG pattern, it is important to carefully explain the situation to the patient. This includes informing them of the advantages of treatment but also that the number of ICD-related complications is relatively high (10–20%) and that, exceptionally, even death related to ICD malfunction has been described.

Some experiences with the use of Quinidine have shown good results (Belhassen *et al.*, 2015; Viskin *et al.*, 2010). Also, the preventive ablation of RV outflow tract has been reported.

In summary, considering all that we have commented on before, and Prognosis (Figure 9.22), **we may conclude that:**

o There is general agreement that asymptomatic patients with fixed type II ECG pattern do not need ICD implant but a close follow-up.

o Patients with a Type II-induced Type I ECG pattern by drugs who are asymptomatic present a low incidence of SD (Garrat and Elliot, 2010). Therefore, the final decision for an ICD implant has to take into consideration the presence of other risk factors. A risk score would be necessary for these cases.

o Patients with a spontaneous Type I ECG pattern, who are asymptomatic, present an incidence of SD that is high in some series (>5% yearly). Therefore, these patients probably require an ICD, although the candidates should be better stratified with a "risk score". Meanwhile, if EPS is negative probably the best option is do not implant an ICD (see before).

o Patients with spontaneous Type I pattern with previous syncope or sustained VT present a real risk of SD.

Therefore, an ICD implant is required. Probably, also, the type II induced type I ECG pattern with previous syncope needs an ICD.

o There is a general agreement with regard to ICD implantation in patients with a Type I and II ECG pattern and true antecedents of previous cardiac arrest (Wilde *et al.*, 2002).

In certain situations, such as in the presence of an electrical storm, patients with or without an ICD may benefit from the administration of β adrenergic stimulating drugs (isoprenaline or orciprena-line) (Maury *et al.*, 2004) (Class II a C).

In selected cases, especially in the presence of an electric storm (see Chapter 5, Ventricular Fibrillation), the possibility of ablation of the VT/VF inducing focus has been considered (Haïssaguerre *et al.*, 2003).

In high-risk patients showing repetitive arrhythmias, quinidine may be useful, as an associated drug, probably because it blocks the Ito current (Belhassen *et al.*, 2004). Furthermore, the use of quinidine empirically has been postulated in cases of asymptomatic Brugada syndrome (Viskin and Rosso, 2010). Probably the administration of quinidine may be a good option in patients with Brugada syndrome where there is not a clear indication for ICD or where there is not the possibility to implant it, as occurs in developing countries.

The future of subcutaneous ICD for the patients, who will often live for decades, as happens in inherited heart diseases, seems very promising (see Appendix A-3).

Brugada's syndrome

- It is an inherited syndrome that is associated with SCN5A gene mutations in at least 20% of cases.
- The ionic mechanism involved consists of an accelerated inactivation of the right ventricle (RV) INa current with transient predominance of the Ito current, generating a heterogeneous dispersion of repolarization between the epicardium and endocardium of the RV.
- An evident electrocardiogram (ECG) phenotype expressed in right precordial leads exists (Type I Brugada pattern). Other morphologies (Type II pattern) with a relatively wide r′ and convex ST elevation have also been described.
- Both ECG patterns, especially type II, have to be differentiated from many other patterns, with r′ in V1–V2 present in different conditions or even in healthy subjects (Figure 9.20) (athletes, patients with thoracic anomalies). However, Type I ECG is very typical.

- The administration of ajmaline as a Na channel blocker in cases with a Type II pattern may help to unmask type I pattern and to determine the diagnosis.
- Other ECG abnormalities (such as conduction disturbances or supraventricular arrhythmias) may be present as well.
- This ECG pattern is frequently associated with severe ventricular arrhythmias (Brugada's syndrome) and may lead to sudden death (SD). Polymorphic ventricular tachycardia/ventricular fibrillation, triggered by a Phase 2 reentry due to a HDR in different zones of the RV, is the most frequent cause of SD.
- To determine whether an ICD implantation is required, we advise following the algorithm shown in Figure 9.22. Despite some controversy, at present we consider implantable cardioverter defibrillator therapy to be necessary in the scenarios described in this figure.

Catecholaminergic Polymorphic Ventricular Tachycardia

Concept, genetic mechanisms, and clinical presentation (Priori et al., 2002a)

This is a familial catecholaminergic autosomal dominant polymorphic ventricular tachycardia (CPVT) that is found especially in children without a long QT interval or structural heart disease. Genetic mutations have recently been shown, both in the ryanodine cardiac receptor genes (RyRz) and in the calsequestrin q2 gene (CASQ2), among others (Blayney *et al.*, 2010). Experimental CPVT models show that the His–Purkinje system is an important source of arrhythmias in these patients (Scheinman 2009).

It has been demonstrated that there are various mechanisms involved. In a first phase, a bidirectional VT is initiated due to triggered activity (late post-potentials). This VT alternatively originates in different ventricular zones (epicardium, endocardium, or M cells) and does not represent a high risk, but often polymorphic VT occurs later as a result of rotors that initiate unstable spiral waves of variable morphology (see Figures 3.13 and 3.15).

Generally, an exercise or emotion-induced syncope constitutes the first clinical manifestation of the disease. Nevertheless, some cases of SD with no previous symptoms have been described.

Electrocardiographic alterations
(*Figure 9.23*)

Generally, after physical exercise or mental stress (Leenhardt *et al.*, 1995), rapid supraventricular arrhythmias occur, followed by frequent PVC, leading to runs of bidirectional VT that may be followed by polymorphic VT, VF, and SD, all despite a normal baseline ECG.

When CPVT is suspected, it is important to perform a Holter ECG, to verify if PVC with bidirectional morphology are present. This information is enough to suspect the

Exercise ▶▶▶   1 sec

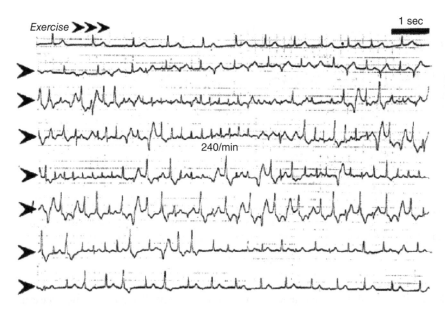
240/min

Figure 9.23 Patient with runs of catecholaminergic multiform ventricular tachycardia (VT). Continuous tracing during an exercise stress test. The sinus tachycardia is accompanied by bigeminal premature ventricular complexes (PVC) along supraventricular tachyarrhythmia with runs of multiform PVC, which lead to a run of bidirectional VT (sixth strip). Arrhythmias disappear shortly after discontinuing exercise in last two strips (taken from Leenhardt *et al.*, 1995).

condition. It has recently been suggested that bradyarrhythmias may also be present. Bidirectional VT, even when it can occur in the context of other conditions, it is considered a "hallmark" of CPVT (Femenia *et al.*; 2012)

Prognostic and Therapeutic Implications

Due to the risk of sudden unexpected death, the prognosis is serious. Therefore, immediate treatment is required.

Beta-blockers should be administered, both in the acute phase to stop the CPVT, as well as during follow-up to prevent new episodes from occurring (Class I C). However, in about 40% of cases β-blockers do not succeed in preventing recurrences during exercise testing. In these patients, as well as in patients with previous syncope and/or family history of syncope, the implantation of an ICD is indicated (Class I C). Administration of β-blockers, however, should not be discontinued, to prevent the occurrence of electrical storms. Published data suggest the usefulness of video-assisted left-sided sympathetic denervation in selected cases, generally associated with ICD or β-blockers (Collura *et al.*, 2009).

Atrial Fibrillation of Genetic Origin

In the past few years, the genetic predisposition to AF has been proven. In fact, familial AF is not considered to be a very rare condition (Arnar *et al.*, 2006).

It is known that familial AF is usually a monogenic disease. First, the locus was reported (Brugada *et al.*, 1997) and later the various genes involved in familial AF (Chen *et al.*, 2003) were described.

In most cases, it is associated with potassium current and occasionally sodium current alterations. Recently, some KCNQI gene mutations that lead to potassium channel changes have been identified. These are manifested as

short or long QT intervals. In fact, short QT syndrome should be ruled out in young patients with AF, especially in the cases of familial AF. Therefore, familial AF may be related to other monogenic channelopathies, such as long or short QT syndrome.

Familial AF appears in young people. Initially, it occurs as short runs of supraventricular tachyarrhythmia or many atrial extrasystoles with very short coupling intervals. However, most of the patients present chronic AF.

Finally, certain evidence suggests that genes related to ionic channels, inflammation and fibrosis play a role in the pathogenesis of non-familial (common) AF (Gudbjartsson *et al.*, 2007).

Familial Torsades de Pointes Ventricular Tachycardia

A rare form of familial Torsades de Pointes VT with a typical QRS complex morphology (Chapter 5, Torsades de Pointes Polymorphic Ventricular Tachycardia), without a long QT interval, and with a short coupling interval has been described (Figure 9.24) (Leenhardt *et al.*, 1994). It has been reported in young people without heart disease and often leads to SD.

The underlying molecular mechanism of this arrhythmia is not known, although family history suggests that it is an inherited disease.

Due to the high incidence of fatal arrhythmias (Torsades de Pointes VT leading to VF), ICD implantation is indicated if the diagnosis is confirmed.

Other Possible Channelopathies

It is possible that in the future new genetic disorders with a characteristic phenotypic ECG pattern will be discovered. These patterns include:

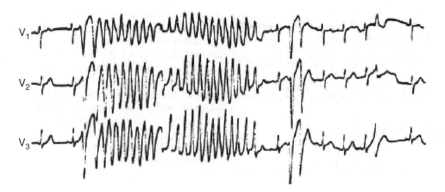

Figure 9.24 Electrocardiogram (V1–V3) of a patient with runs of ventricular tachycardia (VT) with typical Torsades de Pointes morphology, although with a normal QT and a short coupling interval (270 ms). After one run of Torsades de Pointes VT, a second premature ventricular complex (PVC) is observed, but this time the coupling interval is not so short, not leading to another run of Torsades de Pointes VT (taken from Leenhardt *et al.*, 1994).

○ **Some types of pre-excitation** are already genetically determined (Doevendans and Wellens, 2001; Gollob *et al.*, 2001) (see Chapter 8).

○ **Some ECG patterns of early repolarization** (see Chapter 10, Early Repolarization Pattern).

○ **The presence of high and narrow QRS complexes** (Wolpert *et al.*, 2008) (see Chapter 10).

○ **Finally, some other possible patterns include**: (i) cases of familial severe sinus bradycardia (Nof *et al.*, 2007) (see Chapter 10, Severe Sinus Brady-cardia); (ii) some cases of children presenting intraventricular conduction blocks and VT (Iturralde-Torres *et al.*, 2008) (see Chapter 10); and (iii) cases of idiopathic VF in the presence of bradycardia-dependent intraventricular blocks (Aizawa *et al.*, 1993) (see Chapter 10, Other ECG Patterns).

Idiopathic Ventricular Fibrillation

The discovery of the genetic origin of different channelopathies, thanks to the correlation with the ECG phenotype (long and short QT syndromes and Brugada's syndrome) and also the recent discovery of the relationship of early repolarization pattern with SD (Haïssaguerre *et al.*, 2008) (see Chapter 10, Early repolarization pattern), and the possibility that other ECG patterns are related to SD, has led to a dramatic decrease in the number of idiopathic VF cases, although some cases of uncertain origin still exist (Rosso *et al.*, 2008; Haïssaguerre *et al.*, 2009; Nam *et al.*, 2010).

In different pathologic studies (Maron *et al.*, 2009; Subirana *et al.*, 2011), the number of cases that cannot be categorized is already very low (see Table 1.2), although this number could be even smaller because some already known channelopathies without structural heart disease not discovered in the necropsic study may be included in this category.

It has been shown also that approximately 50% of patients with an initial diagnosis of idiopathic VF were identified either as carriers of different types of channelopathies or presenting myocarditis after a systematic study was performed (Krahn *et al.*, 2009).

Self Assessment

A. Describe the electrocardiographic (ECG) findings in hypertrophic cardiomyopathy (HCM).

B. When is implantable cardioverter defibrillator (ICD) therapy necessary in HCM?

C. Describe the ECG findings in arrhythmogenic right ventricle cardiomyopathy (ARVC).

D. What is the best treatment for ARVC?

E. Describe the ECG findings in noncompacted CM.

F. Describe the "score" risk to identify risk of death in patients with heart failure.

G. What is Lenegre syndrome?

H. Describe the concept of channelopathies.

I. Describe the ECG characteristics of long QT syndrome (LQTS).

J. When are β-blockers used in LQTS?

K. What is short QT syndrome?

L. Explain the Type I and II ECG pattern of Brugada's syndrome.

M. What is the prognosis of Brugada Syndrome?

N. What is the role of EPS in Brugada Syndrome?

O. Describe the concept of catecholaminergic polymorphic ventricular tachycardia.

P. Describe the concept of atrial fibrillation of genetic origin.

References

Agarwal S, Tuzcu EM, Desai MY, *et al*. Updated meta-analysis of septal alcohol ablation versus myectomy for hypertrophic cardiomyopathy. J Am Coll Cardiol 2010;55:823.

Aizawa Y, Tamura M, Chinushi M, *et al*. Idiopathic ventricular fibrillation and bradycardia-dependent intraventricular block. Am Heart J 1993;126:1473.

Algra A, Tijssen JG, Roelandt JR, *et al*. QT interval variables from 24 hour electrocardiography and the two year risk of sudden death. Br Heart J 1993;70:43.

Alvarez-Garcia J, Massó-van Roessel A, Vives-Borras M, *et al*. Prevalence, clinical profile and shor-term prognosis of interatrial block in patiens admitted for worsening of heart failure. Abstract accepted in American College of Cardiology Congress, 2016.

Anselm DD, Gottschalk BH, Baranchuk A. Brugada Phenocopies: consideration of morphological criteria and early finding from an International Registry. Can J Cardiol 2014;30(12):1511.

Anttonen O, Väänänen H, Junttila J, *et al*. Electrocardiographic transmural dispersion of repolarization in patients with inherited short QT syndrome. Ann Noninvasive Electrocardiol 2008;13:295.

Anttonen O, Junttila J, Maury F, *et al*. Differences in 12-lead ECG between symptomatic and asymptomatic subjects with short QT interval. Heart Rhythm 2009;6:267.

Antzelevitch C. The Brugada syndrome: ionic basis and arrhythmia mechanisms. J Cardiovasc Electrophysiol 2001;12:268.

Antzelevitch C. Molecular genetics of arrhythmias and cardiovascular conditions associated with arrhythmias. J Cardiovasc Electrophysiol 2003;14:1259.

Antzelevitch C. Heterogeneity and cardiac arrhythmias. An overview. Heart Rhythm 2007;4:964.

Antzelevitch C, Brugada R. Fever and Brugada syndrome. Pacing Clin Electrophysiol 2002;25:1537.

Antzelevitch C, Pollevick GD, Cordeiro JM, *et al*. Loss-of-function mutations in the cardiac calcium channel underlie a new clinical entity characterized by ST-segment elevation, short QT intervals, and sudden cardiac death. Circulation 2007;115:442.

Arad M, Penas-Lado M, Monserrat L, *et al*. Gene mutations in apical hypertrophic cardiomyopathy. Circulation 2005;112:2805.

Ariyarajah V, Tam JW, Khadem A. Inducible malignant ventricular tachyarrhythmia in a patient with genotyped hypertrophic cardiomyopathy in absence of left ventricular hypertrophy or enlargement. Circulation 2009;119:3543.

Arnar D, Throvaldson S, Manolio T, *et al*. Familial aggregation of atrial fibrillation in Iceland. Eur Heart J 2006;27:708.

Asimaki A, Tandri H, Huang H, *et al*. A new diagnostic test for arrhythmogenic right ventricular cardiomyopathy. N Engl J Med 2009;360:1075.

Babai Bigi M, Aslani A, Shahrzad S. aVR sign as a risk factor for life-threatening arrhythmic events in patients with Brugada syndrome. Heart Rhythm 2007;4:1009.

Baldasseroni S, De Biase L, Fresco C, *et al*. Cumulative effect of complete left bundle-branch block and chronic atrial fibrillation on 1-year mortality and hospitalization in patients with congestive heart failure. A report from the Italian network on congestive heart failure (in-CHF database). Eur Heart J 2002;23:1692.

Baranchuk A, Nguyen T, Ryu MH, *et al*. Brugada Phenocopy: new terminology and proposed classification. Ann Noninvasive Electrocardiol 2012;17(4):299.

Baranchuk A, Enriquez A, García-Niebla J, *et al*. Differential diagnosis of rSr′ pattern in leads V1-V2. Comprehensive review and proposed algorithm. Ann Noninvasive Electrocardiol 2015;20:7.

Bayés de Luna A. A non invasive approach to differentiate physiological versus pathological left ventricle hypertrophy. J Med Liban 1999;47(3):190.

Bayés de Luna A. Clinical arrhythmology. John Wiley & Sons, Chichester, 2011.

Bayés de Luna A. Clinical electrocardiography. John Wiley & Sons, Chichester, 2012.

Bayés de Luna A, Furlanello F, Maron BJ, Zipes DP, eds. Arrhythmias and sudden death in athletes. Kluwer Academic Publishers, Dordrecht, 2000.

Bayés de Luna A, Garcia Niebla J, Goldwasser D. The ECG differential diagnosis of Brugada pattern and athletes. Eur Heart J 2010 (E-letter published 14 May 2010).

Bayés de Luna A, Brugada J, Baranchuk A, *et al*. Current electrocardiographic criteria for diagnosis of Brugada pattern: a consensus report. J Electrocardiology, 2012;45:433.

Bayés-Genís A, Lopez L, Viñolas X, *et al*. Distinct left bundle branch block pattern in ischemic and non-ischemic dilated cardiomyopathy. Eur J Heart Failure 2003;5:165.

Belhassen B. Efficacy of quinidine in high-risk patients with Brugada syndrome. Circulation 2004;110:173.

Belhassen B, Rahkovich M, Michowitz Y, *et al*. Management of Brugada Syndrome: thirty-three-year experience using electrophysiologically guided therapy with class IA antiarrhythmic drugs. Circ Arrhythm Electrophysiol. 2015;8(6):1393.

Benito B, Brugada R, Brugada J, Brugada P. Brugada syndrome. Progress Cardiovasc Diseases 2008;51:1.

Benito B, Brugada J, Brugada R, Brugada P. Síndrome de Brugada. Rev Esp Card 2009;62:1297.

Berruezo A, Fernández-Armenta J, Mont L, *et al.* Combined endocardial and epicardial catheter ablation in arrhythmogenic right ventricular dysplasia incorporating scar dechanneling technique. Circ Arrhythm Electrophysiol 2012;5(1):111.

Bezzina C, Veldkamp MW, van Den Berg MP, *et al.* A single Na(+) channel mutation causing both long-QT and Brugada syndromes. Circ Res 1999;85:1206.

Biggi J, Moaref A, Astasi A. Interventricular mechanical dysynchrony: A novel marker of cardiac events in Brugada syndrome. Heart Rhythm 2008;5:79.

Biggi MA, Aslani A, Aslani A. Short QT interval: A novel predictor of androgen abuse in strength trained athletes. Ann Noninvasive Electrocardiol 2009;14:35.

Blayney LM, Jones JL, Griffiths J, *et al.* A mechanism of ryanodine receptor modulation by FKBP12/12.6, protein kinase A, and K201. Cardiovasc Res 2010;85:68.

Borggrefe M, Schimpf R. J-wave syndromes caused by repolarization or depolarization mechanisms a debated issue among experimental and clinical electrophysiologists. J Am Coll Cardiol 2010;55:798.

Bos JM, Towbin JA, Ackerman MJ. Diagnostic, prognostic, and therapeutic implications of genetic testing for hypertrophic cardiomyopathy. J Am Coll Cardiol 2009;54:201.

Brugada P. Commentary on the Brugada ECG pattern. Circ Arrhythm Electrophysiol 2010;3:280.

Brugada P, Brugada J. Right bundle branch block, persistent ST segment elevation and sudden cardiac death: a distinct clinical and electrocardiographic syndrome. A multicenter report. J Am Coll Cardiol 1992;20:1391

Brugada R, Tapscott T, Czernuszewicz GZ, *et al.* Identification of a genetic locus for familial atrial fibrillation. N Engl J Med 1997;336:905.

Brugada P, Brugada R, Mont L, *et al.* Natural history of Brugada syndrome: the prognostic value of programmed electrical stimulation of the heart. J Cardiovasc Electrophysiol 2003;14:455.

Brugada J, Brugada R, Brugada P. Channelopathies: a new category of diseases causing sudden death. Herz 2007;32:185.

Burkett E, Hersberger R. Clinical and genetic issues in familiar dilated cardiomyopathy. J Am Coll Cardiol 2005;45:969.

Casado-Arroyo R, Berne P, Rao JY, *et al.* Long-term trends in newly diagnosed Brugada syndrome: implications for risk stratification. J Am Coll Cardiol 2016;68(6):614.

Castro J, Antzelevitch C, Tornes F. T peak-T and dispersion in a risk factor for VT/VF in patients with Brugada syndrome. J Am Coll Cardiol 2006;47:1828.

Catalano O, Antonaci S, Moro G, *et al.* Magnetic resonance investigations in Brugada syndrome reveal unexpectedly high rate of structural abnormalities. Eur Heart J 2009;30:2241.

Chen Y, Xu SJ, Bendahhou S. KCNQ1 gen of function mutation in familiar atrial fibrillation. Science 2003; 299:251.

Chevallier S, Forclaz A, Tenkorang J, *et al.* New electrocardiographic criteria for discriminating between Brugada types 2 and 3 patterns and incomplete right bundle branch block. J Am Coll Cardiol. 2011;58:2290.

Coats CJ, Quarta G, Flett AS, *et al.* Arrhythmogenic left ventricular cardiomyopathy. Circulation 2009;120:2613.

Collura CA, Johnson JN, Ackerman MJ. Left cardiac sympathetic denervation for the treatment of long QT syndrome and catecholaminergic polymorphic ventricular tachycardia using video-assisted thoracic surgery. Heart Rhythm 2009;6:752.

Coronel R, Casini S, Koopmann TT, *et al.* Right ventricular fibrosis and conduction delay in a patient with clinical signs of Brugada syndrome: a combined electrophysiological, genetic, histopathologic, and computational study. Circulation 2005;112:2769.

Corrado D, Pelliccia A, Heidbuchel H, *et al.* Recommendations for interpretation of 12-lead electrocardiogram in the athlete. Eur Heart J 2010;31:243.

Dalal D, Molin LH. Piccinin J, *et al.* Clinical features of arrhythmogenic right ventricular dysplasia/ cardiomyopathy associated with mutations in plakophilin-2. Circulation 2006;113:1641.

Dalal D, Jain R, Tandri H, *et al.* Long-term efficacy of catheter ablation of ventricular tachycardia in patients with arrhythmogenic right ventricular dysplasia/ cardiomyopathy. J Am Coll Cardiol 2007;50:432.

Doevendans PA, Wellens HJ. Wolff–Parkinson–White syndrome. A genetic disease? Circulation 2001;104:3014.

Dumont CA, Monserrat L, Soler R, *et al.* Interpretation of electrocardiographic abnormalities in hypertrophic cardiomyopathy with cardiac magnetic resonance. Eur Heart J 2006;27:1725.

Elizari MV, Levi R, Acunzo RS, *et al.*, Abnormal expression of cardiac neural crest cells in heart development: a different hypothesis for the etiopathogenesis of Brugada syndrome. Heart Rhythm. 2007;4:359.

Epstein ND, Cohn GM, Cyran F, *et al.* Differences in clinical expression of hypertrophic cardiomyopathy associated with two distinct mutations in the beta-myosin heavy chain gene. A 908Leu-Val mutation and a 403Arg-Gln mutation. Circulation 1992;86:345.

Eriksson MJ, Sonnenberg B, Woo A, *et al.* Long-term outcome in patients with apical hypertrophic cardiomyopathy. J Am Coll Cardiol 2002;39:638.

Extramiana F, Antzelevitch C. Amplified transmural dispersion of repolarization as the basis for arrhythmogenesis in a canine ventricular-wedge model of short-QT syndrome Circulation 2004;110:3661.

Femenía F, Barbosa-Barros R, Vitorino S, *et al.* Bidirectional ventricular tachycardia: a hallmark of catecholaminergis polymorphic ventricular tachycardia. Indian Pacing Electrophysiol J 2012;12(2):65.

Femenía F, Arce M, Van Grieken J, *et al.* Fragmented QRS as a predictor of arrhythmic events in patients with hypertrophic obstructive cardiomyopathy. J Interv Card Electrophisiol 2013;38(3):159.

Fontaine G, Hebert JL, Prost-Squarcioni C, *et al.* Arrhythmogenic right ventricular dysplasia. Arch Mal Coeur Vaiss 2004;97:1155.

Frustaci A, Russo MA, Chimenti C. Structural myocardial abnormalities in asymptomatic family members with Brugada syndrome and SCN5A gene mutation. Eur Heart J 2009;30:1763.

Gaita F, Giustetto C, Bianchi F, *et al.* Short QT syndrome. A familial cause of sudden death. Circulation 2003;108:965.

García-Niebla J, Serra-Autonell G. Effects of inadequate low-pass filter application. J Electrocardiol 2009;42:303.

García-Niebla J, Baranchuk A, Bayés de Luna A. Epsilon wave in the 12-lead electrocardiogram: is it frequency underestimated? Rev Esp Cardiol (Engl Ed) 2016; 69(4):438.

Garrat C, Elliot P. Heart rhythm UK position statement on clinical indications for ICD in adult patients with familial sudden death syndrome. Europace 2010;12:1156.

Gehi AK, Duong TD, Metz LD, *et al.* Risk stratification of individuals with the Brugada electrocardiogram: a meta-analysis. J Cardiovasc Electrophysiol 2006;17:577.

Geisterfer-Lowrance AA, Kass S, Tanigawa G, *et al.* A molecular basis for familial hypertrophic cardiomyopathy: A beta cardiac myosin heavy chain gene missense mutation. Cell 1990;62:999.

Gimeno JR, Tomé-Esteban M, Lofiego C, *et al.* Exercise-induced ventricular arrhythmias and risk of sudden cardiac death in patients with hypertrophic cardiomyopathy. Eur Heart J 2009;30:2599.

Goldberger I, Moss AJ. Long QT syndrome. J Am Coll Cardiol 2008;51:2291.

Gollob MH, Seger JJ, Gollob TN, *et al.* Novel PRKAG2 mutation responsible for the genetic syndrome of ventricular preexcitation and conduction system disease with childhood onset and absence of cardiac hypertrophy. Circulation 2001;104:3030.

Gollob MH, Redpath CJ, Roberts JD. The short QT syndrome: proposed diagnostic criteria. J Am Coll Cardiol 2011;57(7):802.

Gottschalk B, Gysel M, Barbosa-Barros R, *et al.* The use of fontaine leads in the diagnosis of arrhythmogenic right ventricular dysplasia. Ann Noninv Electrocardiol 2014;19(3) 279.

Gottschalk BH, Anselm DD, Brugada J, *et al.* Expert cardiologists cannot distinguish between Brugada Phenocopy and Brugada Syndrome electrocardiogram patterns. Europace 2016a;18(7):1095.

Gottschalk BH, García-Niebla J, Anselm DD, *et al.* New methodologies for measuring Brugada ECG patterns cannot differentiate the ECG pattern of Brugada Syndrome from Brugada Phenocopy. J Electrocardiol 2016;49(2):187.

Grosman KS, *et al.*, Requirements of plakophilin 2 for cardiac function and morphogenesis. J Cell Biol 2004;167:149.

Gudbjartsson DF, Arnar DO, Helgadottir A, *et al.* Variants conferring risk of atrial fibrillation on chromosome 4q25. Nature 2007;448:353.

Gussak I, George S, Bojovic B, Vajdic B. ECG phenomena of the early ventricular repolarization in the 21st century. Indian Pacing Electrophysiol J. 2008;8(3):149.

Haïssaguerre M, Extramiana F, Hocini M, *et al.* Mapping and ablation of ventricular fibrillation associated with long-QT and Brugada syndromes. Circulation 2003;108:925.

Haïssaguerre M, Derval N, Sacher F, *et al.* Sudden cardiac arrest associated with early repolarization. N Eng J Med 2008;358:2016.

Haïssaguerre M, Chatel S, Sacher F, *et al.* Ventricular fibrillation with prominent early repolarization associated with a rare variant of KCNJ8/K_{ATP} channel. J Cardiovasc Electrophysiol 2009;20:93.

Hamid MS, Norman M, Quraishi A, *et al.* Prospective evaluation of relatives for familial arrhythmogenic right ventricular cardiomyopathy/dysplasia reveals a need to broaden diagnostic criteria. J Am Coll Cardiol 2002;40:1445.

Havakuk O, Viskin S. A tale of 2 diseases. The history of long-QT syndrome and Brugada syndrome. J Am Coll Cardiol 2016;67(1):100.

Healey JS, Gula LJ, Birnie DH, *et al.* A randomized-controlled pilot study comparing ICD implantation with and without intraoperative defibrillation testing in patients with heart failure and severer left ventricular dysfunction: a substudy of the RAFT trial. J Cardiovasc Eletrophysiol 2012; 23(12):1313.

Hombach V, Merkle N, Torzewski J, *et al.* Electrocardiographic and cardiac magnetic resonance imaging parameters as predictors of a worse outcome in patients with idiopathic dilated cardiomyopathy. Eur Heart J 2009;30:2011.

Hong EL, Hui-Nam P, Wan Joo S, *et al.* Epicardial ablation of ventricular tachycardia associated with isolated ventricular noncompaction. PACE 2006;29:797.

Hoogendijk MG, Potse M, Linnenbank AC *et al.* Mechanism of right precordial ST-segment elevation in structural heart disease: excitation failure by current-to-load mismatch. Heart Rhythm 2010;7:238.

Horner JM, Kinoshita M, Webster TL, *et al.* Implantable cardioverter defibrillator therapy for congenital long QT syndrome: a single-center experience. Heart Rhythm 2010;7:1616.

Huang Z, Patel C, Li W, *et al.* Role of signal-averaged electrocardiograms in arrhythmic risk stratification of patients with Brugada syndrome: a prospective study. Heart Rhythm 2009;8:1156.

Ikeda H, Maki S, Yoshida N, *et al.* Predictors of death from congestive heart failure in hypertrophic cardiomyopathy. Am J Cardiol 1999;83:1280.

Iturralde-Torres P, Nava-Townsend S, Gómez-Flores J, *et al.* Association of congenital, diffuse electrical disease in children with normal heart: sick sinus syndrome, intraventricular conduction block, and monomorphic ventricular tachycardia. J Cardiovasc Electrophysiol 2008;19:550.

Jain R, Dalal D, Daly A, *et al.* Electrocardiographic features of arrhythmogenic right ventricular dysplasia. Circulation 2009;12:477.

Jervell A, Lange-Nielsen F. Congenital deaf-mutism, functional heart disease with prolongation of the Q-T interval and sudden death. Am Heart J 1957;54:59.

Jons C, Moss AJ, Goldenberg I, *et al.* Risk of fatal arrhythmic events in long QT syndrome patients after syncope. J Am Coll Cardiol 2010;55:783.

Juntilla M, Brugada P, Hong K, *et al.* Differences in 12-lead ECG between symptomatic and asymptomatic Brugada syndrome patients. J Cardiovasc Electrophysiol 2008;19:380.

Kamakura S, Ohe T, Nakazawa K, *et al.* Long-term prognosis of probands with Brugada-pattern ST elevation in leads V1-V3. Circ Arrhythm Electrophysiol 2009;2:495.

Kapplinger JD, Tester DJ, Salisbury BA, *et al.* Spectrum and prevalence of mutations from the first 2,500 consecutive unrelated patients referred for the FAMILION long QT syndrome genetic text. Heart Rhythm 2009;6:1297.

Karaoka H. Electrocardiographic patterns of the Brugada syndrome in two young patients with pectus excavatum. J Electrocardiol 2002;35:169.

Khan IA, Gowda RM. Novel therapeutics for treatment of long-QT syndrome and torsades de pointes. Int J Cardiol 2004;95:1.

Kirchhof P, Franz MR, Bardai A, *et al.* Giant T-U waves precede torsades de pointes in long QT syndrome: a systematic electrocardiographic analysis in patients with acquired and congenital QT prolongation. J Am Coll Cardiol 2009;54:143.

Krahn AD, Healey JS, Chauhan V, *et al.* Systematic assessment of patients with unexplained cardiac arrest: Cardiac Arrest Survivors With Preserved Ejection Fraction Registry (CASPER). Circulation 2009;120:278.

Kurita T, Shimizu W, Inagaki M, *et al.* The electrophysiologic mechanism of ST segment elevation in Brugada syndrome. J Am Coll Cardiol 2002;40: 330.

Lambiase PD, Ahmed AK, Ciaccio EJ, *et al.* High-density substrate mapping in Brugada syndrome: combined role of conduction and repolarization heterogeneities in arrhythmogenesis. Circulation 2009;120:106.

Lambiase PD. T peak-T end interval and T peak-T end/QT ratio as markers of ventricular tachycardia inducibility in subjects with Brugada ECG phenotype. Europace 2010;12:158.

Leenhardt A, Glaser E, Burguera M, *et al.* Short-coupled variant of torsades de pointes. A new electrocardiographic entity in the spectrum of idiopathic ventricular tachyarrhythmias. Circulation 1994;89:206.

Leenhardt A, Lucet V, Denjoy I, *et al.* Catecholaminergic polymorphic ventricular tachycardia in children. A 7-year follow-up of 21 patients. Circulation 1995;91:1512.

Lenegre J. Etiology and pathology of bilateral bundle branch block in relation to complete heart block. Prog Cardiov Dis 1964;6:445.

Leonardi S, Raineri C, De Ferrari GM, *et al.* Usefulness of cardiac magnetic resonance in assessing the risk of ventricular arrhythmias and sudden death in patients with hypertrophic cardiomyopathy. Eur Heart J 2009;30:2003.

Letsas KP, Weber R, Astheimer K, *et al.* T peak-T end interval and T peak-T end/QT ratio as markers of ventricular tachycardia inducibility in subjects with Brugada ECG phenotype. Europace 2010;12:271.

Lev M. Anatomic basis for atrioventricular block. Am J Med 1964;37:742.

Liu N, Ruan Y, Priori SG. Catecholaminergic polymorphic ventricular tachycardia. Prog Cardiovasc Dis 2008;51:23.

Makimoto H, Nakagawa E, Takaki H, *et al.* Augmented ST-segment elevation during recovery from exercise predicts cardiac events in patients with Brugada syndrome. J Am Coll Cardiol 2010;56:1576.

Marbán E. Cardiac channelopathies. Nature 2002;415:213.

Marcus FI, McKenna WJ, Sherrill D *et al.*, Diagnosis of Arrhythmogenic Right Ventricular Cardiomyopathy/Dysplasia. Proposed Modification of the Task Force Criteria. Circulation 2010;121:1533.

Maron BJ. Contemporary considerations for risk stratification, sudden death and prevention in hypertrophic cardiomyopathy. Heart 2003;89:977.

Maron BJ. Contemporary insights and strategies for risk stratification and prevention of sudden death in hypertrophic cardiomyopathy. Circulation 2010;121:445.

Maron BJ, Gottdiener JS, Epstein SE. Patterns and significance of distribution of left ventricular hypertrophy in hypertrophic cardiomyopathy. A wide angle, two dimensional echocardiographic study of 125 patients. Am J Cardiol 1981;48:418.

Maron BJ, Shen WK, Link MS, *et al.*, Efficacy of implantable cardioverter-defibrillators for the prevention of sudden death in patients with hypertrophic cardiomyopathy. N Engl J Med 2000;342:365.

Maron BJ, Towbin JA, Thiene G, *et al.* Contemporary definitions and classification of the cardiomyopathies. An American Heart Association scientific statement from the council on clinical cardiology, heart failure and transplantation committee; quality of care and outcomes research and functional genomics and translational biology interdisciplinary working groups; and Council on epidemiology and prevention. Circulation 2006;113:1807.

Maron BJ, Spirito P, Shen WK, *et al.*, Implantable cardioverter-defibrillators and prevention of sudden cardiac death in hypertrophic cardiomyopathy. JAMA 2007;298:405.

Maron BJ, Maron MS, Wigle ED, Braunwald E. The 50-year history, controversy, and clinical implications of left ventricular outflow tract obstruction in hypertrophic cardiomyopathy from idiopathic hypertrophic subaortic stenosis to hypertrophic cardiomyopathy. J Am Coll Cardiol 2009a;54:191.

Maron BJ, Haas TS, Shannon KM, *et al.* Long-term survival after cardiac arrest in hypertrophic cardiomyopathy. Heart Rhythm 2009b;6:993.

Maury P, Couderc P, Delay M, *et al.* Electrical storm in Brugada syndrome treated with isoprenaline. Europace 2004;6:130.

McKenna WJ, Behr ER. Hypertrophic cardiomyopathy: management, risk stratification, and prevention of sudden death. Heart 2002;87:169.

McKenna WJ, Kaski JP. Pacemaker therapy in hypertrophic obstructive cardiomyopathy: still awaiting the evidence. Rev Esp Cardiol 2009;62:1217.

McKenna WJ, Thiene G, Nava A, *et al.* Diagnosis of arrhythmogenic right ventricular dysplasia/cardiomyopathy. Task Force of the Working Group Myocardial and Pericardial Disease of the European Society of Cardiology and of the Scientific Council on Cardiomyopathies of the International Society and Federation of Cardiology. Br Heart J 1994;71:215.

McLeod CJ, Ackerman MJ, Nishimura RA, *et al.* Outcome of patients with hypertrophic cardiomyopathy and a normal electrocardiogram. J Am Coll Cardiol 2009;54:229.

Medeiros-Domingo A, Iturralde-Torres P, Ackerman MJ. Clinical and genetic characteristics of long QT syndrome. Rev Esp Cardiol 2007;60:739.

Meregalli PG, Tan HL, Probst V, *et al.* Type of SCN5A mutation determines clinical severity and degree of conduction slowing in loss-of-function sodium channelopathies. Heart Rhythm 2009;6:341.

Morita H, Zipes DP, Morita ST, Wu J. Differences in arrhythmogenicity between the canine right ventricular outflow tract and anteroinferior right ventricle in a model of Brugada syndrome. Heart Rhythm 2007;4(1):66.

Morita H, Wu Y, Zipes D. The QT syndromes: long and short. The Lancet 2008a;372:750.

Morita H, Kusano KF, Miura D, *et al.* Fragmented QRS as a marker of conduction abnormality and a predictor of prognosis of Brugada syndrome. Circulation 2008b;118:1697.

Moss AJ. T wave patterns associated with the hereditary QT syndrome. Card Electrophysiol Rev 2002;6:311.

Moss A, Kan RS. Long QT syndrome: From channels to cardiac arrhythmias. J Clin Invest 2005;15:2018.

Moss AJ, Schwartz PJ, Crampton RS, *et al.* The long QT syndrome: A prospective international study. Circulation 1985;71:17.

Moss AJ, Shimizu W, Wilde AA, *et al.* Clinical aspects of type-1 long-QT syndrome by location, coding type, and biophysical function of mutations involving the KCNQ1 gene. Circulation 2007;115:2481.

Murphy RT, Thaman R, Gimeno Blanes J, *et al.* Natural history and familial characteristics of isolated left ventricular non-compaction. Eur Heart J 2005; 26:187.

Nam GB, Ko KH, Kim J, *et al.* Mode of onset of ventricular fibrillation in patients with early repolarization pattern vs. Brugada syndrome. Eur Heart J 2010;31:330.

Nof E, Luria D, Brass D, *et al.* Point mutation in the HCN4 cardiac ion channel pore affecting synthesis, trafficking, and functional expression is associated with familial asymptomatic sinus bradycardia. Circulation 2007;11:463.

Opthof T, Coronel R, *et al.* Dispersion of repolarization in canine ventricle and the ECG T wave: T interval does not reflect transmural dispersion. Heart Rhythm 2007;4:341.

Oto, A. Brugada sign: A normal variant or a bad omen? Insights for risk stratification and prognostication. Eur Heart J 2004;25:810.

Ozeke O, Cavus UY, Atar I, *et al.* Epsilon-like electrocardiographic pattern in a patient with Brugada syndrome. Ann Noninvasive Electrocardiol 2009;14:305.

Paparella G, Capulzini L, de Asmundis C, *et al.* Electro-anatomical mapping in a patient with isolated left ventricular non-compaction and left ventricular tachycardia. Europace 2009;11:1227.

Papavassiliu T, Wolpert C, Flüchter S, *et al.* Magnetic resonance imaging findings in patients with Brugada syndrome. J Cardiovasc Electrophysiol 2004;15:1133.

Pappone C, Radinovic A, Manguso F, *et al.* New-onset atrial fibrillation as first clinical manifestation of latent

Brugada syndrome: prevalence and clinical significance. Eur Heart J 2009;30:2985.

Paul M, Gerss J, Schulze-Bahr E, *et al.* Role of programmed ventricular stimulation in patients with Brugada syndrome: a meta-analysis of worldwide published data. Eur Heart J 2007;28:2126.

Pérez-Riera AR. Learning easily frank vectorcardiogram. Editora e Gráfica Mosteiro, Sao Paulo, Brazil 2009.

Pieroni M, Dello Russo A, Marzo F, *et al.* High prevalence of myocarditis mimicking arrhythmogenic right ventricular cardiomyopathy. J Am Coll Cardiol 2009;53:681.

Pitzalis MV, Anaclerio M, Iacoviello M. QT interval prolongation in right precordial leads in Brugada syndrome. J Am Coll Cardiol 2003;42:1632.

Postema PG, De Jong JS, Van der Bilt IA, *et al.* Accurate electrocardiographic assessment of the QT interval: teach the tangent. Heart Rhythm 2008; 5(7):1015.

Postema PG, Wolpert C, Amin AS, *et al.* Drugs and Brugada syndrome patients: Review of the literature, recommendations, and an up-to-date website (www.brugadadrugs.org). Heart Rhythm 2009;6:1335.

Postema PG, van Dessel PF, Kors JA, *et al.* Local depolarization abnormalities are the dominant pathophysiologic mechanism for type 1 electrocardiogram in brugada syndrome a study of electrocardiograms, vectorcardiograms, and body surface potential maps during ajmaline provocation. J Am Coll Cardiol 2010;55:789.

Priori SG, Napolitano C. Should patients with an asymptomatic Brugada electrocardiogram undergo pharmacological and electrophysiological testing? Circulation 2005;112(2):279.

Priori SG, Napolitano C, Giordano U, *et al.* Brugada syndrome and sudden cardiac death in children. Lancet 2000;355:808.

Priori SG, Napolitano C, Memmi M, *et al.* Clinical and molecular characterization of patients with catecholaminergic polymorphic ventricular tachycardia. Circulation 2002a;106:69.

Priori SG, Napolitano C, Gasparini M, *et al.* Natural history of Brugada syndrome: insights for risk stratification and management. Circulation 2002b;105:1342.

Priori SG, Schwartz PJ, Napolitano C, *et al.* Risk stratification in the long-QT syndrome. N Engl J Med 2003; 348(19):1866.

Probst V, Kyndt F, Potet F, *et al.* Haploinsufficiency in combination with aging causes SCN5A-linked hereditary Lenègre disease. J Am Coll Cardiol 2003;41:643.

Probst V, Veltmann C, Eckardt L, *et al.* Long-term prognosis of patients diagnosed with Brugada syndrome: Results from the FINGER Brugada Syndrome Registry. Circulation 2010;121:635.

Protonotarios N, Tsatsopoulou A, Patsourakos P, *et al.* Cardiac abnormalities in familial palmoplantar keratosis. Br Heart J 1986;56:321.

Rosso R, Kogan E, Belhassen B, *et al.* J-point elevation in survivors of primary ventricular fibrillation and matched control subjects: incidence and clinical significance. J Am Coll Cardiol 2008;52:1231.

Sacher F, Probst V, Iesaka Y, *et al.* Outcome after implantation of a cardioverter-defibrillator in patients with Brugada syndrome: a multicenter study. Circulation 2006;114(22):2317.

Samani K, Wu G, Ai T, *et al.* A novel SCN5A mutation V1340I in Brugada syndrome augmenting arrhythmias during febrile illness. Heart Rhythm 2009;6:1318.

Sarkozy A, Brugada P. Sudden cardiac death and inherited arrhythmia syndromes. J Cardiovasc Electrophysiol 2005;16(Suppl 1):S8.

Sarkozy A, Cherchia G, Paparella G, *et al.* Inferior and lateral ECG repolarization abnormalities in Brugada syndrome. Circ Arrhythmic Electrophysiol 2009;2:154.

Scheinman MM. Role of the His-Purkinje system in the genesis of cardiac arrhythmia. Heart Rhythm 2009;6:1050.

Schimpf R, Giustetto C, Eckardt L, *et al.* Prevalence of supraventricular tachyarrhythmias in a cohort of patients with Brugada syndrome. Ann Noninvasive Electrocardiol 2008;13:266.

Schott JJ, Alshinawi C, Kyndt F, *et al.* Cardiac conduction defects associate with mutations in SCN5A. Nat Genet 1999;23:20.

Schwartz PJ, Spazzolini C, Crotti L, *et al.* The Jervell and Lange-Nielsen syndrome: natural history, molecular basis, and clinical outcome. Circulation 2006;113:783.

Schwartz PJ, Moss AJ, Vincent GM, Crampton RS. Diagnostic criteria for the long QT syndrome. An update. Circulation 1993;88:782.

Sen-Chowdhry S, Syrris P, Ward D, *et al.* Clinical and genetic characterization of families with arrhythmogenic right ventricular dysplasia/cardiomyopathy provides novel insights into patterns of disease expression Circulation 2007;115:1710.

Serra G, Baranchuk A, Bayés de Luna A, *et al.* New electrocardiographic criteria to differentiate the Type-2 Brugada pattern from electrocardiogram of healthy athletes with r'-wave in leads V1/V2. Europace 2014; 16: 1639.

Smits JP, Eckardt L, Probs LV. Genotype-phenotype relationship in Brugada syndrome: ECG features differentiate 8CN5A from non SCN5A related patients. J Am Coll Cardiol 2002;40:350.

Spirito P, Seidman CE, McKenna WJ, *et al.* The management of hypertrophic cardiomyopathy. N Engl J Med 1997;336:775.

Splawsky I, Timothy K. Calcium channel dysfunction causes a multisystemic disorder causes a multisystem disorder including arrhythmia and autism. Cell 2004;119:19.

Steffel J, Kobza R, Oechslin E, *et al*. ECG characteristics at initial diagnosis in patients with isolated left ventricle noncompaction. Am J Cardiol 2009;104:984.

Subirana M, Juan-Babot JO, Puig T, *et al*. Specific characteristics of sudden death in a Mediterranean Spanish population. Am J Cardiol 2011;107(4):622.

Suzuki J, Watanabe F, Takenaka K, *et al*. New subtype of apical hypertrophic cardiomyopathy identified with nuclear magnetic resonance imaging as an underlying cause of markedly inverted T waves. J Am Coll Cardiol 1993;22:1175.

Tada T, Kusano KF, Nagase S. The relationship between the magnitude of T wave alternans and the amplitude of the T wave in Brugada syndrome. J Cardiovasc Electrophysiol 2008;19:56.

Takenaka K, Ai T, Shimizu W, *et al*. Exercise stress test amplifies genotype-phenotype correlation in the LQT1 and LQT2 forms of the long-QT syndrome. Circulation 2003;107:838.

Tiso N, Stephan DA, Nava A, *et al*. Identification of mutations in the cardiac syndrome receptor gene in families affected with ARVD type 2. Human Mol Gen 2001;10:189.

Tops LF, Prakasa K, Tandri H, *et al*. Prevalence and pathophysiologic attributes of ventricular dyssynchrony in arrhythmogenic right ventricular dysplasia/cardiomyopathy. J Am Coll Cardiol 2009;54:445.

Towbin J., Bowles N. The failing heart. Nature 2002; 415:227.

Varnava A, Baboonian C, Davison F, *et al*. A new mutation of the cardiac troponin T gene causing familial hypertrophic cardiomyopathy without left ventricular hypertrophy. Heart 1999;82:621.

Vázquez R, Bayés-Genis A, Cygankiewicz I, *et al*. The MUSIC risk score: a simple method for predicting mortality in ambulatory patients with chronic heart failure. Eur Heart J 2009;30:1088.

Vincent GM. The heart rate of Romano-Ward syndrome patients. Am Heart J 1986l;112(1):61.

Vincent GM, Schwartz P. Denjoy I, *et al*. High efficacy of β-blockers in long-QT syndrome type 1.Contribution of noncompliance and QT-prolonging drugs to the occurrence of β-blocker treatment "failures". Circulation 2009;119:215.

Viskin S, Halkin A. Treating the long-QT syndrome in the era of implantable defibrillators. Circulation 2009; 119:204.

Viskin S, Rosso R. Risk of sudden death in asymptomatic Brugada syndrome: not as high as we thought and not as low as we wished... but the contrary. J Am Coll Cardiol 2010;56:1585.

Viskin S, Rosovski U, Sands AJ, *et al*. Inaccurate electrocardiographic interpretation of long QT: the majority of physicians cannot recognize a long QT when they see one. Heart Rhythm 2005;2:569.

Vyas H, Ackerman MJ. Epinephrine QT stress testing in congenital long QT syndrome. J Electrocardiol 2006;39(4 Suppl):S107.

Watanabe H, Makiyama T, Koyama T, *et al*. High prevalence of early repolarization in short QT syndrome. Heart Rhythm 2010;7(5):647.

Wikoff B, Williamson B, Sterns R, *et al*. Strategic programming of detection and therapy parameters reduces shocks in primary prevention patients. Results from PREPARE study. J Am Coll Cardiol 2008;52:541.

Wilde AA, Antzelevitch C, Borggrefe M, *et al*. Proposed diagnostic criteria for the Brugada syndrome: consensus report. Circulation 2002;106:2514.

Wolpert C, Veltmann C, Schimpf R, *et al*. Is a narrow and tall QRS complex an ECG marker for sudden death? Heart Rhythm 2008;5:1339.

Wordsworth S, Leal J, Blair E. DNA testing for hypertrophic CM: a cost-effectiveness model. Eur Heart J 2010;31:926.

Yamaguchi M, Shimizu M, Ino H, *et al*. T wave peak-to-end interval and QT dispersion in acquired long QT syndrome: a new index for arrhythmogenicity. Clin Sci 2003;105:671.

Yan GX, Antzelevitch C. Cellular basis for the Brugada syndrome and other mechanisms of arrhythmogenesis associated with ST-segment elevation Circulation 1999;100:1660.

Yang T, Chung SK, Zhang W, *et al*. Biophysical properties of 9 KCNQ1 mutations associated with long-QT syndrome. Circ Arrhythm Electrophysiol 2009;2:417.

Yap YG, Behr ER, Camm AJ. Drug-induced Brugada syndrome. Europace 2009;11:989.

Zareba W. Challenges of diagnosing long QT syndrome in patients with non diagnostic resting QTc. J Am Coll Cardiol 2010;53:1692.

Zareba W, Moss AJ, Schwartz PJ, *et al*. Influence of genotype on the clinical course of the long-QT syndrome. International Long-QT Syndrome Registry Research Group. N Engl J Med 1998;339:960.

Zareba W, Moss AJ, Locati EH *et al*., Modulating effects of age and sex on the clinical course of long QT syndrome by genotype. J Am Coll Cardiol 2003;42:103.

Zareba W, Cygankiewicz I. Long QT syndrome and short QT syndrome. Progr Cardiovasc Dis 2008;51:264.

Zhang L, Mmagu O, Liu LW, *et al*. Hypertrophic cardiomyopathy: can the noninvasive diagnostic testing identify high risk patients? World J Cardiol 2014;6(8):764.

10

Other ECG Patterns of Risk

Severe Sinus Bradycardia

When pacemaker activity of the sinus node, or stimulus conduction from the sinus node to the atria, is diminished, passive arrhythmias, such as sinus bradycardia due to a decrease of automaticity and/or a sinoatrial block, occur (see Chapter 6).

In many situations, such as myxedema, the ingestion of many drugs (β-blockers, some other antiarrhythmic agents), and ionic and metabolic disturbances, severe but often asymptomatic sinus bradycardia may be present.

Some asymptomatic cases of inherited severe brady-cardia (related to HCN4 ion channel mutation) have been reported (Nof *et al.*, 2007). These cases are usually associated with a good prognosis and do not require pacemaker implantation in the long term.

If there is a significant sinus bradycardia and symptoms are present (dizziness, syncope), a diagnosis of sick sinus syndrome is confirmed (Figure 10.1). The most important cause of sick sinus syndrome is the idiopathic fibrosis of the sinus node appearing more frequently in elderly people. It is also related to many heart diseases, especially ischemic heart disease. The effects of some drugs must be ruled out at all times (see before). Bradyarrhythmias due to sinus node disease (significant sinus automaticity depression and/or sinoatrial block) are not associated with severe symptoms if a normal junctional escape rhythm exists. Most of the symptoms are caused by other associated alterations: junctional automaticity depression (resulting in a slower escape rhythm) and/or atrioventricular (AV) block. If a normal escape rhythm is found, the patient could be virtually asymptomatic or have only mild symptoms (tiredness, mild dizziness).

Sick sinus syndrome is frequently associated with supraventricular arrhythmias, which alternate with significant bradyarrhythmias (bradycardia-tachycardia syndrome) (Figures 10.2 and 10.3). Indeed, often patients with sick sinus syndrome experience intermittent supraventricular arrhythmias, especially atrial fibrillation (AF), and marked or very marked pauses are frequently found at the end of this crises (Figures 10.2 and 10.3). If this occurs, evident symptoms may be present (pre-syncope or syncope, low cardiac output, paroxysmal dyspnea, etc.). In these cases, the immediate implantation of a pacemaker is recommended. The pacemaker has a dual effect: first, it prevents bradyarrhythmia from occurring and, second, if tachyarrhythmia episodes persist, an appropriate antiarrhythmic treatment may be safely administered to prevent future episodes. The implanted pacemaker should provide: (i) normal ventricular activation whenever possible, (ii) physiologic AV synchrony, and (iii) physiologic chronotropic competence (heart rate increase). This is achieved with an atrial single-chamber pacemaker (AAI) when no AV block is present. As mentioned in Chapter 6, sometimes a DDDR (universal dual chamber rate responsive) pacemaker is finally implanted. This occurs especially when there is uncertainty about the appearance of an AV block in the future. Additionally, if the atrial electrode fails, pacing continues through the ventricular electrode (see Chapter 6, Choosing the Best Pacemaker).

Third-Degree (Advanced) Interatrial Block *(Figures 10.4–10.7)*

This type of interatrial block (p. 214) originates a ± P wave in leads II, III, and VF, with a duration greater than 0.12 s (Bayés de Luna *et al.*, 1985; Ariyarajah *et al.*, 2007a, 2007b) (see Figures 3.19 and 6.14). This morphology is explained due to normal right atrium activation with a craniocaudal direction followed by the left atrium activating retrogradely from the mid-lower part of the septum. This retrograde activation of the left atrium occurs because the Bachmann bundle zone, normally the way to cross the stimulus from the right to the left atrium (see Chapter 3, Depression of Conduction: Blocks), is blocked (Figures 10.4. and 10.5) (Martínez-Sellés *et al.*, 2016a, 2016b). If the first part of the P wave has a very low voltage, due to the increased fibrosis (usually present in these cases), the atrial wave seems negative in II, III, VF, mimicking a junctional rhythm (Figure 10.5).

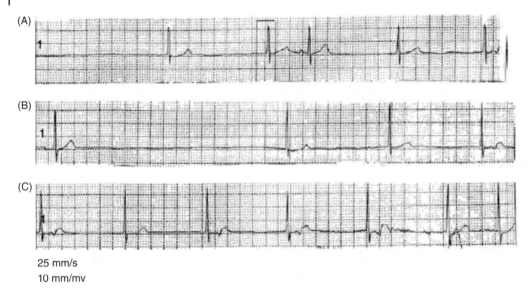

25 mm/s
10 mm/mv

Figure 10.1 Holter recording from a patient with sick sinus syndrome. (A) Note that the escape rhythm is quite slow with some sinus captures. In the first and fourth T waves, a sinus P is probably concealed (see Figure 6.8). The last QRS escape complex is retrogradely conducted to the atria. (B) A pause >3.5 s between the first and second QRS escape complexes. The last QRS complex is also conducted to the atria. (C) Junctional slow escape rhythm, with slow atrial retrograde conduction.

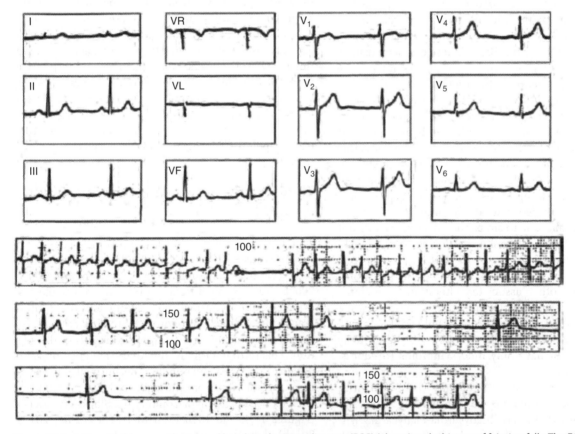

Figure 10.2 A 65-year-old man with a normal baseline electrocardiogram (ECG) (above) and a history of fainting falls. The ECG Holter recording showed a typical bradycardia-tachycardia syndrome (three bottom strips).

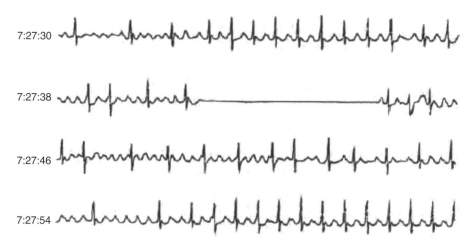

Figure 10.3 A 59-year-old man with typical tachycardia-bradycardia syndrome.

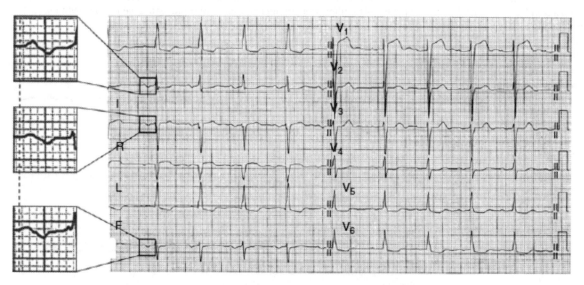

Figure 10.4 A characteristic electrocardiogram (ECG) pattern of advanced interatrial block (P ± in II, III, and VF, and >120 ms) in a patient with ischemic heart disease. See how the onset of P wave (around 180 ms) is seen in lead VF, and the end inn II and III.

In the presence of this type of atrial block with some characteristics (old age, structural heart disease, and ambient arrhythmias) (see later), the incidence of supraventricular tachyarrhythmias, especially atial fibrillation and also atrial flutter usually atypical (Figures 4.6 and 10.6), is very common (Figures 4.6 and 10.7) and the prognosis is poor. Therefore, it has been considered that **the combination of advanced interatrial block** with left atrial retrograde conduction (P wave ± in II, III, and VF) and **supraventricular arrhythmias constitutes a new arrhythmologic syndrome** (Bayés de Luna *et al.*, 1988; Daubert, 1996; Braunwald and Bayés de Luna, 2012) named Bayes syndrome (Conde *et al.*,

2014a, 2014b; Bacharova and Wagner, 2015). The prevalence of A-IAB, which is infrequent in the youth, has been shown to increase with age, being quite frequent in the elderly (8–10%) and reaching up to 25% in centenarians (Martínez-Sellés *et al.*, 2016a). In the latter, it has been associated with a higher prevalence of dementia and previous stroke. Also was previously published (Spodick's group) (Ariyarajah *et al.*, 2007c), there is a high prevalence of interatrial blocks in patients with stroke. It seems clear that aging patients with advanced interatrial block and long P wave duration, evident structural heart disease and ambient arrhythmias (frequent PAC in Holter monitoring), are at high risk of

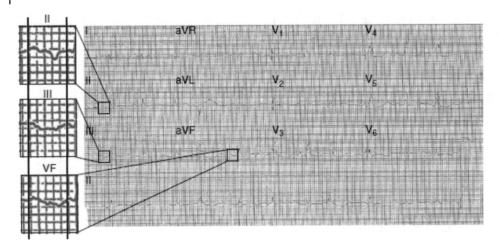

Figure 10.5 A characteristic electrocardiogram (ECG) pattern of advanced interatrial block in a 60-year-old patient with Ebstein's disease. Note that the P ± is very wide in II, and in III it is all negative because in this lead the first and last part of the P wave is isodiphasic. Thus, this may be confused with a junctional rhythm. The patient also suffers from frequent episodes of supraventricular tachyarrhythmia (2×1 and 1×1) flutter that provoke syncope fortunately transient (see Figure 4.65).

Figure 10.6 (A) In this patient with advanced interatrial block, both types of atrial tachyarrhythmias (atrial fibrillation) and atrial flutter are observed. (B) Patient with very important A-IAB (see P wave in II, III, VF) that after a premature atrial complex present a pause followed by an escape junctional complex and a crisis of paroxysmal supraventricular tachyarrhythmia (Dr R Barbosa).

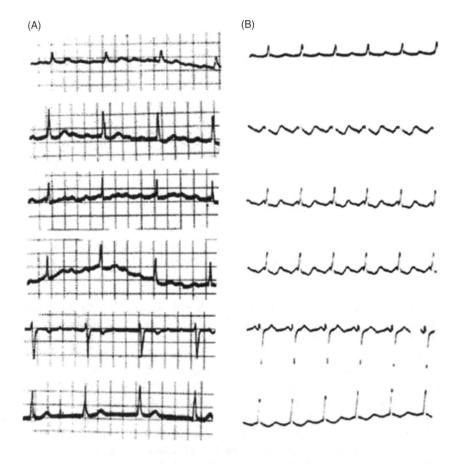

atrial fibrillation/atrial flutter and probably of stroke and cognitive impairment. Even cases of aborted sudden death due to 1×1 atrial flutter have been published (Figures 10.4 and 4.65). Due to this, we consider that it is time to evaluate whether starting anticoagulation earlier (even with no documented AF) in this group of patients would be beneficial to prevent stroke (Bayés de Luna *et al.*, 2017; Martínez-Sellés *et al.*, 2016b). Therefore, to start a registry and, if positive, a clinical trial to demonstrate that seems very convenient.

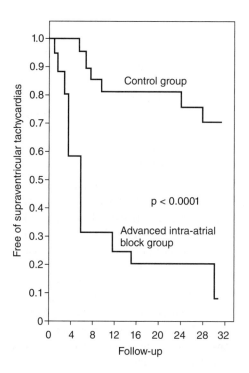

Figure 10.7 Patients with advanced interatrial block and left atrial retrograde activation show many more supraventricular paroxysmal arrhythmias during follow-up when compared with patients from the control group with the same electrocardiographic and clinical characteristics (Bayés de Luna *et al.*, 1988).

High-Risk Ventricular Block

Bundle Branch Block in Patients with Heart Disease

A bundle branch block (BBB) is a marker of bad prognosis in patients with heart disease, especially in cases of left bundle branch block (LBBB). The presence of LBBB, or even right bundle branch block (RBBB), in post-infarction patients with ventricular dysfunction/heart failure (HF) is a marker of higher risk of sudden death (SD), and, in the case of LBBB, it is also a marker for all-cause mortality (Bogale *et al.*, 2007). Patients with HF and LBBB who present AF have the worst prognosis (Baldasseroni *et al.*, 2002; Vázquez *et al.*, 2009) (see Chapter 11, Heart Failure).

A "de novo" advanced RBBB in the course of an acute coronary syndrome constitutes a marker of bad prognosis. This situation obliges us to consider a differential diagnosis between acute coronary syndrome and pulmonary embolism. Naturally, in the course of an acute coronary syndrome with ST segment elevation in precordial leads (STEMI), a RBBB pattern is observed when the left anterior descending coronary artery proximal to the first septal branch is occluded. This is the artery perfusing the right bundle (Figure 10.8) (Bayés de Luna and Fiol, 2008; Wellens *et al.*, 2003). Also, RBBB + SAH usually appears

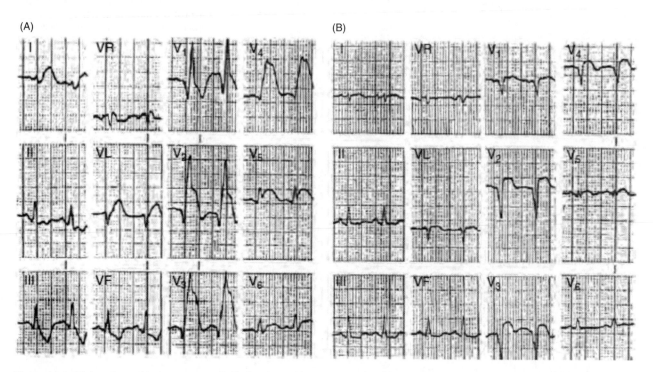

Figure 10.8 (A) A patient with acute myocardial infarction, with anteroseptal and lateral Q waves and advanced right bundle branch block (RBBB) morphology. (B) 24 hours later, the RBBB morphology disappears, although the anteroseptal and lateral Q infarction pattern is still present. In this case, the occluded artery is the anterior left anterior descending (LAD) coronary artery proximal to S_1 because the right bundle branch is perfused by the S_1 branch.

in the rare cases of complete occlusion of main trunk if they are lucky enough to arrive alive to the hospital (Fiol *et al.*, 2012) Meanwhile, we may consider a diagnosis of pulmonary embolism when a new RBBB pattern occurs in patients with an acute episode in which the degree of dyspnea is more significant than that of precordial pain. In this case, the ECG may also show an ST segment elevation in different leads, as well as sinus tachycardia, apart from the advanced RBBB pattern. The presence of a new RBBB is indicative of a massive pulmonary embolism, and thus is associated with a very poor prognosis. The cause of death is not usually a primary arrhythmia, but rather a hemodynamic failure with progressive impairment of automaticity leading to cardiac arrest (Figure 10.9).

It is necessary to rule out that the RBBB pattern may be related to aberrant conduction in relation with sinus tachycardia (tachycardia-dependent block). In this case, the prognosis would not depend on the appearance of RBBB. Therefore, to determine the prognosis, it is important to know whether the patient had previously had an intermittent RBBB related to an increase in heart rate.

Bifascicular Block

Pacemaker implantation is not indicated in cases of bifascicular block in the absence of symptoms and prolonged PR interval. In these conditions it is necessary to study the case carefully (Holter monitoring, EPS, etc.) (see Chapter 6, Clinical, Prognostic, and Therapeutic Implications of Passive Arrhythmias).

Masked bifascicular block is a special type of bifascicular block with a bad prognosis.

o The diagnosis of masked bifascicular block is confirmed when in the presence of a tall and wide R wave in V1 (the ECG pattern suggestive of advanced RBBB), no S wave is recorded in leads I and VL. The presence of extreme left axial deviation is explained by an associated superoanterior hemiblock (Figure 10.10) (Bayés de Luna *et al.*, 1989). At first glance, in an ECG of this type it seems that LBBB is present in the frontal plane (FP), whereas in the horizontal plane (HP), RBBB is observed. The fact that an R wave is recorded in lead V1 but no S wave is seen in leads I and VL is due to a significant left ventricular enlargement and/or associated conduction block in the left ventricular free wall.

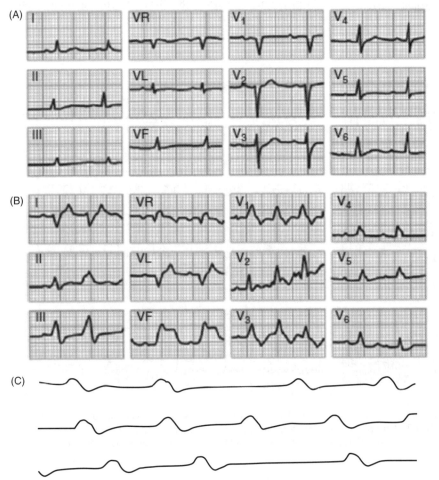

Figure 10.9 (A) Pre-operative electrocardiogram (ECG) in a 58-year-old patient without heart disease. (B) During the post-operative period, the patient suffered a massive pulmonary embolism. The ECG showed a significant right ÂQRS axis deviation, advanced right bundle branch block (RBBB) with ST elevation in V1–V2, III, and VF sinus tachycardia and atrial extrasystoles. (C) The patient died immediately after (continuous ECG strip with agonic rhythm).

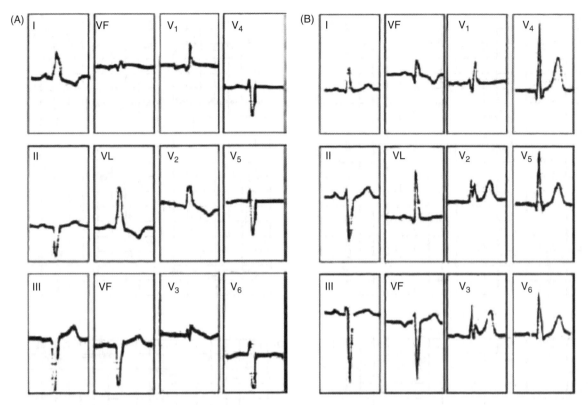

Figure 10.10 Two examples of masked block. (A) Right bundle branch block with anterosuperior hemiblock or, precisely, with partial left bundle branch trunk block, as no "q" is observed in I and VL, with predominant delayed depolarization in the superoanterior area (significant left ÂQRS axis deviation). The left ventricular depolarization is delayed to such an extent that it counteracts the final vectors originated by the RBBB, which, although directed forward, are directed leftwards and not rightwards, thus falling into the positive hemifield of V1 (RBBB pattern in V1). There are no signs of RBBB in the frontal plane, as no S wave is observed in I and VL due to the presence of anterior but leftward forces. (see Figure 10.12) (B) Another example of RBBB + ASH. In this case a "q" wave is observed in I and VL.

The final activation forces (Figure 10.12) are not directed forwards and rightwards, as in the classic bifascicular block (vector 1), but forwards and leftwards (vector 2). The masked bifascicular block rarely occurs intermittently (García-Moll *et al.*, 1994) (Figure 10.11) (see legend). In these cases, prognosis is poor regardless of whether a pacemaker is implanted or not (Bayés de Luna *et al.*, 1989). This occurs because this type of block is usually detected in patients with advanced heart disease. Hence, the diagnosis in itself is a marker for poor prognosis.

Right Bundle Branch Block Plus Alternating Block in the Two Divisions of the Left Bundle Branch

In 1968, Rosenbaum described a type of intraventricular block that could lead to SD and require urgent pacemaker implantation. Several consecutive ECGs showed RBBB and anterosuperior block, alternating with RBBB with posteroinferior hemiblock (Rosenbaum *et al.* 1968) (Figure 10.13). This diagnosis, which usually has evident clinical characteristics (dizziness, near-syncope, etc.), should be named Rosenbaum-Elizari syndrome (Recommended General Bibliography p. xvii). Pacemaker implantation may resolve the problem and improve patient outcome. In the absence of advanced underlying heart disease, the prognosis can be excellent.

Alternating Bundle Branch Block

In this case, the ECG alternatively shows the ECG pattern of LBBB and RBBB, with or without associated hemiblocks, in the same patient (Figure 10.14).

In most cases the patient presents symptoms (dizziness, syncope), and it is necessary to implant a pacemaker as soon as possible because of the potential risk of complete AV block and SD. After the pacemaker is implanted, patients may have a good prognosis in the long-term follow-up when the block is due mainly to the involvement of the specific conduction system.

Advanced Atrioventricular Block

Obviously, the **presence of an acquired AV block requires pacemaker implantation in most cases**. There may be exceptions, such as cases of AV block due to a reversible cause (ischemia, drugs, etc.).

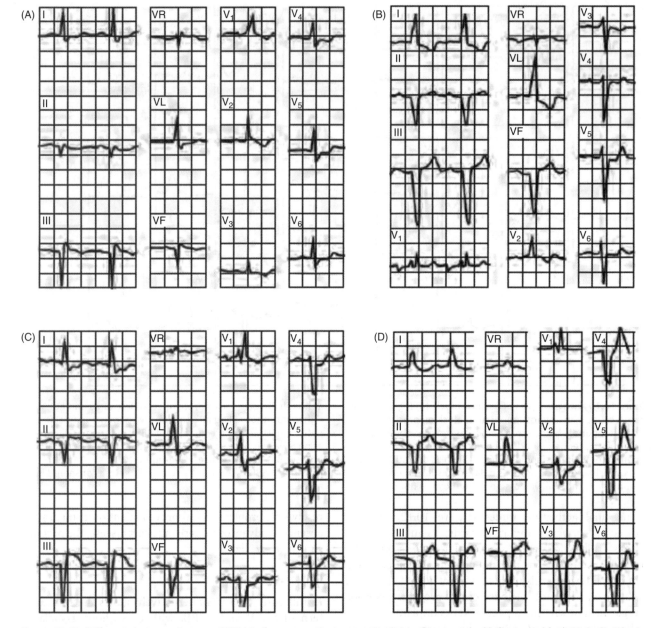

Figure 10.11 Different electrocardiograms (ECGs) in the same patient presenting intermittent masked bifascicular block. Note that the S wave disappears in I and VL (B and D), coinciding with a left ventricular failure episode, and that the R wave in V1 is seen in all ECGs.

The implantation of a pacemaker for **congenital AV blocks is a questionable procedure**. This condition is already present at birth, often related to a systemic disease of the mother during pregnancy (presence of Ro/SS-A and La/SS-B antinuclear antibodies in the mother's blood), which results in fetal myocarditis involving the specific conduction system. Using fetal kinetocardiography, it has been demonstrated (Rein *et al.*, 2009) that 10% of fetuses whose mothers carried these antibodies experienced first-degree AV block at 20–30 weeks' gestation. When dexamethasone was prescribed, AV conduction was normalized and the infant showed no AV block or

evidence of heart disease at birth. This type of AV block has been sometimes found in different members of the same family, although its genetic origin has not been demonstrated to date.

Immune-mediated cardiomyopathy has been recognized in infants born of mothers with antinuclear antibodies. The natural history of patients with isolated congenital AV block that requires pacing depends on their antibody status. If it is positive, it has been demonstrated that it is a predictor of HF and death. The cases with negative antibody status in a long follow-up have a survival free of new HF after pacemaker implant (Sagar *et al.*, 2010).

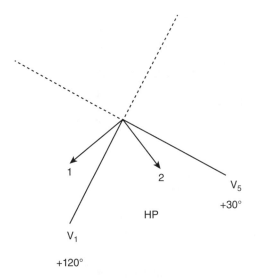

Figure 10.12 In the presence of masked block, the disappearance of the S wave in I, VL, and sometimes V6 is due to the fact that the final activation (2) is directed forward, falling into the positive hemifield of V1 and thus originating an R wave in V1. As it is also directed leftward (due to the significant leftward final forces), it does not, however, originate an S wave in I and VL. Vector 1 is the final vector seen in cases of normal bifascicular block and vector 2 in case of masked block.

Patients with advanced congenital AV block have a certain risk of SD. Although it is difficult to decide the best moment to implant a pacemaker, the tendency is to recommend pacemaker implantation even in the absence of symptoms if the escape rhythm is very slow (Friedman, 1995).

Pacemaker implantation is usually not indicated during childhood: (a) if the baseline rate is ≥50 bpm with a narrow escape rhythm, (b) if the nighttime rate (Holter recording) is never <30–35 bpm with a mean 24-h ventricular rate >45–50 bpm, (c) if the heart rate during an exercise test is >100 bpm, (d) if there is no lengthening of the QT interval, and (e) if there are no important ventricular arrhythmias (see Chapter 6, Figure 6.23). If the previously mentioned parameters worsen during follow-up, or if the patient becomes ymptomatic, pacemaker implantation is recommended (Figure 10.15).

The Presence of Ventricular Arrhythmias in Chronic Heart Disease Patients

The presence of premature ventricular complexes (PVC) in the surface ECG in patients with chronic heart disease, especially ischemic heart disease, indicates that they are probably occurring frequently. In this case, Holter recording and exercise testing to establish their characteristics is recommended. In fact, the presence of any PVC in a routine 10-s ECG in patients with moderate

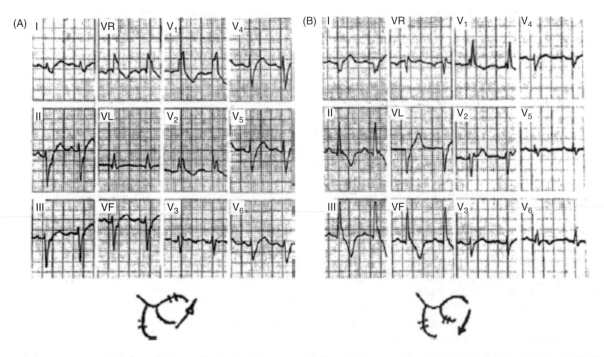

Figure 10.13 Typical pattern of trifascicular block. (A) Right bundle branch block and superoanterior hemiblock (RBBB + SAH). (B) The following day, the frontal ÂQRS turned from −60° to +130° as the result of posteroinferior hemiblock occurring instead of SAH. Below: In both cases the delayed activation of the blocked area of LV originates a leftward or rightward ÂQRS deviation in the frontal plane (A and B, respectively).

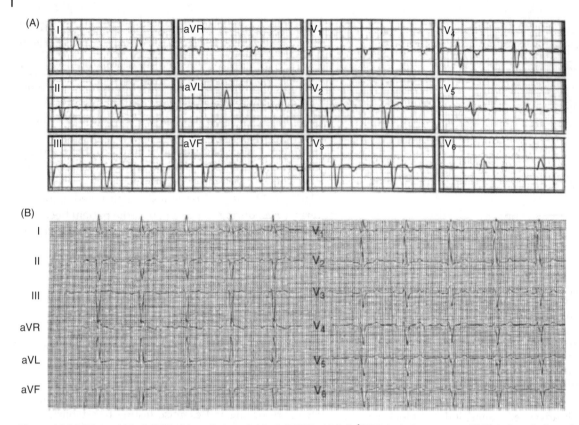

Figure 10.14 Bilateral block. (A) Left bundle branch block (LBBB) with left ÂQRS deviation pattern. (B) Right bundle branch block and superoanterior hemiblock (RBBB + SAH) pattern. The patient suffered from syncope and immediately a pacemaker was implanted.

HF is a powerful predictor of cardiovascular mortality (Van Lee *et al.*, 2010).

Premature ventricular complex morphology may sometimes suggest the presence of necrosis (QR pattern, for example) (see Chapter 5, Premature Ventricular Complexes). It may even be more sensitive than sinus QRS complexes (ST depression) in detecting ischemia (Rasouli and Ellestad, 2001) (Figure 10.16).

Premature ventricular complexes associated with poor prognosis include:

o Those occurring in patients with acute ischemia, mainly with the R/T phenomenon, as they may trigger ventricular fibrillation (VF) (see Figure 5.43).
o Those occurring frequently or repetitively, especially in the presence of advanced heart disease and poor ventricular function mainly in post-infarction patients, as they may lead to sustained ventricular tachycardia (VT) and SD (see Figures 5.12 and 5.13).
o Premature ventricular complexes with a "q" (QR especially with symmetrical T wave) are more often found in patients with associated necrosis and/or a low ejection fraction (dilated cardiomyopathy) and, therefore, have a poor prognosis (see Figure 5.9).
o Very wide and notched >40 ms PVC (see Figure 5.9B).

o Premature ventricular complexes that may present more marked repolarization alterations (ST depression) indicative of ischemia during an exercise testing when compared with QRS complexes of the sinus rhythm (Figure 10.16) (Rasouli and Ellestad, 2001) (see before).

Sustained VT in patients with heart disease is associated with bad outcomes. In cases with low ejection fraction and in patients with inherited heart diseases (Chapter 9), ICD therapy is usually advisable (see Table A-5). The cases of sustained VT in patients without apparent heart disease, if repetitive, must also be considered serious cases. In these cases new episodes usually should first be prevented either with pharmacologic treatment or ablation, if feasible, especially in cases of right ventricular tachycardia or branch–branch reentry. (see Chapter 5 and Appendix A-4.4).

Acquired Long QT
(Figure 10.17)

The acquired long QT interval is more frequent than congenital long QT syndrome. Frequently, there is an evident cause, but a genetic predisposition may also

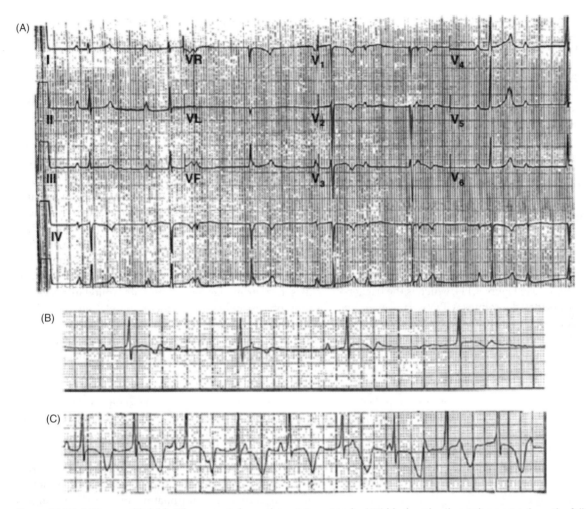

Figure 10.15 A 12-year-old child with congenital complete a trioventricular (AV) block and no heart disease in whom the following findings were observed. (A) At rest, the heart rate, which was always greater than 60 bpm, now decreased to 45 bpm; (C) during the exercise stress testing, it did not exceed 80 bpm; and (B) at night (Holter), it frequently decreased to <35 bpm. These findings, along with the occurrence of exercise dyspnea, recommend pacemaker implantation.

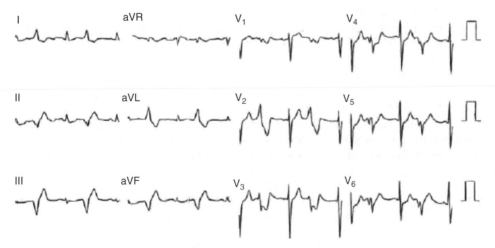

Figure 10.16 Exercise stress testing in a patient with ischemic heart disease. The ST segment of the premature ventricular complex (PVC) shows a more significant alteration than that of sinus complexes (see V3).

Table 10.1 Predisposing factors for QT interval prolongation.

- Heart disease: ischemic heart disease, heart failure, etc.
- Electrocardiogram alterations: baseline prolonged QT, abnormal U wave, T wave alternans, deep and negative
- T wave, significant bradycardia
- Acute neurologic accidents
- Ionic and metabolic alterations: diabetes, anorexia, hypoglycemia, hypothyroidism, obesity
- Septic shock
- Female sex
- Advanced age
- Hypothermia
- Intoxications

exist. Acquired long QT syndrome usually shows a heterogeneous repolarization dispersion, as does congenital long QT syndrome (see Figure 3.11), which is the triggering factor of Torsades de Pointes VT/VF. However, on certain occasions, such as with amiodarone administration, the prolongation of repolarization is homogeneous and the long QT is not associated with a potential risk of arrhythmias.

Table 10.1 shows the most important predisposing factors for long QT syndrome, including other repolarization alterations, which may foster VT/VF. The ECG premonitory signs of TP/VF have already been described (Drew *et al.*, 2010) (Chapter 5, Polymorphic VT: Torsades de Pointes). They occur in patients with bradyarrhythmia, usually with an ionic imbalance and/or the administration of some drugs.

The TP/VF may be seen in different inherited (hypertrophic cardiomyopathy (CM), channelopathies, etc.) and acquired (dilated cardiomyopathy, ischemic heart disease and others) heart diseases, and also as a consequence of septic, toxic, or metabolic shock or associated significant ionic imbalance, and after the administration of certain drugs that may induce abnormal lengthening of QT (Table 10.2). The risk of developing VT/VF is evident when drugs lengthen the QT interval >60 ms and/or QTc is >500 ms. A QT lengthening >30 ms is already considered pathologic.

In most of these cases, long QT syndrome is due to the inhibition of the K currents (Ikr, Iks) by drugs, leading to repolarization delay. This may explain some cases of SD. Torsades de Pointes VT in a drug-induced long QT syndrome usually takes place after the occurrence of a premature complex, followed by a long pause, which is similar to what happens in the LQT2 syndrome (Kirchhof *et al.*, 2009; Drew *et al.*, 2010) (see Chapter 9, Long QT Syndrome).

Due to the potential risk that certain drugs may lengthen the QT interval and initiate arrhythmias such as Torsades de Pointes VT, drug agencies (FDA, EMEA)

now carefully examine a new drug's potential to increase dispersion of repolarization, especially when it concerns the effect on HERG channels (i.e., QT interval). Cases of SD that occurred with two apparently harmless drugs (cisapride and terfenidine) are especially relevant. As already mentioned, Table 10.2 shows some of the drugs that most frequently prolong the QT interval and which have been shown to cause Torsades de Pointes VT. We should remember that the CAST trial (Echt *et al.*, 1991), which assessed the efficacy of different antiarrhythmic drugs (including flecainide and quinidine) for the prevention of post-infarction SD, had to be stopped because more cases of SD were observed in the active treatment group than in the control group. Meanwhile, the majority of the new antiarrhythmic agents studied (azimilide, dofelitide, and ibutilide) are not widely used due to the associated side effects, especially the risk of VT/VF. In this sense, dronedarone, along with amiodarone, is the safest pharmacologic treatment in relation to TV/VF occurrences in spite of possible severe side effects, especially thyroid disfunction, which can usually be avoided with frequent blood thyroid function tests. More information on this subject may be obtained at https://crediblemeds.org/.

Most cases of acquired long QT syndrome recognize a multifactorial reason for delayed cardiac repolarization. The most common causes include polypharmacy impacting the QT interval (for example, the combination of antipsychotics with antibiotics and diuretics), electrolyte disturbances (hypokalemia, hypomagnesemia), ischemia and bradycardia. Discontinuation of all QT prolongers and immediate electrolyte correction is the cornerstone of treatment. Sometimes, in order to prevent or treat Torsades de Pointes, temporary pacing or infusion of isoproterenol is also needed (Digby *et al.*, 2010, 2011).

Table 10.2 Drugs associated with QT prolongation and potential arrhythmogenic risk (for more details, please consult https://crediblemeds.org/).

- Antiarrhythmic drugs: generally, types I and III. Also recently studied drugs (azimilide, ibutilide). Propafenone is probably less risky, in the absence of heart failure.
- Amiodarone has less arrhythmogenic effect despite the fact that significantly prolong the QT interval.
- Type II and IV drugs are safe.
- Macrolide antibiotics: azithromycin, clarithromycin, erythromycin
- Fluoroquinolones: ciprofloxacin, levofloxacin, etc.
- Antidepressants: amitriptyline, fluoxetine, imipramine, paroxetine, etc.
- Antipsychotics: haloperidol, risperidone
- Antihistaminics: terfenadine (withdrawn)
- GI tract: cisapride (withdrawn)

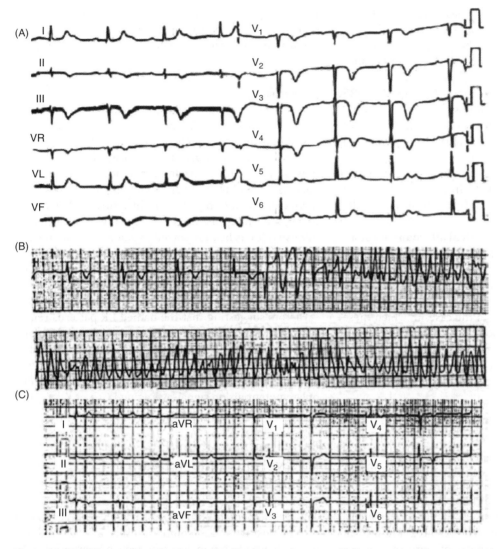

Figure 10.17 A 58-year-old patient hospitalized in an intensive care unit due to sepsis with a very pathologic electrocardiogram (ECG) (A) with a long QT interval and deep negative T wave in anterior and inferior leads. The coronariography showed a normal pattern, whereas the ionogram showed a clear hypomagnesemia. The patient also showed runs of Torsades de Pointes ventricular tachycardia (VT), which led to ventricular fibrillation (VF) (B). Once the clinical and ionic alterations were solved, the QT interval was normalized and the ECG showed only a flat and somewhat negative T wave in inferior leads and in V4–V6 (C).

The use of a long QT interval as a marker of poor prognosis in post-infarction patients is controversial, although more results supporting this hypothesis have been published (Schwartz and Wolf, 1978). It has been reported (Chugh *et al.*, 2009) that an abnormally long QT increases the risk of SD fivefold in chronic ischemic heart disease patients. We have also reported that post-infarction patients showing QT peaks >500 ms in a Holter recording have a poor prognosis (Homs *et al.*, 1997). In all these cases, the QT interval, although long, does not reach the values observed in congenital long QT interval syndrome, nor those related with certain significant ionic or metabolic alterations, such as septic

shock (Figure 10.17). Furthermore, other repolarization alterations (i.e., abnormal or alternating T wave morphology) that may exist in congenital long QT are usually not found (Kirchhof *et al.*, 2009) (see Figure 9.12 and Tables 9.7–9.9).

Electrical Alternans
(see Table 7.1 and Figure 7.5)

This is characterized by a beat-to-beat alternans of ECG morphology on an every-other-beat basis. Electrical alternans occurs when the changes of QRS/T are due to myocardial intrinsic changes, or at least are not explained by periodic changes in ventricular activation, or they are not due to a coincidence with the periodic presence of some arrhythmia. The latter may refer to pseudo-alternans (Table 7.1).

We have already discussed (see Chapter 7, QRS Complexes of Variable Morphology) that QRS electrical alternans may be seen in sinus rhythm in cases of cardiac tamponade and during a narrow AV junctional reentrant tachycardia with an accessory pathway. Some other cases that may be considered pseudo-alternans are: (i) bigeminal PVC in the PR interval, (ii) alternans pre-excitation, and (iii) alternans bundle branch block.

Cases of **repolarization electrical alternans** are associated with a higher risk of developing VT/VF. It has been suggested that microscopic T wave alternans is a risk marker of SD in post-infarction patients (Rosenbaum *et al.*, 1994; Nieminen and Verrier, 2010) and in other situations. Here we will refer to the cases in which these electrical alternans are visible in the surface ECG. In our experience there are three well-defined clinical situations that show evident ST/T alternans in the surface ECG accompanied by VT/VF:

i) T wave alternans sometimes precede a VT Torsades de Pointes episode in patients with long QT syndrome (see Figure 7.5C).
ii) T wave alternans associated with an acquired long QT, as observed in cases of shock and/or significant ionic disorders (see Figure 7.5D).
iii) ST/T alternans indicative of severe and hyperacute ischemia, as observed in cases of acute coronary syndrome involving a large ischemic area and also in cases of severe coronary spasm of a proximal artery (see Figure 7.5B).

Other Electrocardiographic Patterns of Risk for Sudden Death

Early repolarization pattern

Concept

The early repolarization (ER) pattern may be defined as a positive and sharp notch or deflection at the end of QRS/beginning of the ST segment, usually with some elevation of ST (J wave). Some authors (Benito *et al.*, 2010; Myazaki *et al.*, 2010) also consider ER the smooth transition from QRS to ST segment (slurring). Tikkanen (2009) included all cases of J point elevation (>1–2 mm) that were either a notched (clear positive J deflection inscribed on the S wave-typical ER pattern) or a "slurred" pattern in at least two consecutive leads, in

the concept of early repolarization (ER) pattern. The high prevalence of ER in the presence of short QT syndrome has been recently reported (Watanabe *et al.*, 2010).

Mechanisms

It has been postulated that the mechanism of the ER pattern occurs at the beginning of repolarization process and is the consequence of a transient dominant Ito current. When compared with Brugada's syndrome, however, this Ito current is not accompanied by a decrease in an inward sodium current and occurs in all myocardium, not only in the right ventricle. The J wave of hypothermia has similar origin but is of a higher intensity. It has been reported that some transient early Ito currents may participate in the genesis of ST segment elevation in cases of STEMI, and in the triggering of VF in acute myocardial ischemia (Yan *et al.*, 2004) (see later).

Factors suggesting that the named ER patterns represent "early repolarization" rather than "delayed depolarization" are: (i) spontaneous fluctuation of the pattern in the face of stable QRS complexes; (ii) amplitude varying concurrently with the ST segment; and (iii) the absence of late potentials on signal-averaging ECG.

Early Repolarization (ER) Pattern (J Wave) and Sudden Death
(Figure 10.18)

The typical benign ER pattern is usually seen at the end of the positive QRS complex, especially in mid-left precordial leads, but may also be seen in inferior leads. In these cases it is necessary to check carefully the case if the ST segment present down slope pattern (see later) (Figure 10.18A).

Although few reports associated the presence of J waves with SD, especially in patients of South Asia, the first case study demonstrating that ER pattern (J point elevation or J wave >1 mm, especially in inferior leads) presented a higher prevalence among patients with a history of idiopathic VF was published by Haïssaguerre in 2008 (Haïssaguerre *et al.*, 2008). The subjects were mostly men with a mean age of 35 years. Characteristically, PVC origin was concordant with the location of the J wave, (usually J waves in inferior leads and PVC with negative QRS in the same leads), and usually a clear accentuation of ER pattern (J wave) appeared before the final event.

Similar results were obtained by Rosso *et al.* (2008), but Merchant *et al.* (2009) showed some discrepancy because it was found that patients with an ER pattern in

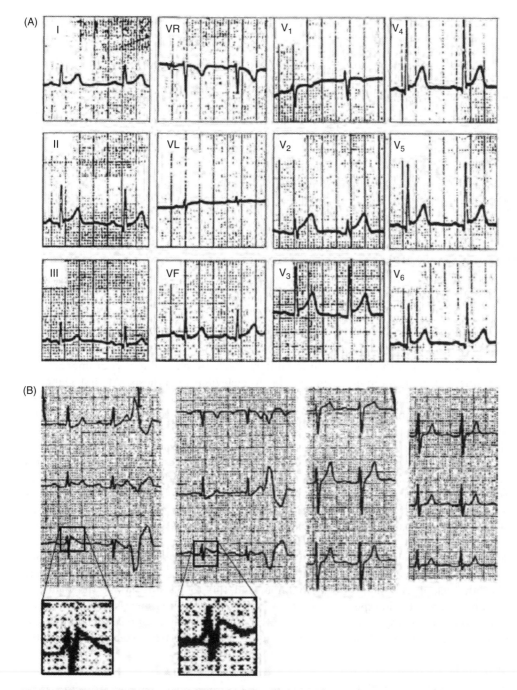

Figure 10.18 (A) Example of an early repolarization pattern in a healthy 40-year-old man. Note the mild pattern (J wave <1 mm) with ascendant ST, seen particularly in the intermediate left precordial and inferior leads. This corresponds to a benign pattern. (B) Example of early repolarization pattern seen especially in inferior leads with a J point of ≥2 mm an descendent ST (compare lead II in A and B). This corresponds to a dangerous pattern (see the PVC with left ÂQRS, arising in inferior wall) (Rosso *et al.*, 2008).

left precordial lateral leads presented a worse prognosis than patients with an ER pattern in inferior leads.

The prognostic significance of the ER pattern (J point elevation) in the general population has been studied (Tikkanen *et al.*, 2009). It has been shown that an ER pattern in inferior leads, especially if ≥2 mm, is associated with risk of death from cardiac causes (P <0.001) and from arrhythmias (P <0.01) in middle-aged subjects (mean age 45 years). However, the absolute risk of death is very small in cases with a J point <2 mm. Death from

Table 10.3 J wave syndromes: similarities and differences (adapted with modifications from Antzelevitch and Yan, 2010).

	Inherited			Acquired		
	ER Pattern I	*ER pattern II*	*ER Pattern III*[*]	*Brugada's syndrome*	*Ischemia-mediated VT/VF*	*Hypothermia-mediated VT/VF*
Leads displaying J point/J wave abnormalities	I, V4–V6		Inferior and sometimes inferolateral leads Global	V1–V3	Any of the 12 leads	N/A
Anatomic location of ECG alterations	Anterolateral left ventricle	Inferior LV	Left and right ventricles	Right ventricle	L and R ventricles	L and R ventricles
Possibility of VF	In marginal cases. Commonly seen in healthy men and athletes	Higher risk specially in some cases (see text)	Yes. Probably Brugada variant	Yes	Yes	Yes

[*]According to some data reported in the Antzelevitch paper – Figure 5 and reference 23 – these cases may correspond to a variant of Brugada's syndrome. ER, early repolarization; VF, ventricular fibrillation; VT, ventricular tachycardia.

cardiac causes occurs late after the baseline ECG. The survival curves started to diverge 15 years after the first ECG, whereas in primary VF this is most commonly observed in younger patients. It is possible that the ER pattern increases vulnerability to fatal arrhythmia in the presence of acute ischemic attack, which is the first cause of death at this age in the Finnish population (Tikkanen *et al.*, 2009). It has recently been suggested (see before) that in early acute STEMI, Phase 2 reentry caused by loss of dome of epicardial transmembrane action potential related to the transient outward potassium current (Ito) that occurs during ischemia can produce a R on T PVC triggering VF (Yan *et al.*, 2004).

More recently, a consensus paper on the value of ER pattern has been published by Macfarlane and colleagues. The authors agreed on the lack of relevance in asymptomatic ER patterns. In summary, we should especially pay attention to this condition when it is symptomatic by syncope or aborted sudden death (Macfarlane *et al.*, 2015).

Antzelevitch and Yan (2010) include ER patterns in the term **J wave syndromes**. This term encompasses all syndromes related to an abnormal J wave: inherited (Brugada's syndrome and three types of early repolarization syndromes) and acquired (ischemia mediated VT/VF and hypothermia mediated VT/VF). As previously discussed (see Chapter 9, Brugada Syndrome: Differential Diagnosis), the ER pattern and Brugada's syndrome may be related to the dominant and transient outward potassium current Ito. It has to be remembered that inferior and lateral repolarization abnormalities in Brugada syndrome have also been reported (Sarkozy

et al., 2009). Table 10.3 summarizes the most important clinical differences between all these syndromes according to the Antzelevitch hypothesis. At first glance, it would seem that the early Type III repolarization patterns of this table represent a variant of Brugada's syndrome, and that the Type II pattern may be also considered dangerous, especially if the J point >2 mm and/or the amplitude changes abruptly. Lastly, it is clear that Type I is very frequently seen in healthy people. However, more information is needed to draw specific conclusions about risk when looking at an ECG with an ER pattern. What we require are: (i) to check the voltage and location of the pattern and also if the pattern is fixed or changes abruptly, (ii) to know the family history, including personal antecedents of syncope or severe arrhythmia, and (iii) to be sure about the technical aspects of ECG recording. It is surprising, for example, that the ER pattern virtually disappears when a 40-Hz low-pass filter is used (García-Niebla *et al.*, 2009) (Figure 10.19).

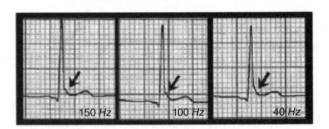

Figure 10.19 A 40-year-old man with a typical early repolarization pattern with small J wave. It should be noted that the low-pass filter at 40 Hz may cause it to disappear.

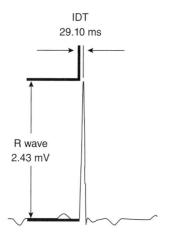

IDT
29.10 ms

R wave
2.43 mV

Figure 10.20 High-voltage QRS complex with abrupt peak of R wave. IDT: intrinsicoid deflection time (Wolpert *et al.*, 2008).

Currently we consider that in the presence of an early repolarization pattern without clear ECG characteristics of possible risk, as previously discussed, and with no previous family or personal history of syncope or SD, it is not necessary to proceed with further investigations, given the considerable amount of cases that despite showing an early repolarization pattern have a good prognosis. Further follow-up studies including patients with early repolarization in inferior leads, especially if ≥2 mm, should be carried out to determine the true significance of this ECG pattern. Remember (see before) that in one study (Tikkanen *et al.*, 2009) it was suggested that VF may be triggered by acute ischemia in the presence of an early repolarization pattern. At present, epidemiologic evidence suggests that the presence of an ER pattern in young adults with no apparent heart disease increases the risk of VF from 4.5/100 000 to 11/100 000 (Rosso *et al.*, 2008). This is a negligible difference. Therefore, the incidental finding of a J wave during screening without specific markers already shown (see before) should not be interpreted as a marker of increased risk. This is reassuring information, both for physicians and patients.

Therefore, we should wait for better clinical–arrhythmic correlation and for the identification of genetic markers of this condition (early repolarization + VF), named Haïssaguerre syndrome (Viskin, 2009). In patients with this syndrome, the association of VF with a genetic variant has already been reported (Haïssaguerre *et al.*, 2009).

Other ECG Patterns

It has also been suggested that a tall and narrow QRS complex with a certain degree of repolarization alteration that is generally nonsignificant could be a marker of

SD (Wolpert *et al.*, 2008) (Figure 10.20). This possible association requires further investigation.

Finally, Aizawa *et al.* (1993) describe the occurrence of idiopathic VF in patients with bradycardia-dependent intraventricular block, and Iturralde *et al.* (2008) also show the association of intraventricular blocks and VT in children (see Chapter 9, Other Possible Channelopathies).

Risk of Serious Arrhythmias and Sudden Death in Patients with Normal or Nearly Normal ECG

We have already stated that SD may occur in people with normal or apparently normal ECG (see Chapter 9, Idiopathic Ventricular Fibrillation). Now we would like to emphasize that a normal ECG does not exclude the presence of advanced heart disease or the risk of SD. On one hand, we see the possible existence of an undiagnosed channelopathy or an idiopathic VF, as already discussed. On the other hand, it is not possible to know when a heart disease patient with a normal ECG will present a significant electrical instability leading to a high risk of SD. This is due to a combination of factors. The ECG does not allow us to determine when a patient has a vulnerable plaque likely to break and trigger an acute coronary syndrome, or when a subtle repolarization abnormality may represent a real danger in an asymptomatic patient. These cases show the limitations of ECG. We should, however, remember that we can get a great deal of information from the ECG if we are able to identify subtle alterations, such as flat or a not-very-deep negative T wave in leads V1 to V3–V4, which, although not posing a risk by itself, may be significant, especially if compared with previous ECGs (Figure 10.21).

We would also like to emphasize that in the presence of precordial pain, normal or nearly normal ECGs, or an unchanged ECG (compared with previous ECGs), should not lead us to rule out the presence of an acute coronary syndrome. The changes may be minor and go unnoticed (Figure 10.22). For this reason, successive ECG recordings are necessary to carefully evaluate how the apparently normal morphologies evolve, especially the T waves in leads V1–V2, as they may be the manifestation of a hyperacute phase of an acute coronary syndrome, eventually evolving into an infarction with ST elevation and a pathologic Q wave (STEMI), triggering VF (Figure 10.22).

Patients with a normal ECG may also suffer from other conditions (aortic rupture, pulmonary embolism, etc.), which may lead to SD (see Chapter 11).

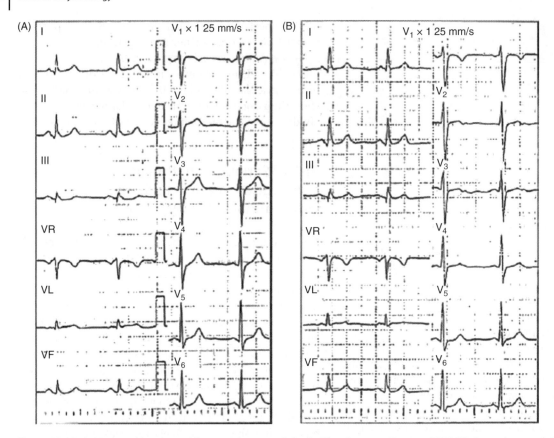

Figure 10.21 A 46-year-old patient with uncertain precordial pain. The electrocardiogram (ECG) (B) showed very subtle repolarization changes in right precordial leads (flat T wave and mild negative U wave), which become more relevant when compared with previous ECGs (A). The exercise stress testing result was positive, and the coronariography showed an important lesion on the left anterior descending coronary artery, which was treated with percutaneous coronary intervention. The subsequent ECG was identical to the previous one (A).

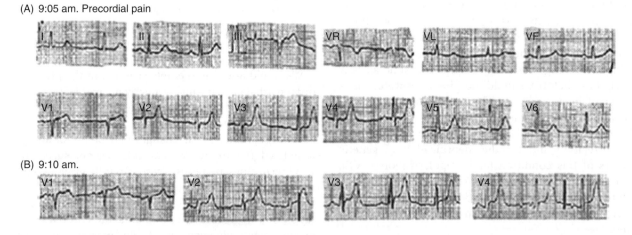

Figure 10.22 A patient with chest pain. (A) Electrocardiogram (ECG) recorded at 9:05 a.m., 20 min after chest pain onset. It shows a slight ST elevation in V1, with ST rectification, followed by tall and symmetrical T wave in V2–V5; a premature ventricular complex (PVC) is observed in III. (B) The ECG recorded 5 min later showed a ST elevation in V1–V4. (C) 5 min later, the patient presented clear ST elevation and sudden ventricular fibrillation (VF), which was treated with electrical cardioversion. In lead II the sequence from ST elevation to VF and recovery of sinus rhythm.

(C) 9:15 am. Continuous recording

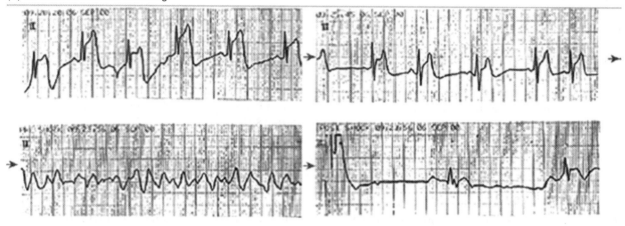

Figure 10.22 (*Continued*)

To summarize, we may say that apparently normal electrocardiograms (ECGs) may, in fact, demonstrate the presence of potentially dangerous pathologies (long or short QT syndrome, spongiform myocardiopathy, Brugada syndrome, early repolarization, etc.).

The correlation of the clinical data with previous ECGs, as well as a detailed analysis of family history, will help to determine the significance of apparently normal ECG morphologies.

In the short-term, the presence of a wide and high T wave in leads V1–V2, especially if the ST segment is rectilinear or slightly depressed, could be a manifestation of the hyperacute phase of an acute coronary syndrome.

Thus, the interpretation of the ECG, taking into account the clinical setting, is very important (see before).

Self Assessment

A. Describe sick sinus syndrome and bradycardia-tachycardia syndrome.
B. What is the P wave morphology most frequently associated with paroxysmal arrhythmias?
C. In which acute heart disease may an advanced right bundle branch block (RBBB) appear and what is its significance?
D. What is a masked bifascicular block?
E. Describe Rosenbaum syndrome.
F. What are the electrocardiogram (ECG) signs associated with a good prognosis in congenital atrioventricular (AV) blocks?

G. Which premature ventricular complexes (PVC) have a poor prognosis?
H. Describe different scenarios where the QT interval is prolonged.
I. List different examples of ECG alternans.
J. What is the relationship between the early repolarization pattern and sudden death (SD)?
K. In which situations may an apparently normal ECG be the expression of a potentially high-risk condition?

References

Aizawa Y, Tamura M, Chinushi M, *et al*. Idiopathic ventricular fibrillation and bradycardia-dependent intraventricular block. Am Heart J 1993;126:1473.

Antzelevitch C, Yan GX. J wave syndromes. Heart Rhythm 2010;7:549.

Ariyarajah V, Puri P, Apiyasawat S, *et al*. Interatrial block: a novel risk factor for embolic stroke? An Noninvasive Electrocardiol 2007a;12(1):15.

Ariyarajah V, Kranis M, Apiyasawat S, *et al*. Potential factors that affect electrocardiographic progression of interatrial block. Ann Noninvasive Electrocardiol 2007b; 12(1):21.

Ariyarajah V, Apiyasawat S, Fernandes J, *et al.* Association of atrial fibrillation in patients with interatrial block over prospectively followed controls with comparable echocardiographic parameters. Am J Cardiol 2007c;99(3):390.

Bacharova L, Wagner G. The time for naming the interatrial block syndrome: Bayes Syndrome. J Electrocardiol 2015;48:133.

Baldasseroni S, De Biase L, Fresco C, *et al.* Cumulative effect of complete left bundle-branch block and chronic atrial fibrillation on 1-year mortality and hospitalization in patients with congestive heart failure. A report from the Italian network on congestive heart failure (in-CHF database).Eur Heart J 2002;23:1692.

Bayés de Luna A, Fiol M. The electrocardiography in ischemic heart disease: clinical and imaging correlations and prognostic implications. Futura-Blackwell, Oxford, 2008.

Bayés de Luna A, Fort de Ribot R, Trilla E. Electrocardiographic and vectorcardiographic study of interatrial conduction disturbances with left atrial retrograde activation. J Electrocardiol 1985;18:1.

Bayés de Luna A, Cladellas M, Oter R, *et al.* Interatrial conduction block and retrograde activation of the left atrium and paroxysmal supraventricular tachyarrhythmia. Eur Heart J 1988;9:1112.

Bayés de Luna A, Cladellas M, Oter R, *et al.* Interatrial conduction block with retrograde activation of the left atrium and paroxysmal supraventricular tachyarrhythmias: influence of preventive antiarrhythmic treatment. Int J Cardiol 1989;22:147.

Bayés de Luna A, Baranchuk A, Martínez-Sellés M, Platonov PG. Anticoagulation in patients at high risk of stroke without documented atrial fibrillation. Time for a paradigm shift? Ann Noninvasive Electrocardiol 2017;22(1). doi: 10.1111/anec.12417.

Benito B, Guasch E, Rivard L, Nattel S. Clinical and mechanistic issues in early repolarization of normal variants and lethal arrhythmia syndromes. J Am Coll Cardiol 2010;56(15):1177. doi: 10.1016/j.jacc.2010.05.037.

Bogale N, Orn S, James M, *et al.* Usefulness of either or both left and right bundle branch block at baseline or during follow-up for predicting death in patients following acute myocardial infarction. Am J Cardiol 2007;99:647.

Braunwald E, Bayés de Luna A. Foreword. Clinical electrocardiography: a textbook. John Wiley & Sons Ltd, Chichester, 2012.

Chugh SS, Reinier K, Singh T, *et al.* Determinants of prolonged QT interval and their contribution to sudden death risk in coronary artery disease: the Oregon

Sudden Unexpected Death Study. Circulation 2009;119:663.

Conde D, Baranchuk A. Bloqueo interauricular como sustrato anatómico-eléctrico de arritmias supraventriculares: syndrome de Bayés. Arch Cardiol Mex 2014a;84(1):32.

Conde D, Baranchuk A. What a cardiologist must know about Bayes's Syndrome. Rev Argent Cardiol 2014b;82:220.

Daubert J. IJC Atrial flutter and interatrial conduction block. In: Waldo A, Touboul P, eds. Atrial flutter: Advances in mechanisms and management. Futura Publishing Company, New York, 1996, p. 331.

Digby G, MacHaalany J, Malik P, *et al.* Multifactorial QT interval prolongation. Cardiol J 2010;17(2):184.

Digby G, Pérez-Riera AR, Barbosa-Barros R, *et al.* Acquired long QT interval: a case series of multifactorial QT prolongation. Clin Cardiol 2011;9(34):577.

Drew BJ, Ackerman MJ, Funk M *et al.,* Prevention of Torsade de Pointes in hospital settings: a scientific statement from the American Heart Association and the American College of Cardiology Foundation. 2010;121(8):1047.

Echt DS, Liebson PR, Mitchell LB, *et al.* Mortality and morbidity in patients receiving encainide, flecainide, or placebo. The Cardiac Arrhythmia Suppression Trial. N Engl J Med 1991;324:781.

Fiol M, Carrillo A, Rodríguez A, *et al.* Electrocardiographic changes of ST-elevation myocardial infarction in patients with complete occlusion of the left main trunk without collateral circulation: differential diagnosis and clinical considerations. J Electrocardiol 2012;45:487.

Friedman RA. Congenital AV block. Pace me now or pace me later? Circulation 1995;92:283.

García-Moll X, Guindo J, Vinolas X, *et al.* Intermittent masked bifascicular block. Am Heart J 1994;127:214.

García-Niebla J, Llontop-García P, Valle-Racero JI, *et al.* Technical mistakes during the acquisition of the electrocardiogram. Ann Noninvasive Electrocardiol 2009;14:389.

Haïssaguerre M, Derval N, Sacher F, *et al.* Sudden cardiac arrest associated with early repolarization. N Engl J Med 2008;358:2016.

Haïssaguerre M, Chatel S, Sacher F, *et al.* Ventricular fibrillation with prominent early repolarization associated with a rare variant of KCN78/KATP channel. J Electrophysiol 2009;20:93.

Homs E, Marti V, Guindo J, *et al.* Automatic measurement of corrected QT interval in Holter recordings: comparison of its dynamic behavior in patients after myocardial infarction with and without life-threatening arrhythmias. Am Heart J 1997;134:181.

Iturralde P, Nava S, Gómez J, *et al.* Association of congenital, diffuse electrical disease in children with normal heart sick sinus syndrome intraventricular conduction block and monomorphic ventricular tachycardia. J Cardiovasc Electrophysiol 2008;5:550.

Kirchhof P, Franz MR, Bardai A, *et al.* Giant T-U waves precede torsades de pointes in long QT syndrome: a systematic electrocardiographic analysis in patients with acquired and congenital QT prolongation. J Am Coll Cardiol 2009;54:143.

Macfarlane PW, Antzelevitch C, Haïssaguerre M, *et al.* The early repolarization pattern. A consensus paper. J Am Coll Cardiol 2015; 66 (4): 470.

Martínez-Sellés M, Massó-van Roessel A, Álvarez-Garcia J, *et al.* Interatrial block and atrial arrhythmias in centenarians: prevalence, associations, and clinical implications. Heart Rhythm 2016a;13(3): 645.

Martínez-Sellés M, Fernández Lozano I, Baranchuk A, *et al.* Should patients at high risk of atrial fibrillation receive anticoagulation? Rev Esp Card 2016b; 69(4):374.

Merchant F, Noseworthy PA, Weiner RB, *et al.* Ability of terminal QRS notching to distinguish benign for malignant ECG forms of early repolarization. Am J Cardiol 2009:104;1402.

Miyazaki S, Shah AJ, Haïssaguerre M. Early repolarization syndrome – a new electrical disorder associated with sudden cardiac death –. Circ J 2010;74(10):2039.

Nieminen T, Verrier RL. Usefulness of T-wave alternans in sudden death risk stratification and guiding medical therapy. Ann Noninvasive Electrocardiol 2010;15276

Nof E, Luria D, Brass D, *et al.* Point mutation in the HCN4 cardiac ion channel pore affecting synthesis, trafficking, and functional expression is associated with familial asymptomatic sinus bradycardia. Circulation 2007;116:463.

Rein AJ, Mevorach D, Perles Z, *et al.* Early diagnosis and treatment of atrioventricular block in the fetus exposed to maternal anti-SSA/Ro-SSB/La antibodies: a prospective, observational, fetal kinetocardiogram-based study. Circulation 2009;119:1867.

Rasouli ML, Ellestad MH. Usefulness of ST depression in ventricular premature complexes to predict myocardial ischemia. Am J Cardiol 2001;87:891.

Rosenbaum M, Eelizari M, Lazzari J. The hemiblocks. Edit Paidos, Buenos Aires, 1968.

Rosenbaum DS, Jackson LE, Smith JM, *et al.* Electrical alternans and vulnerability to ventricular arrhythmias. N Engl J Med 1994;330:235.

Rosso R, Kogan E, Belhassen B, *et al.* J-point elevation in survivors of primary ventricular fibrillation and matched control subjects: incidence and clinical significance. J Am Coll Cardiol 2008;52:1231.

Sagar S, Shen WK, Asirvatham SJ, *et al.* Effect of long-term right ventricular pacing in young adults with structurally normal heart. Circulation 2010;121:1698.

Sarkozy A, Cherchia G, Paparella G, *et al.* Inferior and lateral ECG abnormalities in Brugada syndrome. Circ Arrhythm Electrophysiol 2009;2:154.

Schwartz PJ, Wolf S. QT interval prolongation as predictor of sudden death in patients with myocardial infarction. Circulation 1978;57:1074.

Tikkanen JT, Anttonen O, Juntila MJ, *et al.* Long-term outcome associated with early repolarization on electrocardiography. N Engl J Med 2009;361:2529.

Van Lee V, Mitiku T, Hadley D, *et al.* Rest premature ventricular contractions on routine ECG and prognosis in heart failure patients. Ann Noninvasive Electrocardiol 2010;15:56.

Vázquez R, Bayés-Genis A, Cygankiewicz I, *et al.* The MUSIC risk score: a simple method for predicting mortality in ambulatory patients with chronic heart failure. Eur Heart J 2009;30:1088.

Viskin S. Idiopathic ventricular fibrillation "Le Syndrome d'Haïssaguerre" and the fear of J waves. J Am Coll Cardiol 2009;53:620.

Watanabe H, Makiyama T, Koyama T, *et al.* High prevalence of early repolarization in short QT syndrome. Heart Rhythm 2010;7(5):647.

Wellens HJJ, Gorgels A, Doevedans P. The ECG in acute myocardial infarction and unstable angina. Kluwer Academic Press, Dordrecht, 2003.

Wolpert C, Veltmann C, Schimpf R, *et al.* Is a narrow and tall QRS complex and ECG marker for sudden death? Heart Rhythm 2008;5:1339.

Yan GX, Joshi A, Guo D, *et al.* Phase 2 reentry as a trigger to initiate ventricular fibrillation during early acute myocardial ischemia. Circulation 2004;110:1036.

11

Arrhythmias in Different Heart Diseases and Situations

Briefly discussed in this chapter are the presence of different types of arrhythmias and sudden death (SD) in different heart diseases and situations. We will particularly emphasize the circumstances that lead to serious arrhythmias and especially SD, as well as how SD may be prevented in these patients.

Ischemic Heart Disease

Acute Ischemia

Ventricular Arrhythmias and SD in Acute Myocardial Infarction (AMI) Premature Ventricular Contraction (PVC)

We have already seen (see Chapter 5 Premature Ventricular Complexes: Prognosis) that PVCs are frequent in AMI. However, the number is usually not very high. The number of PVCs and the appearance of runs of ventricular tachycardia (VT) are especially related to the degree and duration of the ischemia. Therefore, the incidence of PVC during MI will decrease if patients receive the fastest and best care to reduce the burden of ischemia. The presence of PVC during AMI in patients admitted to the CCU does not mean that we have to treat them immediately with lidocaine as we did in the past. However, we have to try to stabilize the patient and solve the ionic/metabolic imbalance.

Sustained VT/VF: acute myocardial infarction is the clinical setting that presents the highest risk of SD. The final arrhythmia, especially in patients without previous MI, is usually ventricular fibrillation (VF) (see Figure 1.5) triggered by a PVC with or without previous PVCs (Adgey et al., 1982). VF is considered primary (primary VF) if is not related to recurrent ischemia or severe heart failure.

The appearance of primary VF during acute MI may not necessarily represent a prognosis of bad outcome during the follow-up. In the prefibrinolitic era, primary VF represented an adverse outcome only in cases of anterior MI (Schwartz et al., 1985). Sustained VT in the acute MI phase usually only occurs in patients with prior MI (reentrant circuit).

We have already discussed the great number of SD victims that occur as the first manifestation of acute ischemic attack (see Figure 1.9). They represent a great percentage of the global burden of SD.

In AMI patients, the markers for VF are not absolutely determined. We are going to look at several studies that have been conducted to determine why some patients with acute ischemia (especially those with ST elevation myocardial infarction, STEMI) suffer SD, whereas other patients do not (see Chapter , Early Repolarization and Sudden Death; Tikkanen et al., 2009). Obviously, the degree of acute ischemia plays a very important role.

In the presence of acute ischemia, the grade may be assessed to a great extent by means of the ECG. In STEMI associated with Grade 3 ischemia (Birnbaum et al., 1996; Wellens et al., 2003; Bayés de Luna and Fiol, 2008; Nikus et al., 2010), the ST elevation drags the S wave upwards. In non-ST elevation myocardial infarction (NSTEMI), the cases with significant ischemia present signs of circumferential involvement in the ECG (≥7 leads showing ST segment depression involving the T wave and ST segment elevation in VR). This shows that the main common trunk, or 3-proximal vessels, or LAD + CX or RCA are involved (Bayés de Luna and Fiol, 2008).

It is not just the degree of ischemia, but also its duration, that is important. We have demonstrated (Bayés de Luna et al., 1985) that in patients with coronary spasm, there is a direct relationship between ST segment elevations and the occurrence of ventricular arrhythmias. Despite this, sustained VT rarely occur, given the brevity of the spasm and the absence of scar due to previous MI (Figure 11.1).

It has been shown (Mehta et al., 2009) that, among patients with STEMI and a high-risk ST elevation (global ST changes ≥8 mm), patients with a higher risk of developing VT/VF were characterized by (i) older age, (ii) sinus tachycardia, (iii) a high Killip classification, (iv) low blood pressure, (v) renal impairment, (vi) total sum of ST deviation >13 mm, and (vii) Thrombolysis in Myocardial Infarction (TIMI) flow before percutaneous coronary intervention (PCI) = 0. Meanwhile, patients with the

Clinical Arrhythmology, Second Edition. Antoni Bayés de Luna and Adrian Baranchuk.
© 2017 John Wiley & Sons Ltd. Published 2017 by John Wiley & Sons Ltd.

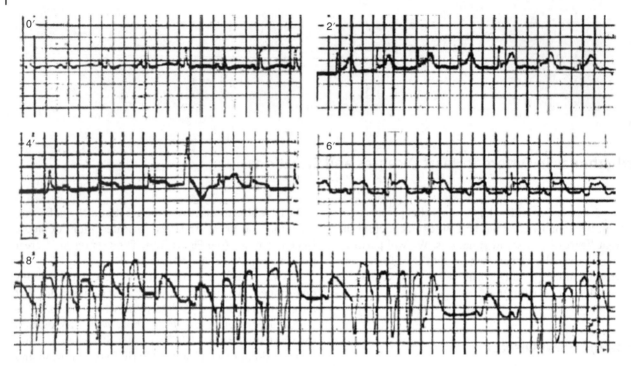

Figure 11.1 A patient with Prinzmetal angina showing an electrocardiogram (ECG) sequence during a crisis. We observe how a peaked T wave is followed by a ST segment elevation (8 min). ST presents a monophasic transmembrane action potential (TAP) and several runs of ventricular tachycardia (VT) appear.

lowest risk of developing late VT/VF were patients who have a TIMI flow = 3 and ≥70% ST resolution post-PCI. Finally, the patients who developed VT/VF after PCI (late VT/VF) had a worse prognosis (30-day mortality rate = 30%) compared with those who experienced VT/VF before PCI (early VT/VF) (30-day mortality rate = 15%). The mortality rate in patients without VT/VF was much lower (≈2.5%). In contrast, in the case of NSTEMI SD is lower than in STEMI. Mortality is especially low in patients with a low-risk score that includes lack of sinus tachycardia and ventricular arrhythmia, among other factors (Briegger *et al.*, 2009).

In another study, the markers of increased risk of VF during the acute phase of STEMI are: (i) a sum of the ST elevations in the three leads >10 mm, (ii) systolic blood pressure <110 mmHg, and (iii) hypokalemia (Fiol *et al.*, 1993).

It has been reported (Scirica *et al.*, 2010) that in the presence of non-STE-acute coronary syndrome (ACS), the presence of nonsustained VT (≥4 beats) in the early phase (7 days Holter) clearly increases the risk of complications.

A published meta-analysis (Gheeraert *et al.*, 2006) showed that the most important risk factors in developing primary VF during AMI are: (i) when the patient is admitted early to hospital after experiencing pain (<2 h) and (ii) evidence of significant abrupt ischemia (significant ST elevation). No major differences have been observed between anteroseptal or inferolateral infarction, or with regard to other markers (hypokalemia or heart rate).

The possible role of genetic factors in the development of VF during STEMI has been published (Hu *et al.*, 2007). In addition, the association of Ito current density, responsible for Brugada's and other J wave syndromes (Antzelevitch and Yan, 2010) and the risk of VF during AMI have been postulated (see Chapter 10, Early Repolarization and Sudden Death). This may explain both the higher incidence of VF in men and in inferior MI with RV involvement. The Ito current is much more prominent in men and in the RV rather than in the LV. We presume that the importance of these genetic interactions in the development of fatal ventricular arrhythmia will be shown to be crucial. In fact, it has been suggested that the fundamental mechanisms responsible for ST elevation and the initiation of VF are similar in the early phase of STEMI and in inherited J wave syndromes. In both cases, heterogeneous dispersion or repolarization and Phase 2 reentry function as a trigger and reentrant substrate for the development of VT/VF (Yan *et al.*, 2004).

During the acute phase of MI, the interaction of ischemia and arrhythmias in the presence of autonomic nervous system (ANS) alterations, LV dysfunction, and genetic–environmental influences (Elosua *et al.*, 2009) are key factors in triggering the final arrhythmias that lead to SD (Figure 11.3).

Ventricular Arrhythmias and Implantable Cardioverter Defibrillator (ICD) Therapy After AMI

We have already discussed the role of ICD in patients at risk for SD in other chapters (Chapters 5 and 10, and the Appendix). Now we would like to simply comment on some aspects with respect to determining the best time for ICD implantation after MI.

It is clear that during the first 4–8 weeks after AMI there is a higher risk of SD (1–2% after 1 month vs 0.12% after 6 months). However, it has been demonstrated that ICD implantation during the first three months after AMI may cause unwanted effects (Goldberger and Passman, 2009). Mortality rate was only reduced if ICD implantation was carried out several months after the occurrence of AMI (Voller, 2009). Patients experiencing VF during the acute phase do not actually benefit from ICD implantation; one month post-AMI they show the same post-infarction mortality rates as patients who had not had VF. The paradox that ICD implantation is not useful during the period of time when SD is more likely to occur is puzzling. However, it has been reported (Pouleur *et al.*, 2010) that SD in the first months after MI is usually due to massive MI or cardiac rupture, and that EP studies may be useful to stratify risk (Kumar *et al.*, 2010) (see Appendix A-4-ICD). However, in high-risk post-MI patients with frequent VT runs or previous sustained VT, it may be beneficial to use a wearable cardioverter defibrillator (WCD) while awaiting the appropriate time for a definitive implant, or perhaps reinforcing the deferral of ICD implantation while awaiting potential improvement of cardiac function (Chung *et al.*, 2010a).

If the patient is a nonresponder to drug therapy for repetitive VT, ablation of VT may be the best alternative treatment (see Appendix A-4 ICD and CRT therapy).

Ventricular Arrhythmias in Episodes of Acute Ischemia Outside AMI

In a coronary spasm the incidence of ventricular arrhythmias is highly related to the duration and severity of the spasm (Bayés de Luna *et al.*, 1985; Stern and Bayés de Luna, 2009) (see before) (Figure 11.1). In our experience (Bayés de Luna *et al.*, 1985), due to the brevity of the episode, even in cases of ST elevation that look like a monophasic transmembrane action potential (TAP), the coronary spasm may trigger runs of VT but not sustained VT leading to SD. However, isolated cases of SD during Prinzmetal angina have been reported (Bayés de Luna *et al.*, 1985), usually in case of R/T PVC leading to VF (Bayés de Luna *et al*, 2014).

During exercise angina, PVCs sometimes appear. However, rarely does the ischemia trigger long runs of VT and even less often VT/VF, due to its brevity. Sometimes, PVCs do not increase in the presence of exercise angina (Figure 11.2). Cases of SD during exercise angina exist but are rare. An episode of sustained VT/VF during positive exercise testing (2 × 10 000 tests, in our experience) is

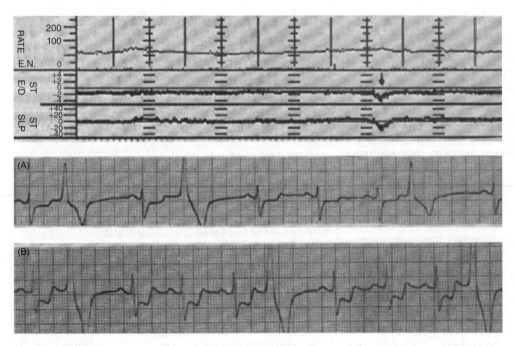

Figure 11.2 Patient with exercise angina who presents ST depression in baseline state that increases during angina crisis. We see this in the Holter recording of the trend of the heart rate and ST segment (see arrrow). The lower part of the figure shows that the number of premature ventricular complexes does not change before (A) and after (B) angina.

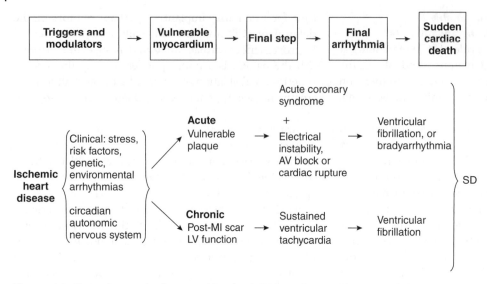

Figure 11.3 Chain of events leading to sudden death (SD) in patients with acute and chronic ischemic heart disease (IHD).

very unusual. Nevertheless, we have to be ready with a cardiac arrest protocol in case this complication appears (see Figure A-5C). One simple measure of caution is to be sure that we do not perform exercise testing on a patient with impending MI, suspicion of acute coronary syndrome, high blood pressure, or frequent PVC that do not disappear promptly. In any case, it is advisable to stop the test in the presence of any complication (presence or increase in the number of PVCs, angina or equivalent symptoms, evident drop in blood pressure or high increase in blood pressure, etc.).

Supraventricular (SV) Arrhythmias

The most frequent supraventricular arrhythmia in AMI is atrial fibrillation (AF) (5–10% of cases), which is lower than 5% in patients treated with statins (Dziewierz *et al.*, 2010). The appearance of AF/atrial flutter usually represents the involvement of the atria by the infarction, and is a marker of large MI and poor prognosis (≈5% vs. 30%). Previous AF was also associated with greater mortality at long-term follow-up (Lau *et al.*, 2009). Other SV arrhythmias are not frequently seen during AMI. However, the presence of sinus tachycardia in AMI is a sign of poor prognosis.

Passive Arrhythmias

In some STEMI with ST elevation in II, III, and VF (inferior infarction), an AV block may be observed as the result of the occlusion of the right coronary artery proximal to the AV node artery. This is usually a suprahisian AV block with a significant vagal component, which generally does not require implantation of a permanent pacemaker because it is often transient. Temporal pacemakers may be necessary in cases of persistent bradycardia or hypotension (Table 11.1). We have already

commented (see Chapter 6, Clinical, Prognostic, and Therapeutic Implications of Passive Arrhythmias) that in cases of anterior AMI the AV block in general is located at an infrahisian level, and is associated with a poor prognosis, not only because it leads to a much slower escape rhythm, but also because of the larger size of the infarction.

Different degrees of sinus bradycardia and/or sinoatrial block may result from sinus dysfunction due to occlusion of the sinus node artery and/or vagal overdrive. Intravenous atropine or, if necessary, pacing generally solve the problem (Table 11.1).

Additionally, coronary spasm of the artery that perfuses the sinus node or AV node may explain the appearance of sinus bradycardia or even transient AV block (see Figure 6.48).

Finally, the appearance of a right bundle branch block (RBBB) during STEMI due to left anterior descending (LAD) artery occlusion is associated with poor prognosis, as it entails a very proximal occlusion before the first septal branch that perfuses the right bundle. If RBBB occurs in presence of total occlusion of left main trunk the prognosis is even worse (Fiol *et al.*, 2012).

Treatment of Arrhythmias in Acute STEMI

We have already commented on some aspects of this. Table 11.1 shows the best treatment (with recommendation classifications and grades of evidence) of the more frequent active and passive arrhythmias included the recommendations for pacemaker implantation in STEMI, according to ESC/AHA guidelines (Recommended General Bibliography p. xvii). These guidelines may be also useful in case of NSTEMI, although in this case the incidence of severe arrhythmias is lower.

Table 11.1 Management of arrhythmias and conduction disturbances in the acute phase of STEMI.

Arrhythmia	Therapy	Class	Level
5) Hemodynamically unstable VT and VF	DC cardioversion	I	C
6) Hemodynamically unstable, sustained monomorphic VT refractory to DC cardioversion	• i.v. amiodarone	IIa	B
	• i.v. lidocaine or sotalol	IIa	C
	• Transvenous catheter pace termination if refractory to cardioversion or frequently recurrent despite antiarrhythmic medication	IIa	C
7) Repetitive symptomatic salvoes of nonsustained monomorphic VT	• i.v. amiodarone, sotalol or other β-blocker	IIa	C
8) Polymorphic VT	• If baseline QT is normal, i.v. sotalol or other β-blocker, amiodarone or lidocaine	I	C
	• If baseline QT is prolonged, correct electrolytes, consider magnesium, overdrive pacing, isoproterenol, or lidocaine	I	C
	• Urgent angiography should be considered	I	C
9) Rate control of atrial fibrillation	• i.v. β-blockers or non-dihydropyridine, calcium antagonists (e.g. diltiazem, verapamil). If no clinical signs of heart failure, bronchospasm (only for β-blockers), or AV block	I / I / IIb	C / C / C
	• i.v. amiodarone to slow a rapid ventricular response and improve LV function	I	C
	• i.v. digitalis if severe LV dysfunction and/or heart failure		
	• Electrical cardioversion if severe hemodynamic compromise or intractable ischemia, or when adequate rate control cannot be achieved with pharmacologic agents		
10) Anticoagulation for atrial fibrillation	• i.v. administration of a therapeutic dose of heparin or a LMWH	I	C
11) Sinus bradycardia associated with hypotension	• i.v. atropine	I	C
	• Temporary pacing if failed response to atropine	I	C
12) AV block II (Mobitz 2) or AV block III with bradycardia that causes hypotension or heart failure	• i.v. atropine	I	C
	• Temporary pacing if atropine fails	I	C

Adapted from ECS practice guidelines: Management of acute myocardial infarction in patients presenting with persistent ST-segment elevation (Van de Werf *et al.*, 2008).

AV, atrioventricular; DC, direct current; i.v., intravenous; LMWH, low molecular weight heparin; LV, left ventricle; VF, ventricular fibrillation; VT, ventricular tachycardia.

Chronic Ischemic Heart Disease

• *Ventricular arrhythmias and sudden death* We will comment on the global prognosis of chronic ischemic heart disease, especially in post-MI patients, and the risk factors that may trigger SD.

Risk factors The risk of severe VA and SD is especially high in the first six months after MI. Although the risk stratification in chronic ischemic patients, especially for SD, evolves continuously (Buxton, 2009), in post-MI patients it is currently related to three main factors (Figure 11.4):

i) **Presence of residual ischemia** (risk of developing another coronary event) (Théroux *et al.*, 1979).

ii) **Ventricular dysfunction** (risk of developing HF) (Moss, 1979).

iii) **Electrical instability** (risk of developing serious ventricular arrhythmias and SD) (Moss, 1979; Bigger *et al.*, 1984) (see Figure 5.12 and 5.13).

The less important these three factors are and the sooner they are identified and controlled, the lower the incidence of SD.

Figure 11.4 summarizes how these factors may interact and which parameters are used to identify the relative importance of these three factors in the development of a chain of events that lead to SD (see Chapter 1, How to Identify Patients at Risk) (Goldstein *et al.*, 1994). The following parameters, among others, have to be considered in the stratification of risk according to the triangle in Figure 11.4.

• **Parameters of electrical instability** are taken from 1) morphofunctional studies (type of scar, presence of

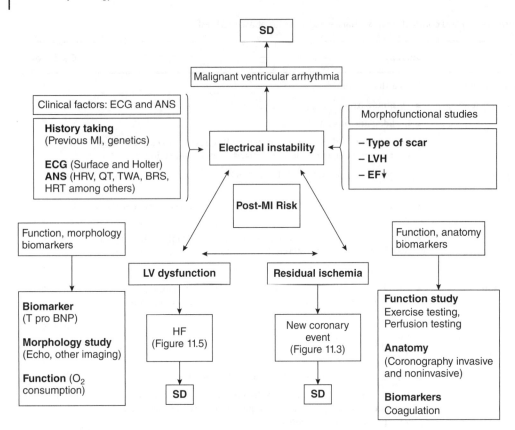

Figure 11.4 Risk stratification in post-infarction patients, according to the presence and interaction of: a) electrical instability, b) ventricular dysfunction, and c) residual ischemia. We see in each of them the different factors that may predict complications and SD, as well as the tests used to detect them. (HRV=heart rate variability; TWA=T wave alternance; BRS=baroreflex sensitivity; HRT=heart rate turbulence; LVH=left ventricular hypertrophy; EF=ejection fraction; HF=heart failure).

left ventricular hypertrophy (LVH) and depressed left ventricular function, atrial size, etc.), 2) history taking and surface ECG, such as previous MI, QRS wideness among others, 3) Holter ECG such as PVC, heart rate, and 4) the study of autonomic nervous system imbalances such as heart rate variability (HRV) and baroreflex sensitivity (BRS) that show decrease of vagal tone and vagal reflexes (Schwartz *et al.*, 1992), an increase of sympathetic overdrive or a decrease in vagal response (see below, Pascale *et al.*, 2009). Other parameters studied include the microvolt–T wave alternans and heart rate turbulence (Figure 11.4).

- **Parameters to study LV function** are taken from: (i) the study of LV function with imaging techniques, (ii) the study of functional state by exercise testing (oxygen consumption), and (iii) a neurohumoral blood test.
- **Parameters of residual ischemia** are taken from anatomic and functional studies, as well as biomarkers.

The study of these parameters emphasizes the importance of the information taken: (i) from history taking, such as familial antecedents, age, and previous MI; and (ii) from the surface ECG, the presence

of wide QRS (Moss, 2002), frequent PVC, fractioned QRS, and ST segment depression during an exercise test (residual ischemia) (Théroux *et al.*, 1979). Even the presence of silent ischemia represents a marker of increased long-term risk of SD (5-year risk) (Schoenenberger *et al.*, 2009).

However, it is surprising that even **in the presence of the same classical triggering factors, such as the number of PVCs, as well as similar clinical characteristics and the size of infarction, some patients experience frequent episodes of sustained VT, whereas others do not.** Undoubtedly, environmental and genetic factors, as well as subtle ANS changes, may influence this, although the current assessment of such parameters shows a low positive predictive value (PPV). It has been demonstrated that some electrophysiologic and anatomical differences in MI scar characteristics may account for the increased likelihood of developing sustained VT. It has been shown (Haqqani *et al.*, 2009) that **in the presence of the same number of PVCs in the Holter monitoring and similar clinical characteristics, sustained VT occurs in patients who have a patched scar, with a greater amount of**

fibrosis, and more fragmented electrograms. This study clearly shows that the anatomic substrate (scar characteristics) is more important than the presence of PVC (triggering and modulating factor) to induce a sustained VT (see Chapter 5, Premature Ventricular Complexes and Classic Ventricular Tachycardia). This study points out the need for noninvasive markers to identify the presence of this substrate. Some of them, such as the presence of a fractioned QRS and intraventricular blocks, have already been mentioned. This study also suggests that the **extensive ablation of scar areas,** including areas of myocardial channels between the scars, is probably a valid and efficient approach (Tung, 2010). Probably, the identification of fibrosis by MRI could be also help to establish a long term prognosis.

It has also been surprising (Pascale *et al.*, 2009) that in patients with old MI without residual ischemia, the presence of significant ventricular arrhythmias was much higher after an old inferior MI when compared to old anterior MI. This unexpected higher incidence of arrhythmias in inferior MI is even more compelling, considering that LVEF was significantly higher after inferior MI than anterior MI. A possible explanation may be that in the inferior wall there is a higher density of receptors with vagal activity that are cardioprotective. Therefore, after an infarction of this area, the protective effect of the vagal response is lowered and thus the risk of ventricular arrhythmia is increased. Perhaps, this increased tendency to ventricular arrhythmias and sudden death in cases of inferior MI have the explanation that happen with early repolarization pattern that are more dangerous if appear in inferior leads.

- *Therapeutic considerations* (see Appendix-A.4, ICD, CRT and ablation) **Implantable cardioverter defibrillator (ICD) is preferable to drug treatment in the prevention of SD, both in secondary prevention** (AVID, CIDS, CASH trials) and **as primary prevention in selected cases** (MADIT I and MADIT II; Moss *et al.*, 1996; Moss 2002). Several parameters (wideness of QRS, preserved autonomic balance, microvolt T-wave alternans) identify patients who would be most likely to benefit from ICD therapy. Recently, the MADIT-CRT trial (Moss *et al.*, 2009) supported the use of double therapy (ICD + cardiac resynchronization therapy (CRT)) in post-MI patients at early stages of HF (see later Heart failure, and Appendix).

In patients with drug-resistant VT or frequent ICD discharges due to sustained VT, the best option is **ablation of the tachycardia** (Tung 2010). Currently, there are series with success rates of 70–80% that will have recurrences lower than 15–20%. Furthermore, the risk of severe complications during the procedure is very small.

Other Arrhythmias

The incidence of AF/flutter is higher in patients with chronic IHD than in the normal population.

Intraventricular blocks and sinoatrial and AV blocks are also more frequent.

Chain of Events Leading to SD

Figure 11.3 summarizes the chain of events that are involved in the triggering of SD in acute and chronic ischemic heart disease (Bayés-Genis *et al.*, 1995).

In the early phase of acute myocardial infarction (AMI), the degree and duration of ischemia shown by the electrocardiogram as an ST elevation helps to identify a group of patients with a higher risk of developing ventricular fibrillation/sudden death (VF/SD).

Several other factors associated with ischemia are involved in the development of SD, such as the presence of premature ventricular complexes (PVCs), autonomic nervous system (ANS) alterations, and possibly some environmental–genetic interactions.

In the early phase of an AMI, different passive arrhythmias may occur as well.

Finally, atrial fibrillation is the most common supraventricular arrhythmia and is associated with poor prognosis.

The most adequate treatment for each type of arrhythmia in cases of ST elevation myocardial infarction may be seen in Table 11.1.

Heart Failure

Concept

Heart failure (HF) is the pathophysiologic state in which the heart is unable to pump blood at the rate required by the metabolizing tissues, or when the heart can do so only with an elevated filling pressure. Heart failure represents a complex clinical syndrome (Recommended General Bibliography p. xvii) that may occur in patients with idiopathic myocardial disease (idiopathic cardiomyopathy) or appear in the course of many heart diseases.

Heart failure frequently presents decreased ejection fraction (DEF) (systolic heart failure) (HF-DEF). However, at least 25–30% of patients with HF present a similar clinical condition with a relatively preserved ventricular function (PEF), (diastolic HF). Diagnosis of HF with PEF is made, even though the ejection fraction is ≥40%, based on (i) the evident presence of HF clinical symptoms and (ii) increased biomarkers (T pro BNP levels). Heart failure with PEF is more frequently observed in hypertensive women than in post-infarction males and although the mortality rate is high, it is lower than in patients with HF-DEF.

In this book, we discuss only those aspects of HF related to cardiac arrhythmias and SD in particular.

Ventricular Arrhythmias and SD

Prognostic Implications

The incidence of PVCs in patients with HF is much higher than in the normal population (see Chapter 5). It has been reported that the presence of one PVC in a routine 10-s ECG in patients with moderate HF is a powerful predictor of CV mortality (Van Lee *et al.*, 2010).

- **Risk markers for SD.** We pointed out in Chapter that SD incidence is higher in the presence of advanced heart disease and heart failure (Figure 1.1). Except for cases of SD in patients with inherited heart disease (see Chapter 9) and those related to AMI, especially in cases of STEMI (see before), most patients who die suddenly show impairment of the ventricular function and HF with DEF (systolic HF) in particular.

Figure 11.5 shows the chain of events leading to ventricular arrhythmia (VT/VF) and SD, especially in functional NYHA Class II–III HF patients (Bayés-Genis *et al.*, 1995). Identification and prevention of these markers, as well as the administration of the most appropriate treatment, may help to reduce the number of cases of SD.

It is estimated that approximately 40% of cardiovascular deaths reported in HF patients are sudden unexpected deaths, whereas the remaining deaths may be attributed to HF progression. The three-year mortality rate in HF patients (NYHA Class II–III) is 20–30%, and half of these deaths can be attributed to SD. Cases of SD in patients with NYHA Class II–III HF are mostly caused by ventricular arrhythmia (VT/VF), whereas in NYHA Class IV patients, bradyarrhythmias play a more important role (see Chapter 1, Arrhythmias and SD, and Figures 1.7 and 1.8). This may explain the inefficacy of antiarrhythmic drugs in preventing SD in Class IV patients.

Although there are some contradictory results, the majority of studies (Vázquez *et al.*, 2009) show that SD is more frequently observed in cases of systolic HF, especially in patients with ischemic dilated cardiomyopathy, than in cases of diastolic HF.

In contrast, there is considerable evidence indicating that several risk markers (heart rate variability (HRV), heart rate turbulence (HRT), sinus tachycardia) reflecting alterations of ANS (Cygankiewicz *et al.*, 2006, 2008) may play a role in the risk stratification of SD in HF patients, although the PPV is low, and now its value has been questioned. At the same time, it has been demonstrated that one of the most extensively studied risk markers (T wave alternans) has been useful in the prediction of SD (Hohnloser *et al.*, 2003; Bloomfield *et al.*, 2004).

Sympathetic innervation increases that can be detected by Im-IBG images correlate with an improvement of HF prognosis and a decrease of ventricular arrhythmias.

A risk score for predicting death in HF patients (MUSIC study) has been published (Vázquez *et al.*, 2009). This study was designed to analyze the prognostic value of different clinical, electrocardiographic (12-lead ECG and Holter), echocardiographic, and biochemical variables in predicting SD in HF patients. This multicenter prospective study enrolled 992 patients with mild to moderate (NYHA Class II–III) HF, with both systolic (75%) and diastolic (25%) HF followed over three years. Seventy-eight percent of patients showed NYHA Class II HF at study entry. Several variables were analyzed to predict all-cause mortality, cardiac death, SD, and HF death. Multivariate analysis identified 10 independent prognostic variables useful for predicting outcome in HF patients (Figure 11.6A), with a different numeric value for each variable. It should be emphasized that only atrial enlargement and T pro BNP levels were found to predict death, regardless of the mechanism involved (cardiac death, SD, and death due to HF progression).

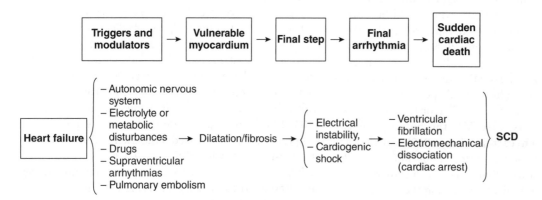

Figure 11.5 Chain of events leading to sudden death in patients with heart failure (Taken from Bayés-Genis, 1995).

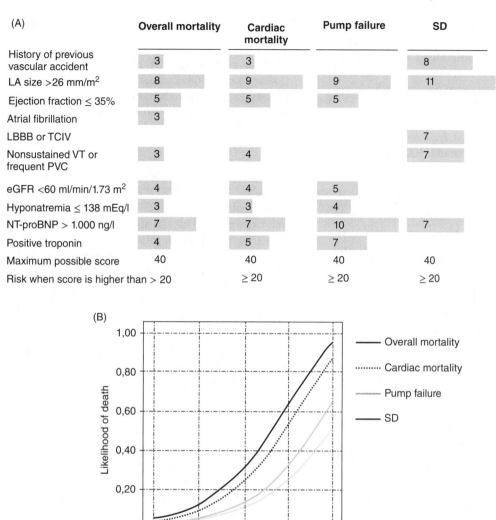

(A)

	Overall mortality	Cardiac mortality	Pump failure	SD
History of previous vascular accident	3	3		8
LA size >26 mm/m²	8	9	9	11
Ejection fraction ≤ 35%	5	5	5	
Atrial fibrillation	3			
LBBB or TCIV				7
Nonsustained VT or frequent PVC	3	4		7
eGFR <60 ml/min/1.73 m²	4	4	5	
Hyponatremia ≤ 138 mEq/l	3	3	4	
NT-proBNP > 1.000 ng/l	7	7	10	7
Positive troponin	4	5	7	
Maximum possible score	40	40	40	40
Risk when score is higher than	> 20	≥ 20	≥ 20	≥ 20

Figure 11.6 (A) Risk score for predicting different types of death. We see the parameters used to determine the score. (B) Mortality curves for the different types of death over a period of 3 years (Vázquez *et al.*, 2009).

A combination of 10 of these variables allowed us to establish a risk score, as shown in Figure 11.6. Figure 11.6B shows the mortality curve according to the type of death studied. With this risk score, two different well-defined populations were found: one population group with a score <20, which is considered a low-risk population, and the other population group with a score >20, considered a high-risk population. A new serum marker of SD has been identified, the ST2 (Pascual *et al.*, 2009), which, jointly with NT-proBNP, is highly predictive of SD. However, further investigation to validate these results is warranted. The economic impact of lowering costs by reducing ICD implantation if we can better predict SD deserves to followed up with studies in the future.

Therapeutic considerations

(see Appendix-A.4 (ICD and Pacemakers-CRT-)(Vardas et al., 2007; Dickstein et al., 2010)

- **ICD implant** in HF patients with important LV dysfunction is highly recommended (Class IB) as **primary prevention therapy** in patients with EF <30–35% or those of NYHA Class II–III despite optimal medical treatment (Moss *et al.*, 1996; Moss, 2002; Bardy *et al.*, 2005). The ICD is effective as **secondary prevention** in patients with EF <35% who have experienced syncope or sustained VT episodes, or those who have undergone resuscitation after a cardiac arrest (Class IA) (AVID, CIDS, CASH trials among others). Currently, ICD implantation in cases of diastolic HF is not considered (see later).

It has been reported that, in HF patients, the benefit from ICD varies depending on the predicted annual mortality defined by the Seattle Heart Failure Model (Levy *et al.*, 2009). The highest benefit (survival increase ≈2 years) was observed in patients with a lower estimated annual mortality (<15%).

Implantable cardioverter defibrillator therapy for the primary prevention of SD in women does not appear to reduce all-cause mortality (Ghanbari *et al.*, 2009). Further studies are needed to corroborate these findings.

It is debatable whether any patient with left ventricle ejection fraction (LVEF) <30% needs an ICD. There are many scientific evidence-based arguments (primary and secondary clinical trials) (see before) and also ethical arguments to support this. However, it is useful to remember that patients have to survive long enough to benefit from an ICD (≈2–3% yearly reduction of mortality). This means that if the patient is very elderly or presents severe diseases that make it unlikely they will survive for long, the benefits of an ICD may be modest. Yet there are no absolute contraindications for ICD implantation except in cases of advanced Alzheimer's or very advanced severe diseases. The patient and the family need to know more about the advantages already explained, the morbidity related to an ICD that is not low, and the financial aspects of its implantation. The final decision has to be taken together and, ideally, should be based only on the clinical state of the patient.

Finally, left ventricular assist devices (LVAD) have recently emerged as an important treatment option for advanced (Phase IV) congestive heart failure, not only as a bridge to cardiac transplantation but also as a destination therapy. However, because patients in this stage often present severe VA (≈30%), the possibility of using ICD + LVAD simultaneously has been considered. This association is safe and clinically feasible. In the six-month follow-up, effective ICD therapies occurred in 16% of patients and inappropriate ICD therapies in only 4% (Kühne *et al.*, 2010). This accounted for the number of all ICD therapies delivered, which was similar to that of other ICD populations.

- **Cardiac resynchronization therapy (CRT)** improves left ventricular function in patients with HF when indicated (LBBB or wide QRS complex ≥150 ms). The best results were obtained when the QRS was ≥150 ms and EF <30–35% (see table Appendix A-4). CRT devices are often (30–50%) implanted with an ICD. However, we have to be sure that both therapies are necessary for the patient (see later and Appendix-A.4, ICD and CRT).

- **Potential expansion of clinical standard indications of CRT**

i) **CRT in early stages of HF.** The REVERSE trial (Linde *et al.*, 2008; Daubert 2009) showed that the use of CRT provides a beneficial response in patients with EF ≤40%, a QRS ≥120 ms with only mild symptoms (NYHA Class I-II), but with a wide QRS and quite severely dilated LV. The likelihood of LV reverse remodeling was highest in patients with nonischemic etiology, or with significant conduction or mechanical delay. Also the MADIT-CRT trial (Moss *et al.*, 2009) demonstrated that CRT is beneficial in the initial stages of HF. This has also been confirmed by the RAFT trial (Tang *et al.*, 2010).

ii) The usefulness of **CRT in some patients with EF >35%** (some diastolic component) has been very promising in one study (Chung *et al.*, 2010b).

iii) One study performed on **patients with QRS <120 ms** has given negative results (Beshai *et al.*, 2007) (see Appendix A.4-CRT).

iv) The indication of **CRT in patients with very advanced HF** has been controversial. When the HF is **very advanced** and the patient presents AF and wide QRS, it has been reported good results with ICD-CRT therapy with (Gasparini *et al.*, 2006) or without (Kahdjooi, 2008) AV node ablation. In these patients, two-year mortality ≈25% decreases to 15% with ICD-CRT, and even more if AV node ablation is performed (see later). Furthermore, AV node ablation substantially reduces the number of inappropriate ICD-CRT discharges. However, it has been reported (Castel *et al.*, 2010) that in patients with Class IV HF, CRT did not significantly improve therapy compared with pharmacologic treatment. In our opinion in an individual patient with very advanced HF and wide QRS that does not respond to pharmacologic treatment and is not a candidate for transplant, a CRT may be very beneficial. We have to try to make this decision more based on ethical and scientific aspects than under economic influences.

Finally we have to remember that not all patients are good responders (see Appendix A-4, Cardiac Resynchronization Therapy (CRT)) and that optimization of CRT ensuring appropriate lead placement, maximizing biventricular pacing, and optimizing AV delay, as well as providing the best HF disease management, are necessary.

Diastolic heart failure (HF) presents a lower mortality, especially sudden death (SD). It is seen more frequently in women with hypertension.

Around 40% of cases of death in patients with HF are SD.

Patients with HF and left bundle branch block plus atrial fibrillation (LBBB+AF) present a higher risk of SD.

The risk score of the MUSIC trial allows us to stratify risk of SD with clinical markers.

When to implant an implantable cardioverter defibrillator (ICD):

- In secondary prevention, in patients with HF and ejection fraction (EF) <35% who have presented syncope, ventricular tachycardia (VT), and, especially, recovered cardiac arrest.
- In primary prevention, in cases of EF <30–35% that do not improve and still remain in HF grade II–III despite full treatment.

To implant a cardiac resynchronization therapy (CRT) alone or with an ICD (CRT-ICD) may be very useful in patients with uncontrolled heart failure.

The current indications for ICD and CRT (CRT-ICD) may be seen in Tables A-4 to A-6 (see Appendix Pacemakers, and Automatic Implantable Cardioverter Defibrillator (ICD)).

Supraventricular Arrhythmias

The SHIFT trial (Swedberg *et al.*, 2010) showed that in patients with HF, reducing heart rate ≤70 bpm with ibabradine decreases (≈25%) both hospitalization and death.

Patients with very advanced heart disease frequently in HF and advanced interatrial block (A-IAB) (Bayés de Luna *et al.*, 1988) present more active supraventricular arrhythmias, especially AF, than the control group without A-IAB (Bayés syndrome) (Bayés de Luna *et al.*, 1988). Also, it has been demonstrated that patients with HF and A-IAB present much higher levels of NT-pro-BNP than the controls (Alvarez *et al.*, 2016); probably, some patients with A-IAB and HF especially aging with ambient arrhythmias may benefit from anticoagulation even without evidence of AF. There is some evidence that supports this hypothesis; however, this needs to be tested in a clinical trial. Currently, AF appears in approximately 20–30% of HF patients and indicates poor prognosis. Therefore, every attempt should be made to revert AF to sinus rhythm (drugs, CV, ablation) and to avoid stroke. Heart failure is one of components of the CHA_2DS_2-V score and increases the risk of stroke. Recovering sinus rhythm not only improves HF but may also reduce the need for ICD implantation if EF is higher than 35% (Bortone *et al.*, 2009). In spite of this, the emphasis on rhythm control in patients with HF and AF has diminished based on neutral data from AF-CHF (Roy *et al.*, 2008). However, we are convinced that we have to make every effort in HF + AF patients to revert AF using new

technology for ablation (Kahn *et al.*, 2008) (see Appendix A-4, Percutaneous Transcatheter Ablation). If this fails, or AF is too advanced for ablation, we advise performing, if the QRS is wide, CRT-ICD approach with AV node ablation (Gasparini *et al.*, 2006) in order to reduce the heart rate during AF, allowing the biventricular pacing to command the heart. Some authors, however, have not found better results when AV node ablation is associated with CRT-ICD (Khadjooi *et al.*, 2008) and permanent AF is now considered an attenuation of the possible beneficial mechanisms of CRT.

Some supraventricular tachyarrhythmias, such as atrial or junctional ectopic focus tachycardia, were quite frequent in the past because they were often induced by digitalis (see later, Special Situations).

Passive Arrhythmias

In HF patients the incidence of passive arrhythmias is higher than in the normal population. Pacemaker implantation is often very necessary, not only in cases of advanced bradycardia due to sick sinus syndrome or AV block, but also in cases of CRT-ICD + AV node ablation to control rapid AF and HF. More recently, septal pacing has demonstrated better results than apical pacing, in patients with moderate LVEF. In patients with low EF requiring permanent pacing (i.e. complete AV block) CRT-ICD should be considered.

In patients with advanced HF, SD is frequently provoked by progressive bradyarrhythmia, usually related to cardiogenic shock (Luu *et al.*, 1989). This is probably why antiarrhythmic agents used to suppress PVC are not useful in this setting and also explain some cases of SD in patients with an ICD.

Valvular Heart Disease

Arrhythmias

Aortic Valve Disease

Ventricular arrhythmias are common in patients with aortic valvular disease. This appears to be a reflection of underlying left ventricular dysfunction and is a factor that should influence the decision to operate (Michel *et al.*, 1992).

Intraventricular or atrioventricular conduction abnormalities are more frequent in aortic stenosis than in aortic regurgitation. When present, they may be caused by severe hypertrophy, extension of calcium from the valve and valve ring into the intraventricular septum, or concomitant heart disease.

Atrial fibrillation (AF) is usually an arrhythmia that appears late in the follow-up, primarily occurring in association with HF. Associated mitral valve disease should be suspected if AF occurs in mild to moderate aortic valve disease.

Mitral Valve Disease

In mitral stenosis, AF is the most common arrhythmia. The overall incidence of AF in this condition is estimated to be 40%. The presence of AF is certain in the long follow-up of patients with severe mitral stenosis (see Figure 4.54). The presence of A-IAB in patients with tight mitral stenosis is a good marker of AF/AFl in a short follow-up (Bayes syndrome) (Bayés de Luna *et al.*, 1988) and may be a candidate for anticoagulation. However, this hypothesis has to be tested in a clinical trial.

In rheumatic mitral regurgitation, AF is again the most common arrhythmia and its presence has an impact on patient outcome.

Several studies report a broad range of incidence of arrhythmias in patients with mitral valve prolapse. Atrial and ventricular premature complexes are frequently found (60–80% of cases) (Figure 11.7) (Kligfield *et al.*, 1987; Zuppiroli *et al.*, 1994). Arrhythmias may be more common in patients with MVP who develop severe mitral regurgitation (Kim *et al.*, 1996).

Sudden Death

Sudden death may occur during the natural follow-up of valvular heart disease, especially in cases of aortic stenosis (Frank *et al.*, 1973). Sudden death is the first manifestation of this disease in about 5% of patients. A history of syncope, or an increase in dyspnea or angina, is a marker of very poor prognosis and requires urgent surgery.

Evidently, the risk of SD, as in all conditions previously discussed, is increased in the presence of HF.

Although the mechanism of SD is not well known, most cases are due to VT/VF or AV blocks (Kulbertus, 1988). After aortic valve replacement, a residual risk remains. Patients with valvular heart disease and inducible sustained VT that present left ventricular volume overload have the highest risk of recurring arrhythmic events (Martinez-Rubio *et al.*, 1997).

In the remaining valvular heart diseases, the incidence of SD is lower and depends on the presence of risk factors such as frequent arrhythmia, concomitant IHD or HF, a history of syncope, or a family history of SD.

Congenital Heart Disease

Arrhythmias

The most characteristic arrhythmias in patients with congenital heart disease are noted here.

Atrial arrhythmias occur in 15% of adults with congenital heart disease and represent a 50% increase in mortality and double the risk of morbidity (Bouchardy *et al.*, 2009). In many cases, atrial arrhythmias (flutter, fibrillation) are related to surgical scars performed during the correction of different congenital heart diseases.

- Patients with an **atrial septal defect** frequently present AF in adulthood, even in the absence of surgical repair. In the presence of a patent foramen oval, even with negligible shunt, some P wave morphology changes in sinus rhythm may be found (sometimes a

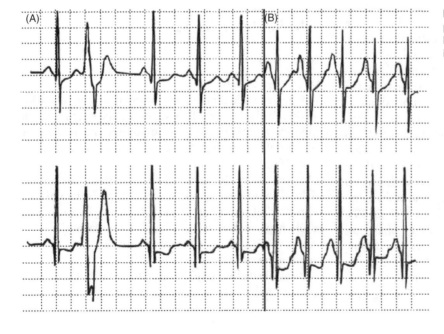

Figure 11.7 Patient with mitral valve prolapse. Holter monitoring shows frequent PVC (A) that disappear when heart rate increases (B).

P± in II, III, VF usually with P wave not as long as in cases of advanced interatrial block) (see Chapter 10, Advanced Interatrial Block With Left Atrial Retrograde Conduction).

- **Ebstein's disease.** Atrial flutter or atrial fibrillation may be seen, especially in adults with or without pre-excitation (WPW). Figure 10.5 shows an example of Ebstein's disease of 60-year-old woman with advanced interatrial block that presents very quick 1×1 atrial flutter, fortunately very transient (see Figure 4.65). Less often, other supraventricular tachycardias and first-degree AV blocks may be seen. The typical ECG characteristics following the ablation of an accessory pathway in patients with Ebstein's disease have been published (Iturralde *et al.*, 2006).
- **Tetralogy of Fallot.** The most important post-operative complications are different types of tachyarrhythmias and, on some occasions, SD.

The development of atrial tachycardias in adults may be associated with an increased morbidity, stroke, or death. Predictors of atrial tachycardias include a greater age at the time of surgical repair and tricuspid regurgitation. Because right bundle branch block pattern appears very frequently due to surgical repair (Figure 11.8), in most tachycardias the QRS is wide after surgery, even in cases with supraventricular origin (Harrison *et al.*, 2001). Ventricular tachycardias, including sustained, monomorphic VT, can occur early after surgery or even years after intracardiac repair. The arrhythmogenic focus is usually along the right ventriculotomy scar (Gatzoulis *et al.*, 2000).

There are many other different congenital heart diseases and procedures performed to repair them, such as Fontan repair for tricuspid artesia or Mustard operation for great vessels transposition that often present different types of SV tachyarrhythmias (Durongpisitkul *et al.*, 1998).

Sudden Death

The risk of SD may occur more frequently in the following congenital heart diseases (Lambert *et al.*, 1974; Driscoll and Edwards, 1985):

- **Anomalous origin of the left coronary artery**. Sudden death occurs especially during exercise, probably due to ischemia that triggers VT/VF.
- **Ebstein's disease**. This is often associated with supraventricular arrhythmias that are sometimes very fast (2×1 or 1×1 atrial flutter), or even ventricular tachycardias that may lead to SD.
- **Pulmonary hypertension and Eisenmenger syndrome**. This may lead to SD during the natural course of the disease, especially after the age of 30, and is probably due to cardiac arrhythmias.
- **Post-operative patients** with different congenital heart defects. Between 1% and 4% of patients with post-operative Tetralogy of Fallot experience SD, probably caused by ventricular arrhythmias. This occurs particularly in patients showing important RV hemodynamic alterations after surgery (Gillette *et al.*, 1977; Garson *et al.*, 1985).

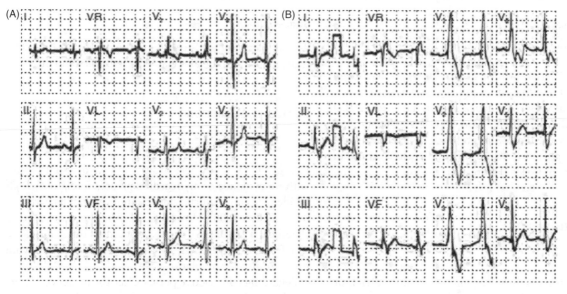

Figure 11.8 (A) Typical electrocardiogram (ECG) in a young child with Tetralogy of Fallot. We see the typical ECG pattern of rsR′ in V1 with QRS <120 ms. (B) After surgery, the patient presents the typical ECG of advanced peripheral right bundle branch block (RBBB).

- Naturally, the presence of **congenital AV block** implies a certain risk of SD, as discussed in Chapter 10 (see Chapter 10, Advanced Atrioventricular Block).

An ICD implantation is indicated in CHD survivors of cardiac arrest, after excluding any reversible causes (Class IB). In cases of spontaneous sustained VT, electrophysiologic study (EPS) is recommended (Class IC).

Hypertensive Heart Disease

Due to the great prevalence of hypertension, the presence of this risk factor in the incidence of arrhythmias and SD is very important.

Arrhythmias

The relationship between left ventricle hypertrophy (LVH) and AF is well established. Data from the Framingham study shows an increased prevalence of AF among patients with hypertensive cardiovascular disease when compared with control subjects, with a risk ratio of about 2.0 (Kannel *et al.*, 1982). In fact, hypertension is part of the CHA_2DS_2-V score. Hypertensive patients with LVH also have an increased incidence of other supraventricular tachycardia.

Patients with electrocardiographic evidence of LVH have a higher prevalence and greater complexity of PVC, and present more serious ventricular arrhythmias than patients without LVH or normotensive subjects (Siegel *et al.*, 1990).

Sudden Death

Hypertensive heart disease, especially when it presents a significant LVH and/or HF, is associated with a higher risk of SD. The presence of sinus tachycardia in hypertensive patients has been described as a risk marker for future SD.

In the LIFE trial (Morin *et al.*, 2009), it has been demonstrated that QRS duration is a marker of SD.

There is pathologic evidence (Subirana *et al.*, 2011) that the number of patients who experience SD and had LVH probably related to the presence of arterial hypertension is higher in Mediterranean regions than in Anglo-Saxon countries (Figure 1.2).

Myocarditis

Arrhythmias

Sinus tachycardia is very frequent. Premature atrial, or more often ventricular, extrasystoles are also common. Sometimes patients with myocarditis can develop both tachy- and bradyarrhythmias. These arrhythmias often resolve themselves after the acute phase. If well tolerated, they usually do not need specific therapy.

Sudden Death

Sudden death is not usually associated with myocarditis, although it may occur in the acute phase and in patients with no previous heart disease, including athletes. In some cases, AV block due to myocarditis has been found in necropsic studies. Some cases of fulminant myocarditis associated with H1N1 influenza A virus have recently been reported (Bratincsák *et al.*, 2010).

Implantable cardioverter defibrillator (ICD) may be recommended in patients with life-threatening VT who are not in the acute phase (Class IIa). If necessary, ablation may be performed. In cases of symptomatic bradycardia or AV block in the acute phase of myocarditis, temporary pacemaker insertion is indicated (Class IC).

Pathologic studies have shown that in some cases the only disease associated with SD is myocarditis (Maron *et al.*, 2009; Subirana *et al.*, 2011).

Cor Pulmonale

Arrhythmias

Both ventricular and supraventricular arrhythmias, especially atrial and ventricular premature complexes, can occur in patients with chronic obstructive pulmonary disease (COPD). Atrial fibrillation and/or atrial flutter are frequently present. Multifocal (Chaotic) atrial tachycardia is not very frequent, but it is characteristic of COPD (see Chapter 4, Chaotic Atrial Tachycardia).

Sudden Death

The incidence of SD is related to the degree of congestive heart failure and the associated arrhythmias and diseases.

Pericardial Disease

Arrhythmias

Patients with acute pericarditis and myocardial biopsy with no evidence of myocarditis present a relatively high incidence of atrial fibrillation, but not ventricular arrhythmias (Ristic, 2000). However, according to other studies (Spodick, 1984, 1998), acute pericarditis does not cause significant arrhythmias in the absence of underlying myocardium or valvular disease.

Regarding constrictive pericarditis, the presence of pericardial calcification appears to be associated with a higher incidence of AF during follow-up (Rezaian *et al.*, 2009).

Sudden Death

Pericardial disease by itself is not related to SD. However, in cases of pericarditis and possible myocardial involvement proven by evidence of myocarditis in an endomyocardial biopsy, the incidence of severe ventricular arrhythmias may increase and the case has to be considered as myocarditis (see Myocarditis). Sudden death may also appear in cases of cardiac tamponade.

Sudden Death in Other Heart Diseases

There are some heart diseases in which SD is specifically related to mechanical problems rather than a primary arrhythmia. This especially occurs in:

- **Cardiac tumors** due to a mechanical obstruction of blood flow.
- **Dissection and/or rupture of the aorta**. This occurs in atherosclerotic aneurisms, especially in those associated with hypertension. It may also be observed in young patients with Marfan syndrome and patients with bicuspid aortic valve and ascending aorta dilatation, sometimes related to an intense isometric exercise (weight lifting).
- **Pulmonary embolism**. Sudden death may occur in patients with massive pulmonary embolism. It is often the cause of death in the post-operative period after surgery, and in other circumstances of excessive rest (tourist airplane syndrome).

Sudden Infant Death Syndrome

This represents a problem of great social impact, with an incidence of 3‰ of births.

The cause of SD has not been clearly determined, although it has been suggested that apart from an incorrect sleeping position it may be associated with some channelopathies, such as long QT syndrome and even Brugada's syndrome (Priori *et al.*, 2000).

It has also been associated with different ANS alterations, such as an increase in vagal tone, and even with pathologic alterations, such as the presence of accessory pathways and different disorders of conduction sometimes associated with ANS alterations.

Bronchopneumonia has also been described as a triggering factor (Morris and Harrison, 2008).

Although prevention is difficult, certain patients have a higher risk of SD, such as newborns with prolonged apnea, or patients with a family history of SD in newborns. These patients should be closely monitored during the weeks following birth.

Athletes
(Figure 11.9)

Surface ECG Morphology
(Corrado et al., 2010)

The morphology of ECG in athletes very frequently presents **findings that may be training-related** and require

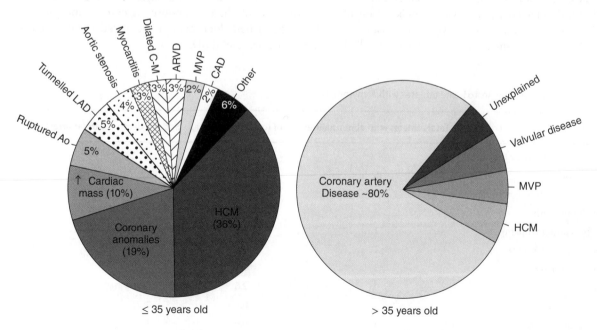

Figure 11.9 Estimated prevalence of cardiovascular diseases responsible for sudden death comparing young (<35 years old) (left) and older (>35 years old) (right) trained athletes. (ARVD = arrhythmogenic RV dysplasia; MVP = mitral valve prolapse; CAD = coronary artery disease; HCM = hypertrophic CM).

no additional evaluation, such as: (i) sinus bradycardia, (ii) first-degree AV block, (iii) partial RBBB pattern, (iv) high voltage of R wave in precordial leads in the absence of other criteria for LVH, and (v) early repolarization pattern. In this case, we have to remember that this pattern has been recently associated with SD (Haïssaguerre *et al.*, 2008) (see Chapter 10, Early Repolarization Pattern). A recent review of the Athlete's ECG has been published and would allow the reader a full comprehensive view of this fascinating topic (Peritz *et al*, 2016).

In contrast, **uncommon and nontraining-related ECG findings** that may indicate further evaluation are: (i) negative T waves ≥ two adjacent leads, (ii) ST segment depression, (iii) pathologic Q waves, (iv) important atrial abnormalities, (v) short or long QT interval, (vi) advanced bundle branch block or hemiblocks, (vii) evident criteria of right or left ventricle hypertrophy, (viii) abnormalities of QRS–ST in V1 suggestive of Brugada pattern, and (ix) the presence of some arrhythmias (runs or sustained VT, AF, advanced second or third degree AV block) (see below).

We have already commented on the differential diagnosis of the rSr′ pattern in V1 frequently seen in athletes with Type II Brugada pattern and pectus excavatum (see Figure 9.21) (Serra *et al.*, 2014). In fact, in this figure is presented Baranchuk's algorithm to differentiate all cases of r′ in V1 (Baranchuk *et al.*, 2015; Koppikar *et al.*, 2015).

Arrhythmias

The most frequent arrhythmias found in athletes are:

- **PVC**. These are not infrequent in healthy athletes, although they usually disappear with exercise. Runs of VT and especially sustained VT have to be considered definitively pathologic and need to be carefully studied

- **Atrial fibrillation** (AF). Whereas paroxysmal AF is rarely seen in young athletes, the incidence of AF in adult athletes is more frequent than in the normal population (Mont *et al.*, 2009);
- **Some benign bradyarrhythmias,** such as sinus bradycardia, often with junctional escapes and/or first-and even second-degree Wenckebach-type AV block may be found, occurring especially at night;
- **Advanced AV block**. This should not be assumed to be training-related and requires further evaluation.

Sudden Death

Although the incidence of SD among athletes is low, it constitutes a serious social problem. In young competitive athletes, the incidence of SD is approximately 1/100 000 people/year (Maron *et al.*, 2009). In athletes over 35 years of age the most frequent cause is ischemic heart disease, whereas in younger athletes the conditions most frequently associated with SD are hypertrophic CM (Moss *et al.*, 2002), coronary anomalies, arrhythmogenic RVD, myocarditis, coronary artery anomalies, and many others (Figure 11.9). It has been demonstrated that the use of doping agents (androgenic-anabolic steroids) may cause a significant shortening of the QT interval (≈350 ms), albeit without reaching the values of short QT syndrome. This is related to the increase in Ito and Ik currents, resulting in a shortened repolarization (Bigi *et al.*, 2009).

Table 11.2 shows cardiac abnormalities found in 161 elite athletes with arrhythmias considered pathologic after arrhythmologic study (Bayés de Luna *et al.*, 2000). More than 40% had an underlying cardiac abnormality, four (2.5%) had documented recovered cardiac arrest, and three presented SD.

Table 11.2 Cardiac abnormalities in 161 elite athletes with arrhythmias.[*]

Disease	Total athletes with abnormalities	% of total elite athletes	Sudden death	Cardiac arrest
Arrhythmogenic ventricular dysplasia	12	7.5		1
Mitral valve prolapse	27	16.7		1
Wolff–Parkinson–White syndrome	15	9.3		1
Dilated cardiomyopathy	3	1.9	1	1
Hypertrophic cardiomyopathy	1	0.6		1
Mitral regurgitation (severe)	1	0.6		
Aortic valvular disease	3	1.9		
Myocarditis	4	2.5		
Coronary artery disease	1	0.6	1	
Unknown cardiomyopathy	1	0.6	1	
Total	68	42.2	3	4

[*] Taken from Bayés de Luna *et al.*, 2000.

Athletes should undergo a cardiology check-up that includes a complete personal and family history and physical examination, a good interpretation of the ECG, and, if feasible, an echocardiogram, a key diagnostic tool in determining the presence of valvular heart disease and cardiomyopathy. In the presence of syncope or other symptoms, especially during exercise, if there is some doubt or if the diagnosis is not clear, imaging techniques, such as a multislice scanner and, especially, a CMR, should be used (see Appendix, Other Nonelectrocardiographic Techniques). If necessary, EPS or even genetic testing and right ventricular biopsy should be performed, especially in the presence of exercise syncope or an "atypical" ECG. Using each of these techniques, HCM, ARVD, other CMs, coronary and aorta anomalies and even channelopathies may be diagnosed.

Alcohol Intake

Arrhythmias

The most common arrhythmias related to alcohol intake are:

- Paroxysmal atrial arrhythmias (holiday heart syndrome) and AF in particular (Menz *et al.*, 1996). Chronic AF is more common in patients with alcoholism (see Chapter , Atrial Fibrillation: Epidemiology and Etiology).
- Ventricular arrhythmias, especially PVC, also frequently occur (Ettinger *et al.*, 1978; Frost and Vestergaard, 2004). Abstinence frequently reduces or even abolishes PVC (Figure 11.10) and episodes of AF.

Sudden Death

Sudden death is more frequent in patients with an unusually high degree of alcohol intake. This often occurs as a consequence of ventricular arrhythmias leading to VF in heavy drinkers (Wannamethee and Shaper, 1992).

Special Situations

Special situations exist where arrhythmias and SD may occur with or without the presence of heart disease. The most important of these situations are described in the following sections.

Administration of Drugs

Drugs and Pro-Arrhythmic Effects

We have already discussed that **some cardiac and non-cardiac agents**, especially Type I antiarrhythmic agents and some chemotherapeutic drugs (see Chapter 4, Atrial Fibrillation: Epidemiology and Eiology, and Chapter 10, Acquired Long QT), **have a pro-arrhythmic effect** and may increase the risk of SD. This depends on the previous cardiovascular state and the dosage and interactions of any drugs, but it is especially related to the lengthening of the QT interval. Currently, drug agencies (FDA, EMEA) strictly monitor new drugs, especially in relation with QTc lengthening and the appearance of Torsades de Pointes VT/VF. To better understand the effects of different drugs on the QT interval, consult https://crediblemeds.org/.

- **Digitalis effect and intoxication:** The digitalis effect induces QT shortening and the effect on the ST segment (concave depression) is very easily detected in the surface ECG. It may be present in the absence or presence of toxic levels of digitalis (Figure 11.11).
  - Digitalis toxicity is expressed frequently by ectopic atrial, junctional tachycardia and ventricular arrhythmias (Kelly and Smith, 1992). Premature ventricular complexes are often the first sign of digitalis toxicity. This may be initially manifest by isolated PVC or ventricular bigeminy. Ventricular tachycardia, sometimes bidirectional (Figure 11.12A), and fatal ventricular fibrillation may occur if digitalis toxicity is not recognized and treated. Digitalis intoxication also triggers atrial and junctional ectopic tachycardia relatively often (Figure 11.13). In both cases, the presence of AV dissociation is relatively frequent (see Figures 4.13, 4.14, and 4.28). The most frequent passive arrhythmias found in digitalis intoxications are slow AV junctional rhythms (Figure 11.11), sinus bradycardia, sinoatrial block, and any degree of AV block.
  - In the past, digitalis intoxication was more common (Bayés de Luna *et al.*, 2011; Recommended General Bibliography p. xvii). The most frequent arrhythmias found were PVC: 80%; VT: 20%; atrial and junctional arrhythmias: 90%; different degrees of AV block: 40%. The presence of digitalis intoxication today is much less frequent than 30–40 years ago. However, it is necessary to be aware that it may still exist and, when in doubt, to proceed to measuring levels of digitalis and start the adequate treatment, if necessary. Patients who present sustained VT, or advanced AV block, considered to be caused by digitalis intoxication must receive antidigitalis antibodies (Class IA). In other cases with less severe arrhythmia, the most appropriate measures are withdrawal of digitalis, rest, restoring normal electrolyte levels, and continuous monitoring of cardiac rhythm. Magnesium and pacing may be prescribed in selected cases (Class II a).
  - Digitalis, like many other drugs that block the AV node more than the accessory pathways, such as verapamil, β-blockers, adenosine, and lidocaine,

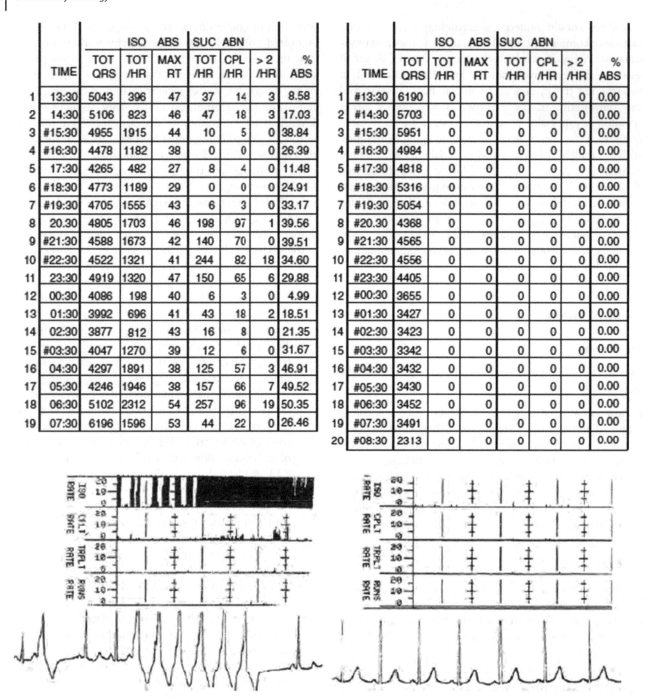

	TIME	TOT QRS	ISO TOT /HR	ABS MAX RT	SUC TOT /HR	ABN CPL /HR	>2 /HR	% ABS
1	13:30	5043	396	47	37	14	3	8.58
2	14:30	5106	823	46	47	18	3	17.03
3	#15:30	4955	1915	44	10	5	0	38.84
4	#16:30	4478	1182	38	0	0	0	26.39
5	17:30	4265	482	27	8	4	0	11.48
6	#18:30	4773	1189	29	0	0	0	24.91
7	#19:30	4705	1555	43	6	3	0	33.17
8	20.30	4805	1703	46	198	97	1	39.56
9	#21:30	4588	1673	42	140	70	0	39.51
10	#22:30	4522	1321	41	244	82	18	34.60
11	23:30	4919	1320	47	150	65	6	29.88
12	00:30	4086	198	40	6	3	0	4.99
13	01:30	3992	696	41	43	18	2	18.51
14	02:30	3877	812	43	16	8	0	21.35
15	#03:30	4047	1270	39	12	6	0	31.67
16	04:30	4297	1891	38	125	57	3	46.91
17	05:30	4246	1946	38	157	66	7	49.52
18	06:30	5102	2312	54	257	96	19	50.35
19	07:30	6196	1596	53	44	22	0	26.46

	TIME	TOT QRS	ISO TOT /HR	ABS MAX RT	SUC TOT /HR	ABN CPL /HR	>2 /HR	% ABS
1	#13:30	6190	0	0	0	0	0	0.00
2	#14:30	5703	0	0	0	0	0	0.00
3	#15:30	5951	0	0	0	0	0	0.00
4	#16:30	4984	0	0	0	0	0	0.00
5	#17:30	4818	0	0	0	0	0	0.00
6	#18:30	5316	0	0	0	0	0	0.00
7	#19:30	5054	0	0	0	0	0	0.00
8	#20.30	4368	0	0	0	0	0	0.00
9	#21:30	4565	0	0	0	0	0	0.00
10	#22:30	4556	0	0	0	0	0	0.00
11	#23:30	4405	0	0	0	0	0	0.00
12	#00:30	3655	0	0	0	0	0	0.00
13	#01:30	3427	0	0	0	0	0	0.00
14	#02:30	3423	0	0	0	0	0	0.00
15	#03:30	3342	0	0	0	0	0	0.00
16	#04:30	3432	0	0	0	0	0	0.00
17	#05:30	3430	0	0	0	0	0	0.00
18	#06:30	3452	0	0	0	0	0	0.00
19	#07:30	3491	0	0	0	0	0	0.00
20	#08:30	2313	0	0	0	0	0	0.00

Figure 11.10 Heavy drinking patient with frequent PVC. After some weeks of abstinence, a complete lack of PVC is shown.

may not be administered for the treatment of junctional reentrant tachycardias or atrial fibrillation (AF) in the presence of WPW pre-excitation. These drugs may be dangerous because they accelerate the accessory pathway conduction in cases of AF (see Chapter 4, AV Junctional Reentrant Tachycardia).

To understand the effects of other drugs on the heart, especially those related with arrhythmias and SD, consult specialized books (see the Recommended General Bibliography p. xvii).

Ionic Alterations

An electrolyte alteration may lead to a Torsades de Pointes VT/VF that triggers SD (see Figure 10.17), especially in the presence of an underlying heart disease. It

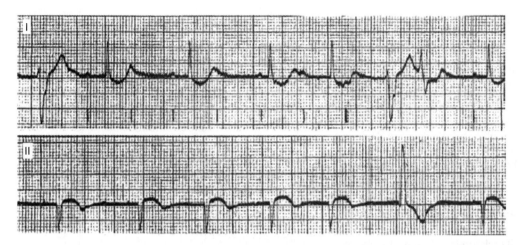

Figure 11.11 Digitalis intoxication: see the typical morphology of ST depression due to the digitalis effect with a shortened QT interval. This is a case of irregular junctional escape rhythm with some sinus and ectopic P waves, premature ventricular complexes (PVC) and ventricular escape complexes.

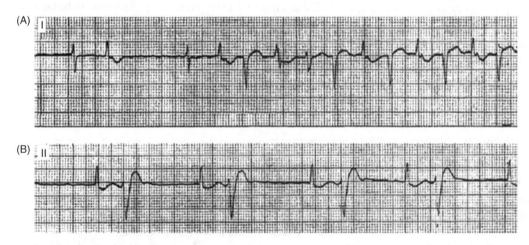

Figure 11.12 Patient with digitalis intoxication and atrial fibrillation (AF). (A) After two bigeminal premature ventricular complexes (PVC), an episode of bidirectional ventricular fibrillation (VF) starts. (B) The same patient presented bigeminal rhythm due to PVC. See the typical ST segment morphology.

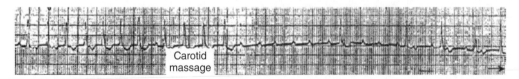

Figure 11.13 Patient with digitalis intoxication and atrial ectopic tachycardia with clear irregular atrial rhythm that is well seen when the atrioventricular (AV) block appears after carotid sinus massage.

has been shown that this mainly occurs in patients with hypokalemia and hypomagnesaemia, increasing sensitivity to digitalis toxicity, especially when taking diuretics (Hollenberg, 1987).

Sleep Apnea Syndrome (SAS)

This syndrome, in both cerebral and obstructive forms, is associated with increased comorbidity and mortality.

The diagnosis is based on overnight polysomnography and the treatment of choice is the application of continuous positive airway pressure (CPAP).

The absolute rate of active (PVC and AF especially) and passive (severe sinus bradycardia or AV block, including advanced) arrhythmias associated with SAS is not very high. However, the odds of an arrhythmia occurring after a respiratory disturbance are nearly 18 times higher than those occurring after normal breathing (Monahan *et al.*, 2009). There is a clear relationship between SAS and AF. Evidently, treating the apnea is the most important and often solves this problem. The presence of SAS increases the risk of AF threefold (Yazdan-Ashoori *et al*, 2011) and it was proposed to be part of the CHADS$_2$ score. The treatment with CPAP induces reversed atrial remodeling and this is visible also as a reduction of the P-wave duration in P-wave signal average (Baranchuk *et al*, 2013). The association of SAS with bradyarrhythmias has proved not to be significant (Baranchuk, 2012).

Ventricular arrhythmias and SD related to other specific pathologies

Cases of VA and even SD related to different processes such as endocrine disorders and diabetes, end-stage renal failure, obesity, dieting, and anorexia have been described. The management of these cases involves removal of triggering factors and treatment of arrhythmia with ICD implantation, if necessary, if the survival expectancy is relatively high (see Heart Failure: Therapeutic Considerations).

Sudden Death in Apparently Healthy People
(see Chapter 9, Idiopathic Ventricular Fibrillation)

In this group we include cases of so-called idiopathic VF comprising progressively fewer numbers of cases due to the discovery of new syndromes related to **channelopathies** (see before). However, the first manifestation of the disease in channelopathies is relatively often the occurrence of syncope or SD (see Chapter 9) (Leenhardt *et al.*, 1994).

We have explained how many cases of SD in apparently healthy adult subjects are due to acute MI (see Chapter 1, Figure 1.9).

Other unexpected causes of SD in apparently healthy people may be the rupture of the aorta, usually associated with an aneurism (see before, Sudden Death in Other Heart Diseases), massive pulmonary embolism, or extracardiac causes, such as serious cerebral or gastrointestinal hemorrhage (Subirana *et al.*, 2011) (see Table 1.2).

Finally, we have already discussed, in Chapter 10, the cases of serious arrhythmias and SD that may appear in patients with normal or near normal ECG.

Self Assessment

A. What is the importance of acute ischemia in sudden death (SD)?

B. What is the role of genetic factors in the triggering of SD in ST elevation myocardial infarction (STEMI)?

C. What is the most frequent supraventricular arrhythmia in acute MI?

D. Explain the most important risk factors in post-MI patients.

E. What is the importance of scar characteristics in the presentation of ventricular tachycardia (VT) in post-MI patients?

F. What are the indications of implantable cardioverter defibrillator (ICD) therapy in heart failure patients?

G. In which congenital heart disease is there more risk of SD?

H. What is the risk of SD in athletes?

I. What is the holiday heart syndrome?

J. Describe the most frequent arrhythmias in digitalis intoxication.

References

Adgey A, Devlin J, Webb SW, Mulholland HC. Initiation of ventricular fibrillation outside the hospital in patients with acute ischemic heart disease. Br Heart J 1982:47;55.

Alvarez- García J, Massó-van Roessel A, Vives-Borrás M, et al. XXXX Prevalence, clinical profile and short-term prognosis of interatrial block in patients admitted for worsening of heart failure. Abstract submitted to ACC'16.

Antzelevitch C, Yan GX. J wave syndromes. Heart Rhythm 2010;7:549.

Baranchuk A, Sleep Apnea, Cardiac Arrhythmias and Conduction Disorders. J Electrocardiol 2012;45:508.

Baranchuk A, Pang H, Seaborn GEJ, et al. Reverse atrial electrical remodelling induced by continuous positive airway pressure in patients with severe obstructive sleep apnea. J Interventional Card Electrophysiol 2013;36(3):247.

Baranchuk A, Enriquez A, García-Niebla J, et al. Differential diagnosis of rSr' pattern in leads V1-V2. Comprehensive review and proposed algorithm. Ann Noninvasive Electrocardiol 2015;20(1):7.

Bardy GH, Lee KL, Mark DB, et al. Amiodarone or an implantable cardioverter-defibrillator for congestive heart failure. N Engl J Med 2005;352:225.

Bayés de Luna A, Fiol M. The electrocardiography in ischemic heart disease: clinical and imaging correlations and prognostic implications. Futura-Blackwell, Oxford, 2008.

Bayés de Luna A, Carreras F, Cladellas M, et al. Holter ECG study of the electrocardiographic phenomena in Prinzmetal angina attacks with emphasis on the study of ventricular arrhythmias. J Electrocardiol 1985;18:267.

Bayés de Luna A, Cladellas R, Oter R, et al. Interatrial conduction block ans retrograde activation of the left atrium and paroxysmal supraventricular tachyarrhythmia. Eur Heart J 1988;9:1112.

Bayés de Luna A, Furinello F, Maron BJ, Zipes DP, eds. Arrhythmias and sudden death in athletes. Kluwer Academic Publishers, Dordrecht, 2000.

Bayés de Luna A, Goldwasser D, de Porta V, et al. Optimizing electrocardiographic interpretation in acute ST-elevation myocardial infarction may be very beneficial. Am Heart J 2011;162(1):e1; author reply e5. doi: 10.1016/j.ahj.2011.02.017.

Bayés de Luna A, Cygankiewicz I, Baranchuk A, et al. Prinzmetal angina: ECG changes and clinical considerations: a consensus paper. Ann Noninvasive Electrocardiol 2014;19(5):442.

Bayés-Genis A, Viñolas X, Guindo J, et al. Electrocardiographic and clinical precursors of ventricular fibrillation: chain of events. J Cardiovasc Electrophysiol 1995;6:410.

Beshai J, Grimm RA, Nagueh SF et al. Cardiac re-synchronization therapy in heart failure with narrow QRS complexes. N Engl J Med 2007;357:2461.

Bigger JT, Fleiss JL, Kleiger R, et al. The relationships among ventricular arrhythmias, left ventricular dysfunction, and mortality in the 2 years after myocardial infarction. Circulation 1984;69:250.

Bigi MA, Aslani A, Aslani A. Short QT interval: A novel predictor of androgen abuse in strength trained athletes. Ann Noninvasive Electrocardiol 2009;14:311.

Birnbaum Y, Herz I, Sclarovsky S, et al. Prognostic significance of the admission electrocardiogram in acute myocardial infarction. J Am Coll Cardiol 1996; 27:1128.

Bloomfield DB, Sgteinman RC, Namerow PB, et al. Microvolt T-wave alternans distinguishes between patients likely and patients not likely to benefit from implanted cardiac defibrillator therapy. Circulation 2004;110:1885.

Bortone A, Boveda S, Pasquié JL, et al. Sinus rhythm restoration by catheter ablation in patients with long-lasting atrial fibrillation and congestive heart failure: impact of the left ventricular ejection fraction improvement on the implantable cardioverter defibrillator insertion indication. Europace 2009;11:1018.

Bouchardy J, Therrien J, Pilote L, et al. Atrial arrhythmias in adults with congenital heart disease. Circulation 2009;120:1679.

Bratincsák A, El-Said HG, Bradley JS, et al. Fulminant myocarditis associated with pandemic H1N1 influenza A virus in children. J Am Coll Cardiol 2010;55:928.

Briegger D, Fox KA, Fitzgerald G, et al. Predicting freedom from clinical events in non-ST-elevation acute coronary syndromes: the Global Registry of Acute Coronary Events. Heart 2009;895:888.

Buxton AE. Risk stratification for sudden death in patients with coronary artery disease. Heart Rhythm 2009;45:969.

Castel MA, Magnani S, Mont L, et al. Survival in New York Heart Association class IV heart failure patients treated with cardiac resynchronization therapy compared with patients on optimal pharmacological treatment. Europace 2010;12:1136.

Corrado D, Pelliccia A, Heidbuchel H, et al. Recommendations for interpretation of 12-lead electrocardiogram in the athlete. Eur Heart J 2010;31:243.

Chung MK, Szymkiewicz SJ, Shao M, et al. Aggregate national experience with the wearable cardioverter-defibrillator: event rates, compliance, and survival. J Am Coll Cardiol 2010a;56:194.

Chung ES, Katra RP, Ghio S, et al. Cardiac resynchronization therapy may benefit patients with left ventricular ejection fraction > 35%: a PROSPECT trial substudy. Eur J Heart Fail 2010b;12(6):581.

Cygankiewicz I, Zareba W, Vazquez R, et al. Relation of heart rate turbulence to severity of heart failure. Am J Cardiol 2006;98:1635.

Cygankiewicz I, Zareba W, Vázquez R et al. Heart rate turbulence predicts all-cause mortality and sudden death in congestive heart failure patients. Heart Rhythm 2008;5:1095.

Daubert C, Gold MR, Abraham WT, et al. Prevention of disease progression by cardiac esynchronization therapy in patients with asymptomatic or mildly symptomatic left ventricular dysfunction: insights from the European cohort of the REVERSE (Resynchronization Reverses Remodeling in Systolic Left Ventricular Dysfunction) trial. J Am Coll Cardiol 2009;54:1837.

Dickstein K, Vardas PE, Auricchio A, et al. 2010 Focused update of ESC guidelines on device therapy in heart failure. Eur Heart J 2010;12(11):1143.

Driscoll DJ, Edwards WD. Sudden unexpected death in children and adolescents. J Am Coll Cardiol 1985;5:118B.

Durongpisitkul K, Porter CJ, Cetta F, et al. Predictors of early- and late-onset supraventricular tachyarrhythmias after Fontan operation. Circulation 1998;98:1099.

Dziewierz A, Siudak Z, Rakowski T, et al. Prognostic significance of new onset atrial fibrillation in acute coronary syndrome patients treated conservatively. Cardiol J 2010;17:57.

Elosua R, Lluisa C, Lucas G. Estudio del componente genético de la cardiopatía isquémica: de los estudios de ligamiento al genotipado integral del genoma. Rev Esp Cardiol 2009;9:24 (English version).

Ettinger PO, Wu CF, DelaCruz C, et al. Arrhythmias and the "holiday heart." Alcohol associated cardiac rhythm disorders. Am Heart J 1978; 95:555.

Fiol M, Marrugat J, Bayés de Luna A, et al. Ventricular fibrillation markers on admission to the hospital for acute myocardial infarction. Am J Cardiol 1993;71:117.

Fiol M, Carrillo A, Rodríguez A, et al. Electrocardiographic changes of ST-elevation myocardial infarction in patients with complete occlusion of the left main trunk without collateral circulation: differential diagnosis and clinical considerations. J Electrocardiol 2012;45:487.

Frank S, Johnson A, Ross Jr J. Natural history of valvular aortic stenosis. Br Heart J 1973;35:41.

Frost, L, Vestergaard, P. Alcohol and risk of atrial fibrillation or flutter: a cohort study. Arch Intern Med 2004;164:1993.

Garson A, Randall DC, Gillette PC, et al. Prevention of sudden death after repair of tetralogy of Fallot: treatment of ventricular arrhythmias. J Am Coll Cardiol 1985;6:221.

Gasparini M, Auricchio A, Regoli F, et al. Four-year efficacy of cardiac resynchronization therapy on exercise tolerance and disease progression: the importance of performing atrioventricular junction ablation in patients with atrial fibrillation. J Am Coll Cardiol 2006;48:734.

Gatzoulis, MA, Balaji, S, Webber, SA, et al. Risk factors for arrhythmia and sudden cardiac death late after repair of tetralogy of Fallot: a multicentre study. Lancet 2000; 356:975.

Ghanbari H, Dalloul G, Hasan R, et al. Effectiveness of implantable cardioverter-defibrillators for the primary prevention of sudden cardiac death in women with advanced heart failure: a meta-analysis of randomized controlled trials. Arch Intern Med 2009;169:1500.

Gheeraert P, Buyzere M, Tacymans Y, et al. Risk factors for primary ventricular fibrillation during acute myocardial infarction. Eur Heart J 2006;27:2499.

Gillette PC, Yeoman MA, Mulins CE, et al. Sudden death after repair of tetralogy of Fallot. Circulation 1977;56:566.

Goldberger JJ, Passman R. Implantable cadioverter-defibrillator therapy after acute myocardial infarction. J Am Coll Cardiol 2009;54:2001.

Goldstein S, Bayés de Luna A, Guindo J. Sudden cardiac death. Futura Publishing, New York, 1994.

Haïssaguerre M, Derval N, Sacher F, et al. Sudden cardiac arrest associated with early repolarization. N Engl J Med 2008;358:2016.

Haqqani HM, Kalman JM, Roberts-Thomson KC, et al. Fundamental differences in electrophysiologic and electroanatomic substrate between ischemic cardiomyopathy patients with and without clinical ventricular tachycardia. J Am Coll Cardiol 2009;54:166.

Harrison DA, Siu SC, Hussain F, et al. Sustained atrial arrhythmias in adults late after repair of tetralogy of Fallot. Am J Cardiol 2001; 87:584.

Hohnloser SH, Ikeda T, Bloomfield DM, et al. T-wave alternans negative coronary patients with low ejection and benefit from defibrillator implantation. Lancet 2003;362:125.

Hollenberg NK. Cardiovascular therapeutics in the 1980s. Am J Med 1987;82:1

Hu D, Viskin S, Oliva A, et al. Novel mutation in the SCN5A gene associated with arrhythmic storm development during acute myocardial infarction. Heart Rhythm 2007;4:1072.

Iturralde P, Nava S, Sálica G, et al. Electrocardiographic characteristics of patients with Ebstein's anomaly before and after ablation of an accessory atrioventricular pathway. J Cardiovasc Electrophysiol 2006;17:1337.

Kannel, WB, Abbott, RD, Savage, DD, McNamara, PM. Epidemiologic features of chronic atrial fibrillation: the Framingham study. N Engl J Med 1982; 306:1018

Kelly, RA, Smith, TW. Recognition and management of digitalis toxicity. Am J Cardiol 1992; 69:108G.

Khadjooi K, Foley PW, Chalil S, et al. Long-term effects of cardiac resynchronisation therapy in patients with atrial fibrillation. Heart 2008;94:879.

Khan MN, Jaïs P, Cummings J, et al. Pulmonary-vein isolation for atrial fibrillation in patients with heart failure. N Engl J Med 2008;359:1778.

Kim S, Kuroda T, Nishinaga M, et al. Relation between severity of mitral regurgitation and prognosis of mitral valve prolapse: echocardiographic follow-up study. Am Heart J 1996;132:348.

Kligfield P, Levy D, Devereux RB, et al. Arrhythmias and sudden death in mitral valve prolapse. Am Heart J 1987;113:1298.

Koppikar S, Barbosa-Barros R, Baranchuk A. A practical approach to the investigation or an rSr′ pattern in leads V1-V2. Can J Cardiol 2015;31(12):1493.

Kühne M, Sakumura M, Reich SS, et al. Simultaneous use of implantable cardioverter-defibrillators and left ventricular assist devices in patients with severe heart failure. Am J Cardiol 2010;105:378.

Kulbertus H. Ventricular arrhythmias, syncope and sudden death in aortic stenosis. Eur Heart J 1988;9(Suppl E):51.

Kumar S, Sivagangabalan G, Zaman S, et al. Electrophysiology-guided defibrillator implantation early after ST-elevation myocardial infarction. Heart Rhythm. 2010;7(11):1589.

Lambert EC, Menon VA, Wagner HR, et al. Sudden unexpected death from cardiovascular disease in children: A cooperative international study. Am J Cardiol 1974;34:89.

Lau DH, Huynh LT, Chew DP, et al. Prognostic impact of types of atrial fibrillation in acute coronary syndromes. Am J Cardiol 2009;104:1317.

Leenhardt A, Glaser E, Burguera M, et al. Short-coupled variant of Torsades de Pointes. A new electrocardiographic entity in the spectrum of idiopathic ventricular tachyarrhythmias. Circulation 1994;89:206.

Levy WC, Lee KL, Hellkamp AS, et al. Maximizing survival benefit with primary prevention implantable cardioverter defibrillator therapy in a heart failure population. Circulation 2009;120:835.

Linde C, Abraham WT, Gold MR, et al. Randomized trial of cardiac resynchronization in mildly symptomatic heart failure patients and in asymptomatic patients with left ventricular dysfunction and previous heart failure. J Am Coll Cardiol 2008;52:1834.

Luu M, Stevenson WG, Stevenson LW, et al. Diverse mechanisms of unexpected cardiac arrest in advanced heart failure. Circulation 1989;80:1675.

Maron BJ, Maron MS, Wigle ED, Braunwald E. The 50-year history, controversy, and clinical implications of left ventricular outflow tract obstruction in hypertrophic cardiomyopathy from idiopathic hypertrophic subaortic stenosis to hypertrophic cardiomyopathy. J Am Coll Cardiol 2009;54:181.

Martinez-Rubio A, Schwammenthal Y, Schwammenthal E, et al. Patients with valvular heart disease presenting with sustained ventricular tachyarrhythmias or syncope: results of programmed ventricular stimulation and long-term follow-up. Circulation 1997;96:500.

Mehta SR, Granger CB, Boden WE, et al. Early versus delayed invasive intervention in acute coronary syndromes. N Engl J Med 2009;360:2165.

Menz V, Grimm W, Hoffmann J, Maisch B. Alcohol and rhythm disturbance: the holiday heart syndrome Herz 1996;21:227.

Michel PL, Mandagout O, Vahanian A, et al. Ventricular arrhythmias in aortic valve disease before and after surgery. J Heart Valve Dis 1992;1:72.

Monahan K, Storfer-Isser A, Mehra R, et al. Triggering of nocturnal arrhythmias by sleep-disordered breathing events. J Am Coll Cardiol 2009;54:1797.

Mont L, Elosua R, Brugada J. Endurance sport practice as a risk factor for atrial fibrillation and atrial flutter. Europace 2009;11:11.

Morin DP, Oikarinen L, Vitasalo M, et al. QRS duration predicts sudden cardiac death in hypertensive patients undergoing intensive medical therapy: the LIFE study. Eur Heart J 2009;30:2908.

Morris JA, Harrison LM. Sudden unexpected death in infancy: evidence of infection. Lancet 2008;371:1815.

Moss AJ. Factors influencing prognosis after myocardial infarction. Curr Probl Cardiol 1979;4:6.

Moss AJ. T wave patterns associated with the hereditary QT syndrome. Card Electrophysiol Rev 2002;6:311.

Moss AJ, Hall WJ, Cannon DS, et al. Improved survival with an implanted defibrillator in patients with coronary disease at high risk for ventricular arrhythmia. N Engl J Med 1996;335:1933.

Moss AJ, Daubert J, Zareba W. MAIDT-II: clinical implications. Card Electrophysiol Rev 2002;6:463.

Moss AJ, Hall WJ, Cannom DS, et al. Cardiac-resynchronization therapy for the prevention of heart-failure events. N Engl J Med 2009;361:1329.

Nikus K, Pahlm O, Wagner G, et al. Electrocardiographic classification of acute coronary syndromes: a review by a committee of the International Society for Holter and Non-Invasive Electrocardiology. J Electrocardiol 2010;43:91.

Pascale P, Schlaepfer J, Oddo M, et al. Ventricular arrhythmia in coronary artery disease: limits of a risk stratification strategy based on the ejection fraction alone and impact of infarct localization. Europace 2009;11:1639

Pascual D, Ordoñez-Llanos J, Tornel PL, et al. Soluble ST2 for predicting sudden cardiac death in patients with chronic heart failure and left ventricular systolic dysfunction. J Am Coll Cardiol 2009;54:2174.

Peritz DC, Chung EH. Criteria for evaluating rSr′ patterns due to high precordial ECG lead placement accurately confirm absence of a Brugada ECG pattern. J Electrocardiol 2016;49(2):182.

Pouleur A, Barkoudah E, Uno H, et al. Pathogenesis of sudden death in a clinical trial of patients post myocardial infarction with left ventricular dysfunction. Circulation 2010;122:597.

Priori SG, Napolitano C, Giordano U, et al. Brugada syndrome and sudden cardiac death in children. Lancet 2000;355:808.

Rezaian GR, Poor-Moghaddas M, Kojuri J, et al. Atrial fibrillation in patients with constrictive pericarditis: the significance of pericardial calcification. Ann Noninvasive Electrocardiol. 2009;14:258.

Ristic AD. Arrhythmias in acute pericarditis. An endomyocardial biopsy study. Herz 2000;25:729.

Roy D, Talajic M, Nattel S, et al. Rhythm control versus rate control for atrial fibrillation and heart failure. N Engl J Med 2008;358:2667.

Schoenenberger AW, Kobza R, Jamshidi P, et al. Sudden cardiac death in patients with silent myocardial ischemia after myocardial infarction (from the Swiss Interventional Study on Silent Ischemia Type II (SWISSI)). Am J Cardiol 2009;104:158.

Schwartz PJ, Zaza A, Grazi S, et al. Effect of ventricular fibrillation complicating acute myocardial infarction on long-term prognosis: importance of the site of infarction. Am J Cardiol 1985;56:384.

Schwartz PJ, La Rovere MT, Vanoli E. Autonomic nervous system and sudden cardiac death. Experimental basis and clinical observations for post-myocardial infarction risk stratification. Circulation 1992;85(1 Suppl):177.

Scirica BM, Braunwald E, Belardinelli L, et al. Relationship between nonsustained ventricular tachycardia after non-ST elevation acute coronary syndrome and sudden cardiac death. Circulation 2010;122:455.

Serra G, Baranchuk A, Bayés de Luna A, et al. New electrocardiographic criteria to differentiate the Type-2 Brugada pattern from electrocardiogram of healthy athletes with r'-wave in leads V1/V2. Europace 2014;16:1639.

Siegel D, Cheitlin MD, Blaek DM, et al. Risk of ventricular arrhythmias in hypertensive men with left ventricular hypertrophy. Am J Cardiol 1990;65:742

Spodick DH. Frequency of arrhythmias in acute pericarditis determined by Holter monitoring. Am J Cardiol 1984;53:842–845.

Spodick DH. Significant arrhythmias during pericarditis are due to concomitant heart disease J Am Coll Cardiol. 1998;32:551.

Stern S, Bayés de Luna A. Coronary artery spasm: A 2009 update. Circulation 2009;119(18):2531.

Subirana MT, JuanBabot JO, Puig T, et al. Specific characteristics of sudden death in a Mediterranean Spanish population. Am J Cardiol 2011;107(4):622.

Swedberg K, Komajda M, Böhm M, et al. Ivabradine and outcomes in chronic heart failure (SHIFT): a randomised placebo-controlled study. Lancet 2010;376:847.

Tang AS, Wells GA, Talajic M., et al. Cardiac-resynchronization therapy for mild-to-moderate heart failure. N Engl J Med 2010;363(25):2385.

Théroux P, Waters DD, Halphen C, et al. Prognostic value of exercise testing soon after myocardial infarction. N Engl J Med 1979;301:341.

Tikkanen JT, Anttonen O, Juntilla MJ, et al. Long-term outcome associated with early repolarization of electrocardiography. N Engl J Med 2009;361:2529.

Tung R, Boyle NG, Shivkumar K. Catheter ablation of ventricular tachycardia. Circulation 2010;122:e389.

Van de Werf F, Bax J, Betriu A, et al. Management of acute myocardial infarction in patients presenting with persistent ST-segment elevation. The Task Force on the management of ST-segment elevation acute myocardial infarction of the European Society of Cardiology. Eur Heart J 2008;29:2909.

Van Lee V, Mitiku T, Hadley D, et al. Rest premature ventricular contractions on routine ECG and prognosis in heart failure patients. Ann Noninvasive Electrocardiol 2010;15:56.

Vardas PE, Auricchio A, Blanc JJ, et al. Guidelines for cardiac pacing and cardiac resynchronization therapy: The Task Force for Cardiac Pacing and Cardiac Resynchronization Therapy of the European Society of Cardiology. Developed in collaboration with the European Heart Rhythm Association. Eur Heart J 2007;28:2256.

Vázquez R, Bayés-Genis A, Cygankiewicz I, et al. The MUSIC risk score: a simple method for predicting mortality in ambulatory patients with chronic heart failure. Eur Heart J 2009;30:1088.

Voller H. PreSCD II trial. ESC session 3591-91. 2009

Wannamethee G, Shaper AG. Alcohol and sudden cardiac death. Br Heart J 1992;68:443.

Wellens HJ, Gorgels A, Doevedans P. The ECG in acute myocardial infarction and unstable angina. Kluwer Academic Publishers, Dordrecht, 2003.

Yan G-X, Joshi A, Guo D, et al. Phase 2 reentry as a trigger to initiate ventricular fibrillation during early acute myocardial ischemia. Circulation 2004; 110:1036.

Yazdan-Ashoori P, Baranchuk A. Obstructive sleep apnea may increase the risk of stroke in AF patients: refining the CHADS$_2$ score. Int J Cardiol 2011;146:131.

Zuppiroli A, Mori F, Favilli S, et al. Arrhythmias in mitral valve prolapse: Relation to anterior mitral leaflet thickening, clinical variables, and color Doppler echocardiographic parameters. Am Heart J 1994;128:919.

Appendix

Introduction

In this appendix we will first deal with the calculation of parameters such as sensitivity (Se), specificity (Sp), and predictive value (PV). These parameters help to determine the actual value of an electrocardiogram (ECG) criterion for the diagnosis of a given arrhythmia, for example, for the differential diagnosis between ventricular tachycardia (VT) and aberrant supraventricular tachycardia in cases of tachycardias with a wide QRS (see Chapter 5, Classic Ventricular Tachycardias). Another example is the importance of the presence of slurring at the end of the QRS complex to differentiate, in cases of paroxysmal junctional reentrant tachycardia, the type of circuit involved (see Chapter 4, Junctional Reentrant Tachycardia: Electrocardiographic Findings).

Later, we will comment on the most useful techniques mentioned throughout the book for the diagnosis of cardiac arrhythmias, along with clinical and surface ECG data.

In this book, we do not go deeply into the pharmacologic and nonpharmacologic technical details of the treatment of different arrhythmias, although we will comment, sometimes extensively, on the most important practical aspects. We recommend consulting the referenced bibliography and the guidelines of different societies (p. xvii). We often include these recommendations in this book. At the end of this Appendix (see A-6), we explain how the guideline recommendations are divided into three groups (I–III) depending on the benefit obtained and also the risk derived from their use. The degree of evidence supporting these recommendations is also described.

Calculation of Sensitivity, Specificity, and Predictive Value
(Table A-1)

The calculation of these parameters is very important in determining the value of any ECG or clinical diagnostic criteria in daily clinical practice.

Conventional electrocardiography may be considered the technique of reference, or gold standard, for the diagnosis of atrial and ventricular blocks, ventricular pre-excitation, most types of cardiac arrhythmia, and some types of acute myocardial infarction (AMI) (in the last instance, when ECG series are performed). It is sometimes necessary, however, to perform other ECG techniques, including invasive techniques, to ascertain the diagnosis. This may be the case in some wide QRS complex tachycardias, or when the localization of an accessory pathway should be confirmed.

In any case, it is very useful to know: (i) the diagnostic value of the criteria applied when interpreting routine ECGs when the ECG is not gold standard (i.e., diagnostic criteria for atrial or ventricular enlargement, necrosis, wide QRS complex tachycardia, etc.); and (ii) the prognostic value of the ECG or other electrocardiographic techniques (i.e., late potentials (LP), T wave alternance, etc.) to predict the occurrence of any particular condition (i.e., ventricular tachycardia/ventricular fibrillation) during the follow-up of post-infarction patients. It is important to apply the concepts of Se, Sp, and PV to both of these considerations.

With this purpose in mind, we can compare the results of the trial test (the presence or absence of determined ECG criteria or a positive or negative result obtained with another ECG technique) with those of the gold standard confirmatory diagnostic technique (reference test). The reference test may be another electrocardiographic test (i.e., intracavitary techniques, in cases of wide QRS complex tachycardia) or another kind of technique (echocardiography, hemodynamics or clinical evaluations, presence or absence of the disease, etc.).

The results from the trial test (presence or absence of a determined ECG criterion, or a positive or negative result in an ECG test) and those from the reference confirmatory diagnostic test (whether it is another electrocardiographic or a different technique, the clinical presence of the disease, etc.) may be presented in a 2×2 table, where the results of the trial test are distributed in

Clinical Arrhythmology, Second Edition. Antoni Bayés de Luna and Adrian Baranchuk.
© 2017 John Wiley & Sons Ltd. Published 2017 by John Wiley & Sons Ltd.

Table A-1 Calculation of Se, Sp, PPV, and NPV.

		Post-myocardial infarction patients (210 pat.)			
		Patients with VT/VF during follow-up	Patients without VT/VF during follow-up		
Late potentials	+	9	40	49	PPV=TP/(TP+FP)= 9/ (9+40)×100=18%
	−	1	160	161	NPV=TN/(TN+FN)= 160/ (160+1)×100=99%
		10	200	210	
		Se=TP/(TP+FN)= 9/(9+1) × 100=90%	Sp=TN/(TN+FP)= 160/ (160+40)×100=80%		

Practical example of the prediction of a clinical event, in this case sudden cardiac death in post-infarction patients, using the information obtained through an electrocardiographic technique (in this case, positivity or negativity of late ventricular potentials). FN, false negative; FP, false positive; NPV, negative predictive value; PPV, positive predictive value; Se, sensitivity; Sp, specificity; TN, true negative; TP, true positive.

the columns, and the real distribution of the process in question, according to the reference test, is distributed in the rows (Table A-1). From this table, Se, Sp, and PV indexes of each trial test may be calculated. Until recently, these concepts were not applied to the ECG diagnosis and, as a result, the ECG diagnosis was intuitive rather than rational in many cases. We will now explain the most important characteristics of these indexes.

o **Specificity (Sp).** The Sp in a trial test (or in this case, specificity of a criterion obtained from a surface ECG or another ECG technique) is defined as the percentage of people without the disease that does not present this ECG criterion. The higher the proportion of persons without a disease who do not show a given ECG criterion, the more specific is this criterion. For instance, if we consider the value of the criterion "QRS with a slow start and high R wave in VR" for the diagnosis of VT (Vereckei *et al.*, 2008) (see Chapter 5, Classic Ventricular Tachycardias) in cases of wide QRS complex tachycardia, the Sp would be 90% if this criterion is found in 10/100 patients without VT. If this criterion is not present in any of the subjects without VT, the Sp would be 100%. The formula used to calculate Sp is:

$$Sp = \frac{True\ negatives\,(TN)}{TN + FP\,(false\ positives)}$$

where FP is false positives and TN is true negatives.

o **Sensitivity (Se).** The Se of an ECG criterion is defined as the percentage of people with a determined disease (i.e., VT) with evidence of an ECG criterion (i.e., QRS with slow inscription and high R waves in VR). If 95%

of patients with VT show this ECG criterion, Se is 95%. The formula to calculate Se is:

$$Se = \frac{True\ positives\,(TP)}{TP + FN\,(false\ negatives)}$$

where FN is false negatives and TP is true positives.

It should be noted that the Sp is determined in a control group (people who do not have the disease under study), whereas the Se is assessed in the group of people with the disease. These two groups have been previously classified using other reference techniques (echocardiography, angiography, clinical outcomes, etc.).

o **Predictive value (PV).** The PV represents the clinical significance of a test. It indicates the actual utility of the test result, whether positive or negative. It shows the likelihood that a positive test result (presence of sign or symptom) indicates disease (positive predictive value (PPV)) or that a negative test result (absent sign of symptom) excludes disease (negative predictive value (NPV)). It is very important to remember that both the Se and Sp of a test or diagnostic criterion depend on the test itself, whereas **the predictive value depends on the prevalence of the disease in the study population** (epidemiology).

We will now give an example of how Se, Sp, and PV are calculated. Let us suppose (Table A-1) that we run a study with a cohort of 210 post-infarction patients to determine the number of patients who will suffer from VT/VF, and we would like to know if the presence of late potentials (LP) will allow us to identify them. Therefore, we should find out the PPV and NPV for the LP technique, or in other words, its value as a marker of poor prognosis in post-infarction patients. We postulate that in a one-year follow-up, 10 out of 210 post-infarction patients will have VT/ VF. Table A-1 shows the Se, Sp, and PV for the LP technique in this particular scenario. Both Se and Sp are high (the latter being 80%), but as there is a large number of patients without VT/VF (200 patients), there are 40 patients without VT/VF that had positive LP. This should be added to the 9/10 patients with VT/VF who also had LP. As a result, only 9/49 patients with positive LP suffered from VT/VF during the follow-up. This explains why the PPV is very low (<20%). On the other hand, the NPV is very high (>99%), because only 1/161 patients with negative LP suffered from VT/VF during the follow-up. This implies that if LP are negative, the risk of VT/VF is very low (<1%), whereas if they are positive, the risk of developing VT/VF is not very high (<20%).

Alternatively, if the number of post-infarction patients who suffered from VT/VF during the follow-up was higher (i.e., ≈50%, or 100 out of 210) with the same Se (90%) and Sp (80%), the number of patients with positive LP would be quite different: 112 (90 (90% of 100 with VT/VF) + 22 (20% of the 110 without VT/VF)). In this situation, the PPV would be much higher:

$$PPV = \frac{(TP)90\left(90\% \text{ of } 100 \text{ cases with VT / VF}\right)}{90 + 22(FP)\left(20\% \text{ of } 110 \text{ cases without VT / VF}\right)} > 85\%,$$

even at the expense of a somewhat lower NPV:

$$NPV = \frac{(TN)88\left(80\% \text{ of } 110 \text{ cases without VT / VF}\right)}{88 + 10(FN)\left(10\% \text{ of } 100 \text{ cases with VT / VF}\right)} \approx 90\%.$$

For this reason, when examining PV, one should consider the epidemiologic reality of each situation.

The procedure to calculate the Se, Sp, PPV, and NPV (as shown in Table A-1) is certainly practical and simple, and there is no need to remember formulas, although we use them indirectly.

It should be noted that the Se and Sp of the different ECG criteria are inversely proportional to each other, in such a way that highly specific criteria are usually not very sensitive. We believe that it is better to use criteria that are highly specific (very few false positives) even at the expense of a lower Se. The ideal scenario would be to have both Se and Sp higher than 90%. Nevertheless, we should remember that depending on the type and size of the sample, even with relatively high Sp and Se (≥80%), the actual utility of a sign (PPV) may be low (Table A-1).

- **Very sensitive ECG signs,** although less specific, **are useful for screening,** whereas the **very specific signs usually confirm the presence of a disease**, but frequently do not appear when the disease is present. The clinician should know the Se, Sp, and PV of the different ECG criteria as well as the different ECG tests, among other types of tests, in order to better determine if a given disease is present or not.

- **Theorem of Bayes.** Finally, we should remember that the reliability of a test (ECG criteria, in this case) increases or decreases according to Bayes' theorem, named after the monk who described it in the eighteenth century. According to this theorem, **the predictive value of a criterion will increase among populations with a higher prevalence of heart disease** (high *a priori* likelihood of suffering from the disease); as prevalence decreases (low *a priori* likelihood of suffering from the disease), the predictive value of the criterion decreases. For example, in a case of wide QRS complex tachycardia, the likelihood of it being ventricular is higher if it is observed in a high-risk group (history of ischemic heart disease (IHD) and other VT episodes) than when observed in non-risk populations (i.e. young adults without documented heart disease).

Diagnostic Techniques

We will give a brief review of the different techniques, including ECG techniques, which, along with clinical history and surface ECGs, are useful to establish a differential diagnosis and to determine both the prognosis and the best therapeutic measures in each case. We will describe the most important indications and the utility of each technique in daily clinical practice.

Holter ECG Monitoring and Related Techniques

Holter ECG monitoring is a continuous ECG recording with accelerated interpretation of data invented by the physicist N. Holter more than 50 years ago. This technique is to the conventional ECG what cinema is to photography. Thanks to this technique we can determine cardiac electrical activity during daily activities (Bayés de Luna *et al.*, 1983).

Holter ECG monitoring is very useful for the diagnosis and evaluation of arrhythmias (Table A-2 and Figures A-1 to A-4). It may be used to quantify the number as well as to determine the characteristics of arrhythmias, the point in time at which they occur, their relationship with exercise, emotions, and sleep, and 24-h (or longer) heart rate behavior, in addition to being used to stratify the risk of sudden death (SD) (Bigger *et al.*, 1984) and to identify the arrhythmia that triggers it (Bayés de Luna *et al.*, 1989). Today, with digital recording systems, data interpretation may be done through the Internet, subsequently saving money and time (Figure A-1). Currently, prolonged recordings of up to seven days are available; they are especially useful to detect the incidence of paroxysmal atrial fibrillation (AF) and to assess whether they have disappeared after ablation. On certain occasions, Holter ECG monitoring may also be useful in studying repolarization alterations (Table A.2).

Holter technology allows us to assess different disturbances of the autonomic nervous system (ANS) based on the study of different parameters, such as RR interval variability (HRV), dynamic QT behavior, and heart rate turbulence (HRT), among others. However, the abovementioned parameters usually have a low PPV. Their real value in daily practice has yet to be completely established. Nevertheless, many published studies show the potential utility of these parameters for risk stratification in postinfarction patients and in heart failure (HF) patients, in addition to other clinical situations (see Chapter 11, Heart Failure). At present, the possibility of using a score from various Holter ECG parameters to increase the PPV of this technology is being investigated. For more information, consult the guidelines of the different scientific societies (Recommended General Bibliography p. xvii).

Event Analyzer

Conventional systems for the telephone transmission of ECG data are available, well known, and obviously useful,

especially if no physician is available or if a pacemaker is to be controlled. Systems related to Holter ECG monitoring, which allow for ECG recording at the time when certain symptoms occur, are particularly interesting (event analyzer). These data are subsequently transmitted by telephone or through the Internet for interpretation. This is of great interest in the study of sporadic symptomatic arrhythmias (Figure A-1).

Currently available implantable loop recorders (Krahn *et al.*, 2004) allow us to more frequently determine the cause of unexplained syncope occurring sporadically in patients who usually have good ventricular function but whose life may be at risk (Reveal Medtronic). In the RAST trial (Krahn *et al.*, 2001), it was demonstrated that the implantable loop recorder is more effective, in terms of diagnosing the cause of unexplained syncope, than the conventional method (conventional event analyzer + tilt table test + intracavitary electrophysiological study (IES)). These loop recorders (REVEAL LINQ, Medtronic) can be implanted subcutaneously in less than three minutes and their battery lasts about three years. The quality of the recordings is identical to other forms of extended cardiac monitoring. Telemetry home monitoring of the implanted device (Ricci *et al.*, 2008) has been shown to be very useful for patient follow-up after pacemaker and implantable cardioverter defibrillator (ICD) implantation, as well as for the detection of paroxysmal arrhythmias (Ricci *et al.*, 2009). Finally, currently long recording ECG monitoring are used in post-stroke cases to help in decision of anticoagulation.

Latest Technologies for Extended Cardiac Monitoring

There is no doubt that extended cardiac monitoring is the future of AF detection and follow-up treatments. For AF detection, only one lead is necessary. Several types of external devices (watches, iPhones, wrist bands) are now available and being tested in different ongoing trials.

Exercise Testing

We will not explain in detail how this test is performed because it is a well-known technique for the reader (Theroux *et al.*, 1979). Conventional exercise testing may be performed according to the Bruce protocol or, in cases where HF is present, according to the Naughton protocol (Bayés de Luna, 2011; Recommended General Bibliography p. xvii). Although generally no major complications occur, very serious ventricular tachyarrhythmias are exceptionally present (Figure A-5C), requiring immediate cardioversion, or advanced AV block due to coronary spasms (see Figure 6.48). Therefore, emergency treatment facilities should be available (cardiopulmonary resuscitation protocol).

Table A-2 Usefulness of Holter monitoring.

Arrhythmias

- Determination of the prevalence of the different arrhythmias in healthy subjects and in the different diseases (Figure A-2)
- Determination of a possible correlation between the symptoms the patient shows (dizziness, palpitations, syncope, etc.) and the presence of arrhythmias (Figure A-3)
- Assessment of the antiarrhythmic pharmacologic treatment and post-ablation treatment
- Assessment of the electrophysiologic mechanism of arrhythmias
- Determination of the arrhythmia responsible for the sudden death (SD) (Bayés de Luna *et al.*, 1989) (see Figure 1.8)
- SD stratification risk (see Figure 11.4)
- Control of the pacemaker function (Figure A-4).

Repolarization alterations

1. Repolarization alterations not due to ischemic heart disease (IHD)
2. Repolarization alterations due to IHD; secondary angina vs. primary angina
3. Silent ischemia
4. Control of treatment for angina
5. Post-infarction risk stratification

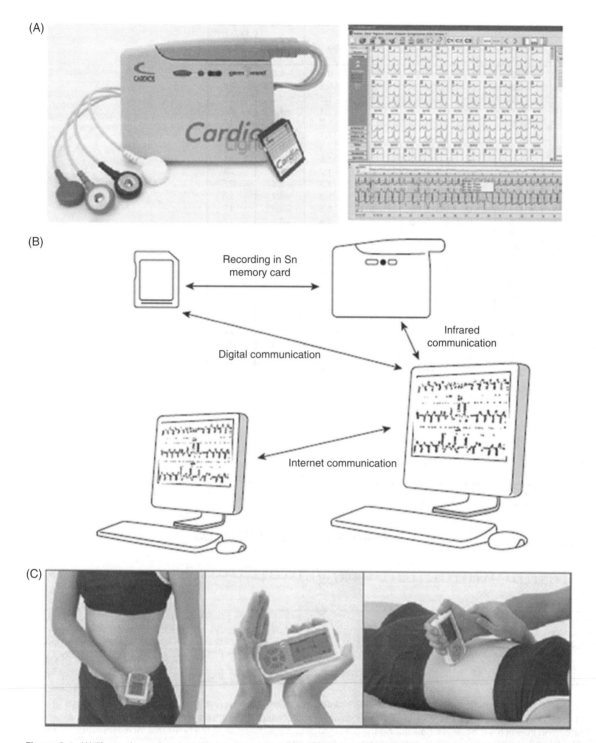

Figure A-1 (A) Three-channel 24-h Holter electrocardiogram (ECG) recorder with software screen. (B) Holter remote acquisition platform. (C) Holter event monitor (www.medicalproductguide.com/companies/14816/gem-med-sl).

In patients with cardiac arrhythmias the exercise test is very useful for:

o Checking whether the premature ventricular complexes (PVC) occur or disappear during exercise and recovery (Figure A-5).

o Assessing the sinus response to exercise in cases of possible inappropriate sinus tachycardia response.

o Checking the response to exercise in a patient with a tachycardia at around 100–120 bpm, when it is uncertain whether the tachycardia is of sinus origin or not (i.e., flutter 2×1 should be ruled out). This may be done

(A)

Time Period	Total PAC	Isolated PAC	Runs of PAC	Beats in Runs of PAC	Total Pauses	Max ST mm	Min ST mm	Max ST Slope degrees
1-13:15	426	255	44	171	2	0.8	−1.5	42
1-14:15	36	33	1	3	2	0.8	−1.1	22
1-15:15	2	2	0	0	2	1.1	−1.3	22
1-16:15	6	6	0	0	2	1.1	−1.1	27
1-17:15	7	3	1	4	5	1.3	−1.3	17
1-18:15	1	1	0	0	5	1.1	−0.8	17
1-19:15	6.093	2	8	6.091	0	1.5	−0.8	35
1-20:15	10.052	0	14	10.052	0	1.5	−0.8	45
1-21:15	1.048	0	13	1.048	0	1.7	−1.7	40
1-22:15	3	3	0	0	0	1.3	−2.1	27
1-23:15	0	0	0	0	0	1.3	−1.7	27
2-00:15	1	1	0	0	0	0.8	−0.6	17
2-01 :15	3	3	0	0	0	0.8	−0.6	17
2-02:15	3	3	0	0	0	1.1	−0.2	11
2-03:15	13	10	1	3	1	1.3	−0.4	11
2-04:15	0	0	0	0	1	1.1	−0.2	14
2-05:15	5	5	0	0	0	0.8	−0.2	11
2-06:15	4	0	1	4	0	1.3	−0.6	17
2-07:15	4	4	0	0	1	1.1	−0.4	22
2-08:15	1	1	0	0	1	1.1	−0.4	17
2-09:15	1	1	0	0	0	0.8	−0.8	22
2-10:15	2	2	0	0	0	0.8	−0.8	27
2-11:15	2	2	0	0	0	0.8	−1.1	22
2-12:15	0	0	0	0	0	0.6	−0.8	17
	17.713	337	83	17.376	22	1.7	2.1	45

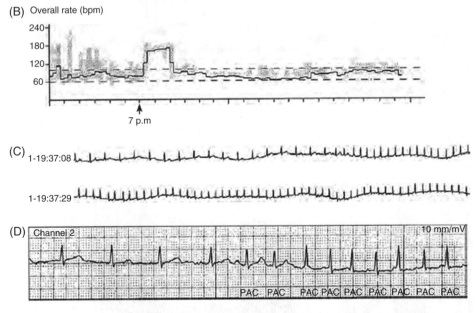

(B) Overall rate (bpm)

7 p.m

(C) 1-19:37:08

1-19:37:29

(D) Channel 2 · 10 mm/mV

PAC PAC PAC PAC PAC PAC PAC PAC PAC

Figure A-2 (A) Time schedule of premature atrial complexes (PAC), isolated or in runs (it is observed that at 7–9 p.m. a paroxysmal tachycardia episode occurs). The number of pauses and ST elevations are also recorded. There are no premature ventricular complexes (PVC). (B) Heart rate trend in which it is observed how during the paroxysmal tachycardia episode the heart rate increases abruptly and stays unchanged for 2 h. (C) and (D) Onset of the paroxysmal tachycardia episode.

by instructing the patient to do a small amount of exercise and checking the heart rate response.

o Determining whether a progressive or sudden heart rate increase is observed in patients with bradycardia. This is a key factor for the differential diagnosis between sinus bradycardia (progressive heart rate increase) and a 2×1 sinoatrial block (sudden heart rate increase).

o Checking the presence of symptoms or ECG changes that may suggest IHD.

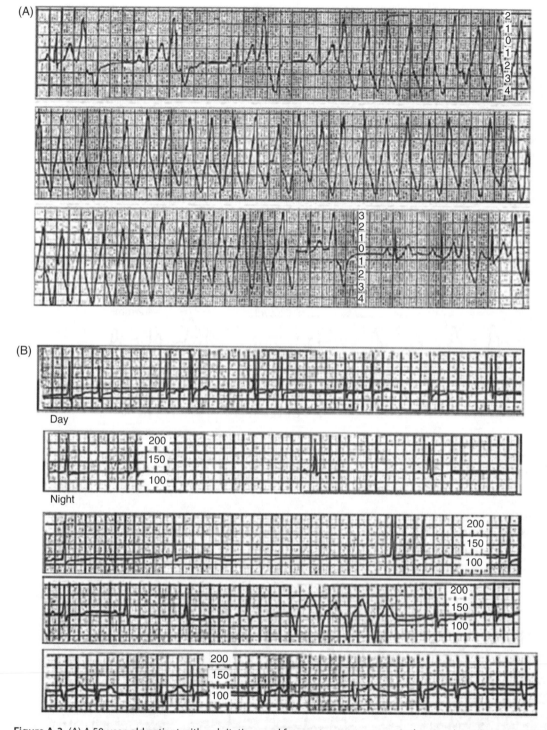

Figure A-3 (A) A 50-year-old patient with palpitations and frequent premature ventricular complexes (PVC, often bigeminal PVC) and runs of ventricular tachycardia (VT), some of which are particularly long (>15″), with a heart rate >150 bpm. (B) A 75-year-old patient with palpitations. The ECG Holter recording showed a sick sinus node (asymptomatic pauses >4″ and frequent premature atrial complexes (PAC), sometimes bigeminal, which are part of a bradycardia-tachycardia syndrome, requiring a pacemaker implantation. Also a run of VT is recorded.

(A)

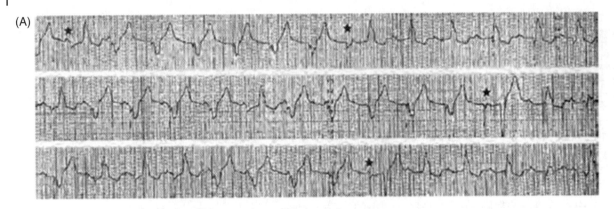

(B)

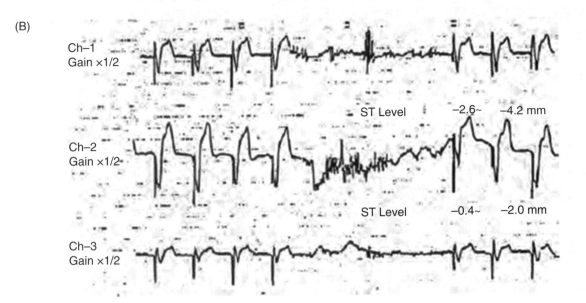

Figure A-4 (A) Stimulation failure (spikes not followed by QRS) (stars) detected by the electrocardiogram (ECG) Holter. (B) Long pause detected by the ECG Holter, due to myopotentials, as a result of interferences caused by muscular contractions (the most frequent cause of oversensing).

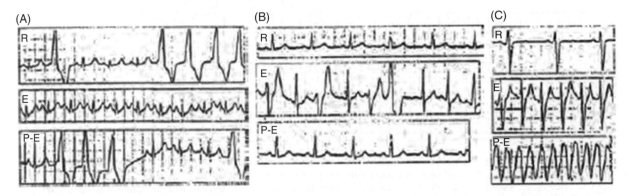

Figure A-5 (A) A young patient without heart disease in whom frequent premature ventricular complexes (PVC) and slow runs of ventricular tachycardia (VT) disappear with exercise (E). (B) Heart disease patient without PVC, who showed frequent PVC during exercise, sometimes repetitive and polymorphic, which disappeared once exercise was discontinued (PE). (C) Even serious arrhythmias may rarely occur. This was a heart disease patient who showed ventricular flutter just after exercise testing, requiring immediate cardioversion R (Rest).

Figure A-6 Catheter location for ablation. Right arterial oblique position (RAO) (right) and left anterior oblique position (LAO) (left). The CS catheter gives us information on electrical activity of the left side without arterial access. CS = coronary sinus; H = His; V = apex RV.

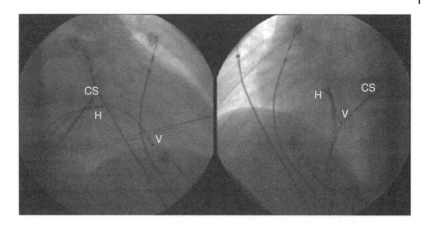

For more information, refer to the guidelines of the different scientific societies (Recommended General Bibliography p. xvii).

Intracavitary ECG and Electrophysiologic Studies

Intracavitary ECG and electrophysiologic studies (EPS) allow for a better assessment of cardiac electrical activity. To perform this study it is necessary to insert various catheters into the heart, which stimulate and record intracavitary electrograms (Figure A-6). These techniques include:

- Electrical activity recording in different areas of the atria and ventricles, including the His bundle and branches. This has allowed us to better understand the activation sequence of the heart, both in normal and pathologic situations.
- Programmed electrical stimulation, including pacing techniques at increasing heart rates, and the application of extra stimulus at progressively shorter intervals with respect to the baseline rhythm, to study the refractory periods of the stimulated area (Figure A-7).

These techniques are very useful in clinical arrhythmology (Table A-3 and Figures A-8–A to A-11). In many situations, despite the great amount of information obtained by the surface ECG, performing an intracavitary ECG and carrying out EPS is essential, not only to confirm the diagnosis but also to determine the best treatment for each type of arrhythmias. Some paradigmatic cases, for example, involve: (i) determining the exact location of an AV block (Figures A-8 and 6.21); (ii) the study of sinus function (Figure A-9); (iii) the mechanisms of a wide QRS tachycardia (Figures A-10 and A-11); (iv) the best area for catheter ablation of a VT (see Figures 5.30 and 5.31), AF (see Figure 4.55), atrial flutter (see Figure 4.68), or precisely identifying the circuit involved in a reentrant AV junctional tachycardia, including WPW syndrome (see Figures 4.25 and 4.26); and (v) they are also very important for guiding the implantation of an automatic ICD or resynchronization pacemaker (CRT), as well as catheter ablation (see later).

Thanks to these techniques, surface ECG diagnosis has advanced considerably so that we are able to apply the data obtained by intracavitary studies to the conventional ECG.

Tilt Table Test

The tilt table test technique is used to unmask the susceptibility to neutrally-mediated (vasovagal) syncope in patients with unexplained syncope. It is useful to confirm the diagnosis of neuromediated syncope, but not for evaluating the efficacy of treatments (see Chapter 1, Syncope). The tilt table test involves placing the patient on a table with a foot support, then tilting the table upward into a complete vertical position. The patient is instructed to remain resting, with the aim of assessing whether syncope occurs spontaneously or after the administration of drugs (i.e., nitroglycerin), at which point the table is returned to a flat (horizontal) position and the syncope disappears (Sutton and Bloomfield, 1999).

It has been reported that during tilt table testing the presence of oscillating systolic blood pressure, varying at ≥30 mm in patients who are nonresponders to the passive head-up tilt and glyceryl trinitrate provocation, may be considered the equivalent to vasovagal syncope, possibly obviating the need for other tests, such as the isoprenaline test (Hausenloy *et al.*, 2009).

Neuromediated syncope may be of a vasodepressor, cardioinhibitory, or mixed type (see Chapter 1, Syncope). Cardioinhibitory response may occur in the form of sinus bradycardia, leading to sinus arrest (20% of the cases in a tilt test) or AV block (4% of the cases) (Figures 1-12 and A-12) (Brignole, 2009). When it is established

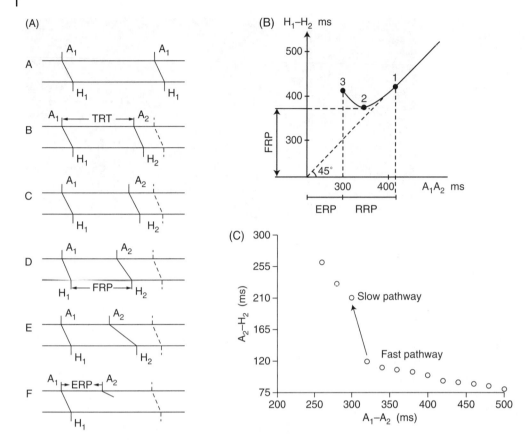

Figure A-7 Diagram showing the different tissue refractory periods, in particular the atrioventricular (AV) node RP. (A) Response sequence to increasingly premature stimuli (A2). (B) Curve obtained from A1–A2 and H1–H2 values under normal conduction conditions. TRT (total recovery time) = shortest distance between the basal impulse (A) and the extra stimulus, with the latter being normally conducted (A2 H2 = A1 H1) (see B in A). FRP (functional refractory period): the shortest H1–H2, regardless of the A1–A2 distance (see D in A and 2 in B) (effective refractory period). ERP: the longest A1–A2 distance that is not followed by a hisian deflection (see F in A and 3 in B). Relative refractory period (RRP) starts when A2–H2 > A1–H1, that is to say, at the end of the TRT, and lasts until the beginning of the ERP (3 in B). (C) Confirmation of AV conduction through both α and β pathways. Note the A2–H2 response (AV conduction), to increasingly shorter A1–A2 (see A). With A1–A2 = 300 ms, the β pathway ERP is reached, resulting in an abrupt and significant A2–H2 increase, as conduction is then only through the α pathway, up to 250 cm, where the ERP of the α pathway is reached.

Table A-3 Utility of intracavitary electrophysiologic studies.

- Study of the refractory periods of the different zones of the heart (Figure A-7)
- Topographic location of the atrioventricular (AV) block (Figures A-8, 6.21)
- Study of the AV (Figure A-7) and VA conduction characteristics
- Study of the sinus function (Figure A-8)
- Study of the accessory pathways characteristics
- Study of the mechanisms of a wide QRS tachycardia and their differential diagnosis (Figures A-10 and A-11)
- Pharmacoelectrophysiology
- Implantable cardioverter defibrillator (ICD) implantation and ablation techniques
- Improvement of diagnostic precision of conventional electrocardiogram (ECG)

that the patient shows the same symptoms as before, the diagnosis is confirmed. A significant cardioinhibitory response, especially if occurring previously to the vasodepressor response, may call for pacemaker implantation, which would become activated when heart rate decreases (Medtronic Venta). However, as syncope usually has a vasodepressor component, a pacemaker implantation does not a guaranteed solution that no more syncope may occur.

Controversy exists about the value of Tilt test for the diagnosis of syncope of unknown origin, given its low specificity and low positive predictive value. In 2006, a group of experts did not include the Tilt Test in its recommendations on an algorithm to determine the cause of syncope (Strickberger *et al.*, 2006). On some occasions, reproducing the symptom during the Tilt Test may help the patients recognizing prodromal symptoms

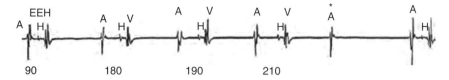

Figure A-8 Electrophysiologic studies (EPS) in a patient with Wenckebach-type 5×4 AV block with pre-hisian block. Note the progressive prolongation of the AH interval, until the fifth A* is not conducted. The more significant conduction delay occurs between the first and second A–H intervals.

Figure A-9 A very long sinus recovery period (SRP). Before the first sinus P wave occurs (A in EHH), two hisian deflexions (H) have been recorded.

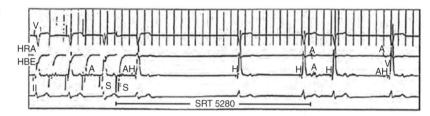

Figure A-10 Ventricular tachycardia (VT) triggered by two extrastimuli separated by 220 ms.

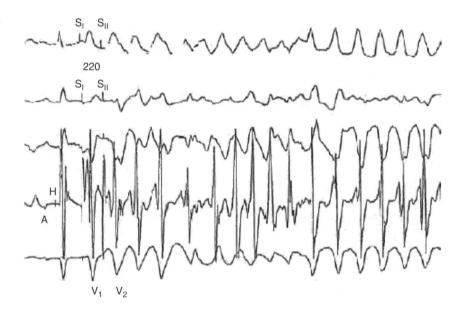

helping them to deal with the real clinical scenarios. As reproducibility is low, serial Tilt Testing is not recommended for the follow-up or for testing drugs or other treatments. Full interrogation using well-validated scores (Sheldon, 2013) can replace the Tilt Test in several cases. The tilt table is still useful as part of the holistic analysis of dysautonomic syndromes.

Analysis of Late Potentials Using a Signal Averaging Electrocardiogram (SAECG)

Late potentials (LP) are low amplitude potentials that are present at the end or after the QRS complex (Figure A-13). They are due to a late activation of myocardial zones where viable muscle tissue alternates with necrotic and/or fibrotic zones. They have been shown to be independent markers of sustained VT (Breithardt *et al.*, 1983).

This technique has been used in coronary patients to detect those at higher risk of developing VT/VF by showing those areas with slow conduction due to the presence of a post-infarction scar. When positive, it is also useful for the diagnosis of arrhythmogenic right ventricular cardiomyopathy and Brugada's syndrome. Generally, Se and Sp are quite high, but in epidemiologic reality, PPV is usually low, whereas NPV is high (see A-1). For example, consider post-infarction patients and the risk of VT/VF (Table A-1). In these cases the PPV is low ($\approx$20%), so that, in theory, only a small percentage of post-infarction patients with positive post-potentials will have sudden cardiac death in the future. However, the clinical practice value is caused by the fact that the

NPV is very high (99%). This means that when LP are negative, the risk of developing sudden cardiac death is very low. Therefore, it is necessary to combine new parameters to increase the PPV. In this sense, the papers published by Gomes *et al.* (1987) and Kuchar *et al.* (1987) are very relevant. The former demonstrated that in patients with positive LP and EF <40%, the number of Holter monitoring ventricular PVC was significant and the prognosis (occurrence of malignant arrhythmias) was poorer. Meanwhile, the latter author showed that patients with positive LP, Lown grade III–IV (Holter), and EF <40% had a 30% possibility of suffering from a severe arrhythmic event during a one-year follow-up. In contrast, patients with only one factor had a much lower chance of suffering from severe arrhythmia (<5%).

Body Surface Potential Mapping

Body surface potential mapping has been used for decades for investigational purposes. Currently, portable and fast electrode placement devices allowing for good quality ECG tracings are available.

These methods generate QRST mappings that allow us to investigate the likelihood of developing arrhythmias and produce risk stratification, although usage in daily clinical practice is very limited (De Ambroggi *et al.*, 1991; Hubley-Kozey *et al.*, 1995; Korhonen *et al.*, 2009). They have been used to demonstrate the importance of late depolarization theory to explain how the typical pattern of coved ST segment in Brugada's syndrome is originated (Postema *et al.*, 2010).

Other Surface Techniques to Record Electrical Cardiac Activity

- **Vectorcardiography** has been a crucial technique in identifying many ECG patterns as atrial (Figures 3.19 and 6.14) and ventricular blocks (Figures 3.26–3.29) (Bayés de Luna *et al.*, 1985). At present it is very useful for educational purposes (Bayés de Luna, 2011; Pérez

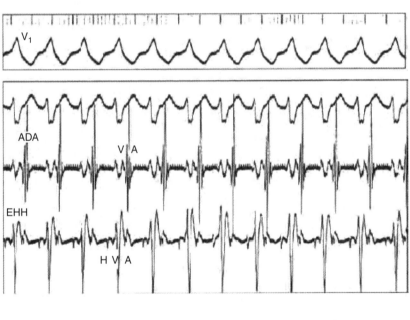

Figure A-11 Wide QRS tachycardia (see V1). The electrophysiologic study showed that the tachycardia was supraventricular in origin, with anterograde activation by the specific conduction system (SCS) (H before V) and retrograde activation through an accessory pathway (A after V). The QRS complex was wide because of an associated right bundle branch block (RBBB) (aberrancy).

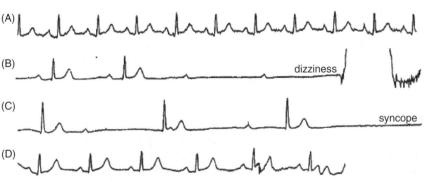

Figure A-12 (A) A young man with syncopal attacks, probably neuromediated (vagal), and a normal electrocardiogram (ECG). Tilt testing was positive, presenting dizziness and cardioinhibitory response with advanced atrioventricular (AV) block (B and C). After recovery in the normal position the AV block completely disappeared.

Riera *et al.*, 2007; Recommended General Bibliography p. xvii). However, the use of vectorcardiography in clinical arrhythmology is very limited. It may be useful in detecting the presence of pre-excitation in uncertain cases, and to better study the cases with atypical pattern of advanced interatrial block, and also along with 12-lead ECG recordings and body mapping, to study the origin of the Brugada pattern (late depolarization hypothesis) (Postema *et al.*, 2010).

- **Wave amplification techniques**, sometimes along with ECG recording at a faster speed, may be useful to better determine atrial activity or make it more visible when not apparent (see Figures 4.38, 4.62, and 5.21) and to diagnose the presence of AV dissociation, which, in turn, is crucial for the differential diagnosis between VT and aberrant supraventricular tachycardia (see Figure 5.21).
- **T wave filtering techniques** allow us to visualize the P wave when it is concealed in the preceding T wave (Goldwasser *et al.*, 2011). We hope this system will be commercialized soon. At present, T wave filtering techniques help to diagnose the location of atrial waves, which may be very useful to better diagnose different types of supraventricular tachyarrhythmias (Figure A-13). There are also promising results showing the possibility to detect AV dissociation in patients with broad QRS tachycardia.

On occasion, the recording of a bipolar precordial lead (Lewis lead) may also be useful. This is obtained by placing the right arm electrode in the second right intercostal space and the left arm electrode in the fourth right intercostal space (Bakker *et al.* 2009).

Other Nonelectrocardiographic Techniques

- **Imaging techniques,** especially **echocardiography**, may be useful to determine left ventricular function and to study right ventricular or aortic pathology. Echocardiography is the first-choice imaging technique for the diagnosis of structural heart disease and the study of dysynchrony between both ventricles that it is useful when deciding if CRT is needed (see later). Currently, echocardiography is used for CRT optimization (looking at mitral regurgitative "jets" or strain) to determine the most efficacious AV delay and V–V delay. It is of less value to identify candidates for CRT as the LVEF and the widening of the QRS represent better markers.
- **CV magnetic resonance** is a key technique to rule out or confirm the diagnosis in some diseases such as arrhythmogenic RVC/D, anomalous origin of coronary arteries, or to better study other diseases such as cardiomyopathies. It is also very useful for detecting atrial fibrosis what is crucial to assess the feasibility of

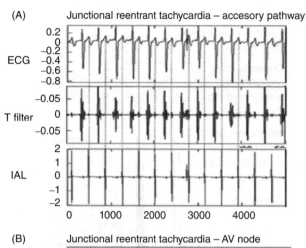

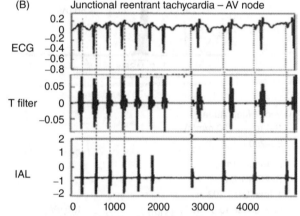

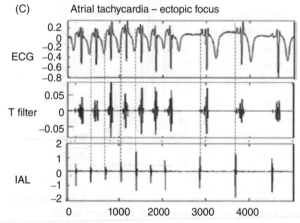

Figure A-13 The technique of T wave filtering allows us to properly locate the atrial wave that is often hidden in the previous T wave. The figure shows three examples with a comparison of surface electrocardiogram (ECG), filtering technique (FT), and intra atrial lead (IAL) to correlate the value of the filtering technique. We can check that FT allows us to identify the appropriate atrial wave in three types of different supraventricular tachyarrhythmias: A = AVRT, B = AVNRT, and C - AT-EF.

CV or AF ablation as demonstrated (Oakes *et al.*, 2009). However, the majority of CV machines cannot offer the possibility to clearly detect atrial fibrosis yet (see Chapter 4, Atrial Fibrillation: Treatment).

(A) Vector Magnitude
400 mm/s 1.00 mm/uV
25–250 Hz

Durations (ms):
Std QRS 105
1 Total QRS 105
LAS under 40 uV 27

MSR Voltages (uV):
Total QRS 532.8
2 Last 40 ms 54.8
Noise 0.2

Cycles 225.0

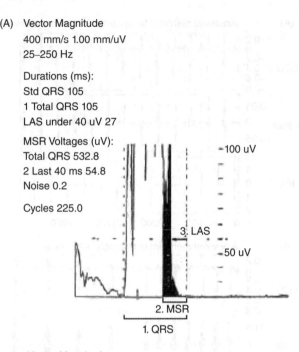

(B) Vector Magnitude
100 mm/s 1.00 mm/uV
25–250 Hz

Durations (ms):
Std QRS 120
1 Total QRS 202
LAS under 40 uV 125

MSR Voltages (uV):
Total QRS 66.4
2 Last 40 ms 2.7
Noise 0.3

Cycles 237.0

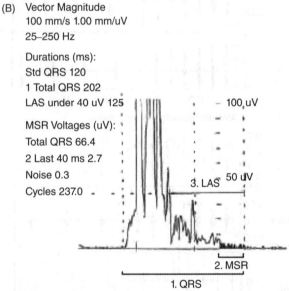

Figure A-14 Late potential normal recording in a patient without heart disease (A) and in a patient with right ventricle (RV) arrhythmogenic dysplasia (B). In the first case, none of the three diagnostic criteria are met: (i) QRS = 105 ms; (ii) MSR (mean square root) voltage of the last 40 ms = 54.8; and (iii) low amplitude signal (LAS) under 40 μV = 27. In the second case the three criteria are met: (i) QRS = 202 ms; (ii) MSR (last 40 ms) = 2.7; and (iii) LAS (<40 μV) = 125.

- Non-invasive (**multislice scanner**) or even invasive coronary angiography may also be necessary to assess the anatomic and functional state of the coronary circulation. The multislice scanner may be used to know the anatomy of pulmonary and coronary veins (AF ablation and CRT).

- Finally, **genetic testing** has become a useful tool to diagnose inherited heart disease in different clinical scenarios. Currently, it is considered to be a first-line diagnostic test only when a genetic disease appears to be responsible for cardiac arrest in clinical test results. Also, it may be useful for the study of relatives of these cases (see Chapter 1, Arrhythmias and Sudden Death).

All these techniques are used with increasing frequency, especially in young patients and athletes with exercise-related syncope or significant arrhythmias, to confirm that no structural heart disease is present (i.e., hypertrophic cardiomyopathy, coronary artery anomalies, arrhythmogenic right ventricular cardiomyopathy, etc.).

Therapeutic Techniques

Cardioversion
(Cakulev et al., 2009)

External electrical cardioversion is based on the delivery of direct current electric shock between two large surface electrodes placed in the right high parasternal position and at the apex (left submammary position). This so-called apex-base position was the most standard position; currently, however, the alternative "anteroposterior" placement is clearly the most effective approach (electrodes are placed in the parasternal and left infrascapular positions). Electrical shock, being painful, has to be delivered under deep sedation.

Electrical cardioversion is used to restore the sinus rhythm in cases of supraventricular and ventricular tachycardias and, as part of the cardiopulmonary resuscitation protocol, in cases of cardiac arrest due to ventricular fibrillation (VF). Even though the exact mechanism of electrical cardioversion is not exactly known, it is hypothesized that the electrical current, passing through the atrial and ventricular myocardium, has a "reset effect" on all cardiac cells, and that this results in the restoration of the sinus rhythm.

The applied energy varies depending on the arrhythmia to be treated. In general, 100–360 J are used to convert atrial arrhythmias, whereas 200– 360 J are applied in cases of VF. In cases of atrial flutter or lower energy VT, a 50-J first shock may be used.

Until recently, defibrillators administered monophasic shocks. Today, most provide biphasic shocks, which require less energy to achieve the same effect, while at the same time minimizing the risk of skin burns.

Because the delivery of shocks during the repolarization phase may induce VF, the apparatus are suited to provide shocks coinciding with a QRS complex (synchronized shock). In the case of VF, shocks are not provided in a synchronized fashion, as rhythm is already chaotic and VF is present.

If elective CV is performed, previous anticoagulation is necessary. The risk of embolic events in the peri-procedure is considered small (Chapter 4, Atrial fibrillation: Prevention of Thromboembolism). There are other risks associated with general anesthesia and possible arrhythmias, but in experienced hands they are very rare and easy to manage.

Pacemakers

Summary of pacemakers

Already discussed in Chapter 6 are: (i) the components of the pacemaker ECG, (ii) the stepwise approach to interpret an unknown ECG pacemaker, and (iii) the evolution of pacemaker technology, including the summary description of a resynchronization pacemaker. In the same chapter we looked at: (i) when a pacemaker has to be implanted and (ii) how to select the best pacemaker in different clinical settings, as well as different implantation protocols.

Figure A-15 shows a conventional dual-chamber pacemaker, an ICD with a dual-chamber pacemaker and, a tri-chamber resynchronizing-defibrillation pacemaker (CRT-ICD). We will now examine the current indications for CRT, and the problem of nonresponders to CRT.

One of the major advances in pacing in the last few years is the leadless pacemaker. Since the first cardiac epicardial pacemaker was implanted in 1958, significant advances have been made on the field. Despite that, the basic design of cardiac pacemaker has remained relatively unchanged: a pulse generator connected to one or more transvenous leads. Current cardiac pacemakers still have several liabilities. The subcutaneous pocket has a potential for local complications such as infections or hematomas. The transvenous leads can lead to acute complications, such as pneumothorax, and the presence of chronic transvenous leads can result in central vein obstruction, infection, and lead failure. Furthermore, the pacemaker leads are considered the Achilles heel of the cardiac pacing system. Studies show that approximately 10% of the patients experience an acute or late complication related to implantation of a pacemaker. Half of them are related with the pacemaker leads (Udo *et al.*, 2012). Because of these limitations, the leadless pacemaker (LPM) has long been of interest to the cardiologists.

- Current technology and indications: There are two LPM currently available, which are delivered through a venous sheath to the right ventricle: the Nanostim (St. Jude Medical, Inc., MN) and the Micra TPS (Medtronic, Inc., MN) (Figure A-16). Both are dime-sized devices with a predicted longevity of 10 years, capable of

single-chamber VVIR pacing. Therefore, these devices are indicated in patients with unicameral pacing requirements, such as chronic atrial fibrillation with atrioventricular block or sinus bradycardia with infrequent pauses. Both of these devices have been evaluated separately in nonrandomized trials (Reddy *et al.*, 2015; Reynolds *et al.*, 2016). The size, design, and results of the two studies were similar. Overall, the LPM have shown a successful implantation rate >95% and adequate pacing measures in more than 90% of the patients at six months follow-up. Major complications occurred in 6.5% of the patients with the Nanostim device and in 4.0% with the Micra device.

The major limitation of the current LPM is their ability to perform single-chamber pacing only. Consequently, these devices would not be appropriate in patients who required dual-chamber pacing or cardiac resynchronization therapy.

Cardiac resynchronization therapy (CRT)

Concept

The history of resynchronization pacemakers began with the pioneering papers by Cazeau *et al.* in 1994, followed by Bakker *et al.* in 2000. It is well known that AV and intraventricular conduction delays provoke or aggravate LV dysfunction, especially in patients with underlying heart disease. Thus, it was thought that solving this problem with biventricular pacing would be a good measure.

Indications

(a) Many trials performed since then (COMPANION, MIRACLE, CARE-HF, and others) (see Table 3.1.2 of the ESC guidelines, Recommended General Bibliography p. xvii) have demonstrated that CRT is particularly effective in patients with heart failure (NYHA III-IV), especially heart failure due to dilated or ischemic cardiomyopathy (CM), a low ejection fraction (EF) <30% and a wide QRS ≥ 120 ms in sinus rhythm (Table A-4). It improves hemodynamic parameters and quality of life, reverses remodeling, and decreases global mortality (Vardas *et al.*, 2007). Recently, CRT efficacy in patients with AF (see Chapters 4 and 9) and also in many other cases of CM, even in specific types, such as adriamycin-induced CM, has been demonstrated.

(b) **Recent trials** (REVERSE, MADIT-CRT, and RAFT) (see Chapter 11, Heart Failure: Therapeutic Considerations) have also shown that CRT is beneficial, reducing the incidence or worsening of HF when implantation is carried out **in the early stages of the disease**.

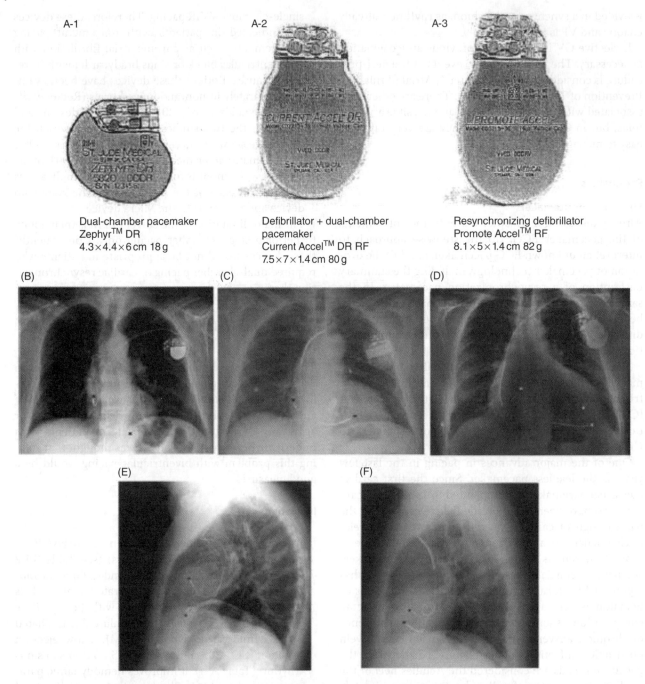

A-1

A-2

A-3

Dual-chamber pacemaker
Zephyr™ DR
4.3×4.4×6 cm 18 g

Defibrillator + dual-chamber
pacemaker
Current Accel™ DR RF
7.5×7×1.4 cm 80 g

Resynchronizing defibrillator
Promote Accel™ RF
8.1×5×1.4 cm 82 g

(B)

(C)

(D)

(E)

(F)

Figure A-15 Model and size of (A-1) dual-chamber pacemaker, (A-2) defibrillator + dual-chamber pacemaker, and (A-3) resynchronizing defibrillator. (B) to (F) show the three types of pacemaker in a frontal and lateral view (courtesy of St. Jude Med).

(c) Different trials are under study to show whether CRT is useful **in cases of EF >35%** (some diastolic component). Already positive results have been published (Chung *et al.*, 2010a). Some cases of hypertrophic CM with predominant HF and EF >35–40% may probably benefit from CRT.

(d) On the contrary, in patients with a **QRS narrower than 120 ms** after some promising results the first

well designed trial (RETHING) (Beshai *et al.*, 2007) shows that **CRT is not beneficial in these patients**. Further studies have to be done in patients with intra-ventricular dysynchrony and QRS ≅ 120 ms.

(e) The value of CRT **in very advanced cases of HF** with wide QRS is controversial. In fact, the benefit of a CRT-ICD (probably associated with AV node ablation) in very advanced HF + AF + wide QRS +

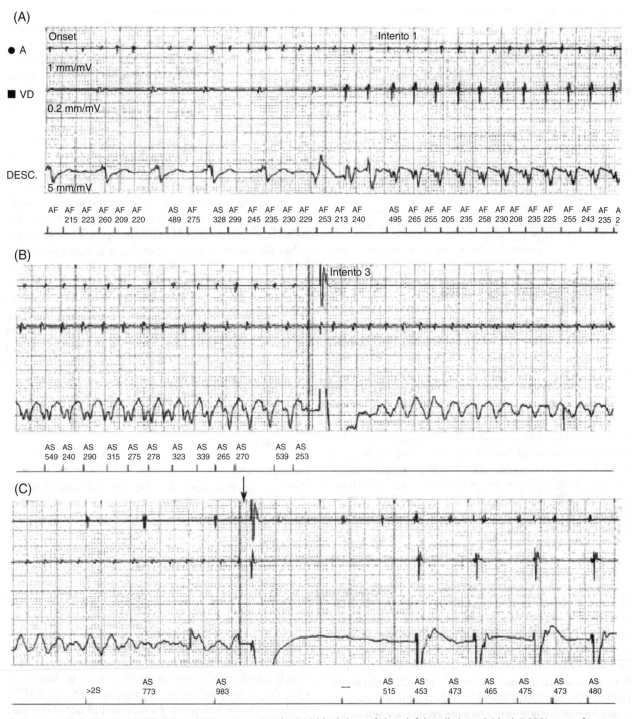

Figure A-16 Patient with atrial fibrillation (AF), atrioventricular (AV) block, heart failure, left bundle branch block (LBBB), runs of ventricular tachycardia (VT) and ejection fraction (EF) <30%, with implanted implantable cardioverter defibrillator-cardiac resynchronization therapy (ICD-CRT). (A) The patient presents a sustained VT, which (B) leads to a VF. In (C) it is observed how pacemaker rhythm is recovered after the fourth ICD discharge (arrow).

low EF has recently been shown (see Chapter 4, Atrial Fibrillation, and Chapter 11, Heart Failure). On the contrary, a study in patients with very advanced HF (Castel *et al.*, 2010) has shown negative results. In our experience CRT may be useful, showing at times very good results in patients with very advanced HF who are nonresponders to the best drug treatment and not candidates for transplant,

Table A-4 Most appropriate indications for cardiac resynchronization therapy (CRT).

Heart failure (HF) patients with sinus rhythm, depressed ejection fraction (EF), and wide QRS (especially true left bundle branch block (LBBB) pattern and QRS ≥140 ms. Often, it is implanted combined with an implantable cardioverter defibrillator (ICD) (CRT-ICD therapy).

However we have also to consider that:

a) CRT may be also useful in HF patients with atrial fibrillation (AF)
b) In severe cases of HF with AF and QRS >120 ms, not solved with atrial ablation, it may be useful to perform AV node ablation + CRT-ICD (Gasparini, 2006)
c) The usefulness of CRT in asymptomatic patients with low EF, and/or patients with HF and EF ≥40% and/or QRS <120 ms, is under study (see text)

---

even without a typical LBBB pattern but with a QRS >120 ms.

Currently, an **ICD may be implanted together with CRT**. This is because CRT does not solve the problem of SD, which is frequent in this group of patients. It is necessary to know which patients will benefit more from combined therapy. If CRT is started in the earlier stages of HF, the number of patients with ICD criteria will probably decrease in accordance with patient improvement, and hence the number of ICD implants would be theoretically reduced. We are not sure which strategy is better from an economic and clinical point of view: to start with CRT-ICD therapy in the early stages of HF, or to implant CRT only and watch for the need for ICD in the future. Reducing the cost of CRT-ICD devices would help in solving this dilemma significantly.

How to Select Candidates for CRT

In the past, some echo parameters used to detect dysynchrony (inter- and intraventricular), together with the duration of the QRS, were the best criteria for CRT eligibility (see Table B-1, ESC guidelines, Recommended General Bibliography p. xvii). Now, after the results of the PROSPECT study (Chung *et al.*, 2008), echo parameters are used much less frequently and QRS duration (QRSd) in a standard 12-lead ECG is the most used criterion for CRT eligibility. The best results are obtained when QRSd >150 ms, the pattern is that of a true LBBB, and the rhythm is sinus with a normal PR interval. However, these ECG parameters are not always synonymous with mechanical dysynchrony, as demonstrated by echocardiography. Thus, some echocardiographic parameters, especially in patients with borderline QRS, are once again used to assist with selection for CRT (Oyenuga *et al.*, 2010). This selection process is done in order to decrease the number of nonresponders.

The Problem of Nonresponders

One of the biggest problems with CRT is that ≅20–30% of patients are nonresponders. We have already commented on which candidates are best. The following parameters may identify nonresponder candidates before implantation: (i) a narrow QRS (≅120 ms), (ii) a large LVD diameter (>75 mm), (iii) a significant MI scar in the lateral wall that may complicate electrode stimulation, and (iv) severe mitral regurgitation. In addition, the parameters in a pre-implant ECG associated with all-cause and cardiac mortality in the follow-up, such as LBBB with a right axis deviation and a long PR interval, are those that express more advanced disease. In addition, the decrease in duration of the QRS after a CRT implant is directly related to a better prognosis. Recently, it has also been demonstrated that a longer QRSd after biventricular pacing was associated with a worse prognosis or need for transplant. Other ECG comparative parameters (before and after CRT) have been reported (Sweeney *et al.*, 2010), which may be useful in predicting response (Gradaus *et al.*, 2008). It has also been shown (Marchant *et al.*, 2010) that patients with LV leads located in an apical position presented more complications/ events than those with leads in a basal ventricular position (48 vs. 21%). Finally, a good implantation technique has to be taken into account (programming, follow-up and control); this is crucial to reduce the number of nonresponders.

Complications

We have to remember that the implantation of resynchronization pacemakers **involves some complications** (see Chapter 6: Pacemaker Complications) that may be acute (coronary sinus dissection perforation, etc.) or chronic (lack of stimulation, electrode problems, infections, etc.). Acute complications do not frequently occur in experienced hands. To avoid or solve chronic problems, when possible, it is necessary to perform a close control test of the device, which may now be done from a distance. Very rarely an endocarditis due to pacemaker infection may unfortunately require the removal of the system, as with all types of pacemakers. All possible benefits and risks of the procedure must be discussed with the patient before proceeding to CRT (CRT-ICD) implant. Ideally, economic factors should not play a part in the final decision.

Automatic Implantable Cardioverter Defibrillator (ICD)
(Figures A-15 and A-16, Tables A-5 and A.6)

Concept

The use of transvenous ICDs began with the pioneering studies performed 30 years ago by Mirowski *et al.* (1980), showing the usefulness of the implanted device in three patients with a high risk of SD (after two recovered cardiac arrests). This follows the previous experiments with animals (Mirowski's dog).

Implantable cardioverter defibrillators are very useful in the prevention of SD because they automatically initiate defibrillation when VT/VF appears. They are also comprised of a back-up VVI low-discharge rate pacemaker to protect the heart from significant bradycardia. Right ventricular pacing, however, should be kept to a minimum as it may be associated with clinical worsening and poorer prognosis (Stockburger *et al.*, 2009). It is advisable to use systems that minimize right ventricular pacing.

Indications

Table A-5 shows the current practical indications for ICD implantation, whereas Table A-6 shows the comparative recommendations for ICD implantation in different clinical situations based on guidelines from the AHA/ACC/

Table A-5 Indication for ICD implantation.*

Primary prevention

- Post-infarction patients (after 12 weeks) with ejection fraction (EF) <30–35%, above all if this does not improve and class II–III heart failure (HF) is present, despite optimum treatment (see Chapter 11)
- Other types of heart diseases with low EF (<30%), which do not improve with pharmacologic treatment (class I B)
- Inherited heart diseases with risk factors (see Chapter 9)

Secondary prevention

1) Cardiac arrest due to ventricular tachycardia (VT)/ ventricular fibrillation (VF) without a cause that may be suppressed (accessory pathway ablation, resolution of serious ischemia, etc.)
2) Syncopal VT or with hemodynamic impairment, especially in patients with inherited heart diseases or HF.

*This is just an approach to the different scenarios. The appropriate indication should be discussed in each case (Chapters 1, 5, 6, and 8. See also Table A-6). Remember that often in presence of HF the association with CRT therapy may be recommended in the appropriate cases.

ESC 2006 and AHA/ACC/ HRS 2008 (Recommended General Bibliography p. xvii). To summarize:

(i) We can state that **ICD implantation is preferable to pharmacological treatment in the prevention of SD**, both as a **secondary preventive measure** (survivors of out-of-hospital cardiac arrest or symptomatic VT) (AVID investigators, 1995) [CIDS (Connolly. *et al.*, 2000)] [CASH (Kuck *et al.*, 2000)] **and also as a primary preventive measure** (patients at high risk due to inherited heart diseases, heart failure, and other heart diseases with EF <30%, [MADIT Trial I and II (Moss *et al.*, 1996; Moss 2002), among others]). A review has been published on ICD indications, side effects, and limitations according to the results of major randomized ICD trials for primary and secondary prevention of SD (Myerburg *et al.*, 2009).

(ii) We have already discussed (see Chapter 11) whether an ICD implant is necessary in all patients with EF <30% and which patients with **ischemic heart disease, HF, and inherited heart disease** will benefit most from ICD implantation (see Chapters 9 and 11; Buxton, 1993).

(iii) **ICD implantation** is not necessary in the presence of primary VF during the acute phase of MI, unless there are other indications (very low EF).

(iv) **ICD implantation** during the first 2–3 months after AMI is not advisable, based on noninvasive parameters such as Holter monitoring (HRV, heart rate or nonsustained VT), that do not show differences in patients with or without these markers (DINAMIT and IRIS trials) (Steker, 2010). The possible explanation was that SD usually occurs due to massive MI or cardiac rupture, not primary arrhythmia (Pouleur *et al.*, 2010) (see Chapter 11, Acute Ischemic Heart Disease: Therapeutic Considerations). However, the

Table A-6 Implantable cardioverter defibrillator therapy: recommendations and guidelines Europe/USA.

Clinical scenario		ACC/AHA/ESC (2006)	AHA/ACC/HRS (2008)
A.	Cardiac arrest due to VT/VF without any reversible cause	IA	IA
B.	Symptomatic sustained VT in heart patients	IB	IB
C.	IHD, (II or III NYHA), EF ≤30% >1–2 months after MI (ICD implant after acute phase)	IB	IA
D.	IHD patients (II or III NHHA). EF 35–40%, >1–2 months after MI	IIa B	IB (EPS+)
E.	IHD patients (INYHA). EF <30% >1–2 months after MI	IB	IA
F.	Dilated CM (idiopathic). EF <30%, II–III NYHA	IB	IB

ACC, American College of Cardiology; AHA, American Heart Association; CM, cardiomyopathy; EF, ejection fraction; EPS, electrophysiologic studies; ESC, European Society for Cardiology; HRS, Heart Rhythm Society; ICD, implantable cardioverter defibrillator; IHD, ischemic heart disease; VF, ventricular fibrillation; VT, ventricular tachycardia.

induction of sustained VT/VF by EPS identifies a subgroup of patients in whom an ICD implant was protective at this critical time (Kumar *et al.*, 2010). These results suggest the need for a randomized trial that compares this strategy with the present primary prevention guidelines that were based on well done randomized trials (DINAMIT and IRIS) trials, but with risk stratification based on noninvasive parameters taken from Holter monitoring (Stecker, 2010) (see before).

(v) **It is known that ICD reduces yearly mortality by 2–3%.** Therefore, its benefit is especially clear if the patient lives for many years (inherited heart diseases).

(vi) **In HF patients with left bundle branch block** (LBBB) or an RV pacemaker with ventricular asynchrony, a resynchronizing pacemaker coupled with an ICD may be implanted (**CRT-ICD therapy**) (see before) (Figures A-15 and A-16). With this therapy, both symptoms and ventricular function usually improve and SD due to VT/VF may be prevented (MADIT-CRT trial) (Moss *et al.*, 2009, among others). CRT-ICD therapy is also useful in cases of AF (see Chapter 4, Atrial Fibrillation: Conversion to Sinus Rhythm and Prevention of Recurrences).

(vii) **In very advanced HF**, simultaneous ICD and left ventricular assisted devices (LVAD) have been shown to be safe and clinically feasible (see Chapter 11, Heart Failure).

(viii) Despite the fact that ICD implantation very efficiently avoids **SD due to VF, SD may still occasionally occur in patients with an ICD implant**. This may be caused not only by a failure in the device but also by many associated pathologies (massive AMI, pulmonary embolism, aortic rupture, etc.).

Complications

ICD patients have to be controlled in specialized units of arrhythmias (pacemakers) (see Chapter 6: The ECG of Pacemakers) not only because of the risk of possible complications of pacemaker implant but also because of the serious problem of inappropriate and unnecessary shocks that may occur in at least 5–10% of cases. This can lead to severe arrhythmias and may cause significant pain and discomfort to patients. One has to be particularly cautious in cases of primary prevention. It has been shown (Tereshchenko *et al.*, 2009) that ICD therapy may result in a detectable local injury current in the ventricular ICD lead electrogram, suggesting a potential mechanism for adverse outcomes, including the occurrence of HF. **Several strategies to reduce the rate of inappropriate defibrillation discharge have been investigated**. To prevent these inappropriate discharges,

T-wave oversensing should be avoided and a proper differentiation between QRS and T waves should be in place (Zareba, 2009). A new dynamic discrimination algorithm has demonstrated the ability to avoid T wave oversensing (Saba *et al.*, 2010). Finally, patients at a relatively low risk for fatal arrhythmias may benefit from a conservative CRT + ICD strategy (fixed long detection intervals) (Gasparini *et al.*, 2009). The administration of antiarrhythmic agents (AAAs) may also be useful to decrease the number of appropriate and inappropriate shocks (see Appendix A-5).

It is important to realize that the number of complications is more evident in younger patients (inherited heart diseases) because they may live several decades more and therefore will be submitted to many generator changes (see Chapter 9).

Before proceeding to ICD implantation, all these somewhat frequent complications, as well as other complications related to pacemaker implantation (see Chapter 6), have to be known to the doctor and must be explained to the patient.

Other Types of ICDs

Wearable cardioverter defibrillators (Chung *et al.*, 2010b) may be useful for transient use in high-risk patients in cases of explantation due to device infection and removal of the pacing system, or in the first months after MI in cases of frequent VT crises, or in post-CABG (see Chapter 11).

A novel subcutaneous ICD that avoids the adverse vascular complications of the transvenous approach but does not have a pacing system is also under study (Bardy *et al.*, 2010). This ICD approach would probably be very useful, especially in patients with no danger of bradycardia and with a good ejection fraction (inherited heart disease). More studies are necessary to confirm this.

Finally, keeping a **semiautomatic external** defibrillator at home for high-risk patients in whom, for whatever reason, an ICD has not been implanted, is becoming more and more common, especially in the United States (see Chapter 6, Cardiac Arrest).

Percutaneous transcatheter ablation

Concept

Percutaneous transcatheter ablation (Recommended General Bibliography p. xvii) has become the technique of choice for the treatment of different types of tachyarrhythmia. In short, it produces a lesion in a circumscribed area of cardiac tissue with a percutaneously catheter placed through either a vein (to obtain access to the right chambers) or an artery for access to the left ventricle (left accessory pathways and left ventricle VT).

Currently, the most frequently used therapeutic modality is radiofrequency ablation (the same energy used in electric scalpels). Energy delivered via radiofrequency is dispersed as heat throughout the surrounding tissue and lesions a few millimeters in diameter and depth are produced. In some cases, cryoablation may be used as an alternative method (ablation by catheter tip freezing of up to –80°C). Cryoablation, a new technique, is discussed separately.

Evolution of the Technique

Catheter ablation was initially used in arrhythmic substrates where it was possible to eliminate the arrhythmia by producing punctual (limited) lesions. For this reason, **accessory pathways** [Wolff–Parkinson–White (WPP) type or concealed accessory pathways] (AVRT) tachycardias **were the first substrates** in which this technique was applied (see Figure 4.25). At present, the efficacy of ablation in these types of arrhythmias is approximately 85–95%, whereas the clinically significant complication rate is lower than 1% (mortality <1‰). This makes ablation a first-line treatment in these patients. **Ablation of the slow pathway (α pathway) in junctional (AV) paroxysmal tachycardias exclusively involving a junctional (AV) circuit** (AVNRT) has achieved even greater success ($\cong$98%). Ablation of the **focus of idiopathic atrial and ventricular tachycardias** is also very successful.

Ablation was later applied to substrates requiring **ablation along lines**, initially in arrhythmic substrates with well-defined circuits. In cases of **typical atrial flutter** where the circuit includes the cavotricuspid isthmus, an ablation line in this location interrupts the flutter circuit in at least 95% of cases and prevents recurrence (see Figure 4.68).

With the appearance of 3D electroanatomic mapping systems, **more complex arrhythmias** requiring a transseptal procedure, **such as atrial fibrillation (AF)**, were addressed. These systems identify the tridimensional location of the catheter and the different areas where triggers (pulmonary veins) are present (**trigger-based ablation**). All this, together with the support of new robotic techniques, has made it possible to perform the ablation of paroxysmal and even chronic AF, reducing risks and providing more benefits to the patient. Burkhardt and Natale (2009) have published a review of the new treatments used in the ablation of AF. Currently, the ablation of VT in heart disease is being performed in many centers with relatively great success.

Current Indications and Technique

In cases of paroxysmal AF, as in many cases of chronic AF, the first step approach involves only the electrical isolation of the pulmonary veins by circumferential ablation of the pulmonary vein openings (**triggers strategy**). Using this approach, the curative rate may reach 70–80% (Haïssaguerre *et al.*, 2000; Pappone and Santinelli, 2006). This approach is best. Adding linear ablations of the left atrium does not usually increase the success rate and may be a source of more left atrial flutter (see Chapter 4, Atrial Fibrillation: Conversion to Sinus Rhythm. Prevention of Recurrence).

In some cases with **repetitive paroxysmal or chronic AF** that show recurrences after trigger-strategy ablation, some groups perform a second step approach based on the addition of "lines" joining the circumferential lesions. There are now new techniques of joining the gaps between these lines that have been shown to increase success rate (Eitel *et al.*, 2010). In addition, to avoid crises of atrial flutter, a cavotricuspid isthmus ablation has to be performed. Currently, in the cases where AF did not stop in the first procedure, or more often in a second, the ablation of atrial areas with complex fragmented electrogram (CFE) and/or greater frequency gradient (H_z) leads to episode reduction, or even discontinuation, in a great number of cases (**added substrate-strategy**). The association of these two strategies, **triggers and substrate**, has been demonstrated to give the best results in difficult cases (Verma *et al.*, 2010). The ablation of any non-PV ectopic focus initiating AF or any type of atrial tachycardia may also be performed.

Some centers that incorporate all these multiple procedures report a long-term success rate of around 80%. This may be even greater in selected cases, for instance, when the patient does not present signs of inflammatory disease (low hs-CRP) (Lin *et al.*, 2010). Currently, the ablation of permanent, long duration AF (AF>1–2 years) and large atria (>5 cm) is becoming more common. However, **long-term results, including series with more cases, are required before this technique may be considered widely accepted** (see Chapter 4, Ablation Techniques).

In cases of **idiopathic VT**, the success of ablation is very high.

It is also good in **sustained monomorphic VT in IHD** patients. In the latter, the objective of ablation is to eliminate the areas with slow conduction (Tung *et al.*, 2010). From an anatomical point of view, this corresponds to the viable myocardium present in scar regions in post MI patients. Therefore the "anatomic" approach is adopted by performing ablation lines joining different scars.

During the past few years, ablation has also established itself as an appropriate treatment aimed at decreasing the occurrence of **VT episodes in ICD implant patients** experiencing multiple ICD discharges.

Ablation is also useful in **other types of VT**, in the presence of different heart diseases and HF and in many inherited heart diseases. Lastly, ablation is very successful

Table A-7 Catheter ablation: Success, recurrences and complications in different arrhythmias.[*]

		Success (%)	Recurrences (%)	Severe complications (<1‰ global mortality) (%)
1	AT-EF	>80	Variable <10	<5
2	AT-MR	≅70	≅10	≅5
3	AVNRT	98–100	<1	<1
4	AVRT	≥90	<5	<2. Especially septal AP
5	AV node ablation	>95	<1	<2
6	JT–EF (children)	80–85	10–15	Pacemaker 4%
7	Atrial fibrillation	P-AF = 70–80	10–25	<5
		C-AF (variable):50–80	30–40	
8	Atrial flutter	90–100	<1	≅1
9	Idiopathic VT	≥80	Variable 10–30	<2
10	VT in HD patients	60–80	Variable 10–30	<3
11	Branch-to-branch VT	95–100	Very low	Very low

[*]See section on respective arrhythmias (Chapters 4, 5, 8, 9, and 11).
AT-EF (atrial tachycardia–ectopic focus), AT-MR (atrial tachycardia–macro-reentrant), AVNRT (AV node junction–reentrant tachycardia);
AVRT (junctional reentrant tachycardia with accessory pathway; JT-EF (junctional tachycardia–ectopic focus); VT (ventricular tachycardia).

in cases of VT due to branch-to-branch reentry (see Chapters 5, 9, and 11).

One of the major advances in the last few years was the development of software that allows the force (pressure) that the operator applies to the tissue to be calculated. This is of utmost importance to achieve deeper lesions, which are associated with better results during pulmonary vein isolation (PVI), the most developed technique to treat AF. Contact force (CF) takes into consideration two variables: (i) average contact force in grams and (ii) forced-time integral (FTI) in grams/seconds. FTI reflects the duration (in seconds) of the average contact force (in grams) during radiofrequency application. Optimum parameters include average contact force of 20 grams with a range between 10 and 30 grams and FTI of 400 gram/seconds that is also considered an indirect surrogate to effective trans-mural lesions. Peak forces exceeding an average CF of 60 g may be potentially hazardous and may lead to perforation, steam pop, and, subsequently, pericardial effusion and cardiac tamponade (Reddy *et al.*, 2015). Currently available force sensor enabled ablation catheters are ThermoCool Smart touch ™ (Biosense-Webster, Inc, Diamond Bar, CA, USA) and Tacticath ™ (St. Jude Medical, St. Paul, MN, USA).

Success Rate, Recurrences and Complications

In general, the success rate of the procedure is high and in many substrates very high, and the number of severe complications is very low (global mortality <1‰). The incidence of recurrences is variable but usually low. The

details about these results in different arrhythmias are summarized in Table A-7 and explained in different sections of the book (Chapters 4, 5, 8, 9, and 11) (consult also Recommended General Bibliography p. xvii).

New Mapping Techniques

The EnSite Array system (St Jude Medical, St Paul, MN, USA) is a noncontact mapping system that uses a multi-electrode array catheter (MEA) with 64 unipolar electrodes mounted on a 7.5-ml inflatable balloon (Kadish *et al.*, 1999). The catheter is introduced via a femoral sheath and positioned in any cardiac chamber. Signals recorded from the MEA derive 3.360 virtual unipolar electrograms simultaneously from a single beat and displays them in a three-dimensional image from the chamber of interest, previously created with a conventional roving catheter.

The major advantage of the EnSite Array system is that a single beat of tachycardia is required to generate an activation map, which makes it especially suited for mapping of nonsustained arrhythmias, including infrequent premature atrial or ventricular complexes, or arrhythmias that are poorly tolerated. High success rates have been described for ablation of RVOT ventricular arrhythmias (Friedman *et al.*, 2002; Zhang *et al.*, 2013). In a large series of 136 patients with idiopathic RVOT PVCs and/or VT, Zhang *et al.* described a success rate after a single procedure of 86.8% at three-year follow-up. The efficacy of MEA has also been reported for other cardiac arrhythmias, including right and left focal atrial tachycardias, atypical atrial flutter and atrial fibrillation. It also has

Figure A-17 The figure illustrates contact force parameters during radiofrequency application (lesion number 61) in the left atrium. The ablation catheter has a green tip indicator to show the direction of the force applied. The data of the contact force shown in the data table (right lower part of the image) with average contact force of 21 g, forced-time integral 455 g/s and duration of application 21.80 seconds. Pink dots represent RF lesions meeting the set up criteria for contact force.

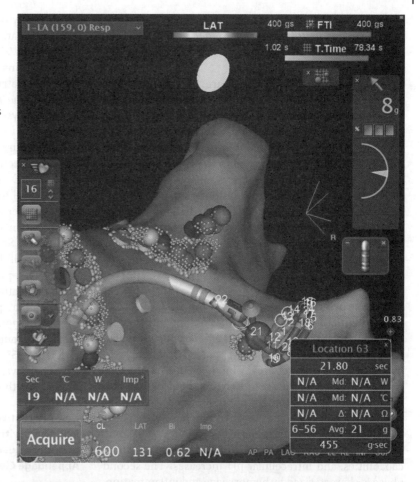

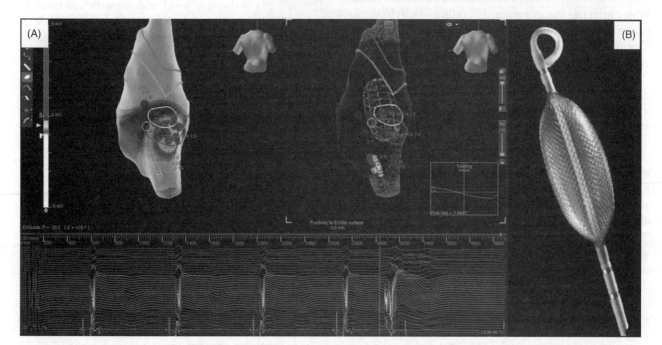

Figure A-18 (A) Noncontact mapping of the right ventricle during RVOT PVC ablation. A single PVC is mapped identifying the site of origin (white dot). In the bottom, the PVC that is being mapped. (B) Balloon array. It is inserted in the right femoral vein an advanced to the chamber of interest.

been used in scar-related VTs, where an endocardial exit region can be identified in more than 90% of cases and a portion of the diastolic pathway can be delineated in 70% (Della Bella *et al.*, 2002).

Some limitations of the system are: (i) the accuracy is reduced in large cardiac chambers, when the distance between the endocardial surface and the center of the balloon exceeds 4 cm; (ii) earliest activation is mapped to the endocardium of the chamber explored, even when the site of origin may be located in the epicardium or an adjacent chamber – in these cases, analysis of unipolar electrograms may be helpful (a unipolar QS pattern suggests successful ablation sites); (iii) the balloon can produce mechanical ectopy that may be confused with clinical PACs or PVCs.

Cryoablation

Heat destroys cells by coagulation and tissue necrosis with potential for thrombus formation and aneurysmal dilation, but cryoablation involves a different pathophysiological process. The objective of cryoablation is to freeze tissue in a target area. The mechanisms of tissue damage involve freezing and thawing, hemorrhage and inflammation, replacement fibrosis, and apoptosis. Cryoablation has two phases. The first phase is transient and the hypothermia causes cardiomyocytes to become less fluid as metabolism slows, ion pumps lose transport capabilities, and intracellular pH increases. The second phase is characterized by hemorrhage and inflammation. Water migrates out of myocardial cells to reestablish the osmotic equilibrium that was disturbed by ice crystals. The fluid traverses damaged microvascular endothelial cells, resulting in ischemic necrosis (Khairy *et al.*, 2008).

Diverse clinical cryoablation applications have been explored as indications continue to be refined. These explored applications include atrioventricular nodal reentrant tachycardia, parahisian accessory pathways, atrial flutter, and atrial fibrillation.

Catheter ablation for atrial fibrillation is centered on electrical isolation of pulmonary veins through circumferential lesions around pulmonary vein ostia. Focal point-by-point radiofrequency ablation has shown considerable success in treating paroxysmal AF.

Balloon-based ablation systems potentially offer a simpler and faster means of achieving pulmonary vein isolation that, theoretically, is less reliant on operator dexterity.

Cryothermal energy offers some advantages over RF energy, including increased catheter stability, less endothelial disruption with lower thromboembolic risk, and minimal tissue contraction with healing, which is thought to result in less esophageal damage and pulmonary vein stenosis.

A recently published meta-analysis on cryoablation of atrial fibrillation showed that a procedural success was achieved in 91.67–100% of patients and 94.87–100% of targeted veins. In the follow-up one-year freedom from recurrence atrial fibrillation was 72.83% (95% CI, 68.79–76.62%). The most common complication was phrenic nerve paralysis, with an overall incidence of 6.38 %. The incidence of thromboembolic complications, including periprocedural stroke, transient ischemic attack, or myocardial infarction, was 0.57% (Andrade *et al.*, 2011).

The FIRE AND ICE trial was a multicenter, randomized trial to determine whether cryoballoon ablation was noninferior to radiofrequency ablation in symptomatic patients with drug-refractory paroxysmal atrial fibrillation. Seven hundred and sixty-two patients were randomized. The mean duration of follow-up was 1.5 years. The primary efficacy endpoint (recurrence of atrial fibrillation, documented occurrence of atrial tachyarrhythmia, prescription of antiarrhythmic drugs, or repeat ablation) occurred in 34.6% of patients in the cryoballoon group and in 35.9% in the radiofrequency group (HR 0.96; 95% CI, 0.76 to 1.22; P <0.001 for noninferiority). There was no significant difference between the two methods with regards to overall safety (Kuck *et al.*, 2016).

New Alternative Treatment for Preventing Stroke in Patients with Absolute Contraindication to Anticoagulation. Endovascular Left Atrial Appendage Closure

The majority of thrombi in AF and, in particular nonvalvular AF, originate from the left atrial appendage (LAA). Although there is significant evidence from randomized trials supporting warfarin and direct oral anticoagulants, there are a considerable number of patients who may gain a benefit from oral anticoagulation who have an absolute contraindication to these agents, principally due to the potential risk of bleeding and occasionally due to patient preference. Several types of device are clinically available with varying degrees of clinical evidence. The main endovascular devices in clinical use are the WATCHMAN (Boston Scientific, Marlborough, MA, USA) and the Amplatzer Cardiac Plug (St Jude Medical, Minneapolis, MN, USA).

- **Watchman Device**: the initial percutaneous device developed and used for closure of the LAA was the PLAATO (Percutaneous Left Atrial Appendage Transcatheter Occlusion) device. This was subsequently replaced by the WATCHMAN device, which is also composed of a nitinol plug. Two randomized controlled trials have been conducted looking at this device. The PROTECT AF trial looked at 707 patients who were able to tolerate warfarin and had a CHADS$_2$ score of greater than 1 (Holmes *et al.*, 2009). This trial was designed to show noninferiority of the device over warfarin in the composite endpoint of ischemic or hemorrhagic stroke, cardiovascular or unexplained death, or systemic embolus. Patients who were enrolled were randomized to either the device or warfarin in a 2:1 ratio. Those who received the device were anticoagulated with warfarin for 45 days post implantation; this was stopped if there was no evidence of flow around the device or if flow was present that the jet width was less than 5 mm in maximum diameter. This was then replaced with dual antiplatelet therapy for six months and then aspirin thereafter. Of those randomized to the device, implantation was successful in 88% of patients. 86% of patients in the device arm were able to discontinue warfarin at 45 days. Although the device was shown to be noninferior, the rate of adverse events in the device group was 4.4%, with a higher incidence for the first three implantations, which then reduced after this. As a result of the high peri-procedural adverse events, the FDA requested more data with more specific endpoints in order to provide a better understanding of the exact benefits and risks of this device.

This resulted in the development of the PREVAIL trial, in which patients with a history of AF and a $CHADS_2$ of greater or equal to 2 were randomized to either the device or warfarin (Holmes *et al.*, 2014). At 18 months the composite of stroke, systemic embolism, and cardiovascular/unexplained death was 6.3% in the control group and 6.4% in those who received the WATCHMAN. The risk of periprocedural complications associated with the WATCHMAN were lower than those in the protect trial, likely reflecting increased physician experience with implantation of the device. Longer follow-up data revealed a significantly higher rate of stroke in patients randomized to the WATCHMAN versus control (13 ischemic strokes in the WATCHMAN arm versus 1 in the control arm; p = 0.044 at a mean of 15 ±8 months post-implant). Long-term follow-up of patients randomized to the WATCHMAN revealed significantly lower rates of hemorrhagic stroke and cardiovascular death than the control group (Reddy *et al.*, 2014). As a result of all of this data combined, the FDA has approved the WATCHMAN device in patients with nonvalvular AF who are at an increased risk of stroke, can take warfarin but have a good reason to be implanted with the device as a suitable alternative.

- **Amplatzer Cardiac Plug (ACP)**: the ACP device used for LAA closure was initially developed for ASD closures with struts added to the device in order to reduce the risk of device embolixation. The device consists of a distal lobe that sits in the body of the LAA and a proximal disk that covers the orifice. In contrast to the WATCHMAN there is limited randomized data for the ACP and most of the data is derived from observational

registries. The largest of these looked at 1047 patients in 22 centers (Tzikas *et al.*, 2016). In this registry implantation success was 97.3% with major adverse periprocedural events at 4.97%. The annual rate of systemic thromboembolism was 2.3%. Although there is very limited evidence this device has been marketed for use with antiplatelet therapy.

Given the significant potential risks of implantation of both of these devices, it is generally considered good practice to have a multidisciplinary approach involving cardiac electrophysiologists, interventional cardiologists, cardiac surgeons, echocardiographers, and radiologists. In order to gain access into the left atrium an inferoposterior trans-septal puncture should be performed. Although the technical factors in implanting these two devices are different, with different measurements being made, it is always important to obtain a high-quality image of the left atrial appendage on fluoroscopy with the injection of contrast through a marker pigtail. An example of the steps involved in the implantation of the ACP is shown on the fluoroscopic images in Figure A-19. Given the need to advance guidewires and sheaths close to and often into the LAA, the hemodynamics should be closely monitored in order to ensure that the patient does not develop a pericardial effusion. This can also be monitored by transesophageal echocardiography (TEE) and fluoroscopy. Other potential periprocedural complications include device embolization and systemic embolism and stroke.

Surgery

A few decades ago, surgery was useful in cases of supraventricular paroxysmal tachycardia (sectioning the accessory pathway and the slow pathway of the AV node in cases of junctional reentrant tachycardia, with the circuit involving the AV node exclusively (AVNRT)) and in cases of severe VT (Recommended General Bibliography p. xvii). Today, ablation techniques now "cure" most supraventricular tachycardias, especially reentrant tachycardias, and even many ectopic tachycardias, as well as flutter and, with less success, AF. Additionally, many cases of VT in healthy subjects or those with heart disease are treated with ablation techniques. Furthermore, implantable cardioverter defibrillator implantation is especially indicated in cases of severe and dangerous VT, provided that the economic situation allows (see before).

Surgical interventions have been reduced to performing ablation lines in chronic AF patients who should undergo valvular and/or coronary surgery. The restoration of the sinus rhythm is sometimes obtained in these cases. As previously discussed (see Chapter 4, Atrial Fibrillation), minimally invasive surgical approaches have been developed to isolate the autonomic ganglion that triggers AF.

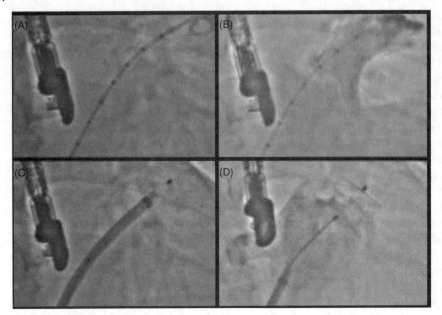

(A) (B) (C) (D)

Figure A-19 Fluroscopic steps in deployment of the ACP. A marker pigatil is seen in image A. This is advanced across the interatrial septum and into the main body of the LAA. Contrast is injected as shown in image B and the image as well as the TEE and CT are examined and measurements made prior to selection of the device type and size. Following this, the device is advanced through the sheath and positioned in the LAA. As shown in image C the lobe is deployed and the location checked on fluoroscopy and TEE. Finally, as shown in image D, the disc is deployed and contrast injected through the sheath in order to ensure a good closure of the orifice of the LAA.

Antiarrhythmic Agents

Classification of Antiarrhythmic Agents

For many years (Vaughan-Williams, 1980), it has been accepted that antiarrhythmic agents (AAA), which are useful for the treatment of supraventricular and ventricular active arrhythmias as well as SD prevention, act by blocking the underlying mechanisms, including alterations of the Na^+, K^+, and Ca^{++} ionic channels and the β adrenergic receptors (Nattel, 1991).

The classification carried out by Vaughan-Williams (1980), which includes four AAA classes, has been the most popular (Table A-8). However, before assessing the actual value of the classical antiarrhythmic drugs according to Vaughan-Williams' classification, we would like to point out the fact that many of these drugs do not have pure mechanisms of action of only one class. For instance, amiodarone has different effects corresponding to Class I, II, III, and IV. In addition, this classification has several limitations:

o It does not include useful antiarrhythmic AAAs for determined cases, such as **adenosine**, atropine, magnesium, or digitalis. In fact, adenosine may be useful in many types of narrow QRS complex regular tachycardias, especially in children. Junctional reentrant tachycardias, with circuits exclusively involving the AV junction, are usually resolved with adenosine (see Chapter 4, AV Junctional Tachycardia: Prognostic and Therapeutic Implications). Additionally, it is helpful in the diagnosis of atrial flutter, allowing for a better identification of the flutter waves by slowing down AV conduction. It should not, however, be administered

Table A-8 Vaughan-Williams' classification of antiarrhythmic agents.

Class I: Na channel blockers
Class I A: quinidine, procainamide, disopiramide
Class I B: mexiletine, lidocaine and fenitoine
Class I C: flecainide, propafenone and morizicine
Class II: β blockers
Class III: K channel blockers, prolonging repolarization: sotalol, bretylium and amiodarone. Dronedarone has recently been included in this group
Class IV: Slow Ca channel blockers: calcium antagonists

in cases of irregular tachycardias or in the presence of pre-excitation. Instead, **magnesium** might be useful in certain Torsades de Pointes VT (see Chapter 5, Torsades de Pointes Polymorphic Ventricular Tachycardia). The **digitalis** slowing effect on AV conduction is well known and, for this reason, it is frequently used in AF with fast ventricular response, except in the presence of pre-excitation.

o It does not take into account the antiarrhythmic effect of other drugs in terms of reducing SD (apart from β-blockers): statins, angiotensin-converting enzyme inhibitors (ACE inhibitors), or even ω-3.

o It does not mention those drugs that, despite some discordant results (Disertori *et al.*, 2009), are used for the prevention and treatment of AF, such as ACE inhibitors and angiotensin-II receptor blockers (ARB II) (Tomoda, 2009).

A more realistic effort to use AAAs has been proposed by the **Sicilian Gambit group** (Schwartz and Zaza, 1992). Their approach consists of trying to identify the underlying mechanism for arrhythmias and determining which parameter is the most vulnerable (the most amenable to change) before selecting the most adequate drug. Table A-9 shows some examples.

Effects on the ECG, Relative Efficacy, and Doses of AAA

Tables A-10 and A-11 show the effects of AAAs, according to Vaughan-Williams' classification, on ECG parameters as well as the relative efficacy in different arrhythmias. The therapeutic doses and concentrations of those used more frequently are shown in Table A-12. We would like to point out that AAAs, especially Class I, have some pro-arrhythmic effects (see later). Ionic and metabolic disturbances, impairment of renal function, advanced heart disease, and all other factors that may prolong the QT interval support this (see Chapter 10, Acquired Long QT). Furthermore, some AAAs given

Table A-9 Sicilian Gambi (Schwartz and Zaza, 1992).

Arrhythmia	Mechanism	Vulnerable parameter	Drugs
Inappropriate sinus tachycardia	Increase of normal automatism	Phase 4 (diastolic depolarization)	B-blockers
Some types of atrial tachycardia	Increase of abnormal automatism	Phase 4 (diastolic depolarization)	Na or Ca channel blockers
Atrial fibrillation	Micro-reentry and others	Prolongation of the atrial refractory period	Amiodarone, sotalol
Torsades de Pointes	Triggered electrical activity	Premature after-potentials	Ca blockers; Mg
Sustained ventricular tachycardia	Reentry	Prolongation of the ventricular refractory period	Amiodarone, procainamide

Table A-10 Effects of antiarrhythmic agents on electrocardiogram parameters.

	I A	I B	I C	II	III	IV
Sinus rhythm	0/+	0	0/–	–	–	0/–
PR interval	0/+	0	0/+	+	+	+
QRS complex duration	+	0	++	0	+	0
QT interval	+	0	0/+	0	++	0
PRE accessory pathway	+	0	+	0/+	+	0/+

+: increase; –: decrease; 0: no change; PRE: longer S_1–S_2 interval, which does not result in a S_2 response.

Table A-11 Relative efficacy of antiarrhythmic agents.

	I A	I B	I C	II	III	IV
Sinus tachycardia	0	0	0	+++	+	0 / ++
Atrial tachycardia	+	0	+	++	++	+
Flutter/atrial fibrillation without pre-excitation						
Prevention of recurrences	++/+++	0	++/+++	+	+++	+
Slowing down the AV conduction	0	0	0	+++	+++	With Ver. and Dilt.
Junctional reentrant tachycardia (in the absence of WPW)						
Stopping the crisis[a]	++	0	++	+++	+++	++ (Verap.)
Premature ventricular complexes (PVC)	+	+	+++	++[b]	+++	0
Ventricular tachycardia	++	++	++	0	+++	0

a) Adenosine is very effective. Not in presence of WPW.
b) It depends: effective in the presence of sympathetic overdrive.

0, no effect; +, minimum effect; ++, moderate; +++, very effective; AV, atrioventricular; Dilt., dilteazen; Ver., verapamil; WPW, Wolff–Parkinson–White.

Table A-12 Therapeutic doses and concentrations of most commonly used antiarrhythmic agents by the authors.

Drug	Dose interval				Time to peak – oral concentration (h)	Elimination (half-life) (h)	Main elimination route
	Intravenous		Oral				
	Loading dose[a]	Maintenance dose[a]	Loading dose[a]	Maintenance dose[a]			
Adenosine	6–12 mg (quick bolus)	–	–	–	–	–	–
Amiodarone	10–15 mg/kg for 10 m. 1 mg/kg for 180 min	0.5–1 mg/min	600 mg/day the first week	200–400 mg, 5 days/week Thyroid control	–	>1 month	Kidney
Digoxin	0.5–1 mg	0.125–0.25 mg/day	0.5–1 mg	0.125–0.25 mg/day	2–6	36–48	Kidney
Dronedarone	–	–	–	400 mg/12 h	3–5	24–40	Fecal
Flecainide	–	–	–	50–100 mg/12 h.	4	3.6	Liver
Lidocaine	1–3 mg/kg at 20–50 mg/min	1–4 mg/min	–	–	–	1–2	Liver
Procainamide	6–12 mg/kg at 0.2–0.5 mg/kg/min	2–4 mg/min	–	–	1	3–5	Kidney
Propafenone	1–2 mg/kg	–	450–750 mg	Maximum 10 mg/kg/day	1–3	5–8	Liver
Propranolol	≤0.20 mg/kg	–	–	10–40 mg/6–8 h	4	3–6	Liver
Sotalol	10 mg in 1–2 min	–	–	40–60 mg/12 h	2.5–4	12	Kidney
Verapamil	5–10 mg in slow bolus (1–2 min)	0.4 mg/min	–	80–120 mg/8 h	1–2	3–8	Liver

a) The initial dose depends on the clinical situation, the patient's weight, the renal function, etc. The lowest dose with the maximum efficacy should be initially provided. Sometimes the dose may be increased (consult the package insert).

without caution may cause or precipitate the appearance of passive arrhythmias (sinus node dysfunction and/or AV block).

It is beyond the scope of this book to analyze the different effects of AAA on ionic channels, receptors, and each electrophysiologic and electrocar diographic effect. We recommend consulting specialized books (see the Recommended General Bibliography p. xvii).

The Current Role and the Future of AAA

We would like to stress the importance of the current role of AAA in the era of pacemakers, ablation, and ICD therapy.

- **Class I AAAs** are currently not used as frequently as in the past. In terms of pro-arrhythmic effects (see before), the CAST trial (Echt *et al.*, 1991) demonstrated that in post-infarction patients with ventricular premature complexes, the group treated with flecainide, encainide, or morizidine had a higher mortality rate than the placebo group due to the pro-arrhythmic effects. Therefore, they are no longer used in post-infarction patients to prevent VT/VF and SD. These drugs, especially propafenone and flecainede, are presently especially used to prevent paroxysmal supraventricular arrhythmias as a first-choice therapy in healthy patients, and also at the onset of an episode (pill-in-the-pocket approach) (Alboni *et al.*, 2004). We use propafenone more often (see Chapter 4, Junctional Reentrant Tachycardia: Prognostic and Therapeutic Implications), although we do not administer it in patients with evident structural heart disease or HF. However, it has been demonstrated (Andersen *et al.*, 2009) that if type I AAAs are given to the appropriate patients, they may be used effectively with reasonable caution. In children, Janousek and Paul (1998) observed that propafenone shows fewer antiarrhythmic effects than flecainide and that antiarrhythmic effects were more frequently observed in patients with structural heart disease (5 vs. 1.5%). Cardiac arrest or SD occurred in 0.6% (5/770) of patients. In general, all AAAs, but especially Class I, should be administered with close monitoring. In the case of frequent PVC, it is interesting to test if Type I AAA suppresses the presence of frequent ectopy (acute drug test) (Bayés de Luna *et al.*, 1987).
- **Class II AAAs (β-blockers)** show, apart from their antiarrhythmic effects, many other properties that make them first-line cardioactive drugs to treat hypertension and HF. They are also useful in situations implying an abnormal increase of automaticity, as well as for extrasystoles due to a sympathetic overdrive. The protective role of β-blockers against SD is also important. In a study of patients who died while wearing a Holter device (Bayés de Luna *et al.*, 1989), we were able to show that VT/VF occurred much more frequently when the baseline rhythm was faster (see Figure 1.4). Beta-blockers are contraindicated to treat AVRT or control heart rate in AF, in the presence of pre-excitation, and have to be administered with caution in other circumstances (see Chapter 4, AV Junctional Reentrant Tachycardia and Atrial Fibrillation). **Sotalol**, a nonspecific β-blocker without intrinsic sympathomimetic activity that also prolongs repolarization (Class III AAA effect), may also be useful.

Out of all **Class III AAAs, amiodarone is the most frequently used** and the one considered as the best AAA, as it is the most effective and produces the fewest number of potentially serious cardiac pro-arrhythmic effects. It is also the most useful in terms of preventing AF recurrences. For patients at risk for SD in whom an ICD cannot be implanted for whatever reason, amiodarone may be administered because it has some protective effect, especially in patients who are also taking β-blockers (Class II b-c) (Janse *et al.*, 1998). Nevertheless, in high-risk patients, amiodarone should not be considered an alternative treatment to ICD implantation (SCD-HeFT) (Bardy *et al.*, 2005). Although it does not have serious secondary effects (especially Torsades de Pointes), its extracardiac effects, especially on the thyroid gland, frequently limit its use.

- **A new AAA called dronedarone** has been commercialized (Hohnloser *et al.*, 2009). It features a similar electropharmacologic profile to amiodarone but does not cause thyroid (it does not contain iodine) or pulmonary side effects. One advantage of dronedarone is that it adequately blocks AV conduction in AF patients (ERATO trial, Davy *et al.*, 2008). Although it is more effective than a placebo at preventing AF recurrences, dronedarone is not as effective as amiodarone (DIONYSOS trial) (Cook *et al.*, 2010; Zimetbaum, 2009). Due to that, according to Singh *et al.* (2010) and Top-Pedersen *et al* (2010), dronedarone does not represent a clear step forward in terms of efficacy with respect to amiodarone for maintenance of sinus rhythm.

After the successful trial with dronaderone in paroxysmal AF (ATHENA), a second trial was conducted (PALLAS Study) in sicker patients with persistent AF (Connolly, 2011). This trial was prematurely terminated due to increased events in the drug arm. Currently, dronaderone is very infrequently used in any form of AF due to the unpredictability of the AF phenotype (Mohajer *et al.*, 2013).

Some case reports have been published showing its efficacy to prevent VT (Fink *et al.*, 2011; Shaaraoui *et al.*, 2010). The efficacy of dronedarone as AAA for

VA is similar to amiodarone in experimental studies (Agelaki *et al.*, 2007). However, in the presence of overt or presumed heart failure the use of dronedarone for VA is not recommended (Coons, 2010).

As in patients with advanced heart failure (high-risk patients) dronedarone may not be recommended; amiodarone, according to the guidelines of AHA/ESC/ACC (Fuster *et al.*, 2011) and the new Guidelines of the European Society of Cardiology (Camm *et al.*, 2010), is still the drug of choice in these cases. However, in patients with low/moderate risk "the safety data" of dronedarone allow it to be considered as a first-line therapy according to the mentioned guidelines, often with other type I or II AAAs.

- **Class IV AAAs (calcium antagonists)** are not frequently used as AAAs, although they may be useful in some supraventricular and ventricular idiopathic arrhythmias, especially to revert an episode (see Chapter 4, Chaotic Atrial Tachycardia).

- It is true that **AAAs are used decreasingly**, not only because of the superior effectiveness of other techniques (pacemakers in passive arrhythmias, ablation techniques in supraventricular tachyarrhythmias, including AF and atrial flutter, and, in some ventricular arrhythmias, ICD implantation for the prevention of SD), but also because of significant side effects, such as negative inotropic and pro-arrhythmic properties. We have already seen that Class I drugs are especially dangerous if administered to advanced heart disease patients. However, some evidence suggests that administration of AAAs (flecainide, propafenone, sotalol, and amiodarone) to AF patients (Andersen *et al.*, 2009) is not associated with a higher mortality rate, when they are given to selected cases, as previously discussed. This at least shows that, at present, there is a deeper knowledge of potentially serious side effects and that in some countries, appropriate patient screening is very well carried out before this treatment is administered (see before).

Meanwhile, it is particularly frustrating to see how the use of most new AAAs (azetimide, dofetilide, ibutilide, etc.) is very limited because of potentially serious side effects. The only new drug evaluated in clinical trials but already approved (Camm *et al.*, 2010) **is vernalakant.** We should not forget, however, the current need for effective AAAs, as patients submitted to successful ablation for AF, as well as those with implanted ICD, frequently suffer from paroxysmal arrhythmias. Generally, these consist of AF recurrences or new atrial arrhythmias in the former case, and AF or VT in the latter. Although ablation of VT is already frequent, it is also important to treat the triggers of new sustained VT crises with the best AAAs. Furthermore, in patients with ICDs the administration of AAAs may be prescribed to limit the number of appropriate shocks. Inappropriate shocks can increase the risk of morbidity and mortality (see Appendix A-4); therefore, the use of AAAs is also beneficial in this scenario. However, it has to be taken into account that sometimes combination therapy may result in some negative secondary effects for the patients due to side effects of the drugs that may include a potential impairment of the arrhythmic recognition capability of the ICD. Therefore, all drug–device interaction has to be considered.

Additionally, in many patients with paroxysmal arrhythmias, invasive techniques are either not the first choice option or not feasible, the latter often being the case in many developing countries. In this scenario, the best option is to administer the most potent and safest AAA. Amiodarone is currently the drug of choice. We hope that another derivative of amiodarone (budiodarone, still in the preliminary research stage) will show some positive results (Arya *et al.*, 2009) and may be the best alternative to amiodarone. One should also be confident that in the future the new drugs under investigation (multichannel blockade, gap junction modulators) for the treatment of AF, in particular, will demonstrate efficacy and a lack of significant side effects (Mazzini and Monahan, 2008; Krishnamoorthy and Lip, 2009; Nattel, 2009).

The aim is that **AAAs have maximum efficacy and minimum side effects**. In future, new drugs will surely be available as a result of deeper knowledge of arrhythmia mechanisms and untoward effects and, above all, advancements in genetic research (pharmacogenetics). Only then will we be able to tailor treatments in such a way that drugs and the corresponding dosages will be selected based on each individual genetic map (Roden, 2003).

Classification of the Recommendations for Diagnostic and Therapeutic Procedures and Level of Evidence (AHA/ESC/ACC Guidelines)

For the reader who likes to delve deep into the knowledge of the diagnostic and therapeutic procedures discussed in this book, it may be useful, apart from reading the original papers (see bibliography), to consult the guidelines of the different scientific societies (in particular, those from AHA/ESC/ACC, Recommended General Bibliography p. xvii). They divide **their recommendations into three categories:**

○ **Class I**: conditions for which there is evidence and/or general agreement that a given procedure or treatment is useful and effective.

○ **Class II**: conditions for which there is conflicting evidence and/or a divergence of opinion about the usefulness/efficacy of a procedure or treatment. It is subclassified into **Class IIa** (the weight of evidence/opinion is in favor of usefulness/efficacy) and **Class IIb** (usefulness/efficacy is not as well established by evidence/opinion).

○ **Class III**: conditions for which there is evidence and/or general agreement that the procedure/treatment is not useful/effective and may, in some cases, be harmful.

Additionally, the **level of evidence** depends on whether data are derived from multiple randomized clinical trials or meta-analysis (**A level of evidence**), or from a single randomized trial or nonrandomized studies (**B level of evidence**). It also depends on whether it is a consensus opinion of experts, based on retrospective studies or submissions (**C level of evidence**). Ideally, the recommendation should, of course, be Class I and based on an A level of evidence.

Although we strongly recommend consulting the guidelines, we emphasize that some express different opinions, and are generally somewhat behind with regard to new discoveries. Sometimes they forget to give advice about habits and maneuvers, such as alcohol intake or Valsalva maneuver, that may trigger or stop some arrhythmic episodes. Furthermore, in general the guidelines do not take into account that the treatment administered also depends on socioeconomic factors, which vary from one country to the next. Bearing this in mind, it is very clear that, even though the guidelines are very useful because they represent the best evidenced treatment, they do not take into account the financial resources of different countries. In fact, the White Book of electrophysiology in Europe (Vardas, 2010) already makes this remark when exposing how differently cardiac arrhythmias are treated in the different countries of Europe. Thus, we believe that the guidelines may give, on some occasions, a more feasible alternative to the best option given in the guidelines. Europe, and obviously the rest of the world, presents so many different economic differences that is very difficult to apply the best guidelines to all countries. Therefore, the criteria of the physician should ultimately prevail when making a decision. This should clearly be based on the guidelines, but also on his/her experience, in the possibilities of his/her country, and taking into consideration what has recently been published or presented on the subject.

Class I and III recommendations of the guidelines should be followed in particular, if possible. Throughout the book we have often included different recommendations based on these guidelines and, in particular cases, also others derived from other committees and societies.

At present, there is a tendency to practice some degree of **defensive medicine** and, in this sense, decision making based on current guidelines is a protective practice. For more information on different guidelines, see www.escardio.org and www.americanheart.org (AHA).

Self Assessment

A. List the diagnoses for which the electrocardiogram (ECG) is the gold standard.	H. Describe the main utility of late potential (LP) recording.
B. How is the 2×2 table used to study the sensitivity (Se), specificity (Sp), and predictive value (PV) of an ECG criterion?	I. Describe the main utility of wave amplification and filtering.
C. What is the statistical relevance of Bayes' theorem?	J. What are the indications for electric cardioversion?
D. Describe the main utility of Holter ECG monitoring in arrhythmias.	K. What are the indications for implantable cardioverter defibrillator (ICD) implantation?
E. Describe the main utility of the exercise test.	L. Discuss the current indications for ablation.
F. Describe the main utility of electrophysiologic studies.	M. Describe the current situation of pharmacologic treatments for arrhythmias.
G. Describe the main utility of the tilt table test.	N. Describe the different recommendation categories of the clinical practice guidelines.

References

Agelaki M, Pantos C, Korantzopoulos P, I. Comparative antiarrhythmic efficacy of dronedarone and amiodarone during acute MI in rats. Eur J Pharmacol 2007;564:150.

Alboni P, Botto GL, Baldi N. Outpatients treatment of recent onset atrial fibrillation with "the pill in the pocket" approach. New Engl J Med 2004;351:2384.

Andersen SS, Hansen LM, Gislason HG, *et al.* Antiarrhythmic therapy and risk of death in patients with atrial fibrillation: a natio wide study. Europace 2009;11:886.

Andrade JG, Khairy P, Guerra PG, *et al.* Efficacy and safety of cryoballoon ablation for atrial fibrillation: A systematic review of published studies. Heart Rhythm 2011;8(9):1444.

Arya A, Silberbauer J, Teichman SL, *et al.* A preliminary assessment of the effects of ATI-2042 in subjects with paroxysmal atrial fibrillation using implanted pacemaker methodology. Europace 2009;11:458.

AVID investigators: Antiarrhythmics Versus Implantable Defibrillators (AVID) – rationale, design, and methods. Am J Cardiol 1995;75:470.

Bakker PF, Meijburg HW, de Vries JW, *et al.* Biventricular pacing in end-stage heart failure improves functional capacity and left ventricular function. J Interv Card Electrophysiol 2000;4:395.

Bakker AL, Nijkerk G, Groenemeijer BE, *et al.* The Lewis lead: making recognition of P waves easy during wide QRS complex tachycardia. Circulation 2009;119:e592.

Bardy GH, Lee KL, Mark DB, *et al.* Sudden cardiac death in heart failure trial (SCD-HeFT) Investigators. Amiodarone or an implantable cardioverter-defibrillator for congestive heart failure. N Engl J Med 2005;352:225.

Bardy G, Smith W, Hood M, *et al.* An entirely subcutaneous implantable cardioverter-defibrillator. N Engl J Med 2010;363:36.

Bayés de Luna A. Clinical electrocardiography. John Wiley & Sons Ltd, Chichester, 2011.

Bayés de Luna A, Serra Grima JR, Oca Navarro F. Electrocardiografia de Holter. Enfoque practico. Editorial Cientifico Medica, Barcelona, 1983.

Bayes de Luna A, Fort de Ribot R, Trilla E, *et al.* Electrocardiographic and vectorcardiographic study of interatrial conduction disturbances with left atrial retrograde activation. J Electrocardiol 1985;18(1):1.

Bayés de Luna A, Guindo J, Torner P, *et al.* Value of effort testing and acute drug testing in the evaluation of antiarrhythmic treatment. Eur Heart J 1987(suppl A):77.

Bayés de Luna A, Coumel P, Leclercq JF. Ambulatory sudden cardiac death: mechanisms of production of fatal arrhythmia on the basis of data from 157 cases. Am Heart J 1989;117:151.

Beshai J, Grimm RA, Nagueh SF, *et al.* Cardioc re-synchronization therapy in heart failure with narrow QRS complexes. New Engl J Med 2007;357:2461.

Bigger JT, Fleiss JL, Kleiger R, *et al.* The relationships among ventricular arrhythmias, left ventricular dysfunction and mortality in the 2 years after myocardial infarction. Circulation 1984;69:250.

Breithardt G, Borgreffe M, Seipel L, *et al.* Prognostic significance of late ventricular potentials after myocardial infarction. Eur Heart J 1983;4:487.

Brignole M. Different electrocardiographic manifestations of the cardioinhibitory vasovagal reflex. Europace 2009;11:144.

Burkhardt D, Natale A. New technologies in atrial fibrillation ablation. Circulation 2009;120:1533.

Buxton AE. Prevention of sudden death in patients with coronary artery disease: the Multicenter Unsustained Tachycardia Trial (MUSTT). Prog Cardiovasc Dis 1993;36:215.

Cakulev I, Efimov IR, Waldo AL. Cardioversion: past, present, and future. Circulation 2009;120:1623.

Camm AJ, Kirchhof P, Lip GYH, *et al.* Guidelines for the management of atrial fibrillation: The Task Force for the Management of Atrial Fibrillation of the European Society of Cardiology (ESC). Eur Heart J 2010;31(19):2369.

Castel MA, Magnani S, Mont L, *et al.* Survival in New York Heart Association class IV heart failure patients treated with cardiac resynchronization therapy compared with patients on optimal pharmacologial treatment. Europace 2010;12:1136.

Cazeau S, Ritter P, Bakdach S, *et al.* Four chamber pacing in dilated cardiomyopathy. Pacing Clin Electrophysiol 1994;17:1974.

Chung ES, Leon AR, Tavazzi L, *et al.* Results of the predictors of response to CRT (PROSPECT) trial. Circulation 2008;117:2608.

Chung ES, Katra RP, Ghio S, *et al.* Cardiac resynchronization therapy may benefit patients with left ventricular ejection fraction >35%: a PROSPECT trial substudy. Eur J Heart Fail 2010a;12:581.

Chung MK, Szymkiewicz SJ, Shao M, *et al.* Aggregate national experience with the wearable cardioverter-defibrillator: event rates, compliance, and survival. J Am Coll Cardiol 2010b;56:194.

Connolly SJ, Gent M, Roberts RS, *et al.* Canadian Implantable Defibrillator Study (CIDS): A randomized trial of the implantable cardioverter defibrillator against amiodarone. Circulation 2000;101:1297.

Cook GE, Sasich LD, Sukkari SR. Atrial fibrillation. DIONYSOS study comparing dronedarone with amiodarone. Br Med J 2010;340:c285.

Connolly SJ, Camm AJ, Halperin JL, *et al.* Dronedarone in high-risk permanent atrial fibrillation. N Engl J Med. 2011;365(24):2268.

Coons JC, Klauger KM, Seybert AL, Sokos GG. Worsening of heart failure in the setting of dronedarone initiation. Ann Pharmacother 2010;44:1496.

Davy J, Herold M, Hoglund C, *et al.* Dronadorone for the control of ventricular rate in permanent atrial fibrillation: The ERATO study. Am Heart J 2008;156:257e1.

De Ambroggi L, Negroni MS, Monza E, *et al.* Dispersion of ventricular repolarization in the long QT syndrome. Am J Cardiol 1991;68:614.

Della Bella P, Pappalardo A, Riva S, *et al.* Non-contact mapping to guide catheter ablation of untolerated ventricular tachycardia. Eur Heart J 2002;23:742.

Disertori M, Latini R, Barlera S, *et al.* GISSI-AF Investigators Valsartan for prevention of recurrent atrial fibrillation. N Engl J Med 2009;360:1606.

Echt DS, Liebson PR, Mitchell LB, *et al.* Mortality and morbidity in patients receiving encainide, flecainide or placebo. The Cardiac Arrhythmia Suppression Trial. N Engl J Med 1991;324:781.

Eitel C, Hindricks G, Sommer P, *et al.* Circumferential pulmonary vein isolation and linear left atrial ablation as a single-catheter technique to achieve bidirectional conduction block: the pace-and-ablate approach. Heart Rhythm 2010;7:157.

Fink A., Duray G., Hohnlosser S. A patient with recurrent atrial fibrillation and monomorphic ventricular tachycardia treated successfully with dronedarone. Europace 2011;13(2):284.

Friedman PA, Asirvatham SJ, Grice S, *et al.* Noncontact mapping to guide ablation of right ventricular outflow tract tachycardia. J Am Coll Cardiol 2002;39:1808.

Fuster V, Rydén LE, Cannom DS, *et al.* 2011 ACCF/AHA/ HRS focused updates incorporated into the ACC/AHA/ ESC 2006 Guidelines for the management of patients with atrial fibrillation: a report of the American College of Cardiology Foundation/American Heart Association Task Force on Practice Guidelines developed in partnership with the European Society of Cardiology and in collaboration with the European Heart Rhythm Association and the Heart Rhythm Society. J Am Coll Cardiol 2011;57(11):e101.

Gasparini M, Lunati M, Santini M, *et al.* Long-term survival in patients treated with cardiac resynchronization therapy: a 3-year follow-up study from the InSync/InSync ICD Italian Registry. Pacing Clin Electrophysiol 2006;29(Suppl 2):S2.

Gasparini M, Menozzi C, Proclemer A, *et al.* A simplified biventricular defibrillator with fixed long detection intervals reduces implantable cardioverter defibrillator (ICD) interventions and heart failure hospitalizations in patients with non-ischaemic cardiomyopathy implanted for primary prevention: the RELEVANT [Role of long dEtection window programming in patients with LEft VentriculAr dysfunction, Non-ischemic eTiology in primary prevention treated with a biventricular ICD] study. Eur Heart J 2009;30:2758.

Gomes JA, Winters SL, Steward D, Horowitz S, *et al.* A new noninvasive index to predict sustained ventricular tachycardia and sudden death in the first year after myocardial infarction. J Am Coll Cardiol 1987;10:349.

Gradaus R, Stuckenborg V, Loher A., *et al.* Diastolic filling pattern and left ventricular diameter predict response and prognosis after cardiac resynchronisation therapy. Heart 2008;94:1026.

Haïssaguerre M, Jais P, Shah DC *et al.* Electrophysiological end point for catheter ablation of atrial fibrillation initiated from multiple pulmonary veins foci. Circulation 2000;101:1409.

Hausenloy DJ, Arhi C, Chandra N *et al.* Blood pressure oscillations during tilt testing as a predictive marker of vasovagal syncope. Europace 2009;11:1696.

Hohnloser SH, Crijns HJ, van Eickels M., *et al.* Effect of dronedarone on cardiovascular events in atrial fibrillation. N Engl J Med 2009;360:668.

Holmes DR, Reddy Y, Turi ZG, *et al.* Percutaneous closure of the left atrial appendage versus warfarin therapy for prevention of stroke in patients with atrial fibrillation: a randomised non-inferiority trial. Lancet. 2009;374:534.

Holmes DR Jr, Kar S, Price MJ, *et al.* Prospective randomized evaluation of the Watchman left atrial appendage closure device in patients with atrial fibrillation versus long-term warfarin therapy: the PREVAIL trial. J Am Coll Cardiol 2014;64:1.

Hubley-Kozey CL, Mitchell LB, Gardner MJ, *et al.* Spatial features in body-surface potential maps can identify patients with a history of sustained ventricular tachycardia. Circulation 1995;92:1825.

Janousek J, Paul T. Safety of oral propafenone in the treatment of arrhythmias in infants and children. Am J Cardiol 1998;81:1121.

Janse MJ, Malik M, Camm AJ, *et al.* Identification of post acute myocardial infarction patients with potential benefit from prophylactic treatment with amiodarone. A substudy of EMIAT (the European Myocardial Infarct Amiodarone Trial). Eur Heart J 1998;19:85.

Kadish A, Hauck J, Pederson B, *et al.* Mapping of atrial activation with a noncontact, multielectrode catheter in dogs. Circulation 1999;99:1906.

Khairy P, Dubuc M. Transcatheter cryoablation part I: preclinical experience. Pacing Clin Electrophysiol 2008;31:112.

Korhonen P, Husa T, Konttila T, *et al.* Complex T-wave morphology in body surface potential mapping in prediction of arrhythmic events in patients with acute myocardial infarction and cardiac dysfunction. Europace 2009;11:514.

Krahn AD, Klein GJ, Yee R, *et al.* Randomized assessment of syncope trial. Conventional diagnostic testing versus a prolonged monitoring strategy. Circulation 2001;104:46.

Krahn AD, Klein GJ, Yee R, Skanes AC. The use of monitoring strategies in patients with unexplained syncope – role of the external and implantable loop recorder. Clin Auton Res 2004;14(Suppl 1):55.

Krishnamoorthy S, Lip G. How is safe the antiarrhythmic drug therapy in atrial fibrillation? PACE 2009;11:837.

Kuchar DL, Thorburn CW, Sammel NL. Prediction of serious arrhythmic events after myocardial infarction: signal-averaged electrocardiogram, Holter monitoring and radionuclide ventriculography. J Am Coll Cardiol 1987;9:531.

Kuck KH, Cappato R, Siebels J, Ruppel R. Randomized comparison of antiarrhythmic drug therapy with implantable defibrillators in patients resuscitated from cardiac arrest. The Cardiac Arrest Study Hamburg (CASH). Circulation 2000;102:748.

Kuck KH, Brugada J, Fürnkranz A, et al. Cryoballoon or radiofrequency ablation for paroxysmal atrial fibrillation. N Engl J Med 2016; 374(23):2235.

Kumar S, Sivagangabalan G, Zaman S, et al. Electrophysiology-guided defibrillator implantation early after ST-elevation myocardial infarction. Heart Rhythm 2010;7:1589.

Lin Y-J, Tsao H-M, Chang S-L, et al. Prognostic implications of the high-sensitive C-reactive protein in the catheter ablation of atrial fibrillation. Am J Cardiol 2010;105:495.

Marchant M, Heist E, McMarty D, et al. Impact of segmented left ventricle lead position on CRT outcomes. Heart Rhythm 2010;7:639.

Mazzini MJ, Monahan KM. Pharmacotherapy for atrial arrhythmias: present and future. Heart Rhythm 2008;5(6 Suppl):S26.

Mirowski M, Reid PR, Mower MM, et al. Termination of malignant ventricular arrhythmias with an implantable automatic defibrillator in human beings. N Engl J Med 1980;303:322.

Mohajer K, Fregeau B, Garg V, et al. Management of atrial fibrillation by Canadian electrophysiologists after early termination of the PALLAS study. Can J Cardiol 2013; 29(1):131.e1-2.

Moss AJ. MADIT-II and implications for noninvasive electrophysiologic testing. Ann Noninvasive Electrocardiol 2002;7:179.

Moss AJ, Hall WJ, Cannom DS, et al. Improved survival with an implanted defibrillator in patients with coronary disease at high risk for ventricular arrhythmia. N Engl J Med 1996;335:1933.

Moss AJ, Hall WJ, Cannom DS, et al. Cardiac-resynchronization therapy for the prevention of heart-failure events. N Engl J Med 2009;361:1329.

Myerburg R, Reddy V, Castellanos A. Indications for implantable cardioverter-defibrillators based on evidence and judgment. J Am Coll Cardiol 2009;54:747.

Nattel S. Antiarrhythmic drug classifications. A critical appraisal of their history, present status, and clinical relevance. Drugs 1991;41:672.

Nattel S. G-protein signaling and arrhythmogenic atrial remodeling: relevance to novel therapeutic targets in atrial fibrillation. Heart Rhythm 2009;6:85.

Oakes RS, Badger TJ, Kholmovski G, et al. Detection and quantification of left atrial structural remodeling with delayed-enhancement magnetic resonance imaging in patients with atrial fibrillation. Circulation 2009;119:1758.

Oyenuga O, Hara H, Tanaka H, et al. Usefulness of echocardiographic dyssynchrony in patients with borderline QRS duration to assist with selection for cardiac resynchronization therapy. JACC Cardiovasc Imaging 2010;3:132.

Pappone C, Santinelli V. Ablation of atrial fibrillation. Curr Cardiol Rep 2006;8:343.

Pérez Riera AR, Uchida AH, Filho CF, et al. Significance of vectorcardiogram in the cardiological diagnosis of the 21st century. Clin Cardiol 2007;30(7):319.

Postema PG, van Dessel PF, Kors JA, et al. Local depolarization abnormalities are the dominant pathophysiologic mechanism for type 1 electrocardiogram in Brugada syndrome a study of electrocardiograms, vectorcardiograms, and body surface potential maps during ajmaline provocation. J Am Coll Cardiol 2010;55:789.

Pouleur A, Barkoudah E, Uno H, et al. Pathogenesis of sudden death in a clinical trial of patients post myocardial infarction with left ventricular dysfunction. Circulation 2010;122:597.

Reddy VY, Exner DV, Cantillon DJ, et al. Percutaneous implantation of an entirely intracardiac leadless pacemaker. N Engl J Med 2015;373:1125.

Reddy VY, Sievert H, Halperin J, et al. Percutaneous left atrial appendage closure vs warfarin for atrial fibrillation: a randomized clinical trial. JAMA 2014;312:1988.

Reddy VY, Dukkipati SR, Neuzil P, et al. Randomized, controlled trial of the safety and effectiveness of a contact force-sensing irrigated catheter for ablation of paroxysmal atrial fibrillation: results of the TactiCath Contact Force Ablation Catheter Study for Atrial Fibrillation (TOCCASTAR) Study. Circulation. 2015;132(10):907.

Reynolds D, Duray GZ, Omar R, et al. A leadless intracardiac transcatheter pacing system. N Engl J Med 2016;374:533.

Ricci RP, Morichelli L, Santini M. Home monitoring remote control of pacemaker and implantable cardioverter defibrillator patients in clinical practice: impact on medical management and health-care resource utilization. Europace 2008;10:164.

Ricci RP, Morichelli L, Santini M. Remote control of implanted devices through home monitoring technology improves detection and clinical management of atrial fibrillation. Europace 2009;11:54.

Roden DM. Cardiovascular pharmacogenomics. Circulation 2003;108:3071.

Saba S, Volosin K, Yee R, *et al*. Combined atrial and ventricular antitachycardia pacing as a novel method of rhythm discrimination: the dynamic discrimination download study. Circulation 2010;121:487.

Schwartz PJ, Zaza A. The Sicilian Gambit revisited – theory and practice. Eur Heart J 1992;13(Suppl F):23.

Shaaraoui M, Freudenberger R, Levin V, *et al*. Suppression of ventricular tachycardia with dronedarone: a case report. J Cardiov Electrophysiol 2011;22(2):201.

Sheldon R. Syncope diagnostic scores. Prog Cardiovasc Dis 2013;55(4):390.

Singh D, Cingoleni E, Diamond G, *et al*. Dronadorone for atrial fibrillation. J Am Coll Cardiol 2010;55:1569.

Stecker E. Is there new hope for sudden cardiac death prevention early after MI. Heart Rhythm 2010;7:1598.

Stockburger M, Krebs A, Nitardy A, *et al*. Survival and appropriate device interventions in recipients of cardioverter defibrillators implanted for the primary versus secondary prevention of sudden cardiac death. Pacing Clin Electrophysiol 2009;32(Suppl 1):S16.

Strickberger SA, Benson DW, Biaggioni I, *et al*. AHA/ACCF Scientific Statement on the evaluation of syncope: from the American Heart Association Councils on Clinical Cardiology, Cardiovascular Nursing, Cardiovascular Disease in the Young, and Stroke, and the Quality of Care and Outcomes Research Interdisciplinary Working Group; and the American College of Cardiology Foundation: in collaboration with the Heart Rhythm Society: endorsed by the American Autonomic Society. Circulation 2006 ;113(2):316.

Sutton R, Bloomfield DM. Indications, methodology, and classification of results of tilt-table testing. Am J Cardiol 1999;84:10Q.

Sweeney MO, van Bommel RJ, Schalij MJ, *et al*. Analysis of ventricular activation using surface electrocardiography to predict left ventricular reverse volumetric remodeling during cardiac resynchronization therapy. Circulation 2010;121:626.

Tereshchenko LG, Faddis MN, Fetics BJ, *et al*. Transient local injury current in right ventricular electrogram after implantable cardioverter-defibrillator shock predicts heart failure progression. J Am Coll Cardiol 2009;54:822.

Theroux P, Waters DD, Halphen C, *et al*. Prognostic value of exercise test soon after myocardial infarction. N Engl J Med 1979;301:341.

Tomoda H. Valsartan and recurrent atrial fibrillation. N Engl J Med 2009;361:532.

Top-Pedersen C, Pedersen OD, Køber L. Antiarrhythmic drugs: safety first. J Am Coll Cardiol 2010;55(15):1577.

Tung R, Boyle NG, Shivkumar K. Catheter ablation of ventricular tachycardia. Circulation 2010;122:e389.

Tzikas A, Shakir S, Gafoor S, *et al*. Left atrial appendage occlusion for stroke prevention in atrial fibrillation: multicenter experience with the AMPLATZER Cardiac Plug. EuroIntervention 2016;11:1170.

Udo EO, Zuithoff NP, van Hemel NM, *et al*. Incidence and predictors of short- and long-term complications in pacemaker therapy: the FOLLOWPACE study. Heart Rhythm 2012;9:728.

Vardas PE, Auricchio A, Blanc JJ, *et al*. Guidelines for cardiac pacing and cardiac resynchronization therapy: the task force for cardiac pacing and cardiac resynchronization therapy of the European Society of Cardiology. Developed in collaboration with the European Heart Rhythm Association. Eur Heart J 2007;28:2256.

Vardas PE. White Book of electrophysiology in Europe. Publication of the European Society of Cardiology 2010.

Vaughan-Williams EM. Review of classification of antiarrhythmic agents. In: Bayés de Luna A, Cosin J, eds, Diagnosis and treatment ofcardiac arrhythnias, Pergamon Press, New York, 1980, p. 125.

Vereckei A, Duray G, Szénási G, *et al*. New algorithm using only lead a VR for differential diagnosis of wide QRS complex tachycardia. Heart Rhythm 2008;5:89.

Verma A, Mantovan R, Macle L, *et al*. Substrate and trigger ablation for reduction of atrial fibrillation (STAR AF): a randomized, multicentre, international trial. Eur Heart J 2010;31:1344.

Zareba W. Inappropriate implantable cardioverter defibrillator therapy. Cardiology J 2009;16:391.

Zhang F, Yang B, Chen H, *et al*. Noncontact mapping to guide ablation of right ventricular outflow tract arrhythmias. Heart Rhythm 2013;10:1895.

Zimetbaum PJ. Dronedarone for atrial fibrillation – an odyssey. N Engl J Med 2009;360:1811.

Index